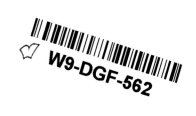

Encyclopedia of
Public Health

Editorial Board

Encyclopedia of Public Health

Edited by Lester Breslow

Volume 3
L-R

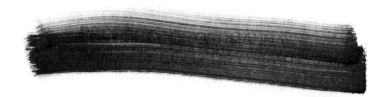

MACMILLAN REFERENCE USA

GALE GROUP
™
THOMSON LEARNING

New York • Detroit • San Diego • San Francisco
Boston • New Haven, Conn. • Waterville, Maine
London • Munich

Macmillan Reference USA
1633 Broadway
New York, NY 10019

Macmillan Reference USA
Gale Group
27500 Drake Road
Farmington Hills, MI 48331-3535

Gale Group and Design is a trademark used herein under license.

Library of Congress Catalog in Publication Data
Encyclopedia of public health / edited by Lester Breslow.
      p. cm.
      Includes bibliographical references and index.
      ISBN 0-02-865354-8 (set : hardcover : alk. paper) — ISBN 0-02-865350-5 (v. 1 : alk. paper) — ISBN 0-02-865351-3 (v. 2 : alk. paper) — ISBN 0-02-865352-1 (v. 3 : alk. paper) — ISBN 0-02-865353-X (v. 4 : alk. paper)
      1. Public health—Encyclopedias.   I. Breslow, Lester.

  RA423 .E53 2001
  362.1'03—dc21   2002031501

Printed in the United States of America

10 9 8 7 6 5 4 3 2 1

L

LABOR UNIONS

Labor unions are the major organizations pursuing the collective interests of workers in the areas of health and safety, especially in the mining, manufacturing, construction, health care, and transportation sectors. Beyond assisting members with their day-to-day needs through contract negotiation and administration, unions actively work for legislative and regulatory remedies for health and safety problems. Union influence extends far beyond the workplaces of the 14 percent of workers in the United States who are unionized. Unions bargain for specific improvements in working conditions; representation and systems for improving conditions, such as health and safety committees; and procedures for members to submit specific complaints to abate hazards. They also provide technical assistance, information, and training to members facing chemical or safety dangers. Additionally, traditional bargaining for hours of work, medical benefits, disability insurance, and job security positively impact the health status of workers.

Unions work politically for the passage and implementation of laws, standards, and regulations designed to improve working conditions and worker health. Early twentieth-century legislation included wage and hour laws, limitations on child labor and industrial home work, workers' compensation, and state labor departments to inspect workplaces for hazards. The labor movement united with public health and public interest groups to pass the Federal Coal Mine Health and Safety Act of 1969 and the Occupational Safety and Health

Act of 1970, greatly expanding the federal presence in these areas. Unions have been the critical force behind most major Occupational Safety and Health Administration (OSHA) standards, providing evidence in the rulemaking record and initiating litigation to force rulemaking and to defend rules against industry opposition. Exposure standards spearheaded by the union movement include those for lead, formaldehyde, benzene, asbestos, blood-borne pathogens, and coke-oven emissions.

In the second half of the twentieth century, union and worker activity in occupational health greatly expanded. The environmental movement of the 1960s led workers to be concerned about the levels of chemical exposure in the workplace. The black lung movement in the coal mines and the white lung movement based in cotton mills spurred the enforcement of exposure limits to chemicals and dusts. The emerging epidemic of asbestos-caused cancer and lung disease defined an approach exposure control and compensation of victims, including those in the general community. Limited rights of workers under the 1970 OSHA law were expanded through collective bargaining, in part due to public recognition of workers' rights to be fully informed of hazards and to fully participate in their abatement. Unions campaigned for and then implemented information rules, such as chemical hazard communication and community right-to-know, to facilitate the control of chemicals.

Unions also defended research institutions such as the National Institute of Occupational

Safety and Health (NIOSH), bargained for joint research programs with employers, and participated in studies that identified many previously unknown chemical hazards. Most recently, unions helped expose underreporting of musculoskeletal disorders, which spurred ergonomics programs and greatly extended the reach of the health and safety paradigm to light industry and the white–collar and service sectors. The expanding health care sector was itself recognized as a high-risk employer, particularly in the areas of infectious disease, chemical exposure, and ergonomic problems. The early twenty-first-century climate of corporate downsizing and off-shore production will challenge union-based and public occupational health and safety institutions.

FRANKLIN E. MIRER

(SEE ALSO: *Asbestos; Carpal Tunnel Syndrome, Cumulative Trauma; Mining; National Institute for Occupational Safety and Health; Occupational Disease; Occupational Lung Disease; Occupational Safety and Health; Occupational Safety and Health Administration*)

LABORATORY PRACTICE STANDARDS AND GUIDELINES

Any laboratory that performs tests which aid in determining an appropriate treatment or action for an illness or disease must establish practice standards and guidelines. Each laboratory procedure should include criteria for acceptable samples or specimens; a list of equipment, supplies, and reagents required; detailed step-by-step instructions for the testing procedure itself; and a list of the quality control procedures to be included, the results to be reported, and the interpretations of those results. Since some tests may require immediate action, protocol should also include directions on reporting details. Guidelines for reporting results to government agencies as required under local or state laws are also established.

In order to protect individuals and sensitive information, strict confidentiality guidelines should be developed for reporting results. These confidentiality guidelines should include disciplinary actions to be taken if protocols are not followed.

Guidelines are also established regarding the interpretation of quality control results and corrections that need to be made if results are not accurate. Additionally, practice standards for the laboratory may include safety procedures to be followed and guidelines for actions to be taken should laboratory accidents occur. In order to document that appropriate actions and procedures have been followed within the laboratory, standard practices should also include guidelines for the length of time that all records and documentation of corrective actions should be kept within the laboratory, and for computer back-up procedures.

KATHLEEN L. MECKSTROTH

(SEE ALSO: *Assurance of Laboratory Testing Quality; Diagnostic Testing for Communicable Disease; Laboratory Services; Laboratory Technician; Reference Laboratory*)

LABORATORY SERVICES

Even though the role of pathogenic bacteria and viruses in human health was defined in the nineteenth century, the first public health laboratories in the United States were called chemical laboratories and only performed elementary analyses of milk, water, and other substances. The Minnesota Board of Health established the first public health chemical laboratory in 1873, and in 1881 the New York legislature established the first state chemical laboratory. By 1869, most of the larger cities in Massachusetts had health boards that were actively involved in the area of sanitary engineering. The state's public health laboratory, established in 1886, was intended primarily to perform chemical analysis, though it was called a "hygienic" laboratory. Michigan followed Massachusetts' lead, moving into the regulation of food and water, and in 1887, the Michigan State Laboratory of Hygiene was established, with Dr. Victor C. Vaughn as director.

Both the Massachusetts and Michigan state hygienic laboratories began working on the connection between the public water supply and typhoid fever. This was probably the first application of bacteriology to sanitary science in the United States. By 1890 a number of state and local laboratories were established, with many of them doing both chemical and bacterial analysis.

The nation's first *diagnostic* public health laboratory was the result of work by Drs. Hermann M. Biggs and T. Mitchell Prudden. In 1887, these two physicians were able to isolate *Vibrio cholerae*, the bacterium that causes cholera, from the feces of ill passengers on an immigrant ship anchored in New York City harbor, and they were anxious to promote their technique as a routine diagnostic measure. It was not until a cholera scare in 1892, however, that they were able to convince the city health department of the need to establish a laboratory to develop and use diagnostic methods. On September 9 of that year, the New York City Department of Health's Division of Pathology, Bacteriology, and Disinfection was created, with Dr. Biggs as the director.

Biggs soon had a second disease upon which to focus his attention. Cases of diphtheria peaked in the 1890s in New York City, and Biggs was ready with a bacteriological diagnostic technique. He used this technique to demonstrate that half the patients in the New York City diphtheria hospital had been misdiagnosed. Because of this high rate of misdiagnosis, he stressed that laboratory testing to confirm a diagnosis would be cheaper than disinfecting and quarantining the homes of every case of suspected diphtheria. The health board agreed, and the first official medical bacteriologist in the United States, Dr. William H. Park, was appointed. Meanwhile, Biggs continued the expansion of the laboratory's diagnostic capabilities. He began routine laboratory bacteriological testing on every suspected tuberculosis case, despite his colleagues' skepticism of its value. In 1895, Biggs added vaccine production to the laboratory. He and his assistant, Park, refined the methods for production of the smallpox vaccine, and of diphtheria and tetanus antitoxins.

The New York City public health laboratory became a model for other public health departments. Within a few years, the diagnostic public health laboratory had become an essential component of an effective health department.

HISTORICAL SCOPE

The laboratory added a new dimension to public health department activities. The ability to isolate and identify disease-producing organisms immeasurably strengthened the prevention and control role of the department. However, this new health department tool of diagnostic bacteriology was not readily accepted by the general medical profession. Duffy, in "The Sanitarians," quoted from an 1884 *JAMA* journal article on Robert Koch and the tuberculosis (TB) bacillus that concludes a "too ready acceptance of the bacillus doctrine" was likely to do more harm than good and that "neither phthisis nor any form of tuberculosis (was) contagious."

Biggs and his associates in New York City met strong resistance from physicians to the city's board of health requirement to report all cases of tuberculosis. The attitude of New York physicians was duplicated around the country as more and more health departments instituted this requirement. Through perseverance and laboratory expertise, health departments were eventually able to convince the public and physicians that tuberculosis was communicable and not an hereditary disease related to environmental conditions.

As the diagnostic expertise of the laboratories grew, the ability of the public health dpeartments to control disease was bolstered. The ability to culture disease-causing organisms from asymptomatic people led to recognition of the carrier state and a reexamination of isolation practice. Laboratory-supported disease control efforts resulted in significant reductions in disease mortality by the early twentieth century.

By mid-century, most of the laboratories had evolved in service provision to the same general scope provided today: testing support of the communicable disease programs, chemical and bacteriologic testing of drinking water, analysis of food and milk, and limited non-communicable disease testing. As continuing advances in technology enhanced the diagnostic capabilities of the laboratories, the public health department core functions of assessment, policy development, and assurance were significantly strengthened.

Development of federal public health laboratories was slower than at the state level, although the nucleus of what would evolve into the National Institutes of Health was established in 1887. In that year Joseph Kinyoun founded the Laboratory of Hygiene, a bacteriology research laboratory at the Marine Hospital on Staten Island. In 1891, this laboratory was moved to Washington, D.C., where it expanded into what became the National Institutes of Health (NIH) forty years later. The NIH laboratories still focus primarily on research and are not usually considered front line public health laboratories. The Centers for Disease Control and Prevention (CDC), which is the acknowledged apex of the public health laboratory system, was established even later than the NIH. In 1942 the Office of Malaria Control in War Areas (MCWA) was established. In 1946 the MCWA was converted to the Communicable Disease Center. It was renamed the Centers for Disease Control in 1980, and in 1992 became the Centers for Disease Control and Prevention. The CDC has since matured into a collective group of laboratories and programs that is dedicated to preserving the health and well-being of the public. The testing performed by CDC, in conjunction with local and state laboratories, has been essential to the provision of safe drinking water, an increased awareness of the importance of environmental health issues, and the decline of communicable diseases such as syphilis.

ROLE OF THE PUBLIC HEALTH LABORATORY

Initially, the role of the public health laboratory (PHL) was simply to serve any of the perceived laboratory needs of the various jurisdictions. Over time this role was defined more precisely, although still ambiguously, under general categories. The PHL became a recognized central part of the public health infrastructure and was charged with supporting this infrastructure in each of the three core public health functions—assessment, assurance, and policy development. Because PHLs differ dramatically in complexity, dependent largely on the population served, the test menus of the laboratories differ greatly. In general, all laboratories support the following core functions: testing information relevant to monitoring the environment; assessing the population's health status; investigating and controlling disease outbreaks; treating and controlling communicable diseases like tuberculosis, syphilis, gonorrhea, and chlamydia; acting as a reference laboratory for private sector laboratories; and assuring the safety of food and water. In addition, many PHLs have ongoing applied research programs directed toward improving the reliability and efficiency of testing, and identifying and controlling emerging problems.

PHL support for assessment and assurance functions are the most diverse. Laboratory testing to support assessment may involve specimens from people, animals, insects, fomites (inert vectors), and environmental sources. Examples of this type of activity are varied, but one of the most common is to support the investigation of disease outbreaks. It is the laboratory's role to isolate and identify the causative agent and to identify the source of the infection, which may be other individuals, insect or animal vectors, water, food, or dirt. For example, in a food poisoning incident associated with restaurant meals, the laboratory is pivotal in the determination of whether the incident is localized (caused by poor food handling procedures or infected staff in a specific restaurant) or widespread (caused by contaminated food distributed to many places locally or nationally).

Population surveillance studies for assessment of disease prevalence in a community also rely on testing and information provided by the PHL. Neonatal screening for metabolic disorders, immune status screening, screening for sexually transmitted diseases, and screening for chronic diseases are examples of this aspect of information gathering by PHLs.

Rabies, botulism, and plague are examples of rare but important diseases of public health significance that are not identified except in public health laboratories. Rabies is routinely identified by dissecting out specific portions of the brain of suspect animals to look for the characteristic lesions produced by the rabies virus. Rabies testing may be performed as routine surveillance of the wild animal population or as a necessary adjunct to contact between an individual and a suspect animal. Testing for *Clostridium botulinum toxin* (which causes botulism) in food or humans requires, at present, the use of animals. This requirement is the basis for the restriction of this assay to PHLs. Plague surveillance is routinely done by PHLs in areas where plague is endemic in the animal population. If antibodies to plague are found in an animal population that may have contact with humans, such as ground squirrels near a picnic area, the area is closed to the public until an eradication effort is successful.

Support of the PHL for the assurance function of public health is probably the most unrecognized and underappreciated facet of its role. Some of the testing cited under the assessment function has elements of assurance, such as the confirmatory reference testing that is offered to all private laboratories without charge. Private sector laboratories having difficulty identifying a microorganism—confirming the true antibody status of a patient or defining the resistance pattern of *Mycobacterium tuberculosis*, for example—are able to request help from a PHL. But the most important role of assurance testing is to assure that community water supplies are safe to drink. In addition to testing drinking water for chemical and microbiological safety, recreational water is tested to insure the safety of swimmers and bathers.

Another assurance function, not readily apparent to the public, is the screening of food handlers in restaurants and other facilities. Food poisoning events trigger this function if an organism is suspected or identified that can be transmitted through contamination of food by a food handler. The food facility staff is screened for suspect pathogens by the PHL, and any individuals found to be infected are removed from the job until subsequent testing assures that they no longer are infected.

The facet of assurance that is most often thought of in connection with PHLs is the provision of certain testing services to the indigent population and to other individuals who might not otherwise be able to afford tests. This aspect of PHL testing varies from state to state depending upon local laboratory resources or the availability of specimen transport to the state laboratory.

Participation of PHLs in the third core function, policy development, is largely through consultation or regulatory services. PHL staff is involved in policy development that impacts research and technology needs as well as health issues such as HIV/AIDS (human immunodeficiency virus/acquired immunodeficiency syndrome), sexually transmitted diseases, and tuberculosis. Policies to solve environmental problems are often developed primarily by PHL staff. Some state PHLs develop and implement regulations that govern all aspects of private clinical and local public laboratory operations within the state. This includes laboratory personnel and facility licensure requirements and environmental monitoring requirements.

In summation, the primary role of PHL is as a service unit providing timely information to facilitate the public health department's mission to protect the health of the community. To adequately perform this role, the laboratory must be functionally integrated within the health department's relevant programs so that the needs and requirements of these programs are met. The unbiased information and laboratory data provided by a PHL are necessary adjuncts to an effective public health department.

COST OF SERVICES

Health care funding continues to increase, but, according to Health and Human Services estimates, public health spending is only about 1 percent of the total, and the expenditure for PHLs is only 3 percent to 5 percent of the public health allocation. This demonstrates that federal, state, and county governments are making a very cost-effective investment in PHLs. The cost savings of population-based interventions based on PHL testing information is estimated to be analogous to the cost savings (ten dollars for every one dollar spent) of an effective immunization program. This estimate is derived from potential medical costs saved versus screening costs for population-based surveillance testing, including that done for rabies, lead poisoning, sexually transmitted diseases, environmental carcinogens and pathogens, and metabolic disorders in newborns.

LABORATORY STRUCTURE AND ORGANIZATION

Because of the wide variability in population between and within states, there is diversity in both the structure and testing services of the PHLs in the individual states. All fifty states and the District of Columbia operate their own PHLs, and some states have local laboratories, which may be autonomous or simply local extensions of the state PHL. The CDC functions primarily as a reference laboratory for the state PHLs, providing confirmatory and esoteric testing services that the state laboratories do not have the resources to perform. The CDC also funds assessment and assurance studies at the local level to investigate issues of particular public health importance. The CDC is an integral part of the PHL system, and plays an important role in national disease surveillance.

Although the Food and Drug Administration (FDA) laboratories are public in the sense of being part of a government organization, they are not public health laboratories because they are not part of a public health department. Both the Environmental Protection Agency (EPA) and the U.S. Department of Agriculture (USDA) also impact PHL operations. Much of the environmental monitoring done by PHLs follows EPA guidelines, and USDA regulations may directly or indirectly play a role in PHL operations. The other federal agency that has recently assumed a major role in PHLs is the Health Care Financing Administration (HCFA), which is involved in the development and implementation of federal regulations that affect all diagnostic laboratories. These regulations are part of the Clinical Laboratory Improvement Amendments of 1988 (CLIA), which supersede all state regulations governing laboratories *unless* the state regulations are more stringent. PHLs that have state regulations governing them in addition to the federally mandated CLIA regulations are subject to inspections on a regular basis to determine if they are in compliance with these laws. The CLIA regulations impact all aspects of laboratory operations. One of the biggest changes for PHLs is the regulation for a laboratory director. All PHLs function in an organization led by a health officer, but the training and academic preparation requirements for the role of laboratory director have varied by jurisdiction. In several states, the laboratory director does not need to have a scientific background or an advanced degree; in others, an advanced degree in a scientific discipline is required. CLIA regulations stipulate that the laboratory director of each PHL must be a physician or a doctoral-level clinical scientist qualified by training, expertise, and experience in the areas of testing offered by the laboratory. In addition, physicians may qualify to direct a laboratory performing high complexity tests (PHLs perform high complexity tests) if they have two years of experience directing or supervising high complexity testing. The only exceptions to these requirements are under a grandfather clause that states that those individuals who are qualified or could have qualified as director before February 28, 1992, under federal regulations or state law are eligible to function as laboratory director.

State population needs and resources largely dictate the size and complexity of state PHLs in terms of staff and test menu. The Lewin Group's report *Public Health Laboratories and Health System Change*, commissioned in 1997 by the United States Department of Health and Human Services, gives figures that illustrate this diversity. According to this report, in fiscal year 1996 the Tennessee state PHL had 186 full-time staff members and a budget of $9.5 million, whereas the Florida state PHL had 354 full-time staff members and a budget of $21 million.

In addition to the state PHL, many states also have regional, county, or city PHLs that provide a quicker response network, but which may forward some samples to the central state laboratory for testing or confirmation of results. The regional laboratories may be extensions of the state PHL or autonomous PHLs funded by the local jurisdiction. For example, Tennessee has four regional state branch laboratories in addition to the central state laboratory located in Nashville. This state PHL organization provides testing services for eighty-nine rural health departments and six metropolitan health departments. One regional laboratory has only two staff members and performs microbiology tests exclusively. In contrast, California operates thirty-nine PHLs in addition to the state laboratory. All of the local laboratories are autonomous and all but three are county health department laboratories. In contrast to this extensive PHL network, other states, such as Oregon and Wyoming, operate only a central state PHL.

Another major difference among state PHLs is the extent to which their resources are utilized in testing primary patient specimens, doing reference testing, training laboratory personnel, monitoring the environment, doing applied research, and functioning as a regulatory agency. Some state laboratories devote a major portion of their resources to direct patient specimen testing; others do very little testing of primary patient specimens and concentrate on reference testing, applied research, and regulatory and epidemiological roles.

Overall, the public health laboratory infrastructure comprises a large number of basically diverse federal, state, and local laboratories that, under the guidance of the CDC, are beginning to function as a network in areas of national public health concern such as food safety and bioterrorism.

Individually, however, state PHLs are the major link between national health initiatives and delivery at the local level, where laboratory information is mandatory for success. Despite the variability in resource focus and complexity, all state health department laboratories have a responsibility to support the core public health functions either directly or in coordination with local or regional PHLs.

CHALLENGES FACED BY PUBLIC HEALTH LABORATORIES

A medical laboratory test is defined as any examination of material derived from the human body for the purpose of providing information for the diagnosis, prevention, or treatment of any disease or impairment. There are two types of laboratories where medical testing is a primary activity: clinical laboratories—including hospital laboratories—and public health laboratories. Although both types of laboratories perform many of the same testing procedures, their primary functions are fundamentally different. Clinical laboratories assist clinicians *only* with individual patients, whereas public health laboratories support the health officer whose responsibility is the community. The clinical laboratory supports primary patient care; the public health laboratory supports programs designed to prevent and control communicable disease and environmental pollution, and plays a key role in epidemiological investigations of disease outbreaks. Clinical laboratories perform testing on specimens from humans; PHLs perform testing on specimens from many different sources—human, animal, insect, environmental, and food.

These are the historical roles of the two types of laboratories and the basis for the establishment of PHLs over a century ago. But there is growing concern in the public health community that the understanding of the significance of the public health laboratory to the public health infrastructure is being lost because of changes in health care systems and a belief that infectious diseases are under control. Former surgeon general William Stewart articulated this belief in 1979 when he declared that it was time to "close the books on infectious diseases" and concentrate on killers such as cancer. Unfortunately, the comfortable conclusion that infectious disease has been vanquished is incorrect. Microorganisms are displaying their ability to subvert our defenses in ways not predicted. New viruses, for which we have no treatment, have emerged; bacteria, once thought conquered with antibiotics, have developed multiple resistance patterns. The U.S. General Accounting Office issued a report in February 1999 that estimates some of the costs associated with infectious diseases. According to this report, there are approximately thirty-three million cases and nine thousand deaths every year from food-borne illnesses, with an associated estimated cost of twenty-two billion dollars per year. Over the past twenty years, international travel has increased threefold along with a substantial increase in the importation of fresh food. These two factors have allowed infectious diseases to spread rapidly across borders. In addition to the incorrect premise that infectious disease has been conquered, rapid changes in the health care environment have profoundly affected traditional services delivered by PHLs.

Until the early 1970s, PHLs were the leaders in microbiology technology. The CDC scientific research laboratories developed improved assays for various organisms and transferred the technology to the PHLs. In turn, the PHLs functioned as training centers for the private clinical laboratory staff. This function, in conjunction with their reference service ability, gave PHLs an elevated status in the community. This status began to erode as private companies entered the biological research and development market. No longer was CDC the leader in reagent and technology development. Biotechnology companies began emerging at a rapid pace as the potential market for improved diagnostic technology became apparent. These companies sell directly to private clinical laboratories, supplying any necessary training along with the new technology. PHLs are no longer the conduit. In addition, private clinical laboratories, because of the highly competitive marketplace in which they operate, have surpassed most PHLs in services and information infrastructure.

These changing dynamics of the laboratory services marketplace accelerated during the 1990s with the growth of managed care, consolidation of laboratories, shrinking of public resources, and the direct competition of clinical laboratories. While more sophisticated technology has raised testing costs, managed care organizations (MCOs) and other providers have demanded that laboratories lower their fees for service. This has served to intensify competition among laboratories and stimulated a quest for more efficient and faster service modes. In general the private laboratories that have survived this competitive pressure have decreased their costs through economies of scale, increased their capacity for quick turnaround of results, and developed better information handling. PHLs have been slow in responding to the need to change, partially because of the resource issues, but also because of bureaucratic inertia. The result is a continuing erosion of stature and a decreasing volume of testing, with a perceived loss in surveillance data for community protection.

FUTURE OF PUBLIC HEALTH LABORATORIES

Image, in the form of perceived importance, is the key to the survival of the public health laboratory system. PHLs must be understood and viewed by the public, by public officials, and by the private sector laboratory professionals as an invaluable resource that contributes in a unique way to the maintenance of health in the population. PHLs must be responsive to changing needs and once again become technological leaders of the laboratory community.

At present, the public health laboratory system is composed of autonomous laboratories linked at the state level, and linked at the federal level to CDC, but not linked to each other or to private diagnostic laboratories. The concept of forming a true national laboratory network, comprised of both private and public laboratories, originated in the late 1960s and is being expressed in a rudimentary way through bioterrorism initiatives and national surveillance for food-borne diseases, antimicrobial resistance patterns, and emerging infectious disease concerns. To continue the momentum to build a strong national network and to focus public awareness on the integral role of public health laboratories in such a system, the Association of Public Health Laboratories (APHL) is developing a strategic plan that will encompass elements of public relations as well as the objectives and steps involved in the development of a national laboratory system. This is a difficult and momentous undertaking, yet it is essential to the provision of health protection at the national as well as at the local level. A critical role for the public health laboratory is to provide the leadership and initiative to create this vital laboratory system.

SYDNEY M. HARVEY

(SEE ALSO *Assurance of Laboratory Testing Quality; Centers for Disease Control and Prevention; Clinical Laboratories Improvement Act; Laboratory Technician; Reference Laboratory; Research in Public Health Laboratories; Screening*)

BIBLIOGRAPHY

Association of Public Health Laboratories (1999). *Core Functions and Capabilities of State Public Health Laboratories.* Washington, DC: Author.

Cordts, J. R. (1995). "The Laboratory as a Model Public Health Function." *CDC/NCID Focus* (March).

Duffy, J. (1996). *The Sanitarians: A History of American Public Health.* Urbana: University of Illinois Press.

Getchell, J. P. (1996). "The Role of the Public Health Laboratory and the Definition of Public Health Laboratory Services." *The Nation's Health* (September):19–21.

Lewin Group (1997). *Public Health Laboratories and Health System Change.*

Skeels, M. R. (1995). "Public Health Laboratories Build Healthy Communities." *Laboratory Medicine* 26:588–592.

U.S. Senate Subcommittee on Public Health (1999). *Emerging Infectious Diseases: Consensus on Needed Laboratory Capacity Could Strengthen Surveillance.* Washington, DC: General Accounting Office.

LABORATORY TECHNICIAN

A laboratory technician is an individual who, under the direct supervision of a laboratory scientist, processes and prepares samples from humans, animals, food, water, soil, and air for examination and testing and who performs routine laboratory tests using written standard testing protocols. In some public health clinics, the laboratory technician is also responsible for collecting the specimens, preparing specimens for shipment to reference laboratories, and for preparing and distributing the reports of the test results. The laboratory technician may also be responsible for routine quality control procedures such as recording temperatures of refrigerators, freezers, and water baths. Additionally, the laboratory technician prepares reagents necessary for testing.

KATHLEEN L. MECKSTROTH

(SEE ALSO: *Assurance of Laboratory Testing Quality; Diagnostic Testing for Communicable Disease; Laboratory Services; Practice Standards; Reference Laboratory*)

LAND USE

Land use regulations that protect public health have a long history. In 1189, England required stone walls (walls that divide two adjoining properties) to be three feet thick and sixteen feet tall. By 1297, front yards were required to be cleared and maintained, and in the fifteenth century all roofs in urban areas were required to be stone, lead, or tile, for fire protection. Public safety was the basis for a 1692 Boston ordinance restricting slaughterhouses, currier houses, and tallow chandler houses to less populous areas of the city.

HISTORY OF LAND USE PLANNING

America's first cities reflected the land planning traditions of the early settlers. The Spanish "Law of the Indies" required central plazas and parks in St. Augustine, Florida, established in 1565. English town planning influenced Sir Francis Nicholson's 1694 radial spoke design for Annapolis, Maryland, and James Ogelthorpe's 1733 neighborhood square plan for Savannah, Georgia. There were twenty-four park squares, with forty families per square in Savannah's grid. Twenty-three of these squares remain, and the original city layout is considered one of America's most lovely and livable.

By the mid-1800s, New York City's crowded, unhealthy environment lacked adequate light and air. In 1858, landscape architects Frederick Law Olmstead and Calvert Vance laid out Central Park in response to the need for open space. The Public Health movement of the 1860s prompted New York and San Francisco to regulate tenements and slaughterhouses, and to separate incompatible land uses to benefit public health. In 1869 Olmstead and Vaux created a design for Riverside, Illinois,

an English garden-style city using curved, tree-lined streets, deep setbacks, and single family detached houses in exclusively residential neighborhoods. This design became the standard suburban streetscape.

At the turn of the twentieth century the City Beautiful movement used parks and public open spaces as centerpieces of the future city as exemplified by the 1893 Columbian Exposition in Chicago, commonly known as the "White City." After the First World War, the movement turned to legal and technical standards for planning. What began as common-sense measures for preserving public safety evolved to include aesthetic, economic, traffic, noise, social, and cultural considerations.

THE PURPOSE OF PLANNING AND ZONING

Daniel Hudson Burnham (1846–1912), the creator of the city plan of Chicago (1909), wrote: "Remember that our sons and grandsons are going to do things that would stagger us. Let your watchword be order and your beacon beauty." Burnham was at the forefront of the City Planning movement, the intent of which was to plan for the future. This was done by the creation of zones with separate land use regulations. In some communities, a plan was the basis for zoning. In most communities, zoning itself was the plan.

A comprehensive plan is the basis for current American land use planning. Such a plan must consider the community's vision for future development; the policies, goals, principles, and standards upon which the development of the community are based; the proposed location, extent, and intensity of future land usage; existing and anticipated future housing needs; the location and types of transportation required; the location of public and private utilities; and the location of educational, recreational, and cultural facilities including libraries, hospitals, and fire and police stations. It is also important to determine how a community's natural resources will be utilized.

After a comprehensive plan is in place, zoning is adopted that conforms to the plan. Zoning is the legal tool used to promote the public health, safety, and welfare of a community. Land is typically divided into zones for different land uses, such as commercial, industrial, and residential. Typically regulated are the location, height, bulk, and number of stories of buildings and other structures. Also regulated are the percentages of lot areas that may be occupied; the set back building lines; the size of yards, courts, and other open spaces; the density of population; and the uses of buildings.

THE EFFECTS OF LAND USE PLANNING ON ENVIRONMENTAL HEALTH

Delaware County was the fastest-growing county in Ohio in the late 1990s. With this growth came increased concerns related to environmental stress. The frequency of road rage, for example, increased due to heavy traffic on what were formerly quiet country roads. A detailed environmental health survey was performed in 1998, which confirmed the concerns of public health professionals that more parks, green space, and wildlife habitat were needed; and that county development, zoning, and land annexation were out of control. The Delaware County Board of Health began working to create environmental health programs that would coordinate with land use planning to reduce the environmental stress. The Delaware County Regional Planning Commission worked with communities to identify an environmentally sound vision for the county, and has assisted them in meeting their goals.

Sustainable, livable cities, like Savannah, Georgia, and Portland, Oregon, have many land use elements in common. Among these are:

1. Central public open spaces (parks, squares, or water) in every neighborhood

2. A variety of architectural styles, with compatible elements

3. Retention of history through restoration of structures

4. Downtown or village centers with intimate, human scale and mixed uses

5. Commercial districts with greenbelts, controlled traffic access points, and sign controls

6. Residential areas with traffic-calming features, low speed limits, and separation of residential uses

7. Industrial parks with wide roads for heavy trucks and landscaped greenbelts

8. Preserved natural features (natural topography, wetlands, floodplains, and water)

9. Preserved agriculture areas

PLANNING RETURNS TO ITS ROOTS

The built environment can affect personal health in ways we are only beginning to measure. Entering the twenty-first century, there was a renewed interest in land use planning and environmental health. Authors like Randall Arendt and Peter Katz have espoused open-space community designs for rural and urban areas. A century after the City Beautiful movement, Americans are once again interested in the quality of life in their communities and in linking land use planning with environmental health.

PHILIP LAURIEN

(SEE ALSO: *Ecosystems; Environmental Determinants of Health; Healthy Communities; Not In My Backyard [NIMBY]; Urban Health; Urban Sprawl*)

BIBLIOGRAPHY

Arendt, R. (1994). *Rural by Design.* Chicago: Planners Press.

Ewing, R. (1996). *Best Development Practices.* Chicago: Planners Press.

Hines, T. S. (1974). *Burnham of Chicago: Architect and Planner.* New York: Oxford University Press.

Katz, P. (1994). *The New Urbanism: Toward an Architecture of Community.* New York: McGraw-Hill.

So, F. S., and Getzels, J., eds. (1988). *The Practice of Local Government Planning,* 2nd edition. Washington, DC: International City Management Association.

Whittick, A., ed. (1980). *Encyclopedia of Urban Planning.* Huntington, NY: Krueger.

LANDFILLS, SANITARY

Sanitary landfills are one of the most popular forms of waste disposal, primarily because they are the least expensive way to dispose of waste. More than four-fifths of municipal solid waste is disposed of in landfills. Landfills are rapidly filling up all around the country, however and the majority of them will close by 2010. Also, many have waste problems that are serious health threats. As of 1983, there were 184 landfills listed, or proposed to be listed, on the Superfund National Priorities List (NPL).

A sanitary landfill is an engineered means of disposing of waste. In a sanitary landfill, waste is spread in layers on a piece of property, usually on marginal or submarginal land. The objective is to spread the layers and then compact them tightly, greatly reducing the volume of the waste. The waste is then covered by soil.

Problems that are encountered in open dumping, including insects, rodents, safety hazards, and fire hazards, can be avoided with landfilling. A landfill should not be located in areas with high groundwater tables. Leachate migration control standards must be followed in the design, construction, and operation of landfills during the use of the facility and during the postclosure period.

Much of the waste in a sanitary landfill will decompose through biological and chemical processes that produce solid, liquid, and gaseous products. Food wastes degrade rapidly, whereas plastics, glass, and construction wastes do not. The most common types of gas produced by the decomposition of the wastes are methane and carbon dioxide. Methane, which is produced by anaerobic decomposition of landfilled materials, is hazardous because it is explosive. Depending on the landfill composition, gases can be recovered and utilized in the generation of power or heat. Landfill recovery science is a new technology that is utilized in many parts of the United States. Sadly, in many places, wetlands and other lands considered to be marginal were used for landfills. Only now are people becoming aware of the value of wetlands and other areas that were used—especially with regard to sensitive habitats, biodiversity, and impacts on groundwater.

After a landfill has reached capacity, it is closed for waste deposition and covered. In some cases it can be used as pasture, as cropland, or for recreational purposes. Maintenance of the closed landfill is important to avoid soil erosion and excess runoff into desirable areas.

MARK G. ROBSON

(SEE ALSO: *Groundwater; Municipal Solid Waste; Sanitation*)

BIBLIOGRAPHY

Herman, K., and Bisesi, M. (1996). *Handbook of Environmental Health and Safety,* 3rd edition, Vol. II. Boca Raton, FL: Lewis Publishers.

Morgan, M. T. (1997). *Environmental Health.* Madison, WI: Brown and Benchmark.

LANDMARK PUBLIC HEALTH LAWS AND COURT DECISIONS

Over the years, public health and medical care services in the United States have expanded incrementally. Modern public health services and medical care programs have emerged from step-by-step actions to deal with specific problems and the needs of specific populations. This article traces the evolution of public health services and medical care programs by describing landmark legislation and court decisions that have strengthened public health and extended medical care to more people. In describing these signal legislative and judicial actions of the twentieth century, many important statutes and judicial decisions are omitted due to the limitations of space. This account is not a substitute for a thorough historical review of the growth of public health and medical care in the United States, but it may illuminate the possibilities of the characteristically American incremental approach for strengthening public health and medical care.

STATE POLICE POWER

In 1905, the U.S. Supreme Court upheld compulsory vaccination as a reasonable exercise of the state police power to protect the health, welfare, and safety of its citizens (*Jacobson v. Massachusetts*). This seminal case on the nature of the police power—the legal basis for state authority in the field of public health—involved a compulsory vaccination regulation of the Cambridge, Massachusetts, Board of Health. The defendant refused to be vaccinated and contended that the requirement invaded his liberty and was hostile to "the right of every freeman to care for his own body and health in such a way as to him sees fit." But the Court held that

the liberty secured by the Constitution to every person . . . does not import an absolute right in each person to be at all times and in all circumstances wholly freed from restraint . . . it was the duty of the constituted authorities primarily to keep in view the welfare, comfort and safety of the many, and not permit the interests of the many to be subordinated to the wishes or convenience of the few.

Acknowledging that there is a sphere in which the individual may dispute the authority of a government, the Court stated

it is equally true that in every well-ordered society charged with the duty of conserving the safety of its members the rights of the individual in respect of his liberty may at times, under the pressure of great dangers, be subjected to such restraint, to be enforced by reasonable regulations, as the safety of the general public may demand . . .

ENVIRONMENTAL HEALTH

One of the basic functions of public health is protection of the environment in which people live and work. The National Environmental Policy Act of 1969 (42 U.S.C.A. §4321 et seq.) marked a watershed in the development of environmental controls. In response to concerns about fragmented environmental programs among diverse federal agencies and lack of effective controls over the multiplicity of antipollution measures, the National Environmental Policy Act provides for an overview of environmental protection efforts and a mechanism for integrating and coordinating the many environmental programs. An important provision of the statute is the requirement for environmental impact statements before any major federal projects expected to have significant impact on the environment can be undertaken. Many states have enacted state environmental policy laws modeled on the federal statutes.

In 1970, Congress enacted the Occupational Safety and Health Act (29 U.S.C.A. §§651–78) "to assure so far as possible to every working man and woman in the Nation safe and healthful working conditions and to preserve our human resources" (651[b]). The act covers every state and territory. It provides for the promulgation of standards by the Secretary of Labor, created the National Institute of Occupational Safety and Health (NIOSH) to conduct studies and research to develop standards, authorizes inspections of workplaces, supports worker training and education, enforces compliance with standards, and encourages state plans that meet the criteria for approval by the Secretary of Labor. In the thirty years that this comprehensive, national law has been in effect, tragic industrial deaths and diseases have been markedly reduced, and workers' health has been protected and advanced.

THE SOCIAL SECURITY ACT

The Social Security Act of 1935 (42 U.S.C.A. §1301 et seq.), according to William Shonick, "was the first substantial entry of the national government into the general field of social welfare and may be viewed as its founding charter." In addition to its provisions on social insurance for retirement benefits and unemployment insurance, the act provides for old age assistance (Title I), aid for dependent children (Title IV), and aid to the blind (Title X). The provision for grants to the states for state and local public health departments (Title VI) and for maternal and child welfare (Title V) led to vastly increased numbers of full-time local health departments, strengthened staffing to provide public health services, and improved support for maternal and child health services.

Over the years, the Social Security Act became the structure for important advances in medical care. In 1965, Congress enacted Medicare (Title XVIII), a social insurance program for hospital and physicians' care for persons over sixty-five and Medicaid (Title XIX), an expanded program paying for medical services for certain categories of low-income people, financed jointly by the federal and state governments. In 1972, Medicare was expanded to include persons of any age with end-stage renal disease and in 1973 disabled persons of any age as defined by Medicare.

Amendments to the Social Security Act have included, among others, the following: (1) measures for peer review of the quality of care (Professional Standards Review Organizations, 1972 and Peer Review Organizations, 42 U.S.C.A. § 1320c-3, §1154 [a][1][A], [B], [C]); (2) the Emergency Medical Treatment and Labor Act (EMTALA 1986, 42

U.S.C.A. §1395dd) requiring hospitals receiving Medicare payments and having an emergency department to serve and stabilize, before transferring, emergency patients and women in labor, regardless of ability to pay; (3) welfare reform (the Personal Responsibility and Work Opportunity Reconciliation Act, 42 U.S.C.A. §603 et seq.), which replaced the entitlement program, Aid to Families with Dependent Children (AFDC), with capped block grants to the states known as Temporary Assistance to Needy Families; and (4) the State Children's Health Insurance Program, enacted in 1997 as Title XXI of the Social Security Act. Much discussed is the expansion of the Social Security Act to add outpatient pharmaceutical benefits to the Medicare program.

THE HILL-BURTON ACT AND HEALTH FACILITIES

During the Depression of the 1930s and continuing through World War II, hospitals in the United States had been neglected and were in great need of repair. The Hill-Burton Hospital Survey and Construction Act of 1946 (42. U.S.C.A. § 291 et seq.) was a brilliant piece of legislation. It provided funds for private and public hospital construction. It launched organized planning of health facilities by requiring states to develop a state hospital plan and by providing funding for planning. It initiated regulation of health facilities by setting standards and requiring licensing of facilities. Thus, this tripartite legislation financed hospital construction on condition of planning and regulation of health facilities by the states.

In 1965, a landmark case established the liability of hospitals for negligence in monitoring and supervising the quality of care in their hospitals. *Darling* v. *Charleston Community Memorial Hospital* involved a malpractice action by an injured football player against the hospital where negligent treatment necessitated amputation of his right leg below the knee. The case held that a hospital has an independent duty to provide medical care to its patients, that it has a duty to provide more than bed and board, and that no longer is the hospital solely the doctor's workshop. *Darling* marked a turning point in the responsibility of hospitals for the quality of care provided in their facilities.

THE FOOD, DRUG, AND COSMETIC ACT

Legislation regulating food, drugs, cosmetics, and equipment is important because these resources essential for assuring health are produced entirely in the private sector. The Pure Food and Drug Act of 1906 prohibited the adulteration and misbranding of drugs. The Federal Food, Drug, and Cosmetic Act of 1938 (21 U.S.C.A. § 301 et seq.) required that the safety of a drug be demonstrated prior to its distribution. The landmark Drug Amendments of 1962 (21 U.S.C.A. § 355) required proof of efficacy before a drug could be marketed. In support of this legislation were the facts that consumers were wasting money on drugs without benefit and that reliance on ineffective drugs could be dangerous when safe and effective alternatives were available.

In 1996, the Food and Drug Administration (FDA) asserted jurisdiction over cigarettes and smokeless tobacco, finding that nicotine is a drug and that cigarettes and smokeless tobacco are drug-delivery devices affecting the structure and function of the body, within the meaning of the Food, Drug, and Cosmetic Act. The FDA issued regulations restricting the sale and distribution of cigarettes and smokeless tobacco in an effort to protect children and adolescents and reduce tobacco addiction in future generations. Although recognizing the great hazards to health posed by tobacco, the U.S. Supreme Court in a five-to-four decision held that the Food and Drug Administration lacked authority to regulate tobacco products and that such regulation was a matter for Congress to decide (*Food and Drug Administration* v. *Brown and Williamson Tobacco Corp.*).

THE CIVIL RIGHTS ACT

Federal antidiscrimination laws have had a major impact on health facilities and, in fact, on all aspects of civil society. Title VI of the 1964 Civil Rights Act (42 U.S.C.A. §§2000d, 2000e) prohibits discrimination on the basis of race, color, or national origin in any program or activity receiving federal financial assistance. Title VII, as amended by the Equal Employment Opportunity Act of 1972, prohibits private employers and state and local governments from discriminating on the basis of age, race, color, religion, sex, or national origin.

The Civil Rights Act of 1964 is the centerpiece of a congeries of antidiscrimination laws that have made the U.S. public health system more ethical and equitable, including the Equal Pay Act of 1963 (29 U.S.C.A. §206 (d)), the Age Discrimination in Employment Act of 1967 (29 U.S.C.A. §621), the Rehabilitation Act of 1973 (29 U.S.C.A. §701 et seq.), the Americans with Disabilities Act of 1990 (42 U.S.C.A. §12101 et seq.), and the Individuals with Disabilities Education Act (20 U.S.C.A. §1400 et. seq.).

LEGALIZATION OF ABORTION

For a century in the United States, desperate women faced with unwanted pregnancies resorted to abortion that was illegal, clandestine, and dangerous. Nearly one-third of all maternal deaths were caused by illegal abortion. In 1973, in a dramatic response to a major health problem and social need, the U.S. Supreme Court held that old-style abortion laws, which made abortion a crime except when performed to save the life of the woman, were a violation of the woman's fundamental right of privacy (*Roe v. Wade*) and also held unconstitutional reformed laws that allowed abortion on categorical grounds (*Doe v. Bolton*).

In 1992, the U.S. Supreme Court reaffirmed its holding, stating that *Roe v. Wade* had acquired "a rare precedential force and could be overturned under fire only at the cost of both profound and unnecessary damage to the Court's legitimacy, and the nation's commitment to the rule of law." But the Court held that the right of privacy is not a fundamental right that requires strict scrutiny of state legislation but rather that restrictive state legislation may be struck down only if it imposes an undue burden on the woman (*Planned Parenthood of Southeast Pennsylvania* v. *Casey*). This is a new test that broadens the right of states to enact legislation restricting the right to choose abortion.

THE NEW YORK MENTAL HYGIENE LAW

Not all landmark legislation is enacted at the federal level of government. State legislation may be of singular importance in protecting the physical and mental health and the legal rights of the people.

The New York Mental Hygiene Law of 1964 revolutionized involuntary admissions to mental hospitals. This statute abolished long-standing judicial procedures for compulsory hospitalization of the mentally ill, which, though legalistic in form, provided only the illusion but not the reality of due process. Instead, the statute provided for initial medical admission on the recommendation of two physicians, like an admission to a hospital for a physical illness, followed by immediate and periodic judicial review so that no patient becomes a forgotten person. A key provision of the law was the establishment and funding of a new agency, the Mental Health Information Service, to inform the court of the patient's condition and to inform the patient of his or her legal rights.

Other states have also modernized their mental hospital admission laws. And, with the decline in hospitalization for mental illness, nearly all states have authorized involuntary outpatient admission to community mental health services.

FLUORIDATION OF PUBLIC WATER SUPPLIES

Fluoridation of public water supplies is an ideal public health measure because it requires minimal action by public health officials, a modest expenditure of funds, and no behavioral change by the public. Adjusting the fluoride content of the water supply to one part of sodium fluoride to a million parts of water yields enormous benefits in dental health—a reduction of sixty percent in dental caries in children who have drunk fluoridated water since birth, a benefit that lasts throughout their lifetime.

In 1965, the Illinois Supreme Court upheld a fluoridation ordinance of the city of Chicago, rejecting the contentions of the plaintiffs that the ordinance was an improper exercise of the police power because tooth decay is not a communicable disease, that the ordinance benefits only a segment of the population (children), and that it is mass medication in violation of the right of each individual to determine whether he or she wishes to be treated (*Schuringa* v. *City of Chicago*). The court held the ordinance a proper exercise of the police power, although tooth decay is not a communicable disease, and not invalid as class legislation because the benefits carry over into adulthood. Even if considered medication, fluoridation is so related to the common good that the rights of the individual must give way. The U.S. Supreme Court refused review of *Schuringa*—the leading case on the constitutionality of fluoridation ordinances.

RUTH ROEMER

(SEE ALSO: *Abortion; Civil Rights Act of 1964; Community Water Fluoridation; Environmental Impact Statement; Environmental Movement; Environmental Protection Agency; History of Public Health; Immunizations; Medicare*)

BIBLIOGRAPHY

Barton, P. L. (1999). *Understanding the U.S. Health Services System*. Chicago, IL: Health Administration Press.

Grad, F. (1985). *Environmental Law*, 3rd edition. New York: Matthew Bender and Company.

McCafferty, G., and Dooley, J. (1990). "Involuntary Outpatient Commitment: An Update." *Mental and Physical Disability Reporter* 14(3):277–287.

McKray, G., and McKray, J. (1980). "Consumer Protection: The Federal Food, Drug, and Cosmetic Act." *Legal Aspects of Health Policy: Issues and Trends*. Westport, CT: Greenwood Press.

New York Mental Hygiene Law (1964). Section 9.01 et seq., *McKinney's* 1996.

Shonick, W. (1995). *Government and Health Services: Government's Role in the Development of U.S. Health Services, 1930–1980*. New York: Oxford University Press.

Smith, D. B. (1999). *Health Care Divided: Race and a Healing Nation*. Ann Arbor: University of Michigan Press.

U.S. Food and Drug Administration (1996). "Nicotine in Cigarettes and Smokeless Tobacco is a Drug and These Products Are Nicotine Delivery Devices under the Federal Food, Drug, and Cosmetic Act: Jurisdictional Determination." 61 Fed. Reg. 44619–45318.

—— (1996). "Regulations Restricting the Sale and Distribution of Cigarettes and Smokeless Tobacco to Protect Children and Adolescents." 61 Fed. Reg. 44396.

CASES

Darling v. *Charleston Community Memorial Hospital*, 33 Ill.2d 326, 211 N.E. 2d 253 (1965).

Doe v. *Bolton*, 410 U.S. 179 (1973).

Food and Drug Administration v. *Brown and Williamson Tobacco Corp.*, U.S., 120 S.Ct. 1291 (2000).

Jacobson v. *Massachusetts*, 197 U.S. 11 (1905).

Planned Parenthood of Southeastern Pennsylvania v. *Casey*, 505 U.S. 833 (1992).

Roe v. *Wade*, 410 U.S. 113 (1973).

Schuringa v. *City of Chicago*, 30Ill.2d 326, cert. den. 379 U.S. 864 (1965).

LANGMUIR, ALEXANDER

Alexander Duncan Langmuir was born in Santa Monica, California, on September 12, 1910, and died on November 22, 1993. Langmuir was visionary, clairvoyant, tenacious, and a dedicated public health leader who gave definition to the science of epidemiology as applied to worldwide public health problems. His academic training led him into public health, and he gained field experience working as a public health officer in New York State and as a member of the Armed Forces Epidemiological Board. He taught for three years at the Johns Hopkins University School of Hygiene and Public Health, and in 1949 assumed the position of chief epidemiologist at what is now the Centers for Disease Control and Prevention (CDC), where he remained for twenty-one years. Upon retirement from the CDC, Langmuir served as a visiting professor at both the Harvard University School of Public Health and Johns Hopkins.

His excellence in the practice of epidemiology was recognized by membership in eleven prestigious societies, including the Institute of Medicine. He received multiple awards, including the Bronfman Award from the American Public Health Association and the Dana Foundation Pioneering Achievements in Health Award. He was a frequent consultant on public health issues both in the United States and throughout the world and the author of over 100 scientific publications.

Langmuir's major contributions include defining the practice of applied epidemiology as a science in public health and preventive medicine; development of the two-year Epidemic Intelligence Service (EIS) training program; developing and promoting public health surveillance as an essential ingredient in the practice of public health; and highlighting the importance of communication in public health. The EIS program is recognized internationally as the premier applied epidemiology training program. Langmuir's hands-on approach to training has spread to more than twenty countries through the development of Field Epidemiology Training Programs, which serve as a vibrant, living memorial to Langmuir's training objectives.

Through his teachings and practice, Langmuir made major contributions to the control and prevention of infectious diseases, including the eradication of smallpox and the control and prevention of poliomyelitis, cholera, vaccine-preventable diseases, and hospital-acquired infections. He was instrumental in carefully defining airborne disease, which led to important mechanisms of control and prevention. An early advocate of the need to apply epidemiological principles to studies of populations and the development of family-planning programs, Langmuir also extended the use of epidemiology in the investigations of cancer and was instrumental in assisting in the development of surveillance programs for birth defects. He was strongly instrumental in assisting in the development of veterinary public health as a discipline, and in the training of veterinarians in applied epidemiology. Langmuir also extended the boundaries of the practice of epidemiology in the control and prevention of public health problems and extended the horizons of the practice of preventive medicine.

PHILIP S. BRACHMAN

(SEE ALSO: *Centers for Disease Control and Prevention; Epidemic Intelligence Service; Epidemiology*)

LATENT PERIOD

A "latent period" is the lag time between exposure to a disease-causing agent and the onset of the disease the agent causes. In infectious diseases it is often identical to the incubation period, but not always. A disease may have incubated but remains latent, or dormant, within the body. For instance, the latent period between exposure to HIV (human immunodeficiency virus) infection and the onset of AIDS (acquired immunodeficiency syndrome) may be many years, although invasion of the body by HIV does cause a transient primary infection two to three weeks after initial exposure. Transmissable spongiform encephalopathy, caused by infectious prions, may have a latent period of up to twenty years or more.

The distinction between latency and incubation is illustrated by the natural history of the asbestos-induced cancer mesothelioma, where there may have been a single finite exposure many years before the onset of malignancy. Exposure to a single large dose of ionizing radiation, such as the exposure of residents of Hiroshima to the atom bomb explosion of 1945, demonstrates the variation in the latent period between exposure to ionizing radiation and the occurrence of malignancies, as well as the relationship between malignancies and radiation dose. In general, there is an inverse relationship between exposure dose and latent period—a high dose generally results in a short latent period, while a low dose means long latency. Leukemia follows exposure to ionizing radiation with an average latency of about five years, while some other malignancies, such as bone cancer, may have a latent period of twenty or more years.

During the latent period between initial exposure and the onset of clinically detectable disease, pathological processes may be progressing slowly and inexorably, and they may be detectable with suitable screening tests. Timely intervention at this stage may arrest the progress of disease. However, much remains to be discovered about the natural history of many disease processes with long latent periods between exposure and the appearance of overt disease.

JOHN M. LAST

(SEE ALSO: *Incubation Period*)

LATINOS

See Hispanic Cultures

LAVERAN, ALPHONSE

Charles-Louis-Alphonse Laveran was born in 1845 in Paris, France, where he also died in 1922. Laveran's father was a distinguished physician in the French military, and Laveran continued the family tradition. He enrolled in l'École du Service de Santé Militaire at Strasbourg in 1863 and served during the Franco-Prussian War. In 1874 he received the post of Professor Agregé des Maladies et Epidemies des Armées. In 1878, Laveran was sent to work in an Algerian hospital outside the city of Constantine. A number of troops had fallen victim to malaria and Laveran began conducting postmortem examinations. Physicians had been familiar with this disease, which is characterized by fever, since ancient times, but its etiology and process of transmission were still unknown. Laveran's initial findings—that the internal organs were discolored—confirmed previous research experiments. When he began to examine blood from the organs, however, he noticed something new. He observed a series of filaments, or parasites, moving independently among the red blood cells.

Laveran presented his discovery at a meeting at the Académie de Médecine in Paris a few weeks later on November 23, 1880. During the next year, Laveran recorded parasites in 148 out of 200 patients believed to have died from malaria. Yet, when Laveran demonstrated his experiment in Italy, a center for the study of malaria, skeptics questioned his deduction that the filaments were independent living organisms. Although he had discovered the parasite that causes malaria, now known as *Plasmodium*, the relationship between the parasite and outbreaks of the disease remained elusive. Laveran returned to Paris in 1884 and published *Traité des Fièvres Palustres*. He continued his studies as a professor of military hygiene at Val-de-Grace Hospital and, after his retirement from the army, at the Pasteur Institute. By the time of his death, Laveran had published approximately six hundred works on the subject of parasites in man and animals and received a Nobel Prize for his work.

JENNIFER KOSLOW

(SEE ALSO: *Malaria; Pathogenic Organisms*)

BIBLIOGRAPHY

Bruce-Chwatt, L. J. (1981). "Alphonse Laveran's Discovery 100 Years Ago and Today's Global Fight Against Malaria." *Journal of the Royal Society of Medicine* 74(7):531–536.

Garnham, P. C. C. (1998). "History of Discoveries of Malaria Parasites." *In History and Philosophy of the Life Sciences* 10(1):93–108.

LAY CONCEPTS OF HEALTH AND ILLNESS

Lay concepts (or folk concepts) of health and illness are conceptual models used by individuals, communities, or cultures in attempting to explain how to maintain health and to provide an explanation for illness. Lay concepts of health and illness often have theoretical underpinnings that arise from the wider theories of illness (e.g., humoral, Ayurvedic, biomedical), but also include locally developed concepts about the body in health and illness that may not directly relate to the major theories of illness.

Lay concepts of health and illness include particular ideas about the way the body functions, and they also highlight particular symptoms as being of special significance. For example, in the Western world, the body is often thought of as an intricate machine which must be kept "tuned-up," and illness is viewed as a breakdown of the machine. This contrasts with the Ayurvedic concept of the body, a concept prevalent in India and South Asia, in which health is seen as a state of balance between the physical, social, and supernatural environment and illness can result from disturbances in many different spheres. In the Western world, a symptom such as chest pain has a particular cultural significance and tends to be regarded with alarm. In Ayurvedic medicine, chest pain is also regarded with concern but as a symptom of emotional upset and not as the organic breakdown of bodily function. In South Asia, the symptom of "semen loss," a symptom generally regarded as innocuous in the Western world, is regarded with alarm. Cultural differences in the meaning of symptoms can lead at times to a delayed diagnosis of potentially serious conditions. For example, abdominal pain associated with appendicitis may not be interpreted to be serious, or a lump in the breast may be attributed to injury rather than to a potentially malignant process.

Lay concepts of illness usually include more than just ideas about the immediate cause of an illness. They also incorporate ideas about gauging the severity of illness, concepts about appropriate treatment for an illness, and ideas about the meaning of illness. Lay concepts of illness differ widely among cultural groups, and also between groups of people from differing socioeconomic strata. A research study done in the United States among members of lower socioeconomic classes revealed that lay concepts of illness in this group tended to have a functional basis—only if a person was ill enough to not be able to work would medical attention be sought. Lay concepts about appropriate treatments for illness may differ from a doctor's concepts; an example from contemporary North America is the commonly held belief that antibiotics are helpful in curing colds and the flu, a notion that most doctors try hard to refute. Lay conceptualization about the meaning of illness is also important. When people fall ill, they need to find an answer to the "why" of the illness as well as to the "how" of the illness. Making sense of serious illness becomes an urgent task that involves the patient at the deepest level.

Lay concepts of illness have been classified as being derived from within the individual, from the natural world, from the social world, or from the supernatural world. For example, lay concepts about illness in rural India often locate the origin of illness within the social world (failure to observe social norms or perform essential rituals) and within the supernatural world (a spirit attack or the "evil eye"). Other lay concepts about illness from India relate to the individual (improper diet) and to the natural world (exposure to extremes of hot or cold). Lay concepts about illness causation in the Western world often locate the origin of ill health within the individual—perhaps the person has behaved inappropriately (wrong diet, lack of exercise); or perhaps the person is vulnerable to illness in some way (hereditary or psychological factors). Lay concepts about illness that locate the cause of illness external to the individual include ideas about infection, exposure to heat or cold, and, increasingly, exposure to environmental contaminants.

Where many people in a culture agree about a pattern of symptoms or signs, and have a conceptual model about the origin and significance of these symptoms and signs, the illness can be termed a folk illness. Folk illnesses have a range of symbolic meanings that have moral, social, and psychological dimensions. A person suffering from a folk illness often expresses emotional distress through the physical body. This emotional distress may arise from conflicts within the family, or from the larger social world that the individual inhabits. Symptoms associated with folk illnesses often have a particular cultural significance, and they are often shaped by the way people in a cultural group think about the body in health and in illness. Traditional healers within a particular culture recognize, interpret, and treat the illness using therapies that are congruent with the particular lay concepts of illness that underpin the condition.

Examples of folk illness include *susto* in Central and South America, *amok* in Malaysia, and *nervios* among Latino populations. Sometimes folk illnesses overlap with serious biomedical disease. For example, a person who complains of weakness, dizziness, and palpitations may be diagnosed by a traditional healer to be suffering from *nervios*, when he or she may be experiencing a serious cardiac or neurological crisis. More often, though, the symptoms do not have a serious organic cause, and are related to the social or emotional stresses the person is experiencing. Biomedical practitioners who are not familiar with *nervios* as a folk illness may misinterpret the condition, and inappropriately overmedicate the patient. Clearly, it is important for biomedical practitioners to learn about local concepts of health and illness and to be alert for symptoms that may reflect emotional and social distress rather than a breakdown in the biomedical functions of the body.

KAREN TROLLOPE-KUMAR
JOHN LAST

(SEE ALSO: *Anthropology in Public Health; Cultural Factors; Ethnicity and Health; Folk Medicine; Theories of Health and Illness*)

BIBLIOGRAPHY

Helman, C. (1990). *Culture, Health and Illness*. Oxford, UK: Butterworth-Heineman.

Kinsley, D. (1996). *Health, Healing and Religion: A Cross-Cultural Perspective*. Englewood Cliffs, NJ: Prentice Hall.

Kleinman, A. (1988). *The Illness Narratives: Suffering, Healing and the Human Condition.* New York: Basic Books.

LDL CHOLESTEROL

Low-density lipoprotein cholesterol (LDL cholesterol) is the "lousy" or "bad" cholesterol carried within a lipoprotein in the blood whose density, when serum is ultracentrifuged, lies between the very low-density (VLDL) and high-density (HDL) lipoproteins. Low-density lipoproteins are deposited by blood beneath the lining of arteries, where they are oxidized and stimulate the formation of cholesterol-containing foam cells, which are the abnormal cells responsible for the development of atherosclerosis. Lowering LDL cholesterol by dietary or pharmacologic means has been shown to decrease the risk of heart attacks, strokes, and death. Eating animal and dairy fat, partially hydrogenated fats used in pastries and fried fast foods, and high levels of dietary cholesterol can all elevate LDL cholesterol.

DONALD A. SMITH

(SEE ALSO: *Atherosclerosis; Blood Lipids; Cholesterol Test; Fats; Foods and Diets; Genetics and Health; HDL Cholesterol; Hyperlipidemia; Triglycerides; VLDL Cholesterol*)

LEAD

Lead (Pb) is a soft, corrosion-resistant gray metal that is a common environmental contaminant in air, food, paint, and water. Lead is recovered from mined sulfide ores, and has been used to fashion items such as statues and tools since at least 6500 B.C.E. The Romans used lead to fashion potable water piping. The relationship between plumbing and lead has become a permanent part of the English language—the word "plumbing" derives from the Latin word for lead, *plumbum*. Besides plumbing, lead has been used to manufacture items such as ceramics, cosmetics, lead batteries, leaded paint, and leaded gasoline. Common chemical species of lead used commercially include lead acetate, lead carbonate, lead chloride, and lead oxide.

Figure 1

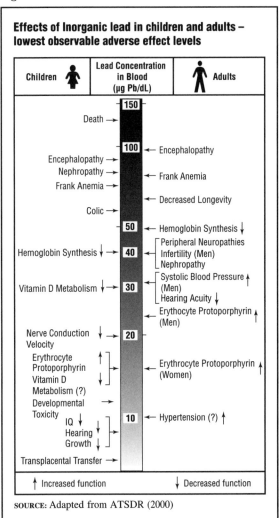

SOURCE: Adapted from ATSDR (2000)

The Agency for Toxic Substances and Disease Registry (ATSDR) estimates that more than one million workers in one hundred occupations are exposed to lead, such as in the lead-battery recycling and lead-smelting industries. Equally important, almost all persons are exposed to lead in residential settings from sources such as paint chips, food, water, cigarettes, and clothing that has been worn in lead-contaminated work environments.

Adverse health effects from lead exposure have been recognized since the time of the Romans. The National Research Council (NRC) traces society's more recent interest in lead poisoning to an 1839 publication by Tanquerel des Planches, who described lead colic in 1,207 occupationally exposed workers. It is now recognized that even low levels of lead exposure are associated with adverse health effects. The U.S. Centers for Disease Control and Prevention (CDC) has identified a lead concentration of ten micrograms per deciliter (μg/dL) of blood as the level of concern above which significant health risks occur. Acute exposure to lead compounds may cause brain damage, kidney damage, and gastrointestinal distress. Chronic exposure to lead results in effects on the blood, the central nervous system, blood pressure, the kidneys, the male reproductive system, and vitamin D metabolism. Children, particularly impoverished children living in homes with lead paint, are particularly at risk from the toxic effects of lead, and may exhibit slowed cognitive development and decreased intelligence after chronic exposure. Figure 1 identifies the health effects of lead at different blood level concentrations.

Because lead does not biodegrade, the approximately 300 million metric tons of lead produced to date remains in the environment. This suggests that humans will continue to be exposed to lead despite the phasing out of lead in consumer products such as gasoline and paint. In the early 1970s, the federal government recognized that steps had to be taken to reduce human exposure to lead, and banned residential leaded paint (1978), and phased out leaded gasoline between 1975 and 1995. The removal of lead from gasoline has proceeded more slowly in the rest of the world. In some countries leaded gasoline remains a significant source of exposure.

The CDC estimates that children's blood lead levels have declined over eighty percent since the mid-1970s. The Lead Contamination Act of 1988 authorized the CDC to initiate programs to eliminate childhood lead poisoning in the United States. The Lead Contamination Act of 1988 authorized the CDC to make grants to state and local agencies for comprehensive programs designed to screen infants and children for elevated blood lead levels, ensure referral for medical and environmental intervention for lead-poisoned infants and children, and provide education about childhood lead poisoning. Despite this impressive decrease in blood lead levels, more than one million children in the United States have blood lead levels above 10 μg/dL, and are at risk of permanent neurological impairment.

MARGARET H. WHITAKER
BRUCE A. FOWLER

(SEE ALSO: *Blood Lead; Environmental Determinants of Health; Heavy Metals; Occupational Disease; Occupational Safety and Health; Regulations Affecting Housing*)

BIBLIOGRAPHY

Agency for Toxic Substances and Disease Registry (ATSDR) (1993). *Toxicological Profile for Lead.* Washington, DC: U.S. Department of Health and Human Services.

—— (2000). *Case Studies in Environmental Medicine: Lead Toxicity.* Available at http://www.atsdr.cdc.gov/HEC/caselead.html.

Centers for Disease Control and Prevention (1997). "Update: Blood Lead Levels—United States 1991–1994." *Morbidity and Mortality Weekly Report* 46(7):141–146 and erratum in 46(26):607.

Lewis, J. (1985). "Lead Poisoning: A Historical Perspective." *EPA Journal.* Available at http://www.epa.gov/history/topics/perspect/lead.htm.

National Research Council, Commission on Life Sciences (1993). *Measuring Lead Exposure in Infants, Children, and Other Sensitive Populations.* Available at http://stills.nap.edu/books/030904927X/html/.

President's Task Force on Environmental Health Risks and Safety Risks to Children (2000). *Eliminating Childhood Lead Poisoning: A Federal Strategy Targeting Lead Paint Hazards.* Available at http://www.epa.gov/children/whatwe/leadhaz.pdf.

U.S. Environmental Protection Agency (U.S. EPA) (1998). *Lead in Your Home: A Parent's Reference Guide.* Office of Prevention, Pesticides, and Toxic Substances. Available at http://www.epa.gov/lead/leadrev.pdf.

LEADERSHIP

Leadership is the process through which an individual tries to influence another individual or a group of individuals to accomplish a goal. Leadership is valued in our culture, especially when it helps to achieve goals that are beneficial to the population, such as the enactment of effective preventive-health policies. An individual with leadership qualities can also improve an organization and the individuals in it, whether it be a teacher who works to get better teaching materials and after-school programs or an employee who develops new ideas and products and influences others to invest in them.

Leadership can be exhibited in a variety of ways and circumstances. Mothers and fathers show leadership in raising their children with good values and encouraging them to develop to their potential. Teachers show it in inspiring students to learn and to develop their intellectual capacity. Health care workers can be leaders and develop services that meet the needs of the communities they serve, or work in collaboration with other organizations to create cost-effective, prevention-oriented programs and services.

Many studies have been done and many books and articles have been published on this subject. Through this work a consistent set of leadership attributes has emerged. An effective leader does most, if not all, of the following:

- *Challenge the Process*—search out challenging opportunities, take risks, and learn from mistakes.

- *Inspire others to come together and agree on a future direction or goal*—create a shared vision by thinking about the future, having a strong positive vision, and encouraging others to participate.

- *Help others to act*—help others to work together, to cooperate and collaborate by developing shared goals and building trust, and help to make others stronger by encouraging them to develop their skills and talents.

- *Set an example*—behave in ways that are consistent with professed values and help others to achieve small gains that keep them motivated, especially when a goal will not be achieved quickly.

- *Encourage others*—recognize each individual's contributions to the success of a project.

Another way of defining leadership is to acknowledge what people value in individuals that are recognized as leaders. Most people can think of individuals they consider to be leaders. Research conducted in the 1980s by James Kouzes and Barry Posner found that a majority of people admire, and willingly follow, people who are honest, forward-looking, inspiring, and competent

An individual who would like to develop leadership skills can profit from the knowledge that leadership is *not* just a set of exceptional skills and attributes possessed by only a few very special people. Rather, leadership is a process and a set of skills that can be learned.

CAROL WOLTRING

(SEE ALSO: *Careers in Public Health; Community Organization; Public Health Leadership Institute*)

BIBLIOGRAPHY

Kouzes, J. M., and Posner, B. Z. (1995). *The Leadership Challenge*, 2nd edition. San Francisco: Jossey-Bass.

Pointer, D. D., and Sanchez, J. P. (1993). "Leadership: A Framework for Thinking and Acting." In *Health Care Management: A Text in Organization Theory and Behavior*, 3rd edition. eds. S. Shortell and A. Kaluzny. New York: Wiley.

LEEUWENHOEK, ANTONI VAN

Antoni van Leeuwenhoek (1632–1723) was born, and also died, in the city of Delft in the Netherlands. Although a linen draper by profession, Leeuwenhoek learned to make lenses and built over five hundred simple microscopes to conduct his numerous personal experiments. With these instruments, Leeuwenhoek investigated the natural world, including water, soil, and human excretions. Because he is considered the first person to have viewed and documented the existence of microscopic organisms, including bacteria, he has been called the first of the microbe hunters.

His lack of formal scientific training led Leeuwenhoek to concentrate on making observations rather than offering theories. Although he never published his work, Leeuwenhoek described his findings in a series of 165 letters to the Royal Society of London, beginning in 1673 and ending only with his death. His first letter, dated April 28, 1673, details his microscopic inspections of mold and bees.

His most famous letter is dated October 9, 1676. This letter communicates the results of a series of experiments on water infused with pepper. Leeuwenhoek began by examining some snow-water that he had kept sealed for three years. He noted no creatures. He then added some peppercorns to the solution, and, after three weeks, he discovered the sudden appearance of a tremendous number of "very little animals." Judging by his calculations of their number and size, historians have surmised that Leeuwenhoek had become the first person to see bacteria. Colleagues reproduced his experiments in the months that followed. Given contemporary medical theories, it did not occur to Leeuwenhoek that what he saw with his microscope was in any way connected to disease, but his observations laid a foundation on which further investigations were born.

JENNIFER KOSLOW

BIBLIOGRAPHY

Dobell, C. (1932). *Anthony van Leeuwenhoek and His "Little Animals."* Reprint. New York: Dover Publications, 1962.

Palm, L. C. (1982). *Antoni van Leeuwenhoek, 1632–1723: Studies on the Life and Work of the Delft Scientist Commemorating the 350th Anniversary of His Birthday.* Amsterdam: Rodopi B.V.

LEGAL LIABILITY OF PUBLIC HEALTH OFFICIALS

Historically, the doctrine of sovereign immunity has prevented lawsuits from being filed against public health officials. Sovereign immunity prevents the states and the federal government, and their officials, from being sued. Most countries have some version of sovereign immunity. In the United States, sovereign immunity does allow lawsuits to prevent the enforcement of unconstitutional laws, but not for injuries to persons. Congress and the states have passed laws called tort claims acts (TCAs) that waive sovereign immunity in certain circumstances. Congress has also passed various civil rights acts that allow suits against persons acting under governmental authority who violate constitutional rights and certain federal laws. Other countries have similar, but usually

much more limited, waivers of sovereign immunity. This article is limited to United States law.

While TCAs and civil rights laws allow lawsuits against public health officials, their liability is still very limited. Public health officials doing core public health policymaking and enforcement are seldom sued successfully in their official capacity, and they are almost never found personally liable. However, not every employee of a public health agency is a protected official, and some activities performed by health departments, such as personal medical services, are not considered core public health activities and are not sheltered from liability. Federal standards for liability are uniform across the states. States, however, have different standards for what is a core public health activity and who is a protected official. The general principles of state liability are similar, but public health officials must become familiar with the laws in their own states.

PRINCIPLES OF LIABILITY

The legal rules for liability for government officials are shaped by three concerns. First, the state generally has no duty to provide services. Second, the government and public officials should be accountable for negligent or intentionally harmful actions. Third, since the state has no duty to provide services, then legal liability will tend to reduce public services, and personal liability for public health officers will make it difficult to attract qualified professionals for public health service. The courts balance the value of the service against the potential harm caused by improper actions. For public health, the potential value of the service is very high because so many persons can be harmed by an epidemic or toxic exposure. The potential risks posed by improper public health actions are relatively low, especially compared to activities such as law enforcement, where deadly force is often at issue. A wrongful quarantine can be quickly reviewed and remedied through a habeas corpus proceeding. Even if the action exceeds the department's legal authority or is based on negligent decision making, the public health officer will be immune, unless the plaintiff can show that the officer knew or should have known the action was illegal or improper. Mistakes alone do not result in liability.

TYPES OF CLAIMS

Public health officials can be sued in their official capacity or as private persons. Official capacity means the public health official is a surrogate for the government and is not personally liable if damages are awarded to the plaintiff. These lawsuits are usually brought to stop enforcement of an alleged unconstitutional law or to stop alleged unconstitutional or otherwise illegal behavior by a health agency. They are governed by sovereign immunity, the principle that the government cannot be sued without its permission.

Private capacity lawsuits assert personal wrongdoing by an official, and, if successful, damages must be paid by the official. This personal wrongdoing may be related to official duties or may be strictly private conduct, such as causing an accident while driving drunk.

LIABILITY UNDER FEDERAL LAW

The Civil Rights Act of 1871 allows citizens to sue persons who, acting under color of state law, deprive them of their constitutional rights. This is the most common basis of federal claims against public health officials. The key section of this law is codified in U.S. law under Title 42, Section 1983, giving the name "1983 actions" to these claims. Since the Eleventh Amendment of the Constitution prohibits most private lawsuits against the states, 1983 actions can be brought against state officials in their personal capacity, but not in their official capacity. City, county, and other nonstate officials can be sued personally and in their official capacity, allowing damages to be obtained from the governmental entity. In 1971, the United States Supreme Court allowed claims against federal officials who violated an individual's constitutional rights in *Bivens v. Six Unknown Named Agents of Federal Bureau of Narcotics*. A "Bivens action" is the federal equivalent of a 1983 action. Bivens actions, 1983 actions, and related actions against public health officials have similar requirements.

1983 actions must allege a violation of the plaintiff's rights arising from the Constitution or certain federal laws. Most public health cases are violations of the constitutional rights of equal protection or due process. Equal protection claims arise from differential treatment that is motivated by improper discrimination, especially discrimination based on race, ethnicity, or religion. Thus the Supreme Court in *Yick Wo v. Hopkins* (1886) held a fire ordinance unconstitutional because it was only applied to Chinese laundries. Differential treatment is constitutional when it is based on nonsuspect classifications or is scientifically appropriate. Thus it would not be an equal protection violation to screen only African Americans for sickle-cell disease, certain Jewish groups for Tay-Sachs disease, or prostitutes for gonorrhea. Refusing to issue a license or permit to a class of persons could be an equal protection violation, unless there were rational grounds for the refusal.

Due process claims arise when a public health official does not provide the procedural safeguards the law requires, or when the law itself may be unconstitutional. If a statute requires thirty-days notice and an opportunity for a hearing before destroying a dangerous building, then it could be a due process violation to destroy such a building without notice. If a defendant has complied with applicable statutes, then the plaintiff can claim that the Constitution requires more process than the state or local law provides. Claims commonly arise when public health officials take action without a pre-deprivation (prior) hearing. If the action is authorized by statute, or the court finds there are exigent circumstances, the court will dismiss the claim.

Section 1983 applies to anyone who acts under color of state law, including those working under the authority of the health department, irrespective of their employment status, and can even be applied to volunteers. It does not provide for vicarious liability, so public health officials can only be held liable for their own actions. They cannot be held liable for the unconstitutional actions of their subordinates, unless they were personally involved in these actions. The courts give public health personnel qualified immunity for their official actions. This means that they will not be held liable unless their conduct violates clearly established statutory or constitutional rights that they should reasonably have known about. Being mistaken about the law is not enough, nor is acting under a law later declared unconstitutional. Since public health officials have broad authority in most jurisdictions, it is difficult to show that a given action is clearly beyond the official's authority if the public health official's actions are consistent with standard public health practices or are intended to manage an immediate threat to the public health. The courts also require that persons bringing 1983 actions show significant harm, which is unusual in public health restrictions because they are easily reviewed and corrected in post-deprivation proceedings.

STATE LAW LIABILITY

State law liability is controlled by the state's constitution and TCAs, which differ among states. State public health officials have official immunity when they are making policy decisions or performing discretionary acts, which are those acts that require the exercise of professional judgment. Inspecting a restaurant and deciding whether it should be cited for health-code violations is a discretionary function. Official immunity for discretionary functions is determined by the nature of the function and not the job title of the employee. It can extend to every employee of the department, although the law is not so clear when tasks are done by private contractors. Tasks that do not require discretion, called ministerial tasks, are either those that follow a predetermined plan and cannot be changed, such as following a checklist, or those that do not involve any special expertise related to public health, such as driving a car. Discretionary immunity applies unless a plaintiff can show that a reasonable person in the official's position would have known that the action was unambiguously beyond the scope of the official's legal authority or was otherwise illegal.

Most states further classify public health functions as governmental or proprietary. There is official immunity for discretionary governmental functions, but not for proprietary functions. The definition of these terms varies greatly between states, with some states holding that almost all public health functions are governmental and others finding that a substantial group are proprietary. Traditional public health services such as restaurant inspection, animal control, health and safety permits and licenses, sanitation, vital statistics, and related functions are considered governmental in almost all states. The biggest exception

is personal medical services, such as prenatal care and general indigent health care. Most states do not consider these as governmental functions and apply ordinary medical malpractice law to them. However, if the medical service is related to protecting the public, rather than just helping an individual, it will be termed governmental. Thus treatment and testing for tuberculosis or sexually transmitted diseases would be a governmental function.

If the function is proprietary or ministerial, then the state TCA will determine the extent of liability and when the official is personally liable. TCAs limit liability—usually between $100,000 and $1,000,000—and generally prevent the recovery of punitive damages. TCAs provide that the state will defend the lawsuit and pay the claim if the official is sued personally. There are usually exceptions if the claim is for intentional wrongdoing that is outside the official's duties. This might include sexual assault charges or criminal conduct such as bribe–taking by an inspector. Depending on state law, the TCA may not apply to nonemployees such as contract physicians in clinics. These individuals may need to have private insurance to defend and pay claims brought against them.

LIMITING LIABILITY

Public health officials should assure that they are well-versed in public health law, and that the personnel in their departments are conversant with the laws that govern their jobs. While many issues are common to all the states and the federal government, it is critical to identify specific state requirements and limitations. Public health officials should work closely with their legal counsel. Protocols should be developed to handle common legal problems such as inspections and warrants. Cooperative agreements should be worked out with other departments and governmental units for handling emergency conditions such as toxic spills or bioterrorism. Local hospitals and medical organizations should be educated about their legal duties and encouraged to work closely with the health department to manage disease outbreaks. Such advance planning reduces the need for public health officials to use coercive legal authority and avoids legal conflicts.

Public health officials should work with legislators at the city, county, and state levels to ensure that public health legislation does not increase their liability. Overly specific legislation, or legislation that provides for excessive pre-deprivation due process, makes it very difficult to respond to emergent conditions or to situations unanticipated by the legislature. It is critical that public health legislation and regulations preserve sufficient flexibility to allow public health officials to act quickly and innovatively. If not, then the officials may be forced to risk potential liability to protect the public's health.

EDWARD P. RICHARDS

(SEE ALSO: *Codes of Conduct and Ethics Guidelines; Landmark Public Health Laws and Court Decisions; Police Powers; Public Health and the Law; Quarantine, and articles on specific diseases mentioned herein*)

BIBLIOGRAPHY

Grad, F. (1990). *The Public Health Law Manual.* APHA Press.

Griffith, L. E., Jr., and Tinio, F. S. (1988). "Municipal, County, School, and State Tort Liability." In *American Jurisprudence*, vol. 57. Lawyers Co-operative Publishing Company.

Nahmod, S. H. (1997). *Civil Rights and Civil Liberties Litigation: The Law of Section 1983*, 4th edition. St. Paul, MN: West Group.

Richards, E. P., and Rathbun, K. C. (1998). "Public Health Law." In *Maxcy-Rosenau-Last Public Health and Preventive Medicine*, ed. R. B. Wallace. Stamford, CT: Appleton and Lange.

—— (1999). *Medical Care Law.* Gaithersburg, VA: Aspen Publishers.

LEGISLATION AND REGULATION

In the United States, public health programs are implemented through governmental agencies at both the state and federal levels. Federal agencies are created by Congress and are part of the executive branch of the government. Some state agencies are created by their state constitution, but most are created though state legislation. State agencies can be part of the governor's office, headed by independently elected officials, or supervised by independent boards that are appointed by the governor or the legislature, or are popularly elected.

ENABLING LEGISLATION

A law establishing an agency is called "enabling legislation." Enabling legislation establishes the mission of an agency and defines its powers. It is the most important limitation on agency action. An agency has only the power it is given in its enabling legislation or by the state constitution. Agencies created by the legislature can have only the powers that the state and federal constitutions allow the legislature to delegate. The legislature can also modify the enabling legislation if it wants to change the agency's mission or powers.

AGENCY REGULATIONS

Enabling legislation may be very specific as to the role of an agency and how the agency is to enforce the law, leaving the agency little discretion in its actions. More commonly, however, the legislature gives an agency a general mandate, such as "protect the public health," and directs the agency to decide the best way to do this. This allows the details to be developed by agency staff, and it makes it easier to respond to new threats and changing conditions because no new legislation is required. When the agency is charged with developing regulations, it must make them available to the public. This can be done through notice and comment rule making, which requires that proposed regulations be published for public comment, that the agency respond to the comments, and that the proposed regulation be revised and republished if necessary. The agency must also publish the information it relied upon to develop the proposed regulation, including whether it relied on private standards such as building codes or standards developed by other agencies. In some circumstances the agency may also have public hearings on proposed regulations. When the regulations are adopted, they are legally binding unless they exceed the agency's authority or conflict with other laws or the state or federal constitution. In emergencies, rules can be published and put into affect without a prior comment period, as long as they are subject to later revision. Thus the agriculture department might publish an emergency rule to block the import of BSE infected beef.

In addition to formal regulations, agencies publish documents that explain how the agency interprets the law, and how to comply with it. These guidance documents do not have the force of law, in that they are not binding on the courts. They are useful because they can provide a plain language explanation of formal regulations and enabling legislation, and thus assist the public with compliance. An agency can also provide guidance by publishing records of enforcement actions. While the agency is not bound to follow past precedent in all cases, it does provide useful information for regulated entities.

JUDICIAL REVIEW

When the courts review a law passed by the legislature, they are obliged to uphold it unless there are constitutional problems with it. When courts review agency regulations, they determine whether the agency is constitutional, whether it is within the powers delegated to the agency, whether the delegation is constitutional, and whether the agency followed the correct procedures for promulgating or enforcing the regulation. If the regulation passes this test, the court will defer to the agency's expertise on nonlegal matters. In a classic public health case, *Jacobson v. Massachusetts* (1905), the United States Supreme Court found that a regulation requiring smallpox vaccination could not be overturned just because some scientists disagreed with it. The Court established the standard that it is the agency's role to choose from available regulatory alternatives, and in the process to balance the needs of the individual and those of the state. The courts will not second-guess such decisions unless they are outside the agency's legal authority, or if the agency acted in an arbitrary and capricious manner in promulgating or enforcing the regulation. Without this deference, public health regulation could often be stalled in the courts. In a modern example, the courts have allowed health departments to require the named reporting of

HIV (human immunodeficiency virus) infection, despite opposition by some public health officials.

EDWARD P. RICHARDS

(SEE ALSO: *Landmark Public Health Laws and Court Decisions; Licensing; Police Powers; Public Health and the Law; Regulatory Authority*)

BIBLIOGRAPHY

Grad, F. (1990). *The Public Health Law Manual.* APHA Press.

Richards, E. P., and Rathbun, K. C. (1998). "Public Health Law." In *Maxcy-Rosenau-Last Public Health and Preventive Medicine,* ed. R. B. Wallace. Stamford, CT: Appleton and Lange.

—— (1999). "The Role of the Police Power in 21st Century Public Health." *Journal of Sexually Transmitted Diseases* 26(6): 350–357.

LEISHMANIASIS

Leishmaniasis is caused by protozoan parasites of the genus *Leishmania* that are spread by the bite of female phlebotomine sand flies of the genus *Phlebotomus* in the Old World and *Lutzomyia* in the New World.

Approximately 350 million people in eighty-eight countries are thought to be at risk for leishmania infection. The true number of infected individuals is unknown, as it is not considered a reportable disease in many of the affected countries. The World Health Organization (WHO) estimates that twelve million people are infected and that there are between 1.5 and 2 million new cases each year.

Leishmania infection occurs in a variety of mammalian hosts, including the domestic dog, rodents, and sloths. When a sand fly, a night-biting insect, takes a blood meal from an infected mammal, it will ingest leishmania parasites, called amastigotes, along with the blood. Over seven days leishmania multiply in the flight muscles and develop into infective, flagellated promastigote forms. When the sand fly next takes a blood meal, these promastigotes are injected into a new mammalian host, where they transform back into the amastigote form and begin to divide. *Leishmania* species are obligate intracellular parasites that infect and replicate in mononuclear phagocytic cells such as macrophages. Infection can also occur via blood transfusion, shared intravenous needles, or, rarely, direct contact with skin lesions. The incubation period in humans is usually from three to eight months, but can be as short as two weeks or as long as several decades.

The spectrum of clinical manifestations caused by leishmania is divided into three broad categories: cutaneous, mucocutaneous, and visceral leishmaniasis. Cutaneous leishmaniasis is found worldwide and results in skin lesions ranging from a single, discrete, self-healing ulcer to diffuse progressive induration. The spectrum of disease is determined by the species of the parasite and the ability of the host to mount a cell-mediated response. A hyper-immune response causes destructive changes such as those seen in mucocutaneous disease, and a hypo-immune response results in visceral and diffuse cutaneous leishmaniasis. In Old World cutaneous leishmaniasis, the usual causative species are *L. major*, *L. tropica*, or *L. aethiopica*. In the Americas, cutaneous lesions are usually the result of infection with *L. braziliensis*, *L. mexicana*, *L. amazonensis*, or *L. panamensis*.

In mucocutaneous leishmaniasis (also called espundia), the infection causes destruction of mucous membranes of the nose, mouth, and throat. This form of *leishmania* is found almost exclusively in the Americas and is seen predominantly in a subset of patients infected with *L. braziliensis*. Diffuse cutaneous leishmaniasisis, caused by *L. aethiopica*, is characterized by induration of skin without ulceration.

Visceral leishmaniasis, or kala-azar, is the most severe form of infection with parasites disseminated throughout the reticuloendothelial system. Patients experience fevers, night sweats, and weight loss. The spleen and liver become enlarged, sometimes massively. Blood work reveals anemia, leucopenia, thrombocytopenia, and a marked increase in gamma-globulin levels. If untreated, visceral leishmaniasis is virtually always fatal.

It used to be thought that each species of *leishmania* resulted in a particular clinical syndrome. However, it is now being recognized that there is considerable overlap in the clinical presentation of each species. Most people bitten by leishmania-infected sand flies will never manifest any evidence of the infection. After recovery from leishmaniasis, a person is immune for life from reinfection by that strain.

Conditions that impair cell-mediated immunity can result in more severe, disseminated leishmanial infections. This has been seen in organ transplant recipients and, most importantly, in persons infected with HIV (human immunodeficiency virus), in whom visceral leishmaniasis has become a frequent opportunistic infection in endemic regions.

Diagnosis is made by microscopic identification of the parasite in tissue samples, by growing the organisms in culture, or by polymerase chain reaction (PCR) of tissue. PCR is a test that will identify even trace amounts of leishmanial DNA in tissue. Samples are taken from the edge or base of a skin ulcer in cutaneous disease. Bone marrow or splenic aspirates are the best tissue samples in cases of visceral disease. Testing for serum antibodies against *leishmania* parasites may be helpful.

Cutaneous lesions often heal spontaneously. Treatment is undertaken when the lesions are in cosmetically disfiguring areas, when the infection is widespread, and for certain *leishmania* spp. that are less likely to heal (e.g., *L. braziliensis*). Pentavalent antimony (sodium stibogluconate, Pentostam), given either systemically or intralesionally, is the drug of choice for cutaneous lesions. Mucocutaneous and visceral leishmaniasis always require intravenous treatment with a pentavalent antimonial. Other effective medications for some species include amphotericin B (HIV-infected individuals) and pentamidine (for *L. panamensis*).

As there are many animal reservoirs of infection, and as elimination of sand flies is unlikely, control of leishmaniasis depends on avoiding exposure to sand flies. This involves a combination of insect repellent, fine-meshed bed nets, and protective clothing, and avoiding areas known to harbor sand flies.

MARTHA FULFORD
JAY KEYSTONE

(SEE ALSO: *Communicable Disease Control; Tropical Infectious Diseases*)

BIBLIOGRAPHY

Arias, J. R.; Monteiro, P. S.; and Zicker, F. (1996). "The Reemergence of Visceral Leishmaniasis in Brazil." *Emerging Infectious Diseases* 2(2):145–146.

Berman, J. D. (1997). "Human Leishmaniasis: Clinical, Diagnostic, and Chemotherapeutic Developments in the Last 10 Years." *Clinical Infectious Diseases* 24:684–703.

Desowitz, R. S. (1991). "Kala Azar: The Long Anguish of the Black Sickness." In *The Malaria Capers.* New York: W. W. Norton & Company.

Evans, T. G. (1993). "Leishmaniasis." *Infectious Disease Clinics of North America* 7(3):527–546.

Hernandez-Perez, J. et al. (1999). "Visceral Leishmaniasis (Kala-azar) in Solid Organ Transplantation: Report of Five Cases and Review." *Clinical Infectious Diseases* 29:918–921.

Herwaldt, B. (1999). "Leishmaniasis." *Lancet* 354:1191–1199.

World Health Organization (2000). "The Leishmaniases and *Leishmania*/HIV Co-Infections—Fact Sheet No. 116." *WHO Information Fact Sheets.* Geneva: Author.

LEPROSY

Evidence of leprosy (Hansen's disease) has been detected in prehistoric human remains, and the disease has been described in Biblical and other historical records dating as far back as the 2nd millennium B.C.E. It was a feared disease, and its victims were shunned because of their disfiguring stigmata—collapsed facial bones, fingers, and toes, with the hands and feet ultimately rotted away. Leprosy was among the first diseases identified as contagious. Early societies took measures to shield their healthy members from contagion: lepers were obliged to wear distinctive clothing and carry a bell to warn others of their presence, or they were segregated in lazarettos, precursors of quarantine stations and isolation hospitals. Segregation remained part of the control measures for leprosy in modern industrial nations until late in the twentieth century, and it still persists in some countries. This is a questionable practice, because the causative acid-fast bacillus that causes leprosy is only sluggishly infective. Transmission usually requires prolonged close personal contact, and children are most vulnerable. Transmission is mainly by nasal secretions, though bedbugs have been suspected as vectors.

The lepra bacillus, *Mycobacterium leprae*, belongs to the same family as tuberculosis. It attacks the skin and peripheral nerves, slowly destroying tissue, deforming the extremities, and disfiguring the face; it runs a natural course over many years, and death is as often due to other infections as to leprosy itself. Worldwide, ten to twelve million people suffer from leprosy, mainly in the Indian subcontinent, parts of the Middle East, and Latin America. Approximately 500,000 new cases are reported annually with about 300 cases per year in the United States, mainly among immigrants who harbored the infection on arrival. Control requires early detection and active treatment with one or more of several effective antibiotics, such as Rifampin. Once treatment is initiated, the risk of transmission is minimized. BCG vaccine confers some resistance to infection, while HIV (human immunodeficiency virus) infection increases the risk of infection with leprosy.

Leprosy is now known as Hanson's disease, named after Armauer Hanson, the Norwegian physician who discovered the cause of the disease in 1873.

JOHN M. LAST

(SEE ALSO: *Contagion; Isolation; Quarantine*)

BIBLIOGRAPHY

Nelson, K. E. (1998). "Leprosy." In *Maxcy-Rosenau-Last Public Health and Preventive Medicine,* 14th edition. ed. R. B. Wallace. Stamford, CT: Appleton & Lange.

LICENSING

A license is a permit granted by a government to carry out a regulated activity. Licensing is the most common form and method of health regulation. Most licensing in the United States is done by the states under their police powers. A state legislature must pass a law requiring a license to engage in a specific activity, such as practicing medicine or preparing food. The statute delegates the power to establish the conditions for licensure to an agency such as a department of health, or to a board such as a board of medical examiners. The agency publishes the conditions for licensure, which are often based on national codes, and every license holder must meet these standards. A license holder can be required to give up certain legal rights as a condition of licensure, such as agreeing to allow inspectors into a restaurant without a warrant. A license can be revoked or limited for not complying with the terms of licensure.

EDWARD P. RICHARDS

(SEE ALSO: *Legislation and Regulation; Police Powers; Public Health and the Law*)

BIBLIOGRAPHY

Richards, E. P., and Rathbun, K. C. (1998). "Public Health Law." In *Maxcy-Rosenau-Last Public Health and Preventive Medicine*, ed. Robert B. Wallace. Stamford, CT: Appleton and Lange.

LIFE EXPECTANCY AND LIFE TABLES

A life table converts a set of age-specific mortality rates into a survival curve, from which summary statistics, such as life expectancy, can be derived. The procedure was developed first for humans, primarily for the purpose of calculating premiums for life insurance and annuities. Later the same approach was used to study the survival of patients, other living species, and inanimate objects.

Crude life tables were produced by the Roman Aemilius Macer in Rome in 225 C.E., and by John Graunt and William Petty in the seventeenth century. The astronomer Edmund Halley, in 1693, was the first to employ correct mathematical methods to calculate a life table, using vital statistics collated by Caspar Neumann of Breslau. Figure 1 shows Halley's Breslau life table, William Farr's life table for England and Wales 150 years later, and a life table for Canada 300 years later.

A life table is easy to calculate if the mortality rates are known for each year of age. Starting with an arbitrary large number, say 1,000, of newborn infants, the number surviving to age one year can be estimated from the mortality rate in the first year of life. Then the number surviving to the age two years can be estimated using the mortality rate in the second year of life, and so on.

In practice, calculations are complicated by the fact that the mortality rates for single years of age cannot be estimated precisely, even in large

Figure 1

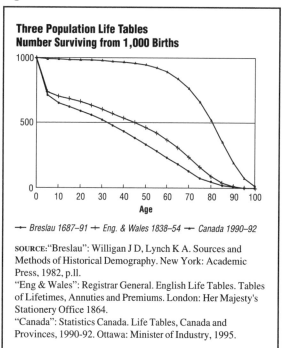

Three Population Life Tables Number Surviving from 1,000 Births

→ Breslau 1687–91 + Eng. & Wales 1838–54 → Canada 1990–92

SOURCE: "Breslau": Willigan J D, Lynch K A. Sources and Methods of Historical Demography. New York: Academic Press, 1982, p.11.
"Eng & Wales": Registrar General. English Life Tables. Tables of Lifetimes, Annuities and Premiums. London: Her Majesty's Stationery Office 1864.
"Canada": Statistics Canada. Life Tables, Canada and Provinces, 1990-92. Ottawa: Minister of Industry, 1995.

populations, and some form of smoothing is required. The sharp decline in mortality during infancy and childhood, and the small numbers in extreme old age, also create problems. However the simple method can be used to calculate abridged life tables, using mortality rates for broader age groups, which are more readily available. Such tables are usually sufficient for public health purposes.

Figure 2 shows the distribution of the ages at death implied by the English and Canadian life tables of Figure 1. In the earlier table the distribution has two peaks, one in the early childhood and the other in the 70–74 age group. In the later table the deaths in childhood have shifted to old age, producing a single peak at 80–84 years. The arithmetic mean of the distribution of ages at death is called life expectancy (i.e., expectation of life at birth), and is widely used as an indicator of the health of the population. The expectation of life at birth is forty-five years for the English life table and eighty-one years for the Canadian life table.

The vast majority of published life tables are period life tables, which are based on mortality rates over a limited time period. Since mortality

Figure 2

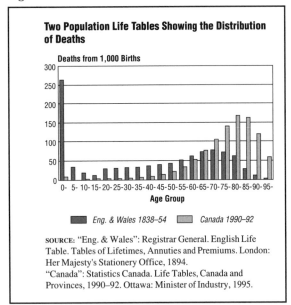

Two Population Life Tables Showing the Distribution of Deaths

Deaths from 1,000 Births

Age Group

■ *Eng. & Wales 1838–54* □ *Canada 1990–92*

SOURCE: "Eng. & Wales": Registrar General. English Life Table. Tables of Lifetimes, Annuities and Premiums. London: Her Majesty's Stationery Office, 1894.
"Canada": Statistics Canada. Life Tables, Canada and Provinces, 1990–92. Ottawa: Minister of Industry, 1995.

Table 1

Mean and Median Survival (Years) in Two Canadian Cohort Life Tables

Cohort Date of Birth:	1831		1891	
	Males	Females	Males	Females
Mean Survival (e_0) 4	0	42	49	54
Median survival	45	48	62	68

SOURCE: Statistics Canada. Report on the Demographic Situation in Canada 1992. Current Demographic Analysis. Ottawa: Minister of Industry, Science and Technology, 1992; p. 150.

changes over time, no actual population experiences the survival depicted in a period life table. Such a table represents, instead, a hypothetical, or synthetic, cohort. Comparing values of life expectancy from different period life tables is really equivalent to comparing age-standardized mortality rates, since reciprocal of life expectancy is a form of age-standardized mortality rate.

True cohort, or generation, life tables require age-specific mortality rates covering nearly 100 years. Table 1 shows the life expectancy for two completed cohorts. Life expectancy is consistently greater for females than for males, and the difference has widened over the sixty-year period between the two groups. Information on the cause of death can be incorporated into the life table calculations in two ways. First, it is possible to calculate the number, out of those alive at a given age, who will die subsequently from a particular cause. Second, the gain in life expectancy which would be obtained by eliminating a particular cause of death can be calculated.

As life expectancy increases toward its natural upper limit, life tables become less useful as indices of the health of a population. Beginning in the 1960s procedures were developed to incorporate information on disability into life tables. The simplest approach is to multiply the number living at a given age, derived from a current life table, by the proportion of the population at that age who are found, in a health survey, to be free of disability. The sum of these products over the life span gives the disability-free life expectation. In such calculations people are considered to be either disabled or not disabled, and the definition is somewhat arbitrary. The method can be expanded to incorporate different levels of disability, which are weighted to give the disability-adjusted life expectancy.

GERRY B. HILL

(SEE ALSO: *Cohort Life Tables; Demography; Graunt, John; Mortality Rates; Rates: Adjusted; Rates: Age-Adjusted; Rates: Age-Specific*)

BIBLIOGRAPHY

Benjamin, B. (1968). *Demographic Analysis.* London: George Allen and Unwin, Ltd.

Chiang, C. L. (1984). *The Life Table and Its Applications.* Malabar, FL: Robert E. Krieger Publishing Company.

Colvez, A., and Blanchet, M. (1983). "Potential Gains in the Life Expectancy Free of Disability: A Tool for Health Planning." *International Journal of Epidemiology* 12:224, 229.

Preston, S. H.; Keyfitz, N.; and Schoen, R. (1972). *Causes of Death. Life Tables for National Populations.* New York and London: Seminar Press.

Statistics Canada (1992). *Report on the Demographic Situation in Canada 1992. Current Demographic Analysis.* Ottawa: Minister of Industry, Science and Technology.

LIFESTYLE

In public health, "lifestyle" generally means a pattern of individual practices and personal behavioral choices that are related to elevated or reduced health risk. Since the mid-1970s, there has been a growing recognition of the significant contribution of personal behavior choices to health risk—in the United States thirty-eight percent of deaths in 1990 were attributed to tobacco, diet and activity patterns, and alcohol. Equally important, illnesses attributable to lifestyle choices play a role in reducing health-related quality of life and in creating health disparities among different segments of the population.

Lifestyles are born of a multitude of causes, from childhood determinants to personality makeup to influences in the cultural, physical, economic, and political environments. Thus, efforts to encourage good health practices should also promote environments that support them. A good resource for lifestyle information is http://www.healthfinder.gov.

DENNIS D. TOLSMA

(SEE ALSO: *Behavior, Health-Related; Behavioral Determinants; Behavioral Risk Factor Surveillance System; Health Promotion and Education*)

BIBLIOGRAPHY

McGinnis, J. M., and Foege, W. H. (1993). "Actual Causes of Death in the United States." *Journal of the American Medical Association* 270:2207–2212.

LIND, JAMES

James Lind (1716–1794) was an Edinburgh Scot, apprenticed to a surgeon at the age of fifteen, who entered the Royal Navy as a ship's surgeon at age twenty-three, serving for nine years. After leaving the navy, he returned to Edinburgh, where he gained a medical degree and went into practice. In 1758 he became consultant physician at a naval hospital and held this position for the next twenty-five years. His experiences at sea had aroused his interest in naval hygiene, and he is recognized as a pioneer in this field.

Lind is remembered mainly for his work on scurvy, the vitamin C deficiency disease. Having observed sailors with scurvy, which was then a prevalent disease among sailors on long sea voyages, he speculated about its likely cause, suspecting that the shortage of fresh food such as fruits and vegetables might be responsible. On his own long voyages he experimented with diets, and he is renowned now among exponents of clinical trials because he reported the first such clinical trial that was systematically designed and conducted. It was a modest trial in which twelve sailors were allocated in groups of two each to receive cider, elixir of vitriol, vinegar, sea water, purgatives, and citrus fruits (oranges, lemons). Those who received the citrus fruits recovered rapidly from their scurvy, while the others did not. Although the sample sizes were grossly inadequate and other aspects of clinical trials were not adopted, this successful demonstration of an effective way to treat and to prevent scurvy immensely enhanced the health prospects of seafarers on long voyages, such as those of the explorer James Cook in the Pacific Ocean a few years later. Cook's sailors had a daily regimen of sucking the juice of a lime, and none of these sailors got scurvy. The slang word "limey" applied to British sailors originated from this practice. Lind wrote several works on naval hygiene, including an *Essay on the Most Effectual Means of Preserving the Health of Seamen in the Royal Navy* (1757); his best known work is *A Treatise of the Scurvy* (1753).

JOHN M. LAST

BIBLIOGRAPHY

Lind, J. (1953). *A Treatise of the Scurvy*. Edinburgh: University Press. (Reprint)

LIPIDS

See Blood Lipids; Hyperlipidemia; *and* Lipoproteins

LIPOPROTEINS

Lipoproteins are particles in the bloodstream that transport fatty substances called lipids between different organs, glands, and tissues. The interior of the lipoprotein contains triglycerides (glycerol esterified with three fatty acids) and cholesterol esterified with fatty acids. The covering membrane of a lipoprotein contains chemicals more easily soluble in blood than those in the interior, such as free cholesterol, phospholipids (e.g., lecithin), and apoproteins. Since the different lipoproteins contain different amounts of triglycerides and cholesterol, they may be separated by centrifuging them into particles with different densities, including low-density (LDL), high-density (HDL), and very low-density (VLDL) particles. Apoproteins (such as apo A in HDL particles and apo B in VLDL and LDL particles) function to direct the lipoproteins to their destinations or to act as coenzymes to activate certain other enzymes that process the lipoproteins.

DONALD A. SMITH

(SEE ALSO: *Atherosclerosis; Blood Lipids; Cholesterol Test; HDL Cholesterol; Hyperlipidemia; LDL Cholesterol; Triglycerides; VLDL Cholesterol*)

LISTER, JOSEPH

Joseph Lister (1827–1912) was an English surgeon. Educated at University College, London, he practiced and taught surgery in Scotland, first in Glasgow and then in Edinburgh, before returning to London in 1877. Lister was concerned about the frequently fatal wound infections that followed surgical operations, and, in search of solutions to this problem, he studied the work of European bacteriologists, notably that of Louis Pasteur. Lister thought that bacteria caused the postoperative infections that were so common, and although the connection between bacteria and infection had not been confirmed beyond doubt at that time, he understood that bacteria could be killed by antiseptics. He came up with the idea of using carbolic acid for this purpose and started the practice of preoperative cleansing of his and his assistants' hands with carbolic acid, as well as spraying carbolic acid liberally in the air in the operating room. The dramatic beneficial results of what amounted to an experimental trial of this regimen were reported in the *Lancet* in 1867. Lister's methods transformed the practice of surgery from a desperate, life-threatening gamble into a relatively safe procedure for many conditions—including the management of childbirth.

Unlike Ignaz Semmelweiss and Oliver Wendell Holmes, who preceded Lister in recognizing the importance of cleanliness in preventing infection during childbirth, Lister offered a method that did not imply that doctors were dirty, and so his message was heeded rather than rejected. Therefore he, more than Semmelweiss or Holmes, deserves much credit for making childbirth safe, as well as for the concept of antiseptic surgical operations. Lister was showered with honors, including elevation to the peerage, the first medical doctor to achieve this distinction. He was buried in Westminster Abbey with the pomp and ceremony reserved for the greatest national heroes.

JOHN M. LAST

(SEE ALSO: *Antisepsis and Sterilization; Holmes, Oliver Wendell; Semmelweiss, Ignaz*)

BIBLIOGRAPHY

Lister, J. (1867). "On a New Method of Treating Compound Fractures, Abscesses, Etc., with Observations on the Conditions of Suppuration." *Lancet* 1:326–329, 357–359, 387–389, 507–509; 2:95–96.

—— (1867). "On the Antiseptic Principle in the Practice of Surgery." *Lancet* 2:353–356, 668–669.

LONGEVITY

See Life Expectancy and Life Tables

LOUIS, PIERRE CHARLES ALEXANDRE

Pierre Charles Alexandre Louis (1787–1872) was a French physician who graduated from the Sorbonne in 1813. He spent several years in Russia, and when he returned to Paris, he worked at l'Hôpital Charité, where he began to collect and numerically analyze information about patients and the treatments they received. His numerical method was quite new to medical practice—no one had ever before counted cases, examined the pathological lesions they had, and classified the outcome of the treatments in such detail. Louis published the results of his studies in a series of monographs, beginning with the one that made him famous, *Récherches Anatomico-Pathologiques sur la Phthisie* (1825). (The first English translation,

Researches in Phthisis–Anatomical, Pathological, Therapeutical, was published by the Sydenham Society of London in 1844.) This is a statistical study of 1,960 clinical cases and 358 autopsy dissections of tuberculosis, and it established his reputation as a distinguished medical scientist. It is now regarded as one of the classic works of medicine.

Louis's statistical analysis of a series of cases of typhoid included evidence enabling him to distinguish it from typhus, and in fact he gave typhoid its name. In 1835, he wrote a scathing polemic on the outcome of bloodletting as a way to treat diseases (*Récherches sur les Effets de la Saignée*), which conclusively proved that far from benefitting patients, this widely used and fashionable procedure harmed, and sometimes even killed them. Aspiring medical scientists who were skeptical about prevailing standards of care and had an interest in Louis's numerical approach, from other countries as well as France, sought him out as a mentor. Among his pupils were William Farr, Oliver Wendell Holmes, and Lemuel Shattuck. Louis founded the Medecine d'Observation in Paris, and he is recognized as the founding father of modern medical statistics.

JOHN M. LAST

(SEE ALSO: *Statistics for Public Health*)

LOVE CANAL

Love Canal is an abandoned canal in Niagara County, New York, where a huge amount of toxic waste was buried. The waste was composed of at least 300 different chemicals, totaling an estimated 20,000 metric tons. The existence of the waste was discovered in the 1970s when families living in homes subsequently built next to the site found chemical wastes seeping up through the ground into their basements, forcing them to eventually abandon their homes.

Love Canal was used from the 1940s through the 1950s by the Hooker Chemical Company and the city of Niagara Falls, among others, to dispose of their hazardous and municipal wastes and other refuse. The canal was surrounded by clay and was thought at the time to be a safe place for disposal—and, in fact, burying chemicals in the canal was probably safer than many other methods and sites used for chemical disposal at the time. In 1953, the Niagara Falls Board of Education bought the landfill for $1 and constructed an elementary school with playing fields on the site. Roads and sewer lines were added and, in the early 1970s, single-family homes were built adjacent to the site.

Following a couple of heavy rains in the mid-1970s, the canal flooded and chemicals were observed on the surface of the site and in the basements of houses abutting the site. Newspaper coverage, investigations by the State of New York and by the U.S. Environmental Protection Agency, combined with pressure from the district's U.S. congressional representative and outrage on the part of local residents, led to the declaration of a health emergency involving "great and imminent peril to the health of the general public." Ultimately, in August, 1978, a decision was made by Governor Hugh Carey, supported by the White House, to evacuate the residents and purchase 240 homes surrounding the site. Shortly thereafter, the residents of nearby homes that did not immediately abut the site also became concerned about their health and conducted a health survey that purported to show an increase in the occurrence of various diseases and problems such as birth defects and miscarriages, which were attributed to chemical exposures. A great controversy ensued over whether the observations were real or reflected normal rates of such problems, and whether chemical exposures had, in fact, occurred. Eventually, political pressure resulted in families being given an opportunity to leave and have their homes purchased by the State. About 70 homes remained occupied in 1989 by families who chose not to move.

The controversy at Love Canal followed on the heels of the heightened awareness that occurred in the 1960s about environmental contamination, and it contributed to public and regulatory concern about hazardous wastes, waste disposal, and disclosure of such practices. Such concerns led Congress to pass the Resource Conservation and Recovery Act (RCRA) and the Toxic Substances Control Act (TSCA) in 1976, and the Comprehensive Environmental Response, Compensation, and Liability Act (CERCLA), also known as the Superfund bill, in 1980. When CERCLA was passed, few were aware of the extent of the problem potentially created by years of inappropriate or inadequate hazardous waste disposal practices. Since implementing CERCLA, the U.S. Environmental Protection Agency has identified more than 40,000 potentially contaminated "Super-fund" sites.

GAIL CHARNLEY

(SEE ALSO: *Environmental Determinants of Health; Environmental Protection Agency; Risk Assessment, Risk Management; Toxic Substances Control Act; Toxicology*)

BIBLIOGRAPHY

Levine, A. (1982). *Love Canal: Science, Politics, and People.* Lexington, MA: Lexington Books.

Mazur, A. (1998). *A Hazardous Inquiry: The Rashemon Effect at Love Canal.* Cambridge, MA: Harvard University Press.

LOW-BIRTHWEIGHT INFANTS

See Infant Mortality Rate; Perinatology; *and* Pregnancy

LUNG CANCER

Lung cancer is a malignant disease in which lung cells become abnormal, characterized by uncontrollable, unlimited growth. These cells can then invade nearby normal tissue and destroy organ structure, a process called "invasion." Lung cancer cells can also break down lung tissue structure and enter the bloodstream or lymphatic system and thus spreads to distant organs in other parts of the body, a process called metastasis. Clinically, lung cancer can be classified into two groups according to its cell types under microscopy: non-small cell lung cancer and small cell lung cancer. Non-small cell lung cancer includes cancers of three cell types: squamous cell carcinoma, adenocarcinoma, and large cell carcinoma. Small cell lung cancer, also called oat cell cancer, is a less common cancer that grows faster, and is more likely to spread to other parts of the body than non-small cell lung cancer.

Lung cancer is a highly lethal disease in the United States and worldwide. According to Parkin et al. (1999), lung cancer was the most frequent cancer in 1990, worldwide, with 1.04 million new cases (771,800 in men and 265,100 in women). It is the most common cancer in men and the fifth most frequent cancer in women. Lung cancer is the leading cause of cancer deaths worldwide, with a total of 921,000 deaths per year (692,600 in men and 228,400 in women) in 1990. In the United States, it was estimated that 169,500 new lung cancer patients (90,700 men and 78,800 women) would be diagnosed and 157,400 (90,100 men and 67,300 women) would die of lung cancer in 2001. The five-year survival rate of lung cancer is 13.7 percent in the United States, 7.8 percent in developing countries, 7 percent in Eastern Europe, 7.9 percent in China, and 6.7 percent in India.

The changes (increase or decrease) of lung cancer incidence corresponds to the alterations of prevalence of smoking in the population twenty to thirty years earlier, representing a latent period between tobacco exposure and the occurrence of lung cancer. A significant decrease in the incidence of lung and bronchus cancer in males in North America started in the late 1980s. Between 1990 and 1996 there was a 2.6 percent decline in incidence per year. Incidence rates of lung and bronchus cancer in females are stabilizing in the United States. Although the death rate from lung cancer in males is decreasing, it is increasing among females, and it has now exceeded the breast cancer death rate among females.

Tobacco smoking is a major cause of lung cancer. Over 4,000 chemical compounds have been identified in the tobacco leaf. Carcinogens in tobacco smoke can damage the cells in the lungs, which may lead to the development of lung cancer. More than fifty chemical compounds in tobacco smoke have been recognized as known or probable human carcinogens, some of which may be formed during combustion (or smoking) and some which may exist naturally in tobacco. Several groups of carcinogens in tobacco smoke are related to lung cancer, including polycyclic aromatic hydrocarbons (PAHs), aromatic amines, benzene, hydrazine, and vinyl chloride. Smoking results in damage to the bronchial and lung epithelium, which leads to lung cell proliferation and finally to lung cancer. Animal studies confirm the carcinogenic potential of tobacco smoke in tissues having smoke contact: in these studies smoke exposure leads to laryngeal tumors and pulmonary adenomas. In humans, cigarette smokers have increased levels of tobacco carcinogen DNA adducts in the lung and bronchus when compared with nonsmokers.

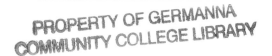

A very strong association between cigarette smoking and lung cancer has been consistently observed in studies done since the early 1950s. These studies have shown that cigarette smoking precedes lung cancer occurrence. It has been estimated that cigarette smokers have a ten-fold higher risk of lung cancer, in comparison with nonsmokers. With the increased number of cigarettes smoked per day, the risk is increased—heavy smokers are at greater risk of lung cancer than moderate smokers; and moderate smokers are at higher risk than light smokers and nonsmokers. The risk for individuals who smoke two or more packs per day is about twenty times that of nonsmokers, and longer smoking duration has a stronger effect on the risk of lung cancer. Beginning to smoke at an early age is also related to an increased risk, and the lung cancer risk declines with an increased duration of cessation. The percentage of reduction in risk after quitting smoking depends on the duration of exposure to smoking. The observed relationship between cigarette smoking and the risk of lung cancer is consistent with different study designs and in studies of different populations all over the world. Over eighty-five percent of deaths from lung cancer can be attributed to cigarette smoking. It is estimated that tobacco smoking accounts for over ninety percent of male lung cancer deaths and seventy-nine percent of female lung cancer deaths in the United States.

Smoking of other tobacco products, such as cigar and pipe smoking, is also associated with an increased risk of lung cancer. Like cigarette smoking, the risk of lung cancer is increased with the frequency and years of cigar and pipe smoking. Environmental tobacco smoke (ETS), also known as secondhand smoke, increases the risk of lung cancer among nonsmokers. It is estimated that ETS may lead to 3,000 new cases of lung cancer per year in nonsmokers in the United States. Other risk factors for lung cancer include race, occupational exposures (e.g., arsenic, asbestos, chromium, mustard gas, PAHs), residential radon exposure, radiation, air pollution, and nutritional factors. The host susceptibility factors for lung cancer include inheritance of different polymorphic genotypes that may interact with tobacco smoke in determining the risk of lung cancer.

Smoking cessation or lifelong abstinence from smoking offer the best opportunities to reduce lung cancer incidence and death rates. Reducing the prevalence of smoking will lead to a dramatic decrease in the incidence of lung cancer in the general population. According to the Centers for Disease Control and Prevention (CDC), cigarette smoking is the single most preventable cause of premature death in the United States. More than 400,000 people die from causes attributable to cigarette smoking each year, including 276,000 men and 142,000 women. The promotion of smoking cessation is the most cost-effective tool against lung and other smoking-related cancers and diseases.

Control of other risk factors, such as workplace exposures associated with the increased risk of lung cancer, environmental tobacco smoke, and radon exposure in residences, may also lead to a reduced risk of lung cancer. Sputum cytology and chest radiographs are not recommended for lung cancer screening because no favorable impact of the screening on lung cancer mortality has been demonstrated. Recent developments have pointed out that the molecular genetic alterations associated with progression toward lung cancer, such as p53 mutations in sputum samples, may help to identify high-risk individuals for early detection and chemoprevention.

ZUO-FENG ZHANG

(SEE ALSO: *Cancer; Causes of Death; Chronic Illness; Environmental Tobacco Smoke; Noncommunicable Disease Control; Smoking Behavior; Smoking Cessation; Women's Health*)

BIBLIOGRAPHY

Baron, J. A., and Rohan, T. (1997). "Tobacco." In *Cancer Epidemiology and Prevention*, ed. D. Schottenfeld. New York: Oxford University Press.

Centers for Disease Control and Prevention (1993). "Smoking-Attributable Mortality and Years of Potential Life Lost—United States, 1990." *Morbidity and Mortality Weekly Report* 42(33):645–648.

Greenlee, R. T.; Hill-Harmon, M. B.; Murray, T.; and Thun, M. (2001). "Cancer Statistics, 2001." *CA: A Cancer Journal for Clinicians* 51:15–36.

International Agency for Research on Cancer (1986). *Evaluation of the Carcinogenic Risk of Chemicals to Humans: Tobacco Smoking*. IARC Monographs, Volume 38. Lyon, France: World Health Organization.

National Cancer Institute (1999). *Health Effects of Exposure to Environmental Tobacco Smoking. The Report of the California Environmental Protection Agency.* Smoking and Tobacco Control Monograph No. 10. Bethesda, MD: National Cancer Institute.

Parkin, D. M.; Pisani, P.; and Ferlay, J. (1999). "Estimates of the Worldwide Incidence of 25 Major Cancers in 1990." *International Journal of Cancer* 80: 827–841.

Pisani, P.; Parkin, D. M.; Bray F.; and Ferlay, J. (1999). "Estimates of the Worldwide Mortality from 25 Cancers in 1990." *International Journal of Cancer* 83:18–29.

Samet, J. M. (1995). "Lung Cancer." In *Cancer Prevention and Control,* eds. P. Greenwald, B. S. Kramer, and D. L. Weed. New York: Marcel Dekker.

M

MAD COW DISEASE

See Bovine Spongiform Encephalopathy *and* Transmissible Spongiform Encephalopathy

MALARIA

Malaria is the most clinically important parasitic disease worldwide. It kills as many as 2.7 million people annually. The human suffering and economic costs are enormous. Although malaria has been eradicated from temperate zones, it continues to pose a major public health threat to more than forty percent of the world's population.

EPIDEMIOLOGY AND TRANSMISSION

Currently, malaria occurs in one hundred countries and territories inhabited by a total of 2.4 billion people (see Figure 1). The World Health Organization estimates that there are 300 million to 500 million clinical cases annually, resulting in approximately 1.5 million to 2.7 million deaths. Ninety percent of the deaths are in children under five years of age living in sub-Saharan Africa. Other risk groups include pregnant women, internally displaced persons and refugees, and international travelers.

Malaria transmission occurs by the bite of an infective female *Anopheles* sp. mosquito. Although most cases are transmitted by mosquito, the infection can be passed from mother to the unborn child, or through contaminated blood products, needle sharing, or organ transplantation.

AGENT AND LIFE CYCLE

Human malaria infection is caused by one or more of four species of the intracellular parasite of the genus plasmodium. *Plasmodium falciparum, P. vivax, P. ovale*, and *P. malariae* differ in geographic distribution, microscopic appearance, clinical characteristics, and potential for conferring immunity in the host. Although *P. vivax* is the most common form of malaria worldwide, *P. falciparum* is the most severe, contributing to most of the morbidity and mortality.

The life cycle of the four species of human malaria consists of two phases: the sexual (sporogony) and asexual phases (schizogony; see Figure 2). Schizogony begins when an infective female anopheline mosquito injects sporozoites into the human host while taking a blood meal. The sporozoite stage of the parasite disappears from circulation within thirty minutes. Those avoiding the host immune system invade the liver and undergo development and multiplication to form schizonts. Over the next five to fifteen days, the schizonts mature, rupture the liver cell, and invade the circulation as merozoites. These merozoites bind to the red blood cell wall. They then penetrate the red blood cell, where they develop as ring forms and grow into trophozoites. Further division creates red blood cell merozoites which form a mature schizont. The blood cell swells and ruptures, releasing merozoites that go on to invade other red blood cells. Clinical symptoms result when the blood cell ruptures and releases cellular debris from infected cells into the bloodstream. The host response to these toxins produces the

Figure 1

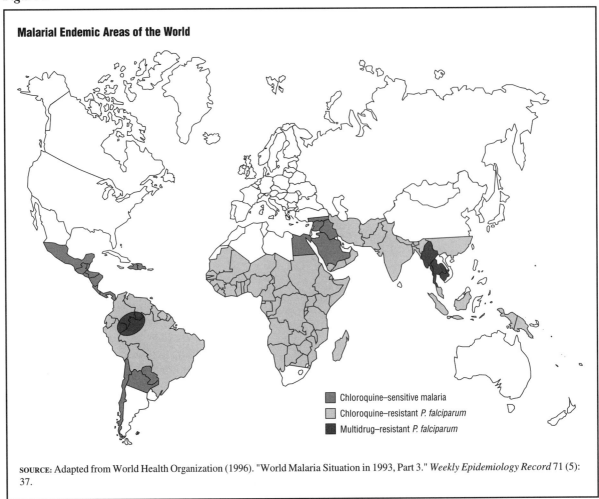

Malarial Endemic Areas of the World

■ Chloroquine–sensitive malaria
■ Chloroquine–resistant *P. falciparum*
■ Multidrug–resistant *P. falciparum*

SOURCE: Adapted from World Health Organization (1996). "World Malaria Situation in 1993, Part 3." *Weekly Epidemiology Record* 71 (5): 37.

classic paroxysms of fever and chills, which are closely timed with the cycles of red blood cell schizogony. The timing of the blood cell phase differs depending on the species of the parasite. *P. vivax* and *P. ovale* classically have cycles of forty-eight hours, *P. malariae* seventy-two hours, and *P. falciparum* forty-eight hours, although this may vary.

After a period of time, some of the merozoites develop into male and female sexual forms called gametocytes. The gametocytes are ingested by the female anopheline mosquito during a blood meal. Inside the mosquito's stomach, the male and female gametocyte fuse to form a zygote, which quickly becomes a mobile oökinete, which penetrates the stomach wall to form an oöcyst. The oöcyst then bursts, releasing sporozoites that migrate to the salivary glands, ready to be injected

into a human host, thus completing the cycle. The parasite generally develops within the mosquito (sporogony) in nine to twelve days, but this time varies according to parasite species and external temperature.

P. vivax and *P. ovale* differ from the other two species in that some hepatic trophozoites, called hypnozoites, may remain dormant and persist in the liver for months to up to four years. Periodic release of merozoites formed from these hypnozoites can produce recurrent parasitemia and clinical symptoms. Recurrent parasitemia can also occur with *P. falciparum* and *P. malariae*, although these species do not form hypnozoites. Infection with these parasites may remain in the blood at subclinical levels because of either the host immune system or use of antimalarial drugs

Figure 2

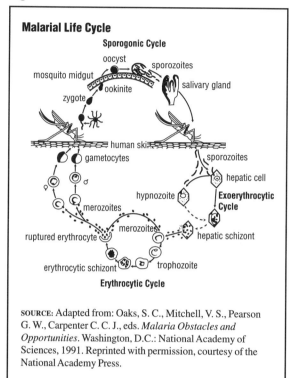

Malarial Life Cycle

SOURCE: Adapted from: Oaks, S. C., Mitchell, V. S., Pearson G. W., Carpenter C. C. J., eds. *Malaria Obstacles and Opportunities*. Washington, D.C.: National Academy of Sciences, 1991. Reprinted with permission, courtesy of the National Academy Press.

that do not completely clear the blood-stage parasites. The level of parasitemia can increase weeks to months later, giving rise to another clinical attack. While *P. falciparum* rarely returns more than several months after the initial infection, *P. malariae* may become active again up to forty years after the infection.

CLINICAL DISEASE AND DIAGNOSIS

The clinical presentation of malaria is very nonspecific. The degree of natural and acquired immunity of the patient can influence the clinical course dramatically. Classic symptoms among nonimmune persons include fever, chills, sweats, body aches, headache, decreased appetite, nausea, vomiting, and diarrhea. Signs of malaria infection may include an enlarged liver and spleen, anemia, jaundice, low blood pressure, fast heart rate, and decreases in the number of white blood cells and platelets. Children may also show fretfulness, unusual crying, and sleep disturbances. The hallmark of malaria is the paroxysms (attacks) of these

symptoms, which recur with predictable periodicity. *P. vivax* and *P. ovale* malaria classically cause symptoms every forty-eight hours, *P. malariae* every seventy-two hours. *P. falciparum* features irregular patterns. The presentation of these classic attacks is highly variable and may not occur at all early in the disease or in partially immune persons.

Life-threatening disease generally occurs only with *P. falciparum* infections and can progress from uncomplicated malaria within hours. Neurologic manifestations are the most common presentation of severe disease, often appearing as altered mental status, drowsiness, coma, or convulsions. Other important severe clinical conditions include renal failure, pulmonary distress, severe anemia, low blood sugar, and shock.

Malaria in pregnancy can have devastating effects, especially when caused by *P. falciparum*. In nonimmune pregnant women, malaria infections can lead to increased risk of maternal and fetal death. Among semi-immune pregnant women, low birth weight due to placental parasitemia represents the greatest risk factor for neonatal death.

Due to the nonspecific nature of malaria symptoms, the diagnosis cannot be made based on clinical signs and symptoms alone. Laboratory diagnostic tests must be performed on any patient suspected of having a malaria infection. The standard for diagnosing malaria is the microscopic visualization of parasites in red blood cells on Giemsa-stained thick and thin smears. Advantages of microscopy include high sensitivity and specificity among properly trained and supervised technicians. Microscopy also offers the ability to identify the infecting species and quantify the level of parasitemia. Immunochromatographic rapid diagnostic tests have been developed that may detect *P. falciparum* and non–*P. falciparum* infections. These require no special equipment and are relatively easy to use. The determination of parasite density is not possible with these dipsticks. Other less common methods used for diagnosing malaria infections include serologic tests using an enzyme-linked immunosorbent assay, radioimmunoassay techniques, and polymerase chain reaction.

TREATMENT

To decrease morbidity and mortality from malaria infections, early diagnosis and prompt treatment with an efficacious drug are important. Unfortunately, due to the increasing spread and intensification of drug resistance, there is a limited number of drugs available to prevent and treat malaria.

Chloroquine has long been the mainstay first-line therapy for uncomplicated *P. falciparum* infection used by malaria control programs; however, resistance to it now exists in most parts of the world. Sulfadoxine-pyrimethamine (SP) has replaced chloroquine in many countries. Resistance to SP has developed in Southeast Asia, parts of South America, and now in certain sites in sub-Saharan Africa. Other drugs commonly used for falciparum infections include quinine, quinidine, amodiaquine, mefloquine, halofantrine, artemisinin compounds, atovaquone, tetracycline, and clindamycin.

Chloroquine is the main drug used for infections with *P. vivax*, *P. ovale*, and *P. malariae*; however, there are reports of chloroquine-resistant *P. vivax* in parts of Oceania. Primaquine is used to eliminate the hypnozoites in *P. vivax* and *P. ovale* infections.

CONTROL MEASURES

Four basic elements of an effective malaria control program include case management, selective and sustainable preventive measures, early detection of epidemics, and the strengthening of local capacity. Appropriate case management is imperative to malaria control programs. It consists of accurate diagnosis followed by rapid, effective treatment. The detection of malaria in children and pregnant women is especially important. Knowledge of mosquito behavior and relevant environmental, social, and economic features is extremely important for malaria prevention programs. These programs often consist of personal protection (e.g., repellents, insecticide-impregnated bednets), chemoprophylaxis (chemical agent to prevent malaria) for travelers or other high-risk persons, and selective mosquito control (e.g., insecticides, larvicides, environmental management). Malaria epidemics can occur when a community with little or no immunity moves into an area of intense malaria transmission. Epidemics often take place in times of socio-political instability (e.g., complex humanitarian emergencies). These may result in high numbers of deaths. Finally, to be able to control transmission, malaria-endemic countries need to integrate control efforts into the national health plan, strengthen in-country scientific capacity to perform malaria research, and mobilize community support for intervention programs.

JOHN R. MACARTHUR
S. PATRICK KACHUR

(SEE ALSO: *Communicable Disease Control; Vector-Borne Diseases*)

BIBLIOGRAPHY

Bloland, P. B.; Lacritz, E. M.; Kazembe, P. N. et al. (1993). "Beyond Chloroquine: Implications of Drug Resistance for Evaluating Malaria Therapy Efficacy and Treatment Policy in Africa." *Journal of Infectious Diseases* 167:932–937.

Bruce-Chwatt, L. J. (1986). *Chemotherapy of Malaria.* Geneva: World Health Organization.

Gilles, H. M., and Warrell, D. A. (1993). *Bruce-Chwatt's Essential Malariology,* 3rd edition. London: Arnold.

Kachur, S. P., and Bloland, P. B. (1998). "Malaria." In *Maxcy-Rosenau-Last's Public Health and Preventive Medicine,* 14th edition, ed. R. B. Wallace. Stamford, CT: Appleton & Lange.

MacArthur, J. R.; Williams, H. A.; and Bloland, P. B. (2000). "Malaria in Complex Humanitarian Emergencies." *Refuge* 18(5):4–11.

Nwanyanwu, O. C.; Ziba, C.; MacHeso, A.; and Kazembe, P. (2000). "Efficacy of Sulphadoxine-pyrimethamine for Acute Uncomplicated Malaria Due to *Plasmodium falciparum* in Malawian Children under Five Years Old." *Tropical Medicine and International Health* 5:355–358.

White, N. J. (1996). "The Treatment of Malaria." *New England Journal of Medicine* 335:800–806.

World Health Organization (1993). *A Global Strategy for Malaria Control.* Geneva: Author.

MALIGNANCY

See Cancer

MALTHUS, THOMAS ROBERT

Thomas Robert Malthus (1766–1834) is remembered primarily for his *Essay on the Principle of Population* (1798). Malthus was a distinguished scholar at Cambridge, where he concentrated on classics and mathematics. Like many others of his time, he entered the church as a clergyman in order to secure a living. His real interest, however, was in the applied mathematics of economics. In the *Essay on the Principle of Population*, Malthus made the mathematical point that while food supplies can increase only in a simple arithmetical progression, populations can increase by geometric progression; and the population must, therefore, inevitably outgrow its food supply, with famine the result. This line of reasoning continues to generate controversy to this day, supported by advocates of environmental sustainability and opposed by advocates of a free market. Malthus's forecasts were not fulfilled in the time frame he envisaged because of a combined effect of colonial expansion, the opening up of vast new areas for agriculture in the Americas, Australasia, and parts of Africa; and the development of increasingly efficient farming and animal husbandry practices. These factors successfully maintained food supplies, even through the hyperexponential population surges of the twentieth century, which saw a quadrupling of the world's population from 1.5 billion in 1900 to 6 billion in 1999. Malthusian population forecasts are not flawed, however, if the time scale is correctly estimated and other factors remain unaltered. Malthus's other works include a treatise much admired by economists, *Principles of Political Economy* (1820).

JOHN M. LAST

(SEE ALSO: *Population Forecasts; Population Growth; Population Policy*)

MAMMOGRAPHY

A mammogram is an X-ray examination of the breast, performed for screening or diagnostic purposes. A screening mammogram is used to detect breast cancer before it is clinically apparent. Two views of the breast tissue are taken: a mediolateral (MLO) view and a craniocaudal (CC) view. A diagnostic mammogram is utilized to evaluate abnormalities seen on a screening mammogram or to further characterize abnormalities on physical examination.

Screening mammography has been shown to decrease breast cancer mortality, particularly for women 40 to 50 years of age and older. The first randomized, controlled trial to evaluate the benefit of mammogram and clinical breast-exam screening was the HIP (Health Insurance Plan) study, initiated in 1963. Approximately 62,000 women between 40 and 64 years of age were assigned at random to either a mammography and clinical breast exam group for four years or to a control group. After ten years of follow-up, the study group had a 30 percent lower mortality from breast cancer in comparison to the control group.

Further randomized controlled trials confirmed the efficacy of screening mammography in decreasing breast cancer mortality. A meta-analysis of nine randomized controlled trials and four case-control studies was reported in 1995. Women aged 50 to 74 who received mammographic screening had a decreased relative risk for breast cancer mortality of 0.74 (95% CI [confidence interval], 0.66–0.83) in comparison to women who did not receive mammographic screening. No reduction in breast cancer mortality with mammographic screening was seen in women aged 40 to 49, after 7 to 9 years of follow-up. With a longer duration of follow-up of 10 to 12 years, there was a 17 percent decrease in breast cancer mortality among women aged 40 to 49 who received screening mammography.

A meta-analyses of eight randomized trials of screening mammography in women aged 40 to 49 was published in 1997. This meta-analysis demonstrated an 18 percent mortality reduction in women aged 40 to 49 who received screening mammography, after 10.5 to 18 years of follow-up.

Based on these results, it is clear that women 50 years old and older benefit from yearly screening mammography in order to decrease their risk of dying from breast cancer; however, there is controversy regarding the utility of screening mammography in women aged 40 to 49. An attempt at resolving this controversy was made at the National Institute of Health Consensus meeting in January 1997, but a consensus could not be reached. Therefore the meeting resulted in two different reports regarding screening mammography in women aged 40 to 49. The majority concluded that screening mammogram was not universally warranted in this age group. A minority report, however, supported the recommendation for screening mammography based on the survival benefit seen at 10 years and longer after screening is initiated. The American Cancer Society supports this recommendation, recommending an annual mammogram for women aged 40 and older.

Another area of controversy is the upper age limit at which to stop performing screening mammography. There is no data from randomized trials regarding the benefits of screening mammography in women older than 75 because of the lack of enrollment of elderly women. This area deserves further study, given that age is the single greatest risk factor for breast cancer and approximately half of all breast cancers occur in women over the age of 65. The American Cancer Society and the National Cancer Institute put no upper age cut-off for screening mammography. The American Geriatric Society has published a position statement regarding breast cancer screening in older women, recommending no upper age limit for breast cancer screening for women with an estimated life expectancy of greater than four years (2000).

Ultimately, the decision regarding screening mammography is up to the patient. Therefore, it is important for a clinician to discuss the benefits and risks of mammographic screening with each individual. The risks of mammographic screening include the risk of a false positive exam, which can lead to further testing, cost, and patient anxiety. Younger women have a higher rate of false positive and false negative exams, a consequence of the exam being less sensitive and specific in this age group. In addition, there is an exceedingly small risk of breast cancer due to radiation exposure from the mammogram. Statistical models indicate that 8 out of 100,000 women who underwent an annual mammogram for 10 years beginning at age 40 develop breast cancer and die from the disease during their lifetime. Women with DNA repair mechanism impairment may be at greater risk.

CLIFFORD HUDIS
ARTI HURRIA

(SEE ALSO: *Breast Cancer; Breast Cancer Screening; Breast Self-Examination; Clinical Breast Examination; Tamoxifen*)

BIBLIOGRAPHY

American Geriatric Society Clinical Practice Committee (2000). "Breast Cancer Screening in Older Women." *Journal of the American Geriatrics Society* 48(7):842–844.

Armstrong, K.; Eisen, A.; and Weber, B. (2000). "Assessing the Risk of Breast Cancer." *New England Journal of Medicine* 342(8):564–571.

Hendrick, R. E.; Smith, R. A.; Rutledge, J. H.; et al. (1997). "Benefit of Screening Mammography in Women Aged 40–49: A New Meta-Analysis of Randomized Controlled Trials." *Journal of the National Cancer Institute Monograph* 22:87–92.

Kerlikowske, K.; Grady, D.; Rubin, S. M.; et al. (1995). "Efficacy of Screening Mammography. A Meta-Analysis." *Journal of the American Medical Association* 273:149–154.

Muss, H. B. (1996). "Breast Cancer in Older Women." *Seminars in Oncology* 23:82–88.

National Institutes of Health Consensus Development Panel (1997). "National Institutes of Health Consensus Development Conference Statement: Breast Cancer Screening for Women Ages 40–49." *Journal of the National Cancer Institute* 89:1015–1026.

Primic-Zakelj, M. (1999). "Screening Mammography for Early Detection of Breast Cancer." *Annals of Oncology* 10(6):S121–S127.

Shapiro, S.; Venet, W.; Strax, P.; et al. (1988). *Periodic Screening for Breast Cancer: The Health Insurance Plan Project and Its Sequelae, 1963–1986.* Baltimore, MD: Johns Hopkins University Press.

—— (1982). "Ten- to Fourteen–Year Effect of Screening on Breast Cancer Mortality." *Journal of the National Cancer Institute* 69:349–355.

MANAGED CARE

Managed care is the enrollment of patients into a plan that makes capitated payments to health care providers on behalf of its members, thus shifting the financial risk for health care from patients and payers to providers. The intent of this shift is to provide incentives to health care professionals to reduce their utilization of resources, ideally through measures such as health promotion and disease prevention among the group's members.

The phrase "managed care" is often loosely used to describe almost any attempt to limit health care expenditures in an increasingly competitive marketplace. Traditionally, however, managed-care plan members are cared for only by doctors who are part of the group. Each member is assigned a primary care physician who acts as that member's main caregiver and care coordinator, thus limiting the member's access to specialists and other more expensive types of care.

In the period following World War II, the predominant American health insurance paradigm was one in which insurance companies sold coverage to employers, who provided coverage to employees as a benefit of employment. Health coverage became an element in contract negotiations between employers and employee unions and during the 1950s and 1960s, when the American workforce was relatively young and healthy, and many industries agreed to provide generous health benefits at little or no direct cost to workers. At the same time, the public sector dramatically expanded its payment for health care with Medicare and Medicaid. In this "unmanaged care" system, patients were free to self-refer to the rapidly growing numbers of specialist physicians, with little or no coordination of their care. With relatively few restrictions, payments were made by insurance companies and government programs to physicians, hospitals, and other health care providers on a fee-for-service or cost basis—the higher the cost or charge, the larger the payment.

Little thought appears to have been given to the predictable effects of the nation's demography (young people of the 1950s and 1960s grew older) or of financial incentives on the cost of care. Patients insulated from the costs of their care by insurance tended to increase their access to, and expectations for, health care; while physicians trained to go to extremes on patients' behalf developed increasingly effective, and expensive, means of doing so. In the 1970s, these two dynamics led to a crisis of rapid and uncontrolled escalation in the costs of care.

Although early managed care plans were first organized in the 1920s, managed care is generally considered as having its origins in the 1940s in not-for-profit organizations such as the Group Health Cooperative of Puget Sound, the Kaiser Foundation Medical Care Program, and the Health Insurance Plan of Greater New York. Managed care spread relatively slowly until the 1970s and 1980s, when the crisis in health care costs began to encourage managed care as a lower-cost alternative to the accepted approach. Increased competition in the health care market led to the adaptation of managed-care techniques by new for-profit health care firms, and at the same time a number of states changed their Medicaid plans to a managed-care approach. This led to rapid increases in managed-care enrollment—as of 1999, more than half of all practicing physicians in the United States, and over 75 percent of the insured population, participated in some form of managed care plan.

Managed care arrangements take many shapes including group- or staff-model health maintenance organizations (HMOs), in which salaried physicians and other providers cared for plan members predominated only among the early managed care plans. These have increasingly been replaced by individual practice associations (IPAs), in which physicians agree to accept managed care patients as part of their existing practices. Point-of-service (POS) plans allow plan members more flexibility than HMOs, but require a higher rate of payment. Preferred provider organizations (PPOs), though often included in the managed care category, are discounted fee-for-service arrangements in which providers accept lower fees in return for a guaranteed patient volume, and are not true managed care efforts.

As noted above, the membership of early HMOs consisted largely of employed workers. Recent attempts to contain costs by enrolling Medicare and Medicaid patients into managed care plans have been only partially successful at best, due to the fact that members of both groups are more likely to have higher-cost health needs than the employed workforce. Some insurers have participated in these plans, only to withdraw when they were unable to meet their financial goals. Other problems have occurred when managed care plans have attempted to improve their competitive position in the marketplace at the cost of their health care mission: misrepresentation of benefits; adverse selection of members; and delaying, limiting, or withholding treatment are some of the problems that have arisen. Problems of this sort have resulted in increased public dissatisfaction and calls for government regulation as the definition of managed care—at one time considered a utopian health-improvement experiment, but now often considered a generic term for cost cutting at human expense—continues to evolve.

JAMES R. BOEX

(SEE ALSO: *Health Maintenance Organization [HMO]; Medicaid; Medicare; Personal Health Services; Primary Care*)

BIBLIOGRAPHY

Breslow, L. "Public Health and Managed Care: A California Perspective." *Health Affairs* 15:92–100.

Enthoven, A. C. (1980). *Health Plan: The Only Practical Solution to the Soaring Cost of Medical Care.* Reading, MA: Addison-Wesley.

Iglehart, J. K. (1992). "The American Health Care System: Managed Care." *The New England Journal of Medicine* 327:742–747.

Starr, P. (1982). *The Social Transformation of American Medicine.* New York: Basic Books.

MANSON, PATRICK

Patrick Manson (1844–1922), the man identified as the "father of tropical medicine," was an Aberdonian Scot who studied medicine in his home city of Aberdeen and in Edinburgh. Following his graduation in 1865, he went straight into the Chinese Imperial Maritime Customs Service, first in Formosa and later in Amoy. His work in China covered a remarkable range and included many original discoveries about the causes and suitable control measures for some of the tropical diseases that were so common at that time. This included work on several intestinal parasites; skin diseases caused by fungus infections; and tropical sprue, a debilitating bowel disease that causes or is associated with vitamin and mineral deficiencies.

In 1877, Manson discovered that the crippling disease known as elephantiasis was caused by a filarial worm and transmitted by mosquitoes—the first demonstration that mosquitoes transmitted diseases. After returning to Britain in 1890 he established a consultant medical practice in London and became a medical teacher and adviser to the British Colonial Office. His work included the reorganization of the West African medical services. In 1898 he published a seminal work, *Tropical Diseases*, and in 1899 he founded the London School of Hygiene and Tropical Medicine. Previously, he had founded a school of tropical medicine in Hong Kong.

Manson influenced a whole generation of British medical scientists who studied and specialized in tropical diseases. The greatest of these was Ronald Ross, to whom he passed on his hypothesis that mosquitoes must be the vector that transmitted malaria. Manson's name is immortalized several times in the taxonomy of the pathogens he identified. He received many honors and awards, including a knighthood.

JOHN M. LAST

(SEE ALSO: *Tropical Infectious Diseases; Vector-Borne Diseases*)

MANTOUX TEST

The Mantoux test is a skin test used to identify individuals who have previously been infected with *Mycobacterium tuberculosis*, the bacterium responsible for tuberculosis infection and disease in humans. The test is performed by injecting 0.1 ml of a solution that contains an extract of cultures of the bacterium, called *tuberculin*, into the dermis layer of the skin of the forearm with a 27-gauge needle. In individuals who previously have been infected with the bacterium, either clinically or subclinically, the test may stimulate a reaction (called "delayed hypersensitivity reaction") if the body's immune system recognizes the antigenic components in the test solution. The skin reaction is "read" forty-eight to seventy-two hours after the injection by measuring the amount of induration (swelling) at the injection site in millimeters. The sensitivity and the specificity of the test depend upon many variables, and false negative results are common.

JOHN L. STAUFFER

(SEE ALSO: *Tuberculosis*)

BIBLIOGRAPHY

American Thoracic Society (2000). "Diagnostic Standards and Classification of Tuberculosis in Adults and Children." *American Journal of Respiratory Critical Care Medicine* 161:1376–1395.

MARGINAL PEOPLE

To be marginal is to be marginalized. Taken broadly, the term "marginalization" evokes a dynamic between two social analytic categories: the "center" (or mainstream), and an area called the "margins." The center is normally associated with dominance, privilege, and power; the margins, with relative powerlessness. To be marginalized is to be placed in the margins, and thus excluded from the privilege and power found at the center. What counts, as marginal, in terms of the characteristics, functions, and meanings of margins, is contested, highly contextual, and historically specific. Marginalization is often based on such notions as gender, culture, language, race, sexual orientation, religion, political affiliation, socioeconomic position or class, and geographic location. Depending on the context and level of analysis, individuals, groups, organizations, communities, and even entire geopolitical systems can be seen as marginalized.

The concept of marginalization is useful in public health to highlight, understand, and ultimately change processes by which social relations mark and maintain boundaries that produce ill health. Social relations, particularly those that have become codified and institutionalized, may not be recognized as problems by all members of a given society, despite being shown to have a determining affect on health. An example of this is social stratification based on ethnicity, class, or income, by which the relative quality of experience in the psychosocial and socioeconomic environment expresses itself through biological mechanisms, as heterogeneity in health and well-being throughout the life cycle.

A focus on social relations in explaining how people come to occupy more or less favorable conditions of living offers a contrast to primarily asocial interpretations of correlative data showing a disproportionate burden of ill health among certain ethnic groups. Instead of viewing these correlative data as a result of an interplay between potentially modifiable behavioral risk factors and presumably nonmodifiable risk markers (e.g., genes), marginalization broadens its theory of causation to include distal factors beyond the individual or group. In this sense, marginalization views ill health as a result of larger forces impinging on populations, rather than as a problem of populations.

Marginalization can be used to appraise these larger forces in numerous ways. One such way has been to focus on a group's distance from the center of society and to highlight marginalized people's exposures to inadequate housing, racism, unemployment, and lack of education. Such conditions of living can be conceptualized as risk conditions—environmental factors that affect the expression of individual-level risk factors, whether behavioral, physiological, or genetic. Risk conditions are the living standards and social conditions that define a marginal group's relations to the mainstream, and can manifest, for example, in a group's cultural history or current economic circumstances. These risk conditions are often more meaningful, yet less convenient, than standard measures of race or ethnicity in understanding population differences in health status.

Another way in which marginalization has been used is to highlight how social processes make individuals and groups feel about themselves, their beliefs, or their place in a greater social order. In this sense, marginalization can invoke feelings of oppression and alienation, with alienation being understood in its general sense as a disassociation of people from meaningful work, their organic social collectivities, or their own identities. At another level, marginalization has been used to conceptualize how ill health is produced through the unequal distribution of power and property, information, patterns of production and consumption, and the biological impact of social inequality. In this regard, the risk conditions or environmental factors that create ill health among marginalized people are understood as products of conflicting social interests among competing groups. To be marginalized, in this sense, is to be distanced from power and resources that enable self-determination in economic, political, and social settings. At yet another level, marginalization has been used to conceptualize how certain groups experience a disease in ways not experienced by mainstream groups. An example of this is the way in which AIDS (acquired immunodeficiency syndrome) is suffered among gay men in Western countries as a condition of shame and moral culpability, characteristics which seldom compound the difficult experiences of AIDS among nonmarginal groups.

Public health interventions suggested by the concept of marginalization have sought policies and environmental regulations to aid healthful living by enabling people, individually and collectively, to gain greater control over their environment, broadly understood. The means for reducing marginalization and its effects on health, through the development of personal skills, the strengthening of communities, and the promotion of more egalitarian social, political, and economic policies, however, continue to be difficult to attain and enforce.

MARK DANIEL
G. FLETCHER LINDER

(SEE ALSO: *Acculturation; Assimilation; Cultural Norms; Ethnicity and Health; Ethnocentrism; Immigrants, Immigration; Minority Rights; Traditional Health Beliefs, Practices; Values in Health Education*)

BIBLIOGRAPHY

Green, L. W., and Kreuter, M. W. (1999). *Health Promotion Planning: An Educational and Ecological Approach.* Toronto: Mayfield.

Hertzman, C.; Frank, J.; and Evans, R. G. (1994). "Heterogeneities in Health Status and the Determinants of Population Health." In *Why Are Some People Healthy and Others Not? The Determinants of Health of Populations,* eds. R. G. Evans, M. L. Barer, and T. R. Marmor. New York: Aldine de Gruyter.

Krieger, N. (1999). "Embodying Inequality: A Review of Concepts, Measures, and Methods for Studying the Health Consequences of Discrimination." *International Journal of Health Services* 29:295–352.

Wallace, R., and Wallace, D. (1997). "Community Marginalisation and the Diffusion of Disease and Disorder in the United States." *British Medical Journal* 314:1341–1345.

MARIJUANA

Marijuana is a dried mixture of the leaves and flowers of *Cannabis sativa*, or hemp plant. Slang words for marijuana include "pot," "weed," "grass," and "dope." The term "cannabis" refers to different psychoactive preparations of the plant, including marijuana, hashish, and hashish oil. Hashish is the resin produced by the flowering tops of the plants; hashish oil is a concentrated form of cannabis extracted from the plant or resin using a solvent. Unpollinated female plants are called sinsemilla (sen-suh-mee-ah) and the flowering tops of these plants produce potent "buds" that do not contain seeds.

The major psychoactive ingredient in cannabis is delta-9-tetrahydrocannabinol (THC), but there are more than sixty related chemicals in marijuana, which are called "cannabinoids." Cannabis also contains other unrelated compounds that have similar psychoactive effects. The World Health Organization reported in 1997 that THC content in marijuana ranges from 0.5 to 4 percent, while concentrations in cannabis oil, hashish, and sinsemilla generally range from 7 to 14 percent, but may be as high as 20 percent. THC concentration depends on the variety, sex, and growing conditions of the plant, and it has increased over the years due to hydroponic cultivation techniques and selective breeding.

Marijuana and other cannabis products are usually smoked as a cigarette (a "joint") or in pipes, but may also be ingested orally. In the 1990s, the use of "blunts" to smoke marijuana became more common. A blunt is made by removing the tobacco from a cigar wrapper and filling it with marijuana, or a mixture of marijuana and some other drug like cocaine.

PSYCHOACTIVE AND PHYSIOLOGICAL EFFECTS

THC is absorbed more quickly into the bloodstream when smoked than when eaten. Effects are felt almost immediately and peak within thirty minutes of smoking. The marijuana "high" results when the THC binds with cannabinoid receptors in the brain. This process slows down regular nerve transmission, interfering with normal function. The cannabinoid receptors are located in the areas of the brain involved in muscle control, sexual functioning, vision and hearing, reasoning, hormone release, and memory.

Short-term effects include a temporary increase in heart rate, blood pressure, and blood flow to parts of the brain. Users generally feel a sense of euphoria, relaxation, hilarity, and heightened sensory perception. Negative psychological reactions may include anxiety, hallucinations, and panic attacks. Many smokers report that they feel unmotivated when they are high. Cannabis intoxication alters perceptions of time and space and impairs reaction time—affecting the performance of psychomotor tasks such as driving, which increases the risk of motor vehicle accidents. Cannabis increases food intake, impairs learning capabilities, and affects short-term memory. Many cannabis effects are subjective and influenced by the social circumstances, but the extent of impairment mainly depends on the potency and dose of the drug, the individual's tolerance to and experience using cannabis, and the difficulty and complexity of the task at hand.

LONG-TERM HEALTH CONSEQUENCES

Many of the studies done on the health consequences of marijuana have been inconclusive, although a picture is emerging of some worrisome long-term health effects. Smoking marijuana affects the respiratory system in much the same way as cigarette smoking. Cannabis smoke contains many of the same toxic chemicals and carcinogens as tobacco, as well as cannabinoids, all of which are respiratory irritants. Frequent marijuana smokers often report laryngitis, hoarseness, and coughing, and they are more likely than infrequent or nonusers to get acute and chronic bronchitis.

In a comprehensive analysis of the health effects of cannabis, the World Health Organization reports that cannabis is known to have adverse effects on the immune system, reproductive system, adrenal hormones, growth hormone, and cognitive function, particularly related to attention and memory processes. The long-term consequences of these effects, however, are not fully known, and further research is warranted. Smoking marijuana during pregnancy reduces oxygen flow to the fetus, which may interfere with growth and result in low birth weight, premature birth, and deficits in verbal ability and memory during childhood.

Preliminary research has demonstrated some positive health benefits of marijuana, including control of nausea and vomiting in people suffering from advanced cancer and AIDS (acquired immunodeficiency syndrome), appetite stimulation for those with wasting diseases, treatment of glaucoma by reducing intraoculer pressure, and control of convulsions and muscle spasms. More research in these areas is needed.

TRENDS IN MARIJUANA USE

Marijuana use by young people in North America peaked at the end of the 1970s, then declined progressively until the early 1990s, when use began to rise again. In the United States, it appears that the rate of increase may have stabilized at the end of the 1990s, although this stabilization was not apparent in Canada. The Monitoring the Future Survey found that lifetime use of marijuana among U.S. high school seniors peaked in 1979 at 60.4 percent, declined to a low of 32.6 percent in 1992, then rose to 49.6 percent in 1997, where it appears to have leveled off. A 1998 Canadian study on marijuana use did not report use among twelfth graders, but did find that approximately 42 percent of tenth graders had used marijuana in the previous year, up from 25 percent in 1991. In comparison, in 1998 only 31.1 percent of tenth graders in U.S. high schools reported use.

Marijuana use across the entire U.S. population was examined in a household survey in 1992 by the National Institute on Drug Abuse, which reported that 33 percent of Americans age 12 years and over had tried marijuana, 9 percent had used it during the previous year, and approximately 4 percent were current users, though the rate of use varied with age. These figures changed little in the 1998 survey. The proportion of Americans who reported having used marijuana at some point in their life was 11 percent among those 12 to 17 years old, 59 percent among those 26 to 34 years old, and 25 percent among people 35 years old and older.

1n 1994, the Canada Alcohol and Other Drug Survey found that 28 percent of Canadians had used cannabis at least once, 7.4 percent used it in the past year, and 3.2 percent were current users. During the early to mid-1990s, the proportion of people in other countries who reported having tried marijuana was 34 percent in Australia, 43 percent in New Zealand, 37 percent in Denmark, 17 percent in Switzerland and 14 percent in the United Kingdom. In general, marijuana use is lower among European, African, Asian, and South American youth than among young people in North America.

Different subgroups in the North American population report different rates of use. In general, males and white youth report higher rates of marijuana use than females, black youth, or young people from other racial or ethnic backgrounds. Young people who have dropped out of school are more likely to use cannabis than those who are in school, and 84.5 percent of students who attended alternative high schools in 1998 said they had tried cannabis.

MARIJUANA AND SUBSTANCE ABUSE

Since the 1970s, research has consistently demonstrated that adolescents progress through a uniform sequence of drug use involvement that begins with alcohol, cigarettes, and marijuana and proceeds to the use of "hard" drugs like hallucinogens, benzodiazepenes, amphetamines, sedatives, cocaine, and heroin. For this reason, marijuana, alcohol, and tobacco have been called "gateway" drugs. Some studies have shown that use of marijuana is almost a necessary condition for cocaine use by youth. The more frequently and intensively that gateway drugs are used, the greater the likelihood of dependence on the drug and progression to a later stage in the sequence of substance use involvement. However, most young people who use marijuana do not progress to dependence, or use harder drugs. The majority of marijuana users do not use other illicit drugs, although they are more likely to smoke cigarettes and drink alcohol than nonusers. Heavy use of marijuana does, however, place users in contact with more diverse networks of drug users and sellers, thereby increasing their exposure to other drugs and to the influence of those who use them. Participation in street culture is related to marijuana use. Those young people who do progress to abuse other illicit drugs and who experience the most harmful consequences are more likely to be socially and economically disadvantaged.

PREVENTION

Most cannabis-use prevention programs are school based, and they tend to focus on illicit drugs in general, not just marijuana. The existence of a stable pattern of drug use suggests that prevention efforts should be directed not only at preventing the initiation of use, but also at curbing the transitions from experimental to regular use of any of the gateway drugs and the transition to other drugs. In reviewing what works in drug-use prevention, D. R. Gerstein and L. W. Green found that no prevention programs were reliably effective in all cases with all groups. However, a number

of principles for effective prevention have been identified. The U.S. National Institute on Drug Abuse suggests that programs should be comprehensive and long-term, with reinforcement over several years; should target all forms of drug abuse; focus on the family, with a parent or caregiver component; include interactive methods, and be age-specific, developmentally appropriate, and culturally sensitive. School programs are best offered in the sixth through tenth grade, and should include components to develop interpersonal social skills, resistance skills, and self-efficacy, and to improve knowledge of health effects. The higher the level of risk in the specific population, the more intensive and targeted the program should be.

MARJORIE A. MACDONALD

(SEE ALSO: *Addiction and Habituation; Behavior, Health-Related; Health Promotion and Education; School Health; Social Determinants; Substance Abuse, Definition of*)

BIBLIOGRAPHY

Adlaf, E. M.; Ivis, F. J.; Smart, R. G.; and Walsh, G. W. (1995). *The Ontario Student Drug Use Survey: 1977–1995*. Toronto: Addiction Research Foundation of Ontario.

Ellickson, P. L.; Hays, R. D.; and Bell, R. M. (1992). "Stepping Through the Drug Use Sequence: Longitudinal Scalogram Analysis of Initiation and Regular Use." *Journal of Abnormal Psychology* 101:441–451.

Gerstein, D. R., and Green, L. W., eds. (1993). *Preventing Drug Abuse: What Do We Know?* Washington, DC: National Academy Press.

Grunbaum, J.; Kann, L.; Kinchen, S.; Ross, J. G.; Gowda, V. R.; Collins, J. L.; and Kolbe, L. J. (1998) "Youth Risk Behavior Surveillance—National Alternative High School Youth Risk Behavior Survey, United States, 1998." *Morbidity and Mortality Weekly Report* 48 (SS07):1–44. Available at http://www.cdc.gov/epo/mmwr/preview/mmwrhtml/ss4807al.htm.

Health Canada (1995). *Canada's Alcohol and Other Drugs Survey: Preview 1995*. Ottawa: Minister of Supply and Services Canada.

Howlett, A. C.; Bidautrussell, M.; Devane, W. A.; Melvin, L. S.; Johnson, M. R.; and Herkenham, M. (1990). "The Cannabinoid Receptor—Biochemical, Anatomical and Behavioral Characterization." *Trends in Neuroscience* 13(10):420–423.

Johnston, L. D.; O'Malley, P. M.; and Bachman, J. G. (2000). *The Monitoring the Future National Survey*

Results on Adolescent Drug Use: Overview of Key Findings, 1999 (NIH Publication No. 00–4690). Rockville, MD: National Institute on Drug Abuse.

Kandel, D. B. (1975). "Stages in Adolescent Involvement in Drug Use." *Science* 73:543–552.

Kandel, D. B., and Yamaguchi, D. B. (1984). "Patterns of Drug Abuse from Adolescence to Early Adulthood: III. Predictor of Progression." *American Journal of Public Health* 74:673–681.

King, A. J. C.; Boyce, W. F.; and King, M. A. (1999). *Trends in the Health of Canadian Youth.* Ottawa: Health Canada. Available at http://www.hsc.gc.ca/hppb/childhood-youth/.

Kozel, N. (1997). *Epidemiological Trends in Drug Abuse: Advance Report.* Washington, DC: National Institute on Drug Abuse. Available at http://www.cdmgroup.com/cewg/doc//697washdc/sum97.advance.html.

National Institute on Drug Abuse (1992). *National Household Survey on Drug Abuse: Population Estimates 1992.* Rockville, MD: National Institute on Drug Abuse.

—— (1999). *National Household Survey on Drug Abuse, National Estimates of Substance Use, 1999.* Bethesda, MD: Substance Abuse and Mental Health Services, National Institute on Drug Abuse. Available at http://www.samhsa.gov/OAS/NHSDA/1999/.

World Health Organization (1997). *Cannabis: A Health Perspective and a Research Agenda.* Geneva: WHO, Division of Mental Health and Prevention of Substance Abuse.

MASS MEDIA

Mass media are tools for the transfer of information, concepts, and ideas to both general and specific audiences. They are important tools in advancing public health goals. Communicating about health through mass media is complex, however, and challenges professionals in diverse disciplines. In an article in the *Journal of Health Communication*, Liana Winett and Lawrence Wallack wrote that "using the mass media to improve public health can be like navigating a vast network of roads without any street signs—if you are not sure *where* you are going and *why*, chances are you will not reach your destination" (1996, p. 173).

Using mass media can be counterproductive if the channels used are not audience-appropriate, or if the message being delivered is too emotional, fear arousing, or controversial. Undesirable side effects usually can be avoided through proper formative research, knowledge of the audience, experience in linking media channels to audiences, and message testing.

TYPES AND FUNCTIONS OF MASS MEDIA

Sophisticated societies are dependent on mass media to deliver health information. Marshall McLuhan calls media "extensions of man." G. L. Kreps and B. C. Thornton believe media extend "people's ability to communicate, to speak to others far away, to hear messages, and to see images that would be unavailable without media" (1992, p. 144).

It follows that employment of mass media to disseminate health news (or other matters) has, in effect, reduced the world's size. The value of health news is related to what gets reported and how it gets reported. According to Ray Moynihan and colleagues:

The news media are an important source of information about health and medical therapies, and there is widespread interest in the quality of reporting. Previous studies have identified inaccurate coverage of published scientific papers, overstatement of adverse effects or risks, and evidence of sensationalism. The media can also have a positive public health role, as they did in communicating simple warnings about the connection between Reye's syndrome and the use of aspirin in children (1999, p. 1645).

Despite the potential of news media to perform valuable health-education functions, Moynihan et al. conclude that media stories about medications continue to be incomplete in their coverage of benefits, risks, and costs of drugs, as well as in reporting financial ties between clinical trial investigators and pharmaceutical manufacturers.

The mass media are capable of facilitating short-term, intermediate-term, and long-term effects on audiences. Short-term objectives include exposing audiences to health concepts; creating awareness and knowledge; altering outdated or incorrect knowledge; and enhancing audience recall of particular advertisements or public service announcements (PSAs), promotions, or program names. Intermediate-term objectives include all of the above, as well as changes in attitudes, behaviors, and perceptions of social norms. Finally, long-term objectives incorporate all of the aforementioned tasks, in addition to focused restructuring of perceived social norms, and maintenance of behavior change. Evidence of achieving these three tiers of objectives is useful in evaluating the effectiveness of mass media.

Mass media performs three key functions: educating, shaping public relations, and advocating for a particular policy or point of view. As education tools, media not only impart knowledge, but can be part of larger efforts (e.g., social marketing) to promote actions having social utility. As public relations tools, media assist organizations in achieving credibility and respect among public health opinion leaders, stakeholders, and other gatekeepers. Finally, as advocacy tools, mass media assist leaders in setting a policy agenda, shaping debates about controversial issues, and gaining support for particular viewpoints.

Television. Television is a powerful medium for appealing to mass audiences—it reaches people regardless of age, sex, income, or educational level. In addition, television offers sight and sound, and it makes dramatic and lifelike representations of people and products. Focused TV coverage of public health has been largely limited to crises. However, for audiences of the late 1950s, the 1960s, and the 1970s, television presented or reinforced certain health messages through product marketing. Some of these messages were related to toothpaste, hand soaps, multiple vitamins, fortified breakfast cereals, and other items.

Public health authorities have expressed concern about the indirect influence of television in promoting false norms about acts of violence, drinking, smoking, and sexual behavior. A hypothetical equation for viewers might be: drinking plus smoking equals sex and a good time. Safe sex practices are rarely portrayed on television. An additional public health concern is that TV viewing promotes sedentariness in a population already known for its multiple risk factors for cardiovascular disease and other chronic illnesses.

A more focused coverage of health matters occurred in the 1990s as a result of two events: (1) an expansion of "health segments" on news broadcasts, which included the hiring of "health" reporters, and (2) the expansion and wider distribution of cable television (CATV) and satellite systems. Television coverage of health issues reveals some of the medium's weaknesses as an educator, however. Health segments incorporated into news broadcasts are typically one to three minutes in length—the consumer receives only a brief report or "sound bite," while the broadcaster remains constrained by the fact that viewers expect the medium to be both visual and entertaining. Fortunately, with the advent and maturation of CATV, more selected audience targeting has become possible. The Health Network is dedicated entirely to health matters, while other cable networks (e.g., Discovery Channel) devote significant amounts of broadcast time to health. This narrowcasting allows the medium to reach particular market segments. However, the proliferation of cable channels decreases the volume of viewers for a given channel at any point in time. According to George and Michael Belch, even networks such as CNN, ESPN, and MTV draw only 1 to 2 percent of prime-time viewers.

Although TV has the potential to deliver messages about HIV/AIDS (human immunodeficiency virus/acquired immunodeficiency syndrome), smoking, cardiovascular disease, cancer, and so on, televised messages have the characteristic of low audience involvement. The main consumer effect of messages occurs through repetition and brand familiarity. Most health messages do not have the exposure level that brands of toothpaste, soap, or antiperspirant receive, for public health groups rarely can sustain the cost of television, thereby limiting their message's penetration.

For all its potential strengths, TV suffers many shortcomings. The cost of placing health messages on TV is high, not only because of the expense of purchasing airtime, but because of production time for PSA creation. Televised messages are fleeting—airing in most instances for only 15 to 30 seconds. Belch and Belch point out that for 13 to 17 minutes of every hour viewers are bombarded with messages, creating a clutter that makes retention difficult.

Radio. Radio also reaches mass and diverse audiences. The specialization of radio stations by listener age, taste, and even gender permits more selectivity in reaching audience segments. Since placement and production costs are less for radio than for TV, radio is able to convey public health messages in greater detail. Thus, radio is sometimes considered to be more efficient.

Radio requires somewhat greater audience involvement than television, creating the need for more mental imagery, or what Belch and Belch call "image transfer." Because of this, radio can reinforce complementary messages portrayed in parallel fashion on TV. However, the large number of radio stations may fragment the audience for health message delivery.

Radio health message campaigns have been effective in developing countries, especially when combined with posters and other mass media. Ronny Adhikarya showed that mass media message targeted at wheat farmers in Bangladesh increased the percentage of those who carried out rat control from 10 percent to 32 percent in 1983. Continuation of the campaign in subsequent years saw rat control efforts rise to 72 percent.

Internet. The advent of the World Wide Web and the massive increase in Internet users offers public health personnel enormous opportunities and challenges. The Internet places users in firmer autonomous control of which messages are accessed and when they are accessed. It is possible to put virtually anything on-line and disseminate it to any location having Internet access, but the user has little control over quality and accuracy. Internet search engines can direct users to tens of thousands of web sites after the user's introduction of one or more keywords. A critical task for public health educators will be to assist people in discriminating among Internet health-information sources. Efforts need to stop short of censorship, thus balancing accuracy, quality, and (in the U.S.) protection of free speech (First Amendment rights).

Unlike TV or radio, which are available in nearly all households, Internet access requires some technical skill, as well as the resources to purchase hardware and Internet subscription services. J. R. Finnegan and K. Viswanath explain that, as with its predecessor technologies, the Internet suffers from a certain "legacy of fear" about its impact on children, youth, and others. As with cinema since the 1940s and TV since the 1950s, the Internet has been accused of promoting mindlessness; exposing people to pornography, violence, and other examples of society's lowest common denominators; and enabling sedentary behavior. The Internet is said to facilitate activities of society's hate groups and to teach children and others how to construct bombs and obtain weapons. Unlike some other mass media, the Internet is presently not universally available across socioeconomic strata due to cost and other barriers. It is possible that this lack of universality has already contributed to existing information gaps between society's "haves" and "have-nots."

The Internet's utility for conveying health information can be illustrated by looking at three sample web sites. Considered by some to be the best source for public health data and information is the web site of the Centers for Disease Control and Prevention (http://www.cdc.gov). From here persons can locate numerous government data sources, obtain facts on chronic and infectious diseases, and gain fingertip access to health updates, including the *Morbidity and Mortality Weekly Report (MMWR)*. Another valuable site is that of the Association for Toxic Substances and Disease Registry (http://www.atsdr.cdc.gov/HEC/primer.html), which includes a primer on health risk communication principles and practice. Through this site, persons learn how to communicate about health risks to a skeptical public, including factors that influence the public's risk perceptions. Finally, Columbia University's health education web site (http://www.goaskalice.columbia.edu) makes it possible to access information on a voluminous array of health topics, with particular relevance to college students. This site also permits individuals to submit questions anonymously, receive responses, and be referred to other Internet links. These items are then archived for use by persons having similar queries.

Speculating about the Internet's future is not easy. However, the Internet offers all of the audio and visual strengths of other electronic media, plus interactivity and frequent updates. The challenge is to increase its availability and augment the skills of Internet users.

Newspapers. Belch and Belch estimate that newspapers are read daily in 70 percent of U.S. households, and in as many as 90 percent of high-income households. Newspapers permit a level of detail in health reporting not feasible with broadcast media. Whereas one can miss a television broadcast about breast cancer, and thus, lose its entire message, one can read the same (and more detailed) message in a newspaper at one's choice of time and venue. Although newspapers permit consumers flexibility concerning what is read, and when, they do have a brief shelf life. In many households, newspapers seldom survive more than one or two days.

Newspapers are available in daily and weekly formats, and local, regional, and national publications exist. In addition, there are numerous special audience newspapers (e.g., various ethnic groups, women and feminist related, gay and lesbian, geography-specific, neighborhood). Consequently, health messages contained in newspapers can reach many people and diverse groups. Newspapers often fall short of their dissemination potential, however. In addition to educating people about public health, deliberate efforts need to be directed at educating other media and politicians (McDermott 2000, p. 269).

Other authorities have illustrated the shortcomings of the newspapers in conveying health information. Few stories call for individual or community policy or action, and even fewer present a local angle.

Magazines. Belch and Belch divide magazines into three varieties: consumer (e.g., *Reader's Digest, Newsweek, People*), farm (e.g., *Farm Journal, National Hog Farmer, Beef*), and business (professional, industrial, trade, and general business publications). Magazines have several strengths, including audience selectivity, reproduction quality, prestige, and reader loyalty. Furthermore, magazines have a relatively long shelf life—they may be saved for weeks or months, and are frequently reread, and passed on to others. Magazine reading also tends to occur at a less hurried pace than newspaper reading. Health messages, therefore, can receive repeated exposure.

Other Print Media. Pamphlets, brochures, and posters constitute other print media used to disseminate health messages. These devices are readily found in most public health agencies, offices of private practitioners, health care institutions, and voluntary health organizations. They are common and familiar educational tools of the American Cancer Society, the American Heart Association, and the American Lung Association. Though widely used, their actual utility is infrequently evaluated (e.g., units distributed vs. changes in awareness, cost analysis). Until the 1990s, few of these print media were developed with the assistance of target audiences, and few contained varied

messages, were culturally tailored, or employed readability and face validity techniques. The extent to which persons read, reread, and keep these devices—or circulate them to other readers—is not well evaluated. Thus, their permanence is unknown.

Outdoor Media. Outdoor media include billboards and signs, placards inside and outside of commercial transportation modes, flying billboards (e.g., signs in tow of airplanes), blimps, and skywriting. Commercial advertisers such as Goodyear, Fuji, Budweiser, Pizza Hut, and Blockbuster all make extensive use of their logo-bearing blimps around sports stadiums. In the United States, none of these outdoor modes are used extensively to convey health messages, although billboards and transit placards are the most likely forms to contain health information. For persons who regularly pass by billboards or use public transportation, these media may provide repeated exposure to messages. Pro-health messages displayed on urban public transportation may suffer, however, from the image problems that afflict urban buses and subways. In addition, the effectiveness of such postings wears out quickly as audiences grow tired of their sameness.

Tobacco and alcohol manufacturers have made extensive use of billboards and other outdoor media. However, the 1998 Master Settlement Agreement between the states and the tobacco industries outlawed billboard advertising of cigarettes. In their 1994 Chicago-based study, Diana Hackbarth and her colleagues revealed how billboards promoting tobacco and alcohol were concentrated in poor neighborhoods. Similar themes were seen in other urban centers (Baltimore, Detroit, St. Louis, New Orleans, Washington, D.C., and San Francisco) where alcohol and tobacco billboards were much more concentrated in African-American neighborhoods than in white neighborhoods. The tobacco industry now pursues the same strategy in developing countries.

MEDIA EFFECTS

Decades of studies on the consequences of mass media exposure demonstrate that effects are varied and reciprocal—the media impact audiences and audiences also impact media by the intensity and frequency of their usage. The results of mass media for promoting social change, especially in developing countries, have become important for public health. J. R. Finnegan Jr. and K. Viswanath (1997) have identified three effects, or functions, of media: (1) the knowledge gap, (2) agenda setting, and (3) cultivation of shared public perceptions.

The Knowledge Gap. Health knowledge is differentially distributed in the population, resulting in knowledge gaps. Unfortunately, mass media are insufficient for distributing information in an egalitarian fashion—changes in social structure and institutions are also necessary for this to occur. Thus, the impact of mass media on audience knowledge gaps is influenced by such factors as the extent to which the content is appealing, the degree to which information channels are accessible and desirable, and the amount of social conflict and diversity there is in a community. Hence, public health media campaigns are more effective when structural factors that impede the distribution of knowledge are addressed.

Agenda Setting. The selective nature of what members of the media choose for public consumption influences how people think about health issues, and what they think about them. When Rudolph Giuliani, the mayor of New York City, publicly disclosed he had prostate cancer prior to the 2000 New York senatorial election, many news media reported the risks of prostate cancer, prompting greater public awareness about the incidence of the disease and the need for screening. A similar episode occurred in the mid-1970s when Betty Ford, wife of President Gerald R. Ford, and Happy Rockefeller, wife of Vice President Nelson Rockefeller, were both diagnosed with breast cancer.

A related theme is the extent to which the media set the public's perception of health risks. According to J. J. Davis, when risks are highlighted in the media, particularly in great detail, the extent of agenda setting is likely to be based on the degree to which a public sense of outrage and threat is provoked. Where mass media can be especially valuable is in the framing of issues. "Framing" means taking a leadership role in the organization of public discourse about an issue. Media, of course, are influenced by pressures to offer balance in coverage, and these pressures may come from persons and groups with particular political action and advocacy positions. According

to Finnegan and Viswanath, "groups, institutions, and advocates compete to identify problems, to move them onto the public agenda, *and* to define the issues symbolically" (1997, p. 324). Thus, persons who desire to access mass media's agenda-setting potential must be aware of the competition.

Cultivation of Perceptions. Cultivation is the extent to which media exposure, over time, shapes audience perceptions. Television is a common experience, especially in the United States, and it serves as what S. W. Littlejohn calls a "homogenizing agent." However, the effect is often based on several conditions, particularly socioeconomic factors. Prolonged exposure to TV or movie violence may affect the extent to which people think community violence is a problem, though that belief is likely moderated by where they live. However, the actual determinants of people's impressions of violence are complex, and consensus in this area is lacking.

THE RELATIONSHIP OF MASS MEDIA TO OTHER FORMS OF COMMUNICATION

The interaction between media messages and interpersonal communication was first described by Elihu Katz and Paul Lazarsfeld in their two-step flow hypothesis. They argued that media effects were moderated principally by interpersonal encounters. Community opinion leaders scan the media for information, then communicate that information to others in interpersonal contexts. It is in this second step, interpersonal interaction, that opinion leaders wield enormous power, influencing others not only by what they choose to reveal but also the slant that they use in conveying the message.

The two-step model has been expanded to include multistep models—most notably information diffusion models. Step models have been limited by their linear assumptions of one-way influence and causation. Media influence is undeniably linked to complex interpersonal dynamics. A shared influence likely results when people are exposed to health messages and then converge together in contexts that influence what they say to one another (and even how they say it), as well as what they selectively think.

George Gerbner describes a three-component framework. The first of these components is semiotics, the study of signs, symbols, and codes. Language comprises one such set of symbols and codes that can be further embellished by sights, sounds, and other visual and aural cues. The second aspect of the framework relates to behaviors and interactions associated with exposure to messages. Psychologists, marketers, and others attempt to predict behavior based on specially designed messages. The third element examines how communication is organized around social systems, and the extent to which history and human experience influence society's institutions.

Designers of health messages need to consider such models and frameworks. Modern views of health behavior change acknowledge eclectic approaches and consider multiple aspects of human experience, from the individual level to the community level. Individual channels of communication (e.g., face-to-face encounters) offer personal support and may invoke trust, but are labor intensive, have limited reach, and may require ancillary materials. Mass media channels transmit information rapidly and to general or specific audiences. Mass media can set agendas, but questions have been raised concerning their impartiality and integrity. Community channels (e.g., coalitions, community action groups, and the like), have less "reach" than mass media, but they reinforce, expand, and localize media messages and offer institutional and social support. Knowledge of the complementary strengths of various channels helps to optimize penetration and effectiveness of health messages.

MASS MEDIA PUBLIC HEALTH CAMPAIGNS—THE RIGHT "MIX"

Because of the inherent properties of various mass media, a U.S. Department of Health and Human Services publication advises that health-message designers consider a series of questions relative to choice of channels:

- Which channels are most appropriate for the health problem/issue and message?

- Which channels are most likely to be credible to and accessible by the target audience?

- Which channels fit the program purpose (e.g., inform, influence attitudes, change behavior)?

- Which and how many channels are feasible, considering your time and budget?

A 1999 article by A. G. Ramirez and colleagues describes a media mix that significantly increased adherence to recommended guidelines concerning cervical cancer screening among women in a predominantly Spanish-speaking Texas border city. The media mix included 82 television segments, 67 newspaper stories, and 48 radio programs, all featuring role models. In a 1998 study by Ramirez and other investigators, programs employing a similar strategy in New York, Florida, and California showed significant change in target behaviors among Hispanic populations.

In Project Northland, Cheryl Perry's team of researchers focused on moderating alcohol use by adolescents, but could not use radio and television spots due to their potential confounding properties (i.e., being heard or viewed by adolescents in a nonintervention comparison group) with respect to evaluation of this school- and community-based intervention. Print media, including posters, brochures, and newsletters, were used in the intervention communities to market health messages and advertise ancillary events, and adolescents and adults were trained in media advocacy to increase media coverage of underage use of alcohol.

The primary health communication tool used by the Centers for Disease Control and Prevention (CDC) is PRIZM, which was developed by Claritas, Inc. PRIZM divides the United States into sixty-two lifestyle clusters, or groups of people with similar "geodemographic characteristics, consumer behaviors, psychosocial beliefs, and media habits" (Parvanta and Freimuth 2000, p. 22). It provides data on 250 sociodemographic census variables and approximately 500 items concerning media preferences, purchasing behaviors, and lifestyle activities.

Following a needs assessment that revealed an abnormally high birth-defect rate in a four-county area of Virginia, mass media were tapped to inform more than 22,000 women of child-bearing age about the health benefits of folic acid supplements and folate-rich foods. The campaign included television and radio PSAs, brochures, posters and display boards, as well as the cooperation of a local grocery store chain that provided other print media (food information cards and special food labels on folate-dense products). In a 1999 evaluation, CDC investigators reported a statistically significant increase in folic acid awareness between 1997 and 1999.

Mass media have been major sources of information about HIV/AIDS and other sexually transmitted infections. In a 2000 study, 96 percent of 1,290 men aged twenty-two to twenty-six reported hearing about these subjects through television advertisements, radio, or magazines. Some authorities have expressed skepticism about the mass media's future motivation to provide positive sex education messages, since portrayal of sex attracts viewers, which in turn, increases revenues.

Other evidence of the media's ability to improve reproductive health and promote population control exists, especially from developing countries. Mass media have made people aware of modern contraception and where to access it, as well as linking family planning to other reproductive health care and to broader roles for women. Communication about family planning and population control creates awareness, increases knowledge, builds approval, and encourages healthful behaviors. In Egypt, where nearly all households have television, population control objectives have been achieved through televised PSAs. Data also support the positive effects of mass media messages on contraception use in Zimbabwe, Ghana, Nigeria, and Kenya. In a 1999 Tanzania-based study, a team of researchers led by Everett M. Rogers showed how the popularity of a radio soap opera promoting family planning increased listeners' self-efficacy with respect to discussing contraception with spouses and peers.

Although mass media are important for disseminating health messages and encouraging an adoption of healthful lifestyles, they currently fall short of their potential. The realization of this potential in the future depends, in part, on increasing the media advocacy skills of public health authorities, improving understanding of competing antihealth media messages, and organizing channels for an optimal media mix.

ROBERT J. MCDERMOTT
TERRANCE L. ALBRECHT

(SEE ALSO: *Advertising of Unhealthy Products; Attitudes; Communication for Health; Communication Theory; Health Books; Health Promotion and Education; Impartiality and Advocacy; Internet; Mass Media and Tobacco Control; Media Advocacy; Patient Educational Media; Radio; Social Marketing*)

BIBLIOGRAPHY

Adhikarya, R. (2001). "The Strategic Extension Campaigns on Rat Control in Bangladesh." In *Public Communication Campaigns,* 3rd edition, eds. R. E. Rice and C. E. Atkin. Thousand Oaks, CA: Sage Publications.

American Academy of Pediatrics Committee on Communications (1995). "Media Violence." *Pediatrics* 95:949–951.

Belch, G. E., and Belch, M. A. (1995). *Introduction to Advertising & Promotion,* 3rd edition. Chicago: Irwin.

Bradner, C. H.; Ku, L.; and Lindberg, L. D. (2000). "Older, but Not Wiser: How Men Get Information About AIDS and Sexually Transmitted Diseases After High School." *Family Planning Perspectives* 32(1):33–38.

Brown, J. D., and Keller, S. N. (2000). "Can the Mass Media Be Healthy Sex Educators?" *Family Planning Perspectives* 32(5):255–256.

Centers for Disease Control and Prevention (1999). "Folic Acid Campaign and Evaluation—Southwestern Virginia, 1997–1999." *Morbidity and Mortality Weekly Report* 48:914–917.

Davis, J. J. (2000). "Riskier Than We Think? The Relationship Between Risk Statement Completeness and Perceptions of Direct to Consumer Advertised Prescription Drugs." *Journal of Health Communication* 5:349–370.

Finnegan, J. R., Jr., and Viswanath, K. (1997). "Communication Theory and Health Behavior Change: The Media Studies Framework." In *Health Behavior and Health Education,* 2nd edition, eds. K. Glanz, F. M. Lewis, and B. K. Rimer. San Francisco: Jossey-Bass Publishers.

Gerbner, G. (1983). "Field Definitions: Communication Theory." In *1984–85 U.S. Directory of Graduate Programs,* 9th edition. Princeton, NJ: Educational Testing Service.

Hackbarth, D. P.; Silvestri, B.; and Cosper, W. (1994). "Tobacco and Alcohol Billboards in 50 Chicago Neighborhoods: Market Segmentation to Sell Dangerous Products to the Poor." *Journal of Public Health Policy* 16(2):213–230.

Katz, E., and Lazarsfeld, P. (1955). *The Part Played by People in the Flow of Mass Communications.* New York: Free Press.

Kreps, G. L., and Thornton, B. C. (1992). *Health Communication Theory & Practice.* Prospect Heights, IL: Waveland Press.

Littlejohn, S. W. (1989). *Theories of Human Communication.* Belmont, CA: Wadsworth Publishing Company.

McDermott, R. J. (2000). "Health Education Research: Evolution or Revolution (or Maybe Both)?" *Journal of Health Education* 33(5):264–271.

Moynihan, R.; Bero, L.; Ross-Degnan, D.; Henry, D.; Lee, K.; Watkins, J.; Mah, C.; and Soumerai, S. B. (1999). "Coverage by the News Media of the Benefits and Risks of Medications." *New England Journal of Medicine* 342:1645–1650.

Parvanta, C. F., and Freimuth, V. (2000). "Health Communication at the Centers for Disease Control and Prevention." *American Journal of Health Behavior* 24:18–25.

Pelletier, A. R.; Quinlan, K. P.; Sacks, J. J.; Van Gilder, T. J.; Gilchrist, J.; and Ahluwalia, H. K. (1999). "Firearm Use in G- and PG-rated Movies." *Journal of the American Medical Association* 282(5):428.

Perry, C. L.; Williams, C. L.; Komro, K. A.; Veblen-Mortenson, S.; Forster, J. L.; Bernstein-Lachter, R.; Pratt, L. K.; Dudovitz, B.; Munson, K. A.; Farbakhsh, K.; Finnegan, J.; and McGovern, P. (2000). "Project Northland High School Interventions: Community Action to Reduce Adolescent Alcohol Use." *Health Education & Behavior* 27(1):29–49.

Ramirez, A. G.; McAlister, A. L.; Villarreal, R.; Suarez, L.; Talavera, G. A.; Perez-Stable, E. J.; Marti, J.; and Trapido, E. J. (1998). "Prevention and Control in Diverse Hispanic Populations: A National Leading Initiative for Research and Action." *Cancer* 83:1825–1829.

Ramirez, A. G.; Villarreal, R.; McAlister, A.; Gallion, K. J.; Suarez, L.; and Gomez, P. (1999). "Advancing the Role of Participatory Communication in the Diffusion of Cancer Screening Among Hispanics." *Journal of Health Communications* 4:31–36.

Robey, B.; Piotrow, P. T.; and Salter, C. (1994). "Family Planning Lessons and Challenges: Making Programs Work." *Population Reports* 22(2):1–27.

Rogers, E. M.; Vaughan, P. W.; Swalehe, R. M. A.; Rao, N.; Svenkerud, P.; and Sood, S. (1999). "Effects of An Entertainment-Education Radio Soap Opera on Family Planning Behavior in Tanzania." *Studies in Family Planning* 30(3):193–211.

U.S. Department of Health and Human Services (1989). *Making Health Communication Programs Work: A Planner's Guide.* Bethesda, MD: National Cancer Institute.

Winett, L. B., and Wallack, L. (1996). "Advancing Public Health Goals through the Mass Media." *Journal of Health Communication* 1:173–196.

MASS MEDIA AND TOBACCO CONTROL

The use of mass media for tobacco control increased in developed countries in the 1990s, particularly in the United States, Canada, Australia, and the United Kingdom. The emergence of significant funding sources, particularly legal statements with tobacco companies and earmarked tobacco taxes, has allowed the implementation of sustained, mass media campaigns with sufficient audience reach to be effective. Media have been used to promote smoking cessation and smoke-free spaces, to raise awareness of health effects and of unethical tobacco industry behavior, and to create support for various policy measures. Although these campaigns have occurred almost exclusively in developed countries, the lessons learned have been consistent enough to be potentially widely applicable.

THE FAIRNESS DOCTRINE

The first mass media tobacco-control campaign in the United States was the result of a federal court judgment. Under U.S. law until 1988, broadcasters were required under the Federal Communications Commission's Fairness Doctrine "to encourage and implement the broadcast of all sides of controversial public issues over their facilities, over and beyond their obligation to make available on demand opportunities for the expression of opposing views." In 1967, in response to a legal challenge by attorney John Banzhaf, the Fairness Doctrine was interpreted as being applicable to tobacco advertising.

As a result, from 1968 to 1970, health ads about cigarette smoking were carried on the airwaves, with about one health ad broadcast for every three cigarette ads. Per capita cigarette sales declined during this period (they increased both before and after), youth smoking prevalence and self-reported consumption declined significantly, and concern by smokers about their health increased significantly. Although it is impossible to isolate the Fairness Doctrine as the major factor influencing these trends, it is reasonable to assume that it was a major contributor. Perhaps a more telling piece of evidence is that when cigarette advertising was banned on broadcast television in the United States in 1971, the tobacco companies did not challenge the ban. The ban resulted in a 80 percent drop in antismoking ads in the broadcast media.

TOBACCO CONTROL MASS MEDIA IN THE UNITED STATES

Public service announcements (PSAs; advertisements for an issue aired free as a public service) have long been a staple of tobacco control and other health promotion strategies. However, there is very little evidence to support the efficacy of PSAs in reducing tobacco use. The airing of PSAs on a voluntary basis does not guarantee exposure to the public at a level sufficient to change attitudes and behavior on a broad scale.

In 1998, California voters passed Proposition 99, a tax on tobacco products dedicated to funding health promotion and tobacco-control activities. Prop 99, as it is commonly known, has paid for a sustained and comprehensive tobacco-control program that includes a mass media campaign. Several other states, including Massachusetts, Oregon, and Florida, have since used funds from tobacco taxes and from legal settlements with tobacco companies to initiate similar programs.

These programs have been associated with significant reductions in tobacco use. Per capita cigarette consumption declined at a far greater rate in California and Massachusetts than it did nationally after initiation of the state programs. In both states, youth smoking rates held steady as they increased in the country as a whole. Oregon's tobacco tax-funded program was associated with an 11.3 percent decline in per capita consumption over two years, far greater than the national rate of decline. Florida showed even more dramatic results. Following implementation of the Florida tobacco-control program, the prevalence of cigarette use dropped 19 percent among middle school students and 8 percent among high school students in a single year. The centerpiece of the Florida campaign was the aggressive, youth-targeted

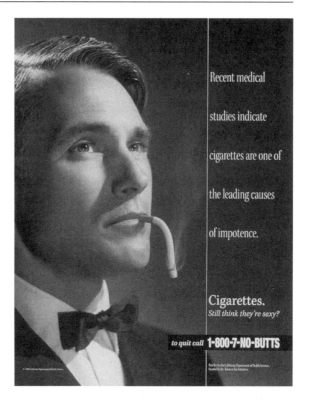

This antismoking advertisement warning men of possible unexpected health risks was published by the California Department of Health. (California Department of Health Services)

"Truth" media and advocacy campaign, which challenged youth to expose the truth behind tobacco marketing and to lead tobacco-control activities in their communities. Further evaluation will be needed to determine whether the Florida declines are sustained.

It is difficult to separate out the effects of mass media relative to other components of these programs, or to broader environmental factors such as the level of spending on tobacco promotion. However, the media campaigns have served to tie together other program components, to raise public awareness of tobacco issues, and to build public support for other tobacco-control measures. In addition, data from California suggest an independent impact of the media campaign. Per capita tobacco sales declined significantly between 1990 and 1992—when the media campaign was the only component of the program that was fully implemented. In addition, consumption declines slowed during a period when spending on media was cut significantly, including the absence of media campaigns for an entire year.

A national paid mass media campaign targeted at youth was launched in 1999 by the American Legacy Foundation. The foundation was established with funds from a 1998 multistate legal settlement and has a mandate to reduce tobacco use through public education and other means. Borrowing from the principles of Florida's Truth campaign, the Legacy campaign has the potential to reduce tobacco use in at least some population segments.

Since 1995, the Campaign for Tobacco-Free Kids has paid for the placement of ads, primarily in the print media, that focus on current political issues. Ads target the public and politicians, and have sometimes focused on one or two individual legislators regarding key decision-making points affecting tobacco-control initiatives. This campaign has not been formally evaluated.

In 1999, the cigarette manufacturer Philip Morris launched a $100 million media campaign ostensibly aimed at discouraging youths from using the products that tobacco companies spend billions of dollars to promote. Focus-group research of youths found that the Philip Morris ads were consistently perceived to be less effective than ads from the successful state campaigns, even before participants were told that the ads were produced by a tobacco company. One of the main points mentioned in the groups was that the ads promoted the choice to smoke or not smoke, but gave no specific reasons why youth should choose not to smoke.

TOBACCO CONTROL AND MASS MEDIA OUTSIDE THE UNITED STATES

Although paid mass media has been used for tobacco control in Canada, Mexico, the United Kingdom, Australia, and Singapore, very few of these campaigns have been evaluated.

In Canada, the federal and provincial governments used paid mass media increasingly in the 1990s to raise public awareness and to promote policy initiatives. The provinces of British Columbia and Ontario received awards for media spots produced as part of a broader tobacco-control strategy. However, none of the recent Canadian campaigns have been evaluated for their effectiveness independently of other policy and program initiatives. These complementary initiatives have been significant.

In Latin America, PSAs remain the most common media tobacco-control tool. There is no evidence to suggest that these campaigns are any more effective that the PSA campaigns in developed countries. Recently, the Pan American Health Organization developed a radio program on smoking cessation in conjunction with radio stations in Columbia and Peru. Although the program has not been formally evaluated, radio listenership and advertising rates increased throughout the broadcast of the multiweek program. Radio is a popular and affordable communication medium in Latin America and has the potential to be a cost-effective tobacco-control tool.

One of the few evaluated campaigns outside of the United States is Australia's 1997 National Tobacco Campaign to promote smoking cessation among adults. The campaign ran for approximately a year with varying levels of intensity, and it utilized graphic images of the physical impact of smoking on the body. The theme, "Every Cigarette is Doing You Damage," aimed to provide smokers with a sense of immediacy about quitting smoking. The campaign also promoted a 24-hour Quitline to give advice and provide references to local resources.

The campaign was associated with increased motivation by smokers to quit and with a 6 percent decline in overall smoking prevalence following a period of little change in smoking prevalence. The lower prevalence was sustained throughout the evaluation period.

Although the campaign was targeted at adults, young teenagers responded more positively to the cessation campaign than to a separate campaign specifically targeted at youth. The campaign has been adapted for use in the United States, Canada, Cambodia, Singapore, Iceland, and Poland.

Tobacco Packages. Although "mass media" usually refers to billboards, magazines and newspapers, and broadcast media outlets, Canada requires that tobacco packages carry health messages that can fairly be described as mass media

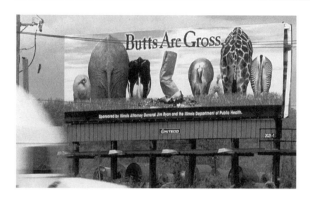

Humor is often used in anti-smoking campaigns targeted at young people. (AP/World Wide Photos)

messages. Beginning in December 2000, all tobacco packages sold in Canada must carry one of sixteen mandated health messages that cover half of the package. The messages draw upon many of the lessons of mass media campaigns, using color photos and graphic images to demonstrate the negative impacts of tobacco use.

Studies commissioned by the federal government to assess potential impact found that messages with pictures are sixty times more effective than text-only messages in encouraging people to stop, or not start, smoking. The messages were found to be 3.5 times more effective than Canada's previous messages, which convinced hundreds of thousands of smokers to try to quit. Further evaluation of the messages will provide insights into the potential of this innovative medium as an effective mass media tool for tobacco control.

STRATEGIES FOR EFFECTIVE MEDIA CAMPAIGNS

Researchers have attempted to identify the conditions under which media campaigns are most successful, including effective messages and themes. First, media campaigns alone are thought to have limited impact, though they can significantly strengthen the effectiveness of other tobacco-control programs such as school programs, community initiatives, and clean indoor-air campaigns. Second, media campaigns must be professionally developed, should rely on a variety of media (electronic, print, and outdoor), and should contain a mix of target audiences and messages.

There is no single magic bullet for effective messages. However, youth seem to respond well to real-life stories and images of the harmful effects of tobacco use, particularly if harm has affected a loved one, if the individual being profiled started smoking when he or she was young, or if the damage took place at a relatively young age. Messages targeted at adults should not contradict youth-targeted messages. Messages should portray nonsmokers as the majority, present realistic tobacco-free lifestyles, and encourage youth empowerment and control. Further research is needed to investigate whether these guidelines hold true in markets outside of North America and Australia, particularly in developing countries.

Substantial evidence exists to support the value of mass media in tobacco-control programs. Although most evidence comes from the United States, there is no evidence to suggest that these campaigns, given adequate funding, would be any less effective in other developed countries or in developing countries. In fact, mass media may have relatively greater impact in countries where the health effects of tobacco use are less well known. Evaluation of mass media campaigns in developing countries is needed to supplement the body of evidence from developed countries.

HEATHER SELIN

(SEE ALSO: *Mass Media; Media Advocacy; Smoking Behavior; Tobacco Control; Tobacco Control Advocacy and Policies–U.S.; Tobacco Sales to Youth, Regulation of*)

BIBLIOGRAPHY

Balbach, E., and Glantz, S. (1998). "Tobacco Control Advocates Must Demand High-Quality Media Campaigns: The California Experience." *Tobacco Control* 7:397–408.

Centers for Disease Control and Prevention (1998). *Best Practices for Comprehensive Tobacco Control Programs.* Atlanta, GA: CDC, National Center for Chronic Disease Prevention and Health Promotion, Office on Smoking and Health.

Commonwealth of Australia (1999). *Australia's National Tobacco Campaign. Evaluation Report,* Vol. 1. Canberra, Australia.

—— (2000). *Australia's National Tobacco Campaign. Evaluation Report,* Vol. 2. Canberra, Australia.

Teenage Research Unlimited (1999). *Counter-Tobacco Advertising Exploratory; Summary Report.* Northbrook, IL: Author.

U.S. Department of Health and Human Services (1989). *Reducing the Health Consequences of Smoking: 25 Years of Progress. A Report of the Surgeon General.* Atlanta, GA: USDHHS, Centers for Disease Control and Prevention, Center for Health Promotion and Education, Office on Smoking and Health.

—— (2000). *Reducing Tobacco Use. A Report of the Surgeon General.* Atlanta, GA: USDHHS, Centers for Disease Control and Prevention, National Center for Chronic Disease Prevention and Health Promotion, Office on Smoking and Health.

MASS MEDICATION

The term "mass medication" describes procedures used to deliver a preventive or therapeutic regimen to a population, rather than to individual members of that population. The implication is that the regimen is delivered unobtrusively. The members of the target population may not be aware that they are receiving the medication, and they have not given individual consent. Examples include the addition of vitamin and mineral supplements to infant formula, iodine to table salt, and fluoride to drinking water. When vitamin and mineral supplements are added to infant formula, the facts are provided on the label, although not everyone reads this; salt that has been enriched with iodine chloride is identified as "iodized salt"; and in most communities where sodium fluoride is added to reservoir water, information about this is kept in the public consciousness by antiflouridationists who make this a political issue. In theory, and usually in practice, individuals can exercise the option to avoid mass medication—they can use infant formula without vitamin and mineral supplements, table salt without added iodine, and drink unfluoridated water. The last of these may require some effort and expense for the individual, but it is feasible.

These situations differ from mass vaccination campaigns against a communicable disease, such as poliomyelitis, when the vaccine is offered to all members of a target population. The distinction is that members of the population usually volunteer to be vaccinated. Thus there are both ethical and political implications of mass medication. In a time when autonomy is the dominant political philosophy, the paternalist philosophy underlying mass medication is less acceptable than it was throughout the twentieth century. Public health authorities who seek to implement a mass medication program, therefore, are wise to do so only after adequate and careful consultation with representatives of the target population.

JOHN M. LAST

(SEE ALSO: *Community Water Fluoridation; Director of Health; Ethics of Public Health*)

MATCHING

Matching is a method used to ensure that two study groups are similar with regards to "nuisance" factors that might distort or confound a relationship that is being studied. Consider a study designed to explore the possible effect of asbestos exposure on the risk of lung cancer. It is known that smoking increases the risk of lung cancer and that asbestos workers are more likely to be smokers than the general public. Smoking, therefore, confuses or confounds the asbestos-lung cancer relationship. In order to eliminate the confounding effect of smoking in a case-control study, one could ensure that the diseased and control groups had equal proportions of smokers.

Matching can be implemented using two main approaches: pair (individual) matching and frequency matching. Pair matching links each member of the case group to a member of the control group with similar characteristics. This type of matching is most commonly seen in studies using twins or paired body parts (e.g., a study of ocular disease in diabetes). Analysis in pair matching often uses the McNemar chi-square method. Frequency matching is more commonly used. The control subjects are chosen to ensure that the frequency of the matching factors is the same as found in the case group. Frequency matching can be implemented in various ways, including category matching, caliper matching, stratified random sampling, or a variant of pair matching.

Matching is most commonly used in case-control studies, although some researchers also use it in cohort studies. Theoretical analysis has shown that matching in cohort studies completely controls for any potential confounding by the matching factors without requiring any special statistical methods. There can be a loss of statistical power, however. On the other hand, in case-control studies matching does not completely control for confounding, thus requiring the use of statistical methods such as the Mantel Hanzel approach, standardization, or logistic regression. There can be substantial loss of power if a case-control study matches on a factor which is not actually a confounder.

The role of matching in epidemiological research is controversial. Many epidemiologists routinely match on age and sex, even when they are not confounders. This practice is to be discouraged. Since a matched case-control study still requires a complex statistical analysis and might reduce statistical power, an argument can be made that matching in case-control studies is not desirable (unless the distribution of the matching factor in the case group is extreme).

As an example of matching, consider a case-control study of the role of dietary factors in the etiology of lung cancer. Given the strong effect of smoking on lung cancer risk, and the relationship of smoking with low intake of fruit and vegetables, one might design a case-control study that matched on smoking status. Each new case would be classified into a smoking category (e.g., never smoked, past smoker, mild, moderate, or heavy smoker). Then, a control subject would be recruited who had a similar smoking history. Although this method appears to be a form of pair matching, it would be analyzed as a frequency matched study.

GEORGE WELLS

(SEE ALSO: *Case-Control Study; Cohort Study; Epidemiology; Statistics for Public Health*)

BIBLIOGRAPHY

Kleinbaum, D. G.; Kupper, L. L.; and Morgenstern, H. (1982). *Epidemiological Research: Principles and Quantitative Methods*. Belmont, CA: Lifetime Learning Publications.

Rothman, K. J., and Greenland, S. (1998). *Modern Epidemiology*, 2nd edition. Philadelphia, PA: Lippincott-Raven.

MATERNAL AND CHILD HEALTH

Maternal and child health (MCH) refers to the health of mothers, infants, children, and adolescents. It also refers to a profession within public health committed to promoting the health status and future challenges of this vulnerable population.

HISTORICAL DEVELOPMENT

One of the greatest achievements of public health in the twentieth century in the United States was the dramatic improvement in the health of mothers and babies: during this period infant mortality declined by greater than 90 percent, and maternal mortality declined by 99 percent. While improvements in living standards, educational levels, and environmental conditions have contributed most to these improvements, public health MCH programs have also played a role.

The development of these MCH programs occurred in the unique political and social landscape of the United States, where a reliance on individualism has shaped the attitude that caring for children is the parents' responsibility, and that government should step in to help only when families and communities are not able to care for their own. The concept of federalism has also played a role in dividing responsibility between the federal government and state and local authorities. Further, the dominance of the biomedical model in the United States has directed most of the monies spent on MCH to the provision of direct clinical services. Some of the major historical developments in MCH are highlighted in Table 1.

Maternal Health. At the beginning of the twentieth century, for every one thousand live births, six to nine women died of pregnancy-related complications. Sepsis was the leading cause of maternal death, with half of the cases following delivery (often performed without following the principles of asepsis), and half associated with illegally induced abortion. Hemorrhage and pre-eclampsia (convulsions) were other leading causes of mortality. In response to the high maternal and infant mortality rates, and to women's suffrage, Congress passed the Maternity and Infancy Act

Table 1

A Chronology of Maternal and Child Health Services in the United States

1909	First White House Conference on Care of Dependent Children
1912	Children's Bureau created
1921	Maternity and Infancy Act (Sheppard-Towner Act) enacted
1929	Sheppard-Towner Act overturned
1930	American Academy of Pediatrics founded
1935	Title V legislation enacted as part of Social Security Act
1935	Crippled Children's Services (CCS) created
1943	Emergency Maternity and Infant Care enacted (P78-156)
1951	American College of Obstetricians and Gynecologists founded
1965	Medicaid (Title XIX) enacted
1965	Head Start Program started
1965	Community and Migrant Health Center Program created
1972	Special Supplemental Food Program for Women, Infants, & Children created
1973	*Roe v. Wade* legalizes abortion before fetal viability
1973	Early and Periodic Screening, Diagnosis and Treatment (EPSDT) created
1976	Supplemental Security Income Program for children with disabilities enacted
1979	Pregnancy-Related Mortality Surveillance System established
1981	Title V MCH Services Block Grant to states created
1984	Emergency Medical Services for Children enacted
1989	OBRA 89 expands coverage of prenatal care for low-income women
1991	Healthy Start Program started
1994	Early Head Start Program started
1996	Temporary Assistance for Needy Families (TANF) program created
1997	State Children's Health Insurance Program created

SOURCE: Courtesy of author.

(also known as the Sheppard-Towner Act) in 1921. The Fetal, Newborn, and Maternal Mortality and Morbidity Report of the 1933 White House Conference on Child Health Protection called attention to the link between poor aseptic practice, excessive and inappropriate obstetrical interventions (induction of labor, use of forceps, episiotomy, and cesarean deliveries), and high maternal mortality. During the 1930s and 1940s, hospital and state maternal mortality review committees were established. At the same time, a shift from home to hospital deliveries was occurring. The proportion of infants born in hospitals increased from 55 percent in 1938 to 90 percent in 1948, which was accompanied by a 71 percent decrease in maternal mortality. Medical advances (including the use of antibiotics, the use of oxytocin to induce labor, safe blood transfusions, and better management of hypertensive disorders) accelerated the declines in maternal mortality. Liberalization of state abortion laws, beginning in the 1960s, contributed to an 89 percent decline in deaths from septic illegal abortions between 1950 and 1973. In 1979, the Centers for Disease Control and Prevention partnered with the American College of Obstetricians and Gynecologists in developing the Pregnancy-Related Mortality Surveillance System, and implementing maternal mortality review boards across the country. At the end of the twentieth century, for every 100,000 live births, only seven to eight women died of pregnancy-related complications—a 99 percent reduction of the rate at the beginning of the century.

Infant Health. At the beginning of the twentieth century, for every one thousand live births, one hundred infants died before age one. Infant mortality began to decline in the early part of the twentieth century, following improvements in urban environments (e.g., sewage and refuse disposal and safe drinking water), milk pasteurization, rising standards of living, and declining fertility rates. The Children's Bureau formed in 1912 called for the establishment of the National Birth Registry in 1915. The Children's Bureau became the primary government agency to work toward improving maternal and infant health and welfare for the next thirty years. In 1935, Congress enacted Title V of the Social Security Act, which authorized and appropriated funds for maternal and child health-services programs. Between 1930 and 1949, infant mortality declined by 52 percent, largely due to antibiotics, development of fluid and electrolyte replacement therapy, and safe blood transfusions. It declined further following the implementation of Medicaid, Community Health Centers, and other federal programs in the 1960s. The Special Supplemental Food Program for Women, Infants, and Children (WIC) was created in 1972. Infant survival continued to improve in the 1970s because of technologic advances in neonatal medicine and the regionalization of perinatal services. Medicaid eligibility for pregnant women and infants was significantly expanded in the 1980s to enhance access to, and utilization of, prenatal care. The development of artificial pulmonary surfactant in the late 1980s and the use of antenatal corticosteroids in the 1990s to prevent and treat respiratory distress syndrome in premature infants also contributed to a decline in infant mortality. Other improvements in infant health in the 1990s include a 50 percent decline in the rates of sudden infant death syndrome, advances in prenatal diagnosis and surgical treatment of birth defects; and national efforts to encourage reproductive-aged women to consume folic acid to reduce the incidence of neural tube defects.

Child Health. Industrialization in the late nineteenth century forced many children into hazardous labor in mills, mines, and factories. In 1909, President Theodore Roosevelt convened the first White House Conference on Care of Dependent Children, which called attention to the unacceptably high rate of infant deaths and the detrimental effects of child labor. This led to the creation of the Children's Bureau in 1912 to "serve all children, to try to work out standards of care and protection which shall give to every child his fair chance in the world." Both the establishment of the Children's Bureau and the passage of the Sheppard-Towner Act met with formidable resistance. They were seen by many as governmental intrusion into the relationship between children and their parents, and they were opposed by the American Medical Association (AMA) because of their potential for governmental interference or control over the practice of medicine—despite an endorsement from the Pediatric Section, which split off from the AMA in 1930 to form the American Academy of Pediatrics. The Sheppard-Towner Act was overturned in 1929. The enactment of Title V in 1935, however, expanded health and social services to mothers and children.

Medicaid was enacted in 1965 as a federal-state partnership to fund health services for low-income families with children. The Head Start program, launched in 1965, provided an intellectually stimulating and healthful environment for preschool children. The Early and Periodic Screening, Diagnosis, and Treatment (EPSDT) program was created in 1967 to fund preventive health services for Medicaid-eligible children, including physical and developmental exams, vision and hearing screening, dental referrals, and immunizations. These advances were followed, however, by a downsizing of federal involvement and the return of power and responsibility for MCH policies to the states in the 1980s. The most significant change was the consolidation of seven categorical MCH programs into the MCH Services Block Grant. Health care coverage for children was re-expanded in 1997 with the creation of the State Children's Health Insurance Program.

Children with Special Health Care Needs. Title V of the 1935 Social Security Act created Crippled Children's Services (CCS), which became the only source of federal funding for the next thirty years for children with special health care needs. Enactment of Medicaid (Title XIX) in 1965 relieved CCS of many of its reimbursement and direct service provision responsibilities. In 1974, the Supplemental Security Income (SSI) Childhood Disability Program began to provide monthly cash payments to low-income children with disabilities and special health care needs. The Omnibus Budget Reconciliation Act of 1989 (OBRA89) directed state Children with Special Health Care Needs programs (CSHCN, formerly CCS) to develop community-based systems of services and to promote and provide family-centered, community-based, comprehensive, and culturally competent services for children with special health care needs. Thirty percent of the MCH Services Block Grant was to be directed toward this use. Alarmed by the rapidly increasing SSI enrollment, Congress redefined disability, restricted eligibility, and reduced cash assistance to children with disabilities in 1996.

CURRENT STATUS

Despite significant improvements in the health of mothers, infants, and children during the twentieth century, the United States compares poorly with other developed nations on most indicators of MCH. In 1997, the United States ranked twenty-fifth in infant mortality and twenty-first in maternal mortality among developed nations. Table 2 presents a report card of selected indicators of MCH in the United States, along with national goals set for the year 2010.

There are also significant disparities in MCH among racial, ethnic, and other sociodemographic categories. For example, African-American infants have twice the chance of dying, of low birth weight, and of being premature, as compared to white infants. Maternal mortality is five times higher among pregnant African–American women than among pregnant white women. The teen pregnancy rate is twice as high among Hispanic women, and three times as high among African-American women, than it is among white women aged fifteen

Table 2

MCH Report Card, United States

Indicator	Current	Goal
Maternal mortality ratio (maternal deaths per 100,000 live births)	7.1	3.3
Percentage of women with adequate prenatal care	73	90
Percentage of women with maternal complications	25.6	20
Percentage of women who smoke cigarettes during pregnancy	13.9	2
Percentage of low-income women with anemia in third trimester	29	23
Percentage of deliveries by cesarean	20.8	15
Infant mortality rate (infant deaths per 1,000 live births)	7.6	5.0
Percentage of low birthweight births (less than 2,500 grams)	7.3	5.0
Percentage of very low birthweight births (less than 1,500 grams)	1.4	1.0
Percentage of premature births (less than 37 weeks)	11.0	7.6
Percentage of women who breast-feed their babies early postpartum	60	75
Percentage of women who breast-feed their babies until 1 year old	8.6	25
Child death rate (deaths per 100,000 children aged 1-14)	35.8	33.7
Percentage of children 19 to 35 months old fully immunized	78	90
Percentage of children under 18 without health care coverage	15.4	0
Percentage of children under 18 who have regular source of care	91	95
Percentage of pregnancies that are planned	49	70
Number of pregnancies per 1,000 females aged 15 to 17	47.6	45
Number of women with fertility problems who had sexually transmitted diseases or pelvic inflammatory disease	800,000	500,000
Percentage of women with *Chlamydia trachomatis* infection	12.3	3.0

SOURCE: U.S. Department of Health and Human Services. *Healthy People 2010.*

to seventeen. Causes of these disparities have not been determined, but they have been attributed to differences in genetics, behavior, culture, socioeconomic class, and access to health care. Recent research on neighborhood and community factors, as well as cumulative life experiences and exposures, may shed light on the persisting disparities in MCH outcomes.

MCH PROGRAMS

A myriad of public health programs have been created over the years to improve the health of disadvantaged mothers, infants, and children, and to reduce disparities in health status and health care access. A few of the major programs are listed below.

MCH Block Grant Program. Title V of the Social Security Act (1935) authorized the use of federal monies for MCH programs. The biggest change to the Title V program came in 1981, when seven MCH programs were consolidated into the MCH block grant. Administration of MCH programs, which support direct delivery of MCH services in the public health setting, devolved to the state level, while state and federal governments share the costs.

Medicaid. Created by Title XIX of Social Security Act in 1965, the objective of Medicaid is to support the provision of health services to low-income Americans. The federal and state governments jointly administer the program and share its costs. Medicaid is really a financing program rather than a service delivery program. States are mandated to cover pregnant women and children six years of age and younger living at up to 133 percent of the federal poverty level, as well as all children up to age nineteen in families with incomes below the poverty level. Medicaid is by far the largest MCH program, funding prenatal and obstetrical care, the EPSDT program, and health services for children with special health care needs. Three out of four Medicaid recipients are women and children, though they consume only one-fourth of total Medicaid expenditures.

Community and Migrant Health Center Program. Created in 1965, the Community and Migrant Health Center Program provides basic primary care to medically underserved (largely rural) areas. It is funded by the federal government and administered at the community level. These centers place a high priority on reducing infant mortality and improving the health of mothers and children. One-third of individuals served by the program are children under age fifteen, and one in four are women of childbearing age.

The Special Supplemental Food Program for Women, Infants, and Children (WIC). Created in 1972, WIC provides supplemental food and nutritional education to low-income pregnant women, nursing mothers, and children diagnosed as being at nutritional risk. It is funded by the federal government and administered by the U.S. Department of Agriculture. Technically speaking, WIC is not a health care program, but evaluations have found WIC to be effective in reducing infant mortality, low birth weight, anemia, and other problems.

Head Start, Early Head Start, and Healthy Start. Project Head Start was created in 1965 to promote social and behavioral competence among preschool children from low-income families and to ensure that the children enter school with a similar foundation as their more economically advantaged peers. The program includes comprehensive health services, including preventive health services. Ten percent of Head Start enrollment is reserved for children with disabilities. Evaluations have shown reduced juvenile delinquency and increased school completion rates among children enrolled in the Head Start program. In 1994, Congress established the Early Head Start program for low-income families with infants and toddlers. Both programs are administered by the Head Start Bureau of the Department of Health and Human Services. The Healthy Start Initiative was created in 1991 to attack the causes of infant mortality and low birthweight using a broad range of community-based interventions in nearly one hundred communities across the United States. The Healthy Start Initiative is administered by the Maternal and Child Health Bureau.

Temporary Assistance for Needy Families (TANF) Program. In 1996, the U.S. Congress passed landmark welfare reform legislation (the Personal Responsibility and Work Opportunity Reconciliation Act) that replaced the Aid to Families with Dependent Children (AFDC) Program with the TANF Program. TANF was intended to give states new opportunities to develop and implement creative and innovative strategies and approaches to removing families from a cycle of dependency on public assistance and creating employment opportunities for them. While reviews of the impact of TANF on the health of women and children have been mixed, TANF has generated additional monies for MCH programs. For example, Los Angeles County created the Long-Term Family Self Sufficiency Plan with its TANF monies. The plan includes programs to help pregnant women gain access prenatal care, and to provide additional support services, such as parenting skills training.

State Children's Health Insurance Program (SCHIP). SCHIP was established in 1997 to provide insurance for children from families with incomes too high to qualify for Medicaid, but too low to afford private health insurance. Of the over 10 million children in the United States who were uninsured in 1997, only 3 million were eligible for Medicaid prior to SCHIP. In its first three years, SCHIP has enrolled over 3 million children. Although enrollment was slow initially, states have responded with innovative strategies to reach out to uninsured children and families to increase enrollment. SCHIP is administered through the Health Care Financing Administration (HCFA).

State Programs. In addition to the programs described above, many state and local governments have developed additional MCH programs of their own. A notable example is the California Children and Families First Initiative, or Proposition 10. Passed in 1998, the initiative has raised approximately $700 million annually from a tobacco surtax to be used to improve early child development for children up to age five. The money will be used to support health care services for children and families, parental education and support services, and child-care programs. Because of the autonomy of its governance structure and its broadly defined goals, it is flexible enough to allow for different approaches that cross the traditional boundaries of MCH, a flexibility that is often not permitted under categorical funding and grant making. Proposition 10 has the potential for providing a model for the rest of the nation.

FUTURE CHALLENGES

At the beginning of the twenty-first century, many challenges in MCH remain. Some of the most important areas of concern are described below.

Maternal Mortality and Morbidity. The decline in maternal mortality in the United States has leveled off since 1982. This does not mean that it has reached an irreducible minimum, as one-third to one-half of the deaths that still occur are probably preventable. Maternal deaths are only the tip of the iceberg, however, as one in four women experience complications during pregnancy, many of which are preventable. An increased effort to assess and assure the quality of health care for pregnant women is needed. Likewise, the connection between maternal health and women's health needs to be better understood. Improving women's health over the life course, and not only during pregnancy, is likely to have the greatest impact on improving maternal and child health.

Infant Mortality and Morbidity. Birth defects are the leading cause of infant death, affecting approximately 3 percent of all live births. Because many birth defects occur in the first three months of pregnancy, they are best prevented by preconceptional and early prenatal care. The causes of most birth defects are still unknown and require further research. Low birthweight and prematurity contribute to most of the infant deaths and congenital neurological disabilities not related to birth defects. They are also the leading cause of infant deaths among African Americans. To date, most interventions during pregnancy designed to prevent low birthweight and prematurity have not been effective.

Prenatal and Preconceptional Care. Although widely accepted, the effectiveness of prenatal care in improving pregnancy outcomes, particularly in preventing low birthweight and prematurity, has not been conclusively demonstrated. While this may reflect methodological flaws in research on prenatal care, it could also suggest that prenatal care is not provided in the proper manner, and some researchers have begun to question the appropriateness of the content of prenatal care. Still others have argued that less than nine months of prenatal care is not enough to reverse the cumulative impact of lifelong habits and exposures on pregnancy outcomes. Most women do not obtain preconceptional care before getting pregnant, and many health care providers do not know how to provide preconceptional care, or they provide it only to women who are actively trying to get pregnant, thereby missing opportunities to improve the outcomes of pregnancies that are unintended.

Breast-Feeding. The benefits of breast-feeding to the health of mothers and infants have been well documented, including enhanced immunity against infections, improved cognitive development, and stronger maternal-infant bonding. Despite these benefits, the initiation and duration of breast-feeding in the United States remains low, particularly among disadvantaged women. Efforts to promote the WHO/UNICEF "Ten Steps to Successful Breast-feeding" in hospitals have met with little success. Changes in cultural norms, workplace practices, and social policy are also needed to encourage breast-feeding among American women.

Immunization. Although the up-to-date immunization rate of children in the United States has been steadily improving, it still falls short of the national goal of 90 percent by age two, particularly for poor children. There is no agreement among public health experts on a strategy to bring this up to the level at which "herd immunity" would protect those children who remain without immunization.

Child Care. Over half of U.S. mothers with children under six work outside the home, and 60 percent of these children receive care outside their homes. In addition to increased risk for infections and injuries, children cared for in day-care centers may receive less support for cognitive and social development than children cared for at home. Support for parents with child-care needs is low, particularly for low-income families.

Family Violence. A U.S. woman has a one-in-five chance of being physically abused at some point in her lifetime. Estimates of the prevalence of physical abuse by an intimate partner during pregnancy range from 4 to 8 percent, but it may be as high as 20 percent. Most communities have inadequate resources to help battered women. Many health care providers do not screen for, or cannot identify, domestic violence. Within communities, a shortage of shelter beds, social workers, and other basic services frequently exists, together with a lack of coordination among health care, social-service, and judicial systems. Children are abused in half of the families where women are abused. While little is known or done about primary prevention of family violence, what is clear is that family violence cannot be overcome without attention to the social and economic conditions that put children and families at risk.

Unintentional and Intentional Injury. Injury is the leading cause of death among children and adolescents, with motor-vehicle injury being the single leading cause. Other causes include fires/burns and drowning. Homicides and suicides account for one-fourth of injury-related deaths among adolescents. While progress has been made in preventing deaths related to motor-vehicle injury, largely attributable to a reduction in alcohol-related fatalities, little progress has been made in preventing deaths related to homicides and suicides.

Tobacco, Alcohol, and Other Drugs. Nearly one-third of teens are current smokers, and half have drunk alcohol within the last month. Nearly one-third have used marijuana, and 5 percent have used cocaine. Alcohol and other drugs contribute significantly to unintentional and intentional injuries among adolescents, including motor-vehicle accidents, homicide, suicide, as well as unintended pregnancies, sexually transmitted infections, and a host of other medical and social problems. Success of clinical interventions at the individual level is modest; and the effectiveness of neighborhood- and community-level interventions remains to be demonstrated.

Sexual Behavior and Unintended Pregnancy. One-third of girls and nearly one-half of boys in the United States have had sexual intercourse by the ninth grade, and 20 percent of all youth in grades nine through twelve have had four or more sexual partners. While these rates are similar to European rates, the rates of sexually transmitted infections and unintended pregnancies are much higher among U.S. teens. One in four sexually active adolescents will get a sexually transmitted infection by age twenty. Nearly one million adolescent women become pregnant each year in the United States, with half of these pregnancies resulting in live births. Teen mothers have lower educational attainment, lower future earnings, and higher welfare dependency. Two-thirds of these teen births occur outside of marriage.

CONCLUSION

Much of the advancement in maternal and child health has been made outside of public health. Progress in medicine, education, environment (both physical and social), gender and race relations, public policy, and many social areas have made, and will continue to make, important contributions to MCH. An important challenge for MCH as a profession is to promote change outside the traditional boundaries of MCH in order to improve the health of mothers, infants, children, and adolescents.

MICHAEL C. LU

J. ROBERT BRAGONIER

(SEE ALSO: *Alcohol Use and Abuse; Child Care, Daycare; Child Health Services; Domestic Violence; Head Start Program; Immunizations; Infant Mortality Rate; Perinatology; Pregnancy; Prenatal Care; Reproduction; Sexually Transmitted Diseases; Teenage Pregnancy; Title V; Tobacco Control; Women, Infants, and Children Program [WIC]; Women's Health*)

BIBLIOGRAPHY

Binkin, N. J.; Williams, R. L.; Hogue, C. J. R.; and Chen, P. M. (1985). "Reducing Black Neonatal Mortality: Will Improvement in Birth Weight Be Enough?" *Journal of the American Medical Association* 253:372–375.

Centers for Disease Control and Prevention (1999). "Achievements in Public Health, 1900–1999: Healthier Mothers and Babies." *Morbidity and Mortality Weekly Report* 48:849–858.

Hoffman, J. D., and Ward, K. (1999). "Genetic Factors in Preterm Delivery." *Obstetrics and Gynecological Survey* 54:203.

Hutchins, V. L. (1997). "Maternal and Child Health Bureau: Roots." *Pediatrics* 94:695–699.

Kotch, J. B.; Blakely, C. H.; Brown, S. S.; and Wong, F. Y., eds. (1992). *A Pound of Prevention: The Case for Universal Maternity Care in the U.S.* Washington, DC: American Public Health Association.

Kotch, J. B., ed. (1997). *Maternal and Child Health: Programs, Problems and Policy in Public Health.* Gaithersburg, MD: Aspen Publishers.

Naylor, A. F., and Myrianthopoulos, N. C. (1967). "The Relation of Ethnic and Selected Socio-Economic Factors to Human Birth-Weight." *Annual of Human Genetics* 37:71–83.

U.S. Department of Health and Human Services, Maternal and Child Health Bureau (1999). *Title V: A Snapshot of Maternal and Child Health 1997.* Rockville, MD: Health Resources and Services Administration.

U.S. Department of Health and Human Services, Office of Disease Prevention and Health Promotion (2000). *Healthy People 2010,* 2nd edition. Washington, DC: US Government Printing Office.

MATERNAL AND CHILD HEALTH BLOCK GRANT

The Maternal and Child Health Block Grant (MCHBG) is a U.S. federal program designed to improve the health of mothers and children. It was created under the Omnibus Budget Reconciliation Act of 1981. In federal fiscal year 2000, the MCHBG amounted to $709 million. Each state's share is calculated on a formula based on the state's share of the seven programs that Congress consolidated under Title V of the Social Security Act. These programs dealt with specific conditions such as adolescent pregnancy, lead poisoning, sudden infant death, and hemophilia and other genetic conditions. States must provide three dollars to match every four dollars in federal MCHBG funds they receive.

The MCHBG enables the federal and state governments to address issues like infant mortality, access to health care for mothers and children, rehabilitation services for blind and disabled children, and coordinated care for children with special health care needs (e.g., children with disabilities). States must spend at least 30 percent of their MCHBG funds for prevention and primary-care services for children, and at least 30 percent for children with special health care needs.

A portion of the MCHBG is set aside at the federal level for Special Projects of Regional and National Significance (SPRANS) grants, the Traumatic Brain Injury Demonstration Grant Program, and other specialized purposes. The program is administered by the Maternal and Child Health Bureau of the Health Resources and Services Administration. About 17 million women and children receive services funded, at least in part, by the MCHBG.

RICK DAVIS

(SEE ALSO: *Child Health Services; Health Resources and Services Administration; Maternal and Child Health*)

MATHEMATICAL MODEL

See Probability Model

MAXIMUM TOLERATED DOSE

The maximum tolerated dose (MTD) is operationally defined in toxicology as the highest daily dose of a chemical that does not cause overt toxicity in a ninety-day study in laboratory mice or rats. This dose is then used for longer-term safety assessment in the same species, usually lasting two years or a lifetime. The rationale for using the MTD is to maximize the likelihood of detecting any chronic disease effects of a chemical, including cancer. Using higher doses also increases the statistical likelihood of detecting the intrinsic hazards of chemicals.

The MTD is controversial, however, in part because of difficulties in extrapolating findings to more realistic doses, and in extrapolating from animals to humans. Its detractors also point out that subtle physiological changes occur at higher doses that can alter the metabolism and disposition of chemicals in ways that make the findings irrelevant to more realistic dose levels. The MTD has been retained, in part, because its long-term use provides a comparative benchmark for the study of additional chemicals. It is supplemented, however, by parallel studies of lower doses, and by a greater emphasis on predictive approaches dependent upon understanding the underlying mechanisms of chemical toxicity.

BERNARD D. GOLDSTEIN

(SEE ALSO: *Risk Assessment, Risk Management; Safety Assessment; Toxicology*)

BIBLIOGRAPHY

National Research Council Committee on Risk Assessment Methodology (1993). *Issues in Risk Assessment.* Washington, DC: National Academy of Sciences.

Rodricks, J. V.; Starr, T. B.; and Taylor, M. R. (1991). "Evaluating the Safety of Carcinogens in Food—Current Practices and Emerging Developments." *Food Drug Cosmetic Law Journal* 46(5):513–552.

MEASLES

Measles is a viral respiratory illness characterized by high fever and generalized rash. Symptoms start ten to twelve days after airborne exposure and include fever, malaise, conjunctivitis, runny nose, and cough. About fourteen days after exposure, a maculopapular rash appears at the hairline, extends to the face and upper neck, and, over the next three days, spreads down the body to the hands and feet. Although measles is usually not severe in developed countries, it can lead to serious complications including diarrhea (8% of cases), ear infections (7%), pneumonia (6%), encephalitis (0.1%), subacute sclerosing panencephalitis (SSPE) (0.001%), and death (0.2%). Measles is much more serious in developing countries, causing about one million deaths annually during the 1990s. The case fatality rate can be as high as 25 percent, with deaths often caused by secondary infections such as diarrhea or pneumonia. Measles is also a common cause of blindness in the developing world.

Measles is one of the most contagious diseases in the world. The virus, a paramyxovirus containing a single strand of RNA, is normally spread through respiratory droplets and can be transmitted from four days before to four days after rash onset. Before vaccines were introduced, nearly everyone was infected by age ten to twelve years. Immunity is lifelong following infection.

A live attenuated vaccine was licensed in 1963, and further attenuated vaccines are now used around the world. The vaccine is about 95 percent effective in the United States when administered at the recommended age of twelve to fifteen months, and immunity is considered lifelong. It is usually given in conjunction with the mumps and rubella vaccines. Children in developing countries are vaccinated at nine months of age because of the higher risk of infection in infancy.

Routine treatment of measles includes supportive care such as oral rehydration therapy for diarrhea and respiratory care for patients with pneumonia. Antibiotics are used to treat secondary bacterial infections. Although antiviral medications have been used to treat complex measles infections, there are few studies to confirm their effectiveness. High-dose vitamin A therapy reduces mortality and prevents blindness and is recommended by the World Health Organization for children in developing countries.

Global measles eradication has been a goal since the development of an effective vaccine.

Humans are the only reservoir for the measles virus, which can survive only hours in the environment. Endemic measles can be eliminated from large geographic areas using intensive vaccination programs, as seen in the United States in the late 1990s. However, measles is so infectious that immunization rates of at least 90 to 95 percent must be attained to interrupt transmission. In addition, the billions of doses required to achieve eradication highlight the need for injection safety and the potential development of needle-free vaccination methods. Finally, the HIV (human immunodeficiency virus) epidemic presents several barriers to measles eradication. HIV-infected persons have a lower response to measles vaccination, develop more severe cases of the disease, and, theoretically, may be infectious for longer periods of time. There is hope that these challenges will be surmounted and measles will be eradicated, following smallpox into the history books.

SONIA KLEMPERER-JOHNSON
MARK PAPANIA

(SEE ALSO: *Communicable Disease Control; Disease Prevention; Eradication of Disease; Immunizations*)

BIBLIOGRAPHY

Atkinson, W.; Wolfe, C.; Humizter, S.; and Nelson, R., eds. (2000). "Measles." In *Epidemiology and Prevention of Vaccine-Preventable Diseases: The Pink Book*. Atlanta, GA.: U.S. Department of Health and Human Services.

Redd, S. C.; Markowitz, L. E.; and Katz, S. L. (1999). "Measles Vaccine." In *Vaccines*, eds. S. A. Plotkin and W. A. Orenstein. Philadelphia, PA: W. B. Sanders.

MÉDICINS SANS FRONTIÈRES

See International Nongovernmental Organizations

MEDIA ADVOCACY

Media advocacy is the process of disseminating policy-related information through the communications media, especially where the aim is to effect action, a change of policy, or to alter the public's view of an issues. While a strict definition of "media" advocacy is limited to the strategic use of mass media in regard to a policy initiative, public health views the term more broadly. Almost identical techniques are often used to encourage people to change health behaviors as those directed towards changing policy; and media advocacy may be a single element of a specific campaign as well as an ongoing process. Media advocacy is practiced at all levels, from national to community-based campaigns. The ultimate targets of most media advocacy are politicians and other decision makers.

Media advocacy activities may be proactive and initiated by public health workers, or they may be reactive. Reactive media advocacy involves taking action when required, especially when opponents of health policy actively seek to mislead, change the agenda, or divert attention to other issues.

Media advocacy may be used for an ongoing campaign, perhaps to ensure that the need for a new health screening service is kept on the political agenda. Similarly, a health organization may use media advocacy over a short period—to launch a campaign to increase the uptake of a new screening service, for example, or to publicize a new report on health inequalities.

An example of media advocacy with several different interim goals is an ongoing campaign against tobacco. Certain information is directed towards politicians and other opinion leaders whose support is needed for antitobacco measures, while different but related information is aimed at current or potential smokers. While the first is aimed at changing policy, the second seeks a behavior change. Both, however, share the overall goal of reducing tobacco-induced disease. In addition, an ongoing media advocacy program on tobacco will also involve monitoring the media for misleading information put out by those with vested interests in selling tobacco, and offering a prompt rebuttal.

Media advocacy is opportunistic. It exploits opportunities to use the media to convey information to large numbers of people, including special target groups. Those who work in media advocacy have a good understanding of the way the press and broadcasting organizations work; and they maintain good relationships with journalists, so as to be readily accessible to supply information and comment, and work with suitable experts who can give interviews and assist jounalists whenever necessary.

It is important to differentiate between media advocacy, an essential part of what is often termed "public information" work, and paid media campaigns, such as television spots or informational advertisements in newspapers, which are a common feature of "public education" programs. In contrast to the opportunistic and ongoing nature of media advocacy, paid media campaigns involve a more programmed delivery of education-oriented information, based on prior research, to specific target audiences. A public-education program may sometimes be supported by media advocacy, and vice-versa, but more often media advocacy is practiced on its own.

HOW MEDIA ADVOCACY WORKS

Media advocacy for public health assumes that public health advocates and journalists have something to offer each other, that there is a convenient symbiosis between their professions. Those on the health side have potential stories, and they want to get coverage for them as part of a campaign to bring about change, and journalists want new stories to fill time or editorial (i.e., nonadvertising) space in their media. Journalists often rely on specialists to help them gather, analyze, and comment on the material they use, and sometimes to suggest stories in the first place. Public health advocates either are such specialists, or they can provide access to them. They also provide ideas for new stories, new angles on old topics, and substantive information to help the journalist to produce an article or story.

Furthermore, health is a popular topic. Most people have a personal interest in anything affecting what is, as many see it, their most cherished gift—their health. Public health leaders, therefore, by the very nature of their subject, have a head start when competing for the attention of journalists and for space in their media.

Anyone can do media advocacy—from an individual or members of a small, community-based health organization to the largest state or federal government health agency. Few tools are needed other than a telephone and, preferably, personal computing equipment. In larger organizations, a press and public affairs department will usually carry out much of the work, involving others as required. In a smaller organization the functions may be part of an information officer's duties, or, in a very small unit, they may be performed by one person, perhaps the chief executive.

Among the most common activities of media advocacy are the following:

- Monitoring media for coverage of relevant topics; this service is often contracted to specialist agencies, or may be achieved via Internet-based services.

- Identifying and disseminating interesting news stories that support public health policies.

- Responding to journalists' inquiries and information requests.

- Supplying access to experts who can assist journalists.

- Preparing press releases and background papers.

- Arranging press conferences.

- Planning a media diary, including identification of special dates and opportunities.

- Responding to misleading or erroneous items in the media.

- Listing and training individuals to act as experts and spokespersons on particular health issues.

- Searching for new angles on existing stories, and new spokespersons and organizations to back and to speak publicly for the policy—a wide variety of professionals and organizations may be recruited to support public health policy.

To maximize the effectiveness of media advocacy, journalists should be treated with a certain priority; and everyone who can help with a story, such as the chief executive, key experts, and other contacts should observe this policy. It is easier to contact journalists than many other professionals—most are dependent on keeping in touch with their sources and other key contacts, so they tend to be readily accessible.

Where a coalition of health agencies and individuals is working in pursuit of the same goal, it is essential to coordinate activities and information. Disparities in facts and figures provided by different coalition partners may be seized upon by opponents of the policy being proposed, not only damaging the public credibility of those supporting the policy, but discouraging journalists from trusting, or even approaching them again in the future.

For most public health topics, special opportunities will arise for attracting the attention of journalists, and thus getting coverage. In particular, special occasions such as key meetings, publication dates of new statistics or reports, and other important dates (such as anniversaries) should be examined in advance to see whether they can serve as pegs on which news stories can be hung.

Among the pegs and material that can attract media coverage are:

- Publication of a new government policy affecting a health issue.

- New research, such as a study of a disease or of a health care procedure.

- Changes in trends of a disease, or of a factor causing ill health.

- Official action on a health issue.

- Special considerations of women, children, and ethnic groups with regards to a health issue.

- Latest trends in health status or health behaviors among exemplar groups, such as doctors, teachers, or athletes.

- Schools activities about certain health problems.

- Civil-rights issues associated with health.

- Special days or weeks designated as a focus for health issues.

Public health advocates can also make good use of physicians and other health professionals as experts to provide journalists with comments, information, and analysis. In the age of mass communications, with opinions constantly being heard from people described as "experts" on many topical issues, public cynicism may devalue what experts say, as few may be perceived as neutral. However, physicians and other health professionals tend to be perceived as primarily interested in people's health, especially when opposing those with obvious vested interests.

Medical and health publications offer special opportunities for coverage of public health stories. Apart from their potential subject interest, journalists on health publications will tend to have more relevant background knowledge and contacts than those in other media. In addition, some of these journals, especially the leading medical scientific publications, are themselves highly influential with the general media. Most health correspondents on newspapers and in broadcast media scan the leading medical journals, which often serve as the source or inspiration for their own stories.

BENEFITS OF MEDIA ADVOCACY IN PUBLIC HEALTH

There are many benefits of the creative and energetic use of media advocacy in public health. Many public health issues are closely integrated with other aspects of public policy, and therefore part of public debate. It is thus appropriate for public health leaders to inform the debate and ensure that appropriate issues are raised and that accurate information is published.

Among the advantages of media advocacy is that it can reach a wide audience, including key decision makers, and that issues and information presented within news items in the media tend to carry more credibility than those presented in paid media advertisements or in public relations material. It is also inexpensive: apart from the participants' time, there are relatively few costs. In addition, media advocacy on one issue can develop a closer rapport with journalists, which in turn may later benefit coverage of a separate, unrelated health issue. Similarly, it can build the capacity of public health agencies to treat strategic media initiatives as an integral component of health campaigns.

Media advocacy on any area of policy, including public health, can face certain problems, some being a function of success. For example, journalists may feel that coverage of a particular issue has reached saturation. Among other common problems are individual events (and people) are often more attractive as elements in a story than the policy issues underlying the story; health may be seen as a personal responsibility, with public health policy viewed as irrelevant, superfluous, unwanted, or costly to the taxpayer; in libertarian terms, public health policy involving the regulation of certain commercial activities may be seen as politically undesirable; and mass media can trivialize serious issues. As with all aspects of media advocacy, creative thinking and constant reevaluation of strategy are likely to offer the best solutions to these problems.

DAVID SIMPSON

(SEE ALSO: *Health Promotion and Education; Mass Media; Mass Media and Tobacco Control*)

MEDICAID

Enacted in 1965, Medicaid is the major public financing program for providing health and long-term care coverage to the low-income population of the United States. It was originally enacted as a means of providing funds to help states provide health care for welfare recipients and has evolved into a program that finances care for more than one in seven Americans. Medicaid enables millions of Americans to gain access to needed health services, helping to close the gaps in care between the poor and nonpoor, ease the financial burdens of health care, and provide a health care safety net for the nation.

Authorized under Title XIX of the Social Security Act, Medicaid is a means-tested entitlement program financed by the states and the federal government and administered by the states. Federal financial assistance is provided to states for coverage of specific groups of people, and benefits are paid for by the states and through federal matching payments based on each state's per capita income. The federal share ranges from 50 to 80 percent of Medicaid expenditures and averaged 56.5 percent in 1998. State participation in the Medicaid program is voluntary, but all states have chosen to participate.

MEDICAID COVERAGE

Although Medicaid was created to assist low-income Americans, coverage is dependent upon several other criteria in addition to income. Eligibility is primarily for those persons falling into particular categories, such as low-income children, pregnant women, elderly people, people with disabilities, and parents not exceeding specific income thresholds. Single adults are generally ineligible, no matter how poor, unless they are disabled. Within federal guidelines, states set their own income and asset eligibility criteria for Medicaid, resulting in large variations in coverage among states.

In 1998, 40.4 million people were enrolled in Medicaid. This included 20.7 million low-income children and 8.6 million low-income adults in families with children. The vast majority of adults were women. Historically, most women and children have been eligible for Medicaid because they received cash assistance through Aid to Families with Dependent Children (AFDC). Over time, eligibility was expanded to women and children not receiving welfare. The Temporary Assistance to Needy Families (TANF) welfare reforms implemented in 1996 officially severed the automatic link between Medicaid coverage and cash assistance for families.

There were 4.1 million elderly persons covered by Medicaid in 1998. Some elderly persons are eligible because they receive cash assistance through Supplemental Security Income (SSI), and others have incomes too high to qualify for cash assistance but spend-down to Medicaid by incurring high health care expenses. Many elderly Medicaid beneficiaries are "dual eligibles," or people who receive both Medicare and Medicaid. These people rely on Medicaid for assistance with Medicare's cost-sharing requirements and premiums, and sometimes for coverage of services not included in the Medicare benefits package (i.e., long-term care or prescription drugs).

Medicaid also covered 7.0 million blind and disabled persons in 1998. Most disabled persons

Figure 1

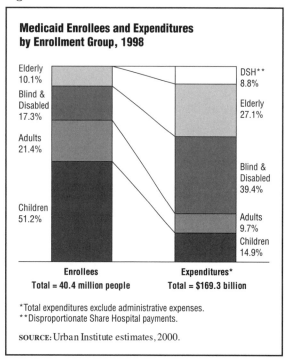

Medicaid Enrollees and Expenditures by Enrollment Group, 1998

Enrollees
Total = 40.4 million people

Elderly 10.1%
Blind & Disabled 17.3%
Adults 21.4%
Children 51.2%

Expenditures*
Total = $169.3 billion

DSH** 8.8%
Elderly 27.1%
Blind & Disabled 39.4%
Adults 9.7%
Children 14.9%

*Total expenditures exclude administrative expenses.
**Disproportionate Share Hospital payments.

SOURCE: Urban Institute estimates, 2000.

are eligible for Medicaid because they receive SSI cash assistance, though some spend-down to eligibility. Some disabled Medicaid beneficiaries are also dual eligibles.

From the perspective of whom is served, Medicaid is predominantly a program assisting low-income families, but from the perspective of how Medicaid dollars are spent, Medicaid funds primarily serve the low-income aged and low-income disabled populations. Adults and children in low-income families make up nearly three quarters (73%) of enrollees, but account for only 25 percent of spending (see Figure 1). In contrast, the elderly and disabled account for 27 percent of enrollees and the majority (67%) of spending, largely due to their intensive use of acute care services and the costliness of long-term care in institutional settings. In 1998, the average per capita cost for a child on Medicaid was $1,225, almost all of which went to basic acute care, while the corresponding figures for the disabled and elderly were $9,558 and $11,235, respectively, a significant portion of which went to long-term care services.

Although Medicaid is a key source of coverage for the low-income population, in 1998 it covered

Figure 2

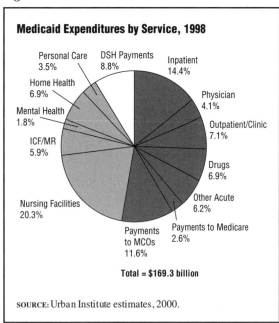

Medicaid Expenditures by Service, 1998

Personal Care 3.5%
DSH Payments 8.8%
Inpatient 14.4%
Home Health 6.9%
Physician 4.1%
Mental Health 1.8%
Outpatient/Clinic 7.1%
ICF/MR 5.9%
Drugs 6.9%
Nursing Facilities 20.3%
Other Acute 6.2%
Payments to MCOs 11.6%
Payments to Medicare 2.6%

Total = $169.3 billion

SOURCE: Urban Institute estimates, 2000.

Figure 3

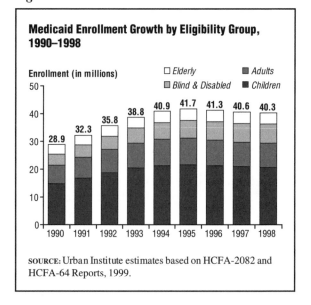

Medicaid Enrollment Growth by Eligibility Group, 1990–1998

Enrollment (in millions)
☐ Elderly   ■ Adults
▨ Blind & Disabled   ■ Children

28.9 32.3 35.8 38.8 40.9 41.7 41.3 40.6 40.3
1990 1991 1992 1993 1994 1995 1996 1997 1998

SOURCE: Urban Institute estimates based on HCFA-2082 and HCFA-64 Reports, 1999.

only about a quarter of nonelderly Americans with incomes below 200 percent of the poverty level. Limits on coverage were largely due to limits on eligibility, especially for adults, and enrollment obstacles for those who are eligible. The decoupling of Medicaid and welfare, as well as the 1997 State Children's Health Insurance Program to extend coverage additional low-income children, offers states new opportunities to extend Medicaid coverage to millions of low-income children and their parents. Many states, however, have yet to draw on this new flexibility to extend Medicaid.

COVERED SERVICES

Medicaid covers a broad range of services with nominal, if any, cost sharing by beneficiaries. Every individual entitled to Medicaid is guaranteed a minimum package of federally mandated services, including:

- Inpatient and outpatient hospital care

- Physician, midwife, and certified nurse practitioner services

- Laboratory and X-ray services

- Nursing home care and home health care

- Early and periodic screening, diagnosis, and treatment (EPSDT) for children under twenty-one years of age

- Family planning

- Rural health clinic/federally qualified health center services

States also have the option to cover additional services and still receive federal matching funds. Commonly offered services include prescription drugs, clinic services, case management, hearing aids, dental care, and intermediate care facilities for the mentally retarded (ICF/MR).

Because they are so costly, long-term care services account for a significant amount of Medicaid spending. Of the $169.3 billion spent in 1998 (see Figure 2), 38 percent was spent on long-term care services, primarily nursing home care. Acute-care services were about half (53%) of total spending, with nearly half of all acute-care spending allocated for premiums to managed care organizations (MCOs). About 9 percent of Medicaid spending does not go directly to benefits for enrollees, but provides supplemental payments for hospitals with a disproportionately large population of indigent patients; these are called disproportionate share hospital payments (DSH). These additional payments are intended to enable these hospitals to

Figure 4

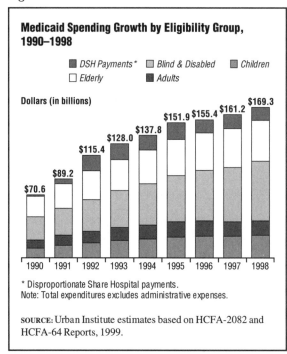

Medicaid Spending Growth by Eligibility Group, 1990–1998

■ DSH Payments* ▨ Blind & Disabled ▨ Children
□ Elderly ■ Adults

Dollars (in billions)

$70.6 $89.2 $115.4 $128.0 $137.8 $151.9 $155.4 $161.2 $169.3

1990 1991 1992 1993 1994 1995 1996 1997 1998

* Disproportionate Share Hospital payments.
Note: Total expenditures excludes administrative expenses.

SOURCE: Urban Institute estimates based on HCFA-2082 and HCFA-64 Reports, 1999.

offset some of the costs of providing services to uninsured patients.

CARE DELIVERY

Traditionally, Medicaid services have been delivered on a fee-for-service basis. Beginning in the 1990s, however, many states began to look to managed care as a model of service delivery in an effort to decrease costs and emphasize primary care and care coordination. Medicaid managed-care models range from health maintenance organizations (HMOs) that use prepaid capitated contracts to loosely structured networks that contract with selected providers for discounted services and use gatekeeping to control utilization.

States initially targeted low-income families for managed-care enrollment, but efforts to enroll aged or disabled beneficiaries increased in the late 1990s. In 1997, states were given more latitude in using Medicaid managed care under the Balanced Budget Act (BBA) of 1997, including the authority to mandate managed-care enrollment for most Medicaid populations. AS of June 1999, 17.8 million Medicaid beneficiaries—over half of all Medicaid beneficiaries—were enrolled in managed care, a sixfold increase from the 2.7 million enrolled in 1991.

States may also seek waivers of federal Medicaid rules to design new service delivery models for Medicaid beneficiaries. Home and community-based service (HCBS) waivers (also called 1915(c) waivers) are often used by states to deliver targeted community-based care for frail elderly or disabled individuals. Although all states have such waivers, the population served remains small.

TRENDS IN ENROLLEE AND EXPENDITURE GROWTH

Medicaid enrollment rose dramatically in the early 1990s, peaking at 41.7 million beneficiaries in 1995 (see Figure 3). This growth was mostly attributable to expanded coverage of low-income pregnant women and young children and increases in the number of blind and disabled beneficiaries. However, from 1995 to 1998, enrollment declined, especially for low-income adults and children eligible for Medicaid based on receipt of cash assistance under welfare programs, due in part to state and federal changes in welfare and immigration policy.

During the early 1990s, Medicaid expenditures grew nearly 30 percent annually, due to a combination of health care inflation, state use of alternative financing mechanisms, and an increase in enrollment. Only a small fraction of spending growth was due to the expansions in coverage of low-income pregnant women and children (see Figure 4). Legislation enacted to limit the states' capacity to raise funds through provider taxes and to limit DSH payments played a role in slowing Medicaid spending growth during these years. By 1995, growth in annual expenditures had dropped to under 10 percent, and it had nearly leveled off by 1998 rising less than 4 percent annually from 1995 to 1998.

MEDICAID'S IMPACT

Since the mid-1960s, Medicaid has been a major force in shaping health and long-term care services for the most vulnerable and needy Americans. In the year 2000, Medicaid covered more Americans than any other health insurer, accounted for 15 percent of the nation's spending on health care, and was the major source of federal financial assistance to the states, accounting for 40 percent of all federal grant-in-aid payments to states. It covers one-quarter of all American children, 40 percent of all births, and is the single largest source of public financing for HIV/AIDS (human immunodeficiency virus/acquired immunodeficiency syndrome) care. Medicaid is also the only significant public program providing financing for long-term care, covering 70 percent of nursing home residents and nearly half of nursing home costs nationwide. It has impacted every sector of health care in America, from hospital care to nonmedical support services.

More importantly, Medicaid has a significant impact on the individuals it serves. Before Medicaid, the poor saw providers less often than the nonpoor, and they faced serious financial burdens in obtaining care. Medicaid has reshaped the availability and provision of care to the poor, raising access to levels similar to those with private coverage. In contrast, poor Americans who do not have Medicaid coverage continue to face significant barriers to care.

DIANE ROWLAND
RACHEL GARFIELD

(SEE ALSO: *Access to Health Services; Medicare; National Health Systems; Poverty and Health; Uninsurance*)

BIBLIOGRAPHY

Coughlin, T. A.; Ku, L..; and Holahan, J. (1994). *Medicaid Since 1980*. Washington, DC: The Urban Institute Press.

Hurley, R.; Freund, D.; and Paul, J. (1993). *Managed Care in Medicaid: Lessons for Policy and Program Design*. Chicago: The Health Administration Press.

Iglehart, J. (1994). "The American Health Care System—Medicaid." *New England Journal of Medicine* 340(5): 403–408.

—— (1995). "Medicaid and Managed Care." *New England Journal of Medicine* 332(25):1727–1731.

Kaiser Commission on Medicaid and the Uninsured (1999). *Medicaid: A Primer*. Washington, DC: The Kaiser Family Foundation.

Lillie-Blanton, M.; Martinez, R. M.; Lyons, B.; and Rowland, D., eds. (1999). *Access to Health Care: Promises and Prospects for Low-Income Americans*. Washington, DC: The Kaiser Family Foundation.

Riley, T. (1995). "Medicaid: The Role of the States." *Journal of the American Medical Association* 274(3):267–270.

Rogers, D. E.; Blendon, R. J.; and Moloney, T. W. (1982). "Who Needs Medicaid?" *New England Journal of Medicine* 307(1):13–18.

Rowland, D. (1995). "Medicaid at 30." *Journal of the American Medical Association* 274(3):271–273.

Rowland, D.; Salganicoff, A.; and Keenan, P. S. (1999). "The Key to the Door: Medicaid's Role in Improving Health Care for Women and Children." *Annual Review of Public Health* 20:403–426.

MEDICAL CARE

See Personal Health Services

MEDICAL GENETICS

Public health and medical genetics are strongly linked. The applications of both begin at preconception, when folic acid supplementation can be used to reduce birth defects, and continue through pregnancy, when testing is often done to detect abnormalities. At birth, screening of newborns for biochemical disorders enables the prevention of morbidity associated with diseases such as phenylketonuria. The use of genetic screening for disorders expressed at older ages is expanding as a result of advances in molecular biology and cancer monitoring. With knowledge of the human genetic code, there will be acceleration in the diagnosis and treatment of genetic conditions and, consequently, the need for its incorporation into public health.

CLASSIFICATION OF GENETIC DISORDERS

The types of genetic disorders that may occur in any population can be classified into five categories:

1. Chromosome disorders are caused by the loss, gain, or abnormal arrangement of one or more chromosomes. Their frequency in the population is about 0.2 percent. Examples include Down syndrome and Turner's syndrome.

2. Mendelian disorders come from the mutation of a single gene. The transmission pattern is divided further into autosomal dominant, autosomal recessive, X-linked dominant, and X-linked recessive. The frequency is about 0.35 percent.

3. Multifactorial disorders involve interactions between genes and environmental factors. The nature of these interactions is poorly understood. The risks of transmission can be estimated empirically, and the estimated frequency in the population is about 5 percent. Examples include cleft lip and neural tube defects.

4. Somatic genetic disorders are not inherited but occur after conception. They often give rise to malignancies and involve environmental and genetic influences.

5. Mitochondrial disorders arise from mutations in the genetic material in mitochondria. Mitochondrial DNA is transmitted only through the maternal line. These conditions are rare.

CHROMOSOME DISORDERS

Down Syndrome. The most frequent chromosome disorder (1 in 800 births in the United States) is the one associated with Down syndrome (also called Down's syndrome or trisomy 21). A common cause of mental retardation, Down syndrome is caused, in most instances, by an extra chromosome being segregated in an egg during development. The event is random. Another cause (3 to 4% of cases) is a robertsonian translocation, in which chromosome 21 attaches to another chromosome. In this case, although the amount of genetic material is normal, the number of chromosomes is 45 instead of 46. The offspring of a parent with a robertsonian translocation have a 25 percent chance of having Down syndrome. Accordingly, karyotyping (the examination of chromosomes) is required for all children born with Down syndrome.

Down syndrome can be diagnosed during the prenatal period with amniocentesis and chorionic villous sampling. These tests involve obtaining either amniotic fluid or a sample from the placenta. Risks for Down syndrome increase with robertsonian translocation and previous birth of a child with Down syndrome; increasing maternal age; and low serum levels of maternal alpha (α)-fetoprotein (because the liver of a fetus with Down syndrome is immature, α-fetoprotein levels are lower than normal). Further risk for Down syndrome can be ascertained by measuring the serum levels of α-fetoprotein, estrogen, and human chorionic gonadotropin (hCG) in the blood.

Turner's Syndrome. Turner's syndrome is a disorder of growth and development occurring in about 1 in 2,000 births. The syndrome involves errors in one of the X chromosomes and is often associated with heart defects, osteoporosis, infertility, and short stature. Diabetes, hypothyroidism, and congenital urinary-tract abnormalities are also more common among patients with Turner's syndrome (35 to 70%) than in the general population. Edema before birth may cause webbing of the neck, a low posterior hairline, and ear abnormalities.

Klinefelter's Syndrome. Klinefelter's syndrome, characterized by a 47, XXY karyotype, is a disorder of growth and development, occurring in about 1.7 per 1,000 male infants. The disorder usually is diagnosed at puberty or during an infertility evaluation. In adolescents, its characteristics include gynecomastia (40%), small testicles, tall stature, and an arm span that is greater than the person's height. Klinefelter's syndrome is the most common cause of hypogonadism in males, and testosterone levels are about half the normal value, while follicle-stimulating hormone and lactate dehydrogenase levels are increased. Treatment includes testosterone, and occasionally mastectomy for gynecomastia.

MENDELIAN DISORDERS

Dominant Disorders. With classic dominant inheritance, an affected person has a parent with the same disorder. The parent usually mates with someone who does not have the genetic disorder, and the offspring have a 50 percent chance of having the disorder. Typically, predisposition for the disorder is carried on one chromosome, and expression of the disorder is modified by the chromosome makeup of the other parent. The dominant condition usually does not alter the ability to reproduce but tends to alter proteins that provide structure to a body. Examples of dominant disorders include Marfan syndrome (this has changes in the materials that give tissues strength), Huntington's disease (a degenerative nerve disease), neurofibromatosis (a disease that changes nerve structure), achondroplasia (a condition that alters cartilage), and familial hypercholesterolemia (a condition causing atherosclerosis because of increased cholesterol level). About 6 percent of cases of breast cancer are inherited dominantly.

Recessive Disorders. With classic recessive disorder inheritance, both mates have a gene for the disorder. The offspring have a 25 percent chance of having a normal gene pattern, a 50 percent chance of being a carrier, and a 25 percent chance of having the disorder. Carriers tend to have a reproductive advantage in certain environments; for example, sickle cell trait carriers are more resistant to falciparum malaria than noncarriers. The disorders tend to involve enzymes, and if siblings have the disorder it tends to be of the same severity because there is no modifying gene, as in a dominant disorder. If untreated, recessive disorders tend to cause death at an early age.

Certain nationalities are associated with recessive disorders. For example, people of Caribbean, Latin American, Mediterranean, or African descent have higher rates of sickle cell anemia or thalassemia, and those of Ashkenazi Jewish origin have higher rates of Tay-Sachs disease—and possibly Gaucher's disease (1 in 450 births). Screening is important for each of these groups.

In addition to the medical history, laboratory screening tests performed on newborns can detect recessive disorders. States require that many of these tests be performed. Examples are phenylketonuria, galactosemia, and hemoglobinopathy tests. The ideal time for conducting these laboratory studies is seventy-two hours after birth, although with early hospital dismissal of newborns, this timing is difficult. The American Academy of Pediatrics recommends that screening tests be performed in all infants before dismissal from the hospital. If the infant is dismissed less than twenty-four hours after birth, the screening tests should be repeated before the infant is two weeks old. Many medical clinics recommend rescreening if dismissal occurs at forty-eight hours, as the diagnoses of phenylketonuria and hypothyroidism may be missed if the infant is not retested after early dismissal. In some states, other screening tests are performed in newborns to detect galactosemia (with an incidence of 1 in 50,000 births, this disorder involves a defect in the enzyme for converting glucose to galactose), hemoglobinopathies, and congenital adrenal hyperplasia.

Nearly 30,000 people in the United States have cystic fibrosis, a recessive disorder. It is carried by about 1 in 25 Caucasians in the United States, and these carriers often do not have a family history of cystic fibrosis. The clinical characteristics include pancreatic insufficiency (85% of patients), pulmonary disease characterized by recurrent infections and bronchiectasis, and failure to grow. In more than 60 percent of patients, the diagnosis is made during the first year of life. The gene associated with cystic fibrosis was identified in 1989 on chromosome 7, and encodes the protein cystic fibrosis transmembrane conductance regulator (CFTR), which is a chloride channel in cells. The failure of this channel to work properly causes excess chloride in sweat and changes in fluid balance, which in turn cause thickened mucus in the lungs. The most common defect in cystic fibrosis cells is the absence of phenylalanine in the protein. Testing is recommended for patients with a family history of cystic fibrosis and their partners. There are more than 150 mutations of the cystic fibrosis gene, and testing can detect 85 percent of the carriers.

MULTIFACTORIAL DISORDERS

Neural Tube Defects. Neural tube defects (NTDs) are the disorders most commonly screened for prenatally. The incidence of NTDs is between 1 in 1,000 and 2 in 1,000 births. A family history of NTDs and diabetes in the mother increases the risk significantly. If the mother's diet is supplemented with folic acid before conception, however, the incidence of NTDs decreases. These defects are associated with high mortality, high morbidity, and long-term developmental disability. They involve structural abnormalities of the spine, spinal cord, head, and brain.

In the United States, of every 1,000 pregnant females who are tested between 16 and 18 weeks' gestation, about 25 to 50 will have increased levels of maternal serum alpha-fetoprotein (msAFP) and 40 to 50 have low levels. The mothers with high levels of msAFP can undergo ultrasonography to assess gestational age, the presence of a multiple gestation, or significant abnormality. An alternative is to repeat the test within one to two weeks for mothers with abnormally high or low levels of the protein. If the repeat studies confirm the previous abnormal results, ultrasonography is then performed. After screening with ultrasonography, about 17 of the patients with increased levels of msAFP and 20 to 30 with low levels will have no findings that explain the abnormal values. Amniocentesis should be performed in these patients. Of the 17 patients with high levels, 1 or 2 will have a fetus with a significant NTD, whereas 1 in 65 of those with a low msAFP will have a fetus with a chromosome abnormality (1 in 90 chance of Down syndrome). For a pregnant female with an abnormally high msAFP level and a fetus with no NTD, the risk of stillbirth, low birth weight, neonatal death, and congenital anomalies is increased.

Other Disorders. The overall risk for recurrent cleft lip, with or without cleft palate, is 4 percent if a sibling or parent has the abnormality and 10 percent if it is present in two previous siblings. Lip pits or depressions on the lower lip of a newborn may be the manifestation of an autosomal dominant trait, and the recurrence rate for a sibling is 50 percent.

Generally, the incidence of multifactorial congenital disorders is less than 5 percent. The incidence of recurrence is 2 to 5 percent for cardiac anomalies, 1 to 2 percent for tracheoesophageal fistula, 1 to 2 percent for diaphragmatic hernia, 6 to 10 percent for hypospadias, and 4 to 8 percent for hip dislocation.

PRENATAL TESTING

In North America, about 8 percent of pregnancies meet the criteria for performing amniocentesis or chorionic villous sampling. The following are basic points for prenatal testing:

1. All patients have the right to receive information about the genetic risk associated with a pregnancy. This allows parents to make an informed choice about having a child with an abnormality.

2. All patients have the right to refuse testing. What a patient decides to do about any given risk factor is entirely up to the patient. Genetic testing is voluntary except for what the state requires (e.g., neonatal screening for phenylketonuria, hypothyroidism, and other inborn errors of metabolism).

3. Genetic screening is not expected to detect all genetic disorders in a given population.

CANCER AND GENETICS

Certain families have an increased risk for specific cancers. Many of these families have an identifiable gene associated with the disorder. Possession of the gene does not automatically mean that cancer will develop in the patient. The expression of most genes can be altered by environmental factors and by other genes. Consequently, a risk can be predicted only on the basis of the history of the gene being found in other families. If a family has a tendency for cancer, it is prudent to consult a geneticist (a list is available from the National Society of Genetic Counselors, 233 Canterbury Drive, Wallingford, PA 19080).

Breast Cancer Genes. BRCA1, a tumor-suppressor gene, accounts for 5 to 10 percent of all cases of breast cancer. It is autosomal dominant. A woman from a family prone to breast or ovarian cancer who carries certain mutations of BRCA1 has about an 80 percent chance that breast cancer will develop and a 40 to 60 percent chance of getting ovarian cancer. Members of a family with multiple cases of breast or ovarian cancer can be tested to determine whether they have a genetic alteration in BRCA1. If such an alteration is found, presymptomatic screening could be performed on other family members as part of a research protocol. Routine screening for mutations is not reasonable because nearly 100 different mutations of this gene have been identified, many of which are unique to specific families. Certain races, such as Ashkenazi Jews (European descent), have a high incidence of a site-specific mutation on BRCA1. Screening a specific population is not feasible because the patient may have other mutations in the gene, and even if a mutation were found, the implication of a mutated BRCA1 gene in a family not prone to cancer is not known.

A BRCA2 gene has been discovered and is thought to account for other genetically linked cases of breast cancer. This gene is associated with families with a history of cancer that have a high incidence of breast cancer among male family members. Patients with the genes need follow-up. The studies include breast self-examination monthly, breast examination by a physician semiannually, and mammography annually. Ovarian surveillance includes pelvic examination, ultrasonographic visualization of the ovaries, and measurement of the serum level of CA 125 for this cancer antigen. Prophylactic bilateral mastectomy and oophorectomy also can be considered as alternatives. One study revealed a 10 percent incidence of primary peritoneal cancers after prophylactic oophorectomy.

Colorectal Cancer. The two major forms of hereditary colon cancer are hereditary nonpolyposis colon cancer (HNPCC) and familial adenomatous polyposis (FAP). Four separate genes are associated with colon cancer. Management includes annual colonoscopy beginning at age twenty-five, or when the patient is ten years younger than the youngest relative discovered to have colon cancer. Flexible sigmoidoscopy is inadequate. Women should undergo transvaginal ultrasonography or endometrial biopsy annually. FAP, characterized by the appearance of hundreds of adenomas in the large bowel, accounts for 0.5 percent of colon cancers. Colon cancer develops in virtually 100 percent of patients with untreated FAP. Removal of the colon decreases the risk to 10 percent.

THE FUTURE OF MEDICAL GENETICS

Sequencing of the human genome was completed in 2000. The completion of this task will speed the development of molecular genetic recognition and treatment. Readers can obtain useful information from the list of Internet sites included.

JOHN W. BACHMAN

(SEE ALSO: *Environmental Determinants of Health; Genes; Genetic Disorders; Genetics and Health; Human Genome Project; Newborn Screening; Prenatal Care; Risk Assessment, Risk Management*)

BIBLIOGRAPHY

Centers for Disease Control and Prevention. *Translating Advances in Human Genetics into Public Health Action: A Strategic Plan.* Available at http://www.cdc.gov/genetics/publications/strategic.htm.

Columbia-Presbyterian Medical Center. "Congenital Disorders. Screening for Neural Tube Defects—Including Folic Acid/Folate Prophylaxis." In *Guide to Clinical Preventive Services,* 2nd edition. Available at http://www.cpmcnet.columbia.edu/texts/gcps/gcps0052.html.

Cystic Fibrosis Foundation. *Facts about Cystic Fibrosis.* Available at http://www.cff.org/facts.htm.

Horowitz, M., ed. (2000). *Basic Concepts in Medical Genetics: A Student's Survival Guide.* New York: McGraw-Hill.

Human Genome Program of the U.S. Department of Energy. "Human Genome Project Information." Available at http://www.ornl.gov/hgmis/.

National Down Syndrome Society. *Education. Research. Advocacy: One Vision, One Voice.* Available at http://www.ndss.org/index.html.

National Institutes of Health. "Office of Rare Diseases." Available at http://www.cancernet.nci.nih.gov/ord/genetics-info.html.

National Library of Medicine and HRSA. *Gene Tests.* Available at http://www.genetests.org/.

Nussbaum, R. L.; McInnes, R. R.; and Willard, H. F. *Thompson and Thompson Genetics in Medicine,* 6th edition. St. Louis, MO: W. B. Sanders.

Robert H. Lurie Comprehensive Cancer Center of Northwestern University. *The Genetics of Cancer.* Available at http://www.cancergenetics.org/home.htm.

Turner's Syndrome Society of the United States. Available at http://www.turner-syndrome-us.org/.

University of Kansas Medical Center. *Genetics and Rare Conditions Site.* Available at http://www.kumc.edu/gec/support/.

MEDICAL SOCIOLOGY

Some have argued that medical sociology should be thought of as a loosely connected network of disparate subgroups rather than as a single discipline. Many medical sociologists tend to argue against certain axioms in the biomedical model of health and illness. They reject the reductivist approach of biomedicine, which claims that health and disease are natural phenomena that exist in the individual body rather than in the interaction of the individual and the social world; they reject the doctrine of specific etiology, the vision that disease can be induced by introducing a single specific factor into a healthy animal; and they reject biomedicine's claim to scientific neutrality. Like sociology in general, subgroups within medical sociology vary according to dichotomies such as human agency versus social structure, conflict versus consensus, and idealism versus realism. Subgroups also vary according to subject matter, thus the sociology of medicine can be distinguished from the sociology of health and illness, the sociology of healers, and the sociology of the health care system. Medical sociologists also distinguish between the sociology of health, the study of health, illness, and health care to further sociological theory; and sociology in health, the use of sociological insights to complement biomedicine's objectives and priorities. There are four often interrelated areas of research in medical sociology: the social production of health and illness, the social construction of health and illness, postmodern perspectives on health and illness, and the study of the health care system and its constituent parts.

Research in the social production of health and illness tends to explore variations in biomedical indicators of health such as self-reported health status and morbidity or mortality statistics. Social epidemiology shows that the distribution of disease is related to the structure of social inequalities (i.e., to occupational class, socioeconomic status, gender, marital status, age, ethnicity, area of residence, housing, family structure, and employment status), although it does little to explain these microlevel relationships.

The political economy perspective incorporates a broader political and economic framework, arguing that relations of domination within patriarchal capitalism create conditions of deprivation within which some people must struggle to maintain health. It claims that there is a contradiction between the pursuit of health and the pursuit of profit. It notes the large differentials in health found among social classes, sometimes pointing to unhealthy work environments of the lower classes as an explanation, and also notes the strong relationship found among Western countries between aggregate health and degree of income inequality. This perspective has been criticized, however, for failing to recognize the substantial health gains that have accompanied capitalist development and for proposing a scenario with little opportunity for intervention or change.

Social relations (such as social support for individuals and social capital or social cohesion for communities) have been investigated as determinants of the health of individuals and communities. There is also strong empirical support for the importance of lifestyle practices and behaviors embedded in social environments and cultural contexts. On a global scale, some authors argue that capitalist imperialism influences the presence and distribution of illness in developing nations, through the transfer of modern medicine, industry, and technology from the West, which is motivated in part by profit-driven pharmaceutical companies, for example. Finally, some authors investigate the role of Western medicine in creating as well as preventing illness. They argue that improvements in health have come mainly from nonmedical factors, and that medicine reproduces the legitimacy of the dominant social order by serving as a means of social control.

Social construction research views illness behaviors and the experience of health and illness as social states. Interactionist theory argues that people bestow meaning on their interactions with others—that selves are emergent and socially constructed. An early sociological contribution was the distinction between disease (an objective state), illness (the subjective experience of disorder), and sickness (the social state associated with being ill). Talcott Parsons's sick role, a social role with certain rights and obligations for those so labeled, shows the power of medicine to define illness and shows that illness is a form of social deviance. Subsequent work has introduced core sociological concepts such as deviance, labeling, career, medicalization, socialization, self, and identity to the field. Interactionist approaches have been criticized for neglecting the hard realities of power and politics and for their cognitivist bias, sharply separating the mind and body.

Postmodernist thought rejects binary oppositions, instead focusing on a shifting reality with multiple truths. Foucauldian social constructionism of claims that diseases are fabrications of powerful discourses wherein individuals explore the boundaries of their self-identity, engaging in the endless task of self-transformation. Others argue that the body is a liquid commodity, an object of circulating capital, in a new world of hyperreality filled with new forms of technology. The sociology of the body stresses the re-entrance of the physical body within sociological discourse, exploring how socially structured physiology affects social behavior and vice versa. These perspectives are criticized for their lack of an ethic, extreme relativism and abstraction, and lack of attention to the greater political context.

Some micro-level concerns when studying the health care system are entry into and experience with the health care system and patient-practitioner relationships, which have shifted focus from the provider's interest in compliance to a power-based perspective. Some argue that medicalization (providers defining needs) impinges on patient autonomy and acts as a form of social control directing deviance into controllable channels. Others explore the behaviors of providers, the management of uncertainty in practice, and implicit theories of professional knowledge. A prevailing theme at the meso-level, the interactional region between the face-to-face encounter and the wider social structure, is medical dominance, the power of medicine to define matters in its own interests, applied to the study of professions, occupations, hospitals, and medical schools, for example. Some have studied the adoption of a cloak of competence in the socialization of medical students. Community involvement in planning and decision making—the democratization of medical care—received attention in the late 1990s. Finally, some macro-level concerns are the role of multinational pharmaceutical companies in shaping the nature of health care and the reasons for and historical development of health insurance.

GERRY VEENSTRA

(SEE ALSO: *Cultural Norms; Social Networks and Social Support; Sociology in Public Health; Values in Health Education*)

BIBLIOGRAPHY

Annandale, E. (1998). *The Sociology of Health and Medicine: A Critical Introduction.* Malden, MA: Polity Press.

Evans, R. G.; Barer, M. L.; and Marmor, T. R., eds. (1994). *Why Are Some People Healthy and Others Not? The Determinants of Health of Populations.* New York: Aldine de Gruyter.

Freidson, E. (1970). *Professional Dominance: The Social Structure of Medical Care.* New York: Atherton Press.

Illich, I. (1976). *Limits to Medicine.* Toronto: McClelland and Stewart.

Martin, E. (1987). *The Woman in the Body.* Boston: Beacon Press.

McKeown, T. (1976). *The Role of Medicine: Dream, Mirage or Nemesis?* London: Nutfield Provincial Hospitals Trust.

Parsons, T. (1951). *The Social System.* Glencoe, IL: Free Press.

Starr, P. (1982). *The Social Transformation of American Medicine.* New York: Basic Books.

Veenstra, G. (2000). "Social Capital, SES and Health: An Individual-level Analysis." *Social Science and Medicine* 50:619–629.

Wilkinson, R. G. (1997). *Unhealthy Societies: The Afflictions of Inequality.* New York: Routledge.

MEDICAL WASTE

Medical waste is generally defined as any solid waste generated during the medical diagnosis or treatment of humans or animals, in related research, or in the production of biologicals used in clinical activities. Concern about medical waste streams has been growing. Syringes washing up on New Jersey beaches in the 1980s following massive illegal dumping of medical wastes into New York harbor threw a spotlight on the issue. Similar beach problems have occurred in Britain and have been suggested to be a cause of hepatitis B among users of recreational waters.

A number of factors make management of medical wastes more difficult than other waste streams. Standard landfill disposal is complicated by the potential for infection of workers and of the general public. On-site incineration of hospital wastes, a common practice that effectively destroys infective organisms, is of increasing concern as a source of dioxins due to the high chlorine content of many of the disposable plastics in common medical use. Local opposition has made it more difficult to site and plan hospital incinerators. Mercury from amalgam fillings discarded in dental offices has been suggested to be a cause of mercury discharge into surface water from publicly owned water-treatment works.

While there are federal guidelines concerning medical wastes, including a 1989 Medical Waste

Tracking Act administered by the U.S. Environmental Protection Agency (EPA), the major regulatory control is by state and local authorities. The increased cost of safe disposal of medical waste has led to efforts to reduce the size of the waste stream, including consideration of a return to reusable syringes, endoscopy tubes, and other medical devices. This requires a careful assessment of the tradeoff with simplicity of use, certainty of sterility, and lower costs provided by the disposable items. There is also a tradeoff between increased medical-waste disposal costs and the likelihood of illegal dumping. Clinically useful plastics formulated without chlorine are also being actively sought to decrease the risk of dioxins from incineration.

Not all medical waste comes from obvious point sources such as hospitals, doctors' offices, clinical laboratories, and research facilities. Over a million syringes are used at home by diabetics and others on a daily basis. This has led to community-based approaches to collect and safely dispose of these syringes and needles. Similarly, the trend toward shorter hospital stays means postoperative patients are more frequently discharged to their homes with surgical dressings and other potentially contaminated medical paraphernalia. Chronic infectious diseases are also now more likely to be treated at home than in a hospital. Patients, families, and visiting nurses should be instructed in the proper handling of these wastes. Landfilling of medical wastes is a particular problem in many developing countries, where scavenging of landfills is an organized activity among the poor. In addition to exposure to infectious agents, there have been instances where discarded radioactivity sources, such as cobalt used in the treatment of cancer, have been recycled into the community with devastating effects.

BERNARD D. GOLDSTEIN

(SEE ALSO: *Environmental Protection Agency; Municipal Solid Waste; Ocean Dumping; Sewage System*)

BIBLIOGRAPHY

Phillip, R.; Pond, K.; and Rees, G. (1997). "Research and the Problems of Litter and Medical Wastes on the U.K. Coastline." *British Journal of Clinical Practice* 51(3):164–168.

Phillips, G. (1999). "Microbial Aspects of Clinical Waste." *Journal of Hospital Infection* 41:1–6.

Thomas, C. S. (1977). "Management of Infectious Waste in the Home Care Setting." *Journal of Intravenous Nursing* 20(4):188–192.

MEDICARE

As the largest publicly funded health care program, Medicare plays an essential role in insuring the needs of America's elderly and disabled populations. It remains one of the most popular federal programs, although it has been under considerable scrutiny since the 1980s because of its large share of the federal budget and rapid rates of expenditure growth. Initially, the program covered about 19 million persons who were sixty-five years of age and older. In 2000, over 39 million persons, nearly one in every eight Americans, were enrolled, and that number is projected to rise to nearly 78 million by 2030.

As enacted in 1965, Medicare offered coverage to all persons aged sixty-five and older. After that, eligibility was limited to persons sixty-five years of age and older who were eligible for some type of Social Security benefit, usually as a worker or dependent. In 1972, the program's scope was expanded to include persons who receive Social Security Disability Insurance, after meeting a two-year waiting period. Persons with permanent kidney failure who face costly kidney dialysis treatments were also added to the program. Despite warnings about creating a "disease of the month" approach to Medicare eligibility, no other groups have been added since 1972.

Because of its size—nearly $213 billion in spending in 1999—Medicare plays an important role in the overall health care system. Changes in Medicare's payment systems are often adopted by other insurers, and decisions by Medicare about coverage of new technologies are also closely watched. Further, subsidies for medical education and for hospitals serving a disproportionate number of low income patients or located in rural areas are provided through the Medicare program, even though these reflect broader health care issues.

MEDICARE'S COVERAGE

Medicare's benefit package has changed little since 1965, although changes in the way care is delivered have affected the size of the various components of that benefit package. Part A of Medicare, also called Hospital Insurance, covers inpatient hospital services, up to one hundred days of care in a skilled nursing facility following a hospital stay, and some hospice services. Part B of Medicare, Supplementary Medical Insurance, covers physician services, outpatient hospital care, laboratory services, and other ambulatory services. Home health care services—skilled care such as rehabilitation provided to persons who are homebound—have been subject to a number of changes in recent years; as of 2000 they were divided between the two parts of the program.

When Medicare began, it was dominated by inpatient hospital care, which accounted for about two-thirds of all spending under the program. But as care has moved out of the inpatient setting, Part B has expanded and now represents over 40 percent of spending, about the same as spending on inpatient hospital care. In addition, post-acute care—skilled nursing-facility care services and home health—has also increased in importance. But these benefits have also come under increased criticism for moving Medicare into the domain of long-term care services.

Part B is voluntary and requires a premium from those who choose to enroll. Because that premium represents only 25 percent of the costs of the benefit, however, most who are eligible choose to enroll in Part B. In addition to the premium, Medicare beneficiaries are required to pay an array of cost-sharing charges. Both parts have a deductible, and most services are subject to some type of coinsurance. This cost sharing, and the exclusion of some benefits (such as prescription drugs) from coverage, results in a benefit package that is less comprehensive than that available to many younger families. Consequently, a market for supplemental insurance has arisen, either supported by employers as part of a retirement package or purchased specifically by beneficiaries. This latter supplemental insurance is referred to as "Medigap."

Gaps in coverage for low-income beneficiaries are made up through Medicaid, a joint federal/state program for which most Medicare beneficiaries can qualify if they have limited financial resources. In addition, legislation passed in 1988 established a Qualified Medicare Beneficiary program to use Medicaid to further fill in the gaps. Later programs include the Specified Low Income Medicare Beneficiary program and a program for Qualified Individuals. These programs help fill in Medicare's cost sharing or premium requirements for persons with low incomes but who do not qualify for full Medicaid benefits. But participation is relatively low and varies across the states. Thus, the comprehensiveness of coverage for older Americans and eligible disabled persons varies considerably via this complicated environment of patchwork supplemental benefits.

Another way in which beneficiaries can obtain supplemental benefits is to opt out of traditional Medicare and enroll in a managed care plan. This option has been available for many years, but the Balanced Budget Act (BBA) of 1997 expanded its scope by creating a new Part C of Medicare—Medicare+Choice. In early 2000, about 6.2 million beneficiaries—nearly 16 percent of all beneficiaries—participated in Medicare+Choice plans. Medicare+Choice moves Medicare away from its traditional role as the insurer and into a role as a purchaser of insurance. Beneficiaries who enroll in Medicare+Choice agree to get all of their care from a private plan. This plan, which is paid a fixed monthly amount on behalf of each enrollee, is usually a health maintenance organization (HMO) although other types of plans may also participate. These plans may offer benefits in addition to the basic Medicare benefit package, and they can afford to do so in part because of savings that arise from requiring beneficiaries to abide by a stricter set of rules, such as using only doctors, hospitals, and other health care providers who are on a prescribed list.

Most studies of Medicare's HMO program have suggested that plans have been overpaid, so that Medicare's contributions implicitly help subsidize additional benefits for those in private plans. As a result, some beneficiaries are better off, but Medicare then loses money on each enrollee. Changes made under the BBA were intended to reduce these overpayments, but the new restrictions have been controversial and may have contributed to a number of plans withdrawing from the Medicare+Choice system. Reforms of Medicare+Choice are likely to continue to be controversial.

Another consequence of the absence of a comprehensive Medicare benefit is the financial burden that beneficiaries face in paying for their own care. When the premiums that they pay for Part B and supplemental insurance are added to the direct expenses for care not covered by any insurance, older Americans pay about 20 percent of their incomes for health care (even excluding the costs of long-term care for persons in institutions). Enrollees in the Medicare+Choice program face smaller but not insignificant burdens. In 1965, when Medicare was instituted, the share of income that individuals paid for their care was about 19 percent. Medicare initially reduced that share, but it has gradually risen again over time as the costs of health care have gone up faster than the incomes of older Americans. Even with no changes in policy, the share of income spent on health will likely rise over time if health costs continue to outpace retirement incomes.

REFORM ISSUES

Because Medicare is projected to grow substantially as the baby boom generation reaches sixty-five years of age, it is likely to become an ever larger share of the federal budget and need additional revenues. Efforts to find ways to reduce spending on Medicare have been a high priority for politicians who do not wish to raise taxes. The urgency behind various reform efforts has diminished, however, as projections of spending growth moderated at the end of the 1990s.

Nonetheless, several competing approaches to reform remain under discussion. They usually focus on reducing per capita spending and range from incremental changes to major structural reforms that would shift Medicare more under the control of private plans. Incremental approaches usually seek to modernize the existing Medicare program, largely by changing payment policies for services and for private plans. Critics of this approach worry that it focuses more on prices charged for services and less on controlling the amount of care being used.

One of the principal Medicare restructuring plans is a variant of the 1999 plan of the co-chairs of the National Bipartisan Commission on the Future of Medicare. It has since been offered in an amended form by Senators John Breaux (D-Louisiana) and Bill Frist (R-Tennessee). Termed "premium support," this approach would require that beneficiaries choose among an array of private plans (with traditional Medicare being just one choice). If the plan chosen is more expensive than the national average, the beneficiary would have to pay a higher premium. This would presumably result in greater awareness by beneficiaries of the costs of health care and a greater incentive for private plans to hold the line on costs so as to be competitive. Traditional Medicare, which is now effectively the default plan for most persons, would become much more expensive and perhaps would be eliminated over time. This and other proposals to expand competition in Medicare are controversial because they are based more on theory than on practice, and because many supporters of Medicare are skeptical of the level of savings likely to be generated and fearful of what protections for beneficiaries might be lost if private plans take over.

Other proposed reforms that are sometimes combined with changes aimed at the efficient operation of Medicare include increases in the age of eligibility and income-testing the program, either through higher premiums or eliminating eligibility entirely for persons at high income levels. All of these proposals, and any new ones, will likely continue to be debated as baby boomers move inexorably toward eligibility for Medicare and as the projected costs of Medicare continue to grow.

MARILYN MOON

(SEE ALSO: *Access to Health Services; Economics of Health; Health Care Financing; Landmark Public Health Laws and Court Decisions; Managed Care; Medicaid; National Health Insurance; Retirement; Uninsurance*)

BIBLIOGRAPHY

Aaron, H. J., and Reischauer, R. D. (1995). "The Medicare Reform Debate: What Is the Next Step?" *Health Affairs* 14:8–30.

Feder, J., and Moon, M. (1999). "Can Medicare Survive its Saviors?" *American Prospect* May–June:56–60.

Fuchs, V. (1999). "Health Care for the Elderly: How Much? Who Will Pay for It?" *Health Affairs* 18:1–21.

Health Care Financing Administration (2000). *Medicare & You 2000.* Washington, DC: U.S. Government Printing Office.

Moon, M. (1996). *Medicare Now and in the Future,* 2nd edition. Washington, DC: The Urban Institute Press.

Vladeck, B. (1996). "The Political Economy of Medicare." *Health Affairs* 18:22–36.

Wilensky, G., and Newhouse, J. (1999). "Medicare: What's Right? What's Wrong? What's Next?" *Health Affairs* 18:92–106.

MEDICATION ABUSE, ELDERLY

Medication abuse occurs when patients do not take medication in the prescribed manner, when they use other people's medication, or when they combine prescribed medication with over-the-counter, traditional, or herbal medicines. Such medication misuse among the elderly is responsible for one out of every ten dollars spent in the health care systems of North America. Medication use increases with age, and incidence of drug-related illness is higher in the elderly than in the general population. The public health importance of medication abuse is due to the progression and negative outcome of disease, loss of productivity, and diminished quality of life that often results from such abuse. There are also economic consequences due to increased treatment in ambulatory settings and more frequent hospital and nursing home admissions.

PATRICK MCGOWAN

(SEE ALSO: *Geriatrics; Gerontology; Medicare*)

MEDLINE

Medical Literature Analysis and Retrieval System (MEDLARS) on Line, or MEDLINE, is a bibliographic database that contains citations to medical literature. It is based on the United States National Library of Medicine's *Index Medicus*, an index for medical journals, and it gives access to authoritative, published medical articles.

MEDLINE is the most comprehensive database for health and medicine and includes citations from more than 4,300 journals from around the world. The complete database covers literature from 1966 to the present. More than 80 percent of the 9 million referenced articles are in English, and 75 percent of the articles have abstracts or short summaries.

MEDLINE is used primarily by medical and scientific professionals as a primary source for seeking information pertaining to disease, illness, and biomedical research. MEDLINE has been diversified and developed in various forms to be searchable for free over the World Wide Web in databases such as PubMED and Medline*plus.* This database is also available through public and academic libraries where professional librarians are willing to assist individuals in learning how to retrieve relevant information from this service.

LARRY S. ELLIS

(SEE ALSO: *Data Sources and Collection Methods; Information Systems; Information Technology*)

BIBLIOGRAPHY

Department of Health and Human Services, National Institutes of Health, United States National Library of Medicine. *NLM's Databases & Electronic Information Sources.* Bethesda, MD: United States National Library of Medicine. http://www.nlm.nih.gov/databases/databases.html.

Hutchinson, R. N., David (1998). *Medline for Health Professionals: How to Search PubMed on the Internet.* Sacramento: New Wind Publishing.

Katcher, B. S. (1999). *Medline: A Guide to Effective Searching.* San Francisco: The Ashbury Press.

MELANOMA

Melanoma is a cancer that forms in the pigment cells (melanocytes) of the skin. There were approximately forty-seven thousand new cases in the United States in the year 2000, nearly eight thousand of which were fatal, mostly due to metastases. Reports of melanoma cases doubled in frequency during the last decade of the twentieth century. Solar exposure and genetic factors are responsible for the majority of cases.

Reduction in exposure to ultraviolet light, especially early in life, and regular screening of those at increased risk are the best approaches to reducing mortality from melanomas. The overall five-year survival rate is 85 percent, and surgical excision of early tumors is usually curative. More effective treatment for advanced malignant melanoma is needed, however.

ARTHUR J. SOBER

(SEE ALSO: *Cancer; Skin Cancer; Ultraviolet Radiation*)

BIBLIOGRAPHY

Balch, C. M.; Houghton, A.; Sober, A. J.; and Soong, S. J., eds. (1998). *Cutaneous Melanoma*, 3rd edition. St. Louis, MO: Quality Medical Publishing.

MENSTRUAL CYCLE

The menstrual cycle encompasses approximately four weeks framed by two menstrual flows (called "periods"). Though few population-based, hormonally valid prospective studies of menstrual cycle intervals and ovulation are available, normal menstrual cycles are twenty-one to thirty-five days long with flow lasting three to five days. The menstrual cycle occurs during approximately thirty to forty-five years of a woman's life beginning with menarche (the first flow) at ages ten to sixteen. The menstrual cycles permanently end with menopause (one year following the final menstrual period), which occurs between ages forty and fifty-eight.

Within each normal menstrual cycle a complex, highly coordinated series of hormonal, physiological and physical changes occur in a predictable fashion. The cycle is divided by ovulation into two phases called follicular and the luteal phase. The start of flow is cycle day 1. The follicular phase leads to increased sexual interest at midcycle, slippery (like egg white) cervical mucous, and release of an egg (ovulation). Ovulation marks the end of the follicular and start of the luteal phase that itself ends with flow. Luteal phase length is ten to sixteen days, during which changes occur in the endometrium (lining of the uterus), breasts, fluid balance, exercise physiology, metabolism, and women's experiences (molimina). If fertilization does not occur, the thickened endometrium starts

to shed and a new cycle begins. The normal menstrual flow entails approximately 43 ± 2.3 (median 32) milliliters of blood loss and will soak two to eight regular-sized pads or tampons.

Menstrual interval and ovulatory disturbances (see below) are most common in adolescence (young gynecological age) and in the years prior to menopause (perimenopau). In general, they are reversible and treatable and thus represent disturbances of physiology rather than diseases.

DISTURBANCES OF MENSTRUAL FLOW

Menorrhagia, abnormally heavy flow, occurs at the extremes of menstrual life when ovulation disturbances are also common. Women older than forty-five or fifty tend to have greater blood loss with more variability than women of other ages. The cause of menorrhagia is often unclear but it entails soaking over eleven to sixteen pads or tampons and is associated with clots, cramping (dysmenorrhea), and anemia.

DISTURBANCES OF CYCLE INTERVAL

Amenorrhea, no vaginal bleeding for six or more months, indicates a rare anatomical abnormality (of uterus or vagina), very low or noncyclic, normal estrogen production. Primary amenorrhea means delay of menarche beyond fifteen years of age in 6.4 percent of the population.

Secondary amenorrhea, after menarche, is rare—it occurs in about 1 to 2 percent of the population. The most common causes are (undiagnosed) pregnancy, lactation, young gynecological age (years after menarche), undernutrition or weight loss, and emotional stress (including depression, anxiety, and eating disorders [anorexia and bulimia]). Although amenorrhea is attributed to exercise, it is more likely related to coexistent emotional stress, nutritional deficiencies, and young age.

Oligomenorrhea, flow at intervals longer than thirty-six (but less than 180) days, is more common than amenorrhea and also occurs at the extremes of reproductive life. However, 30 percent of women twenty to forty-nine years old had cycle intervals

Figure 1

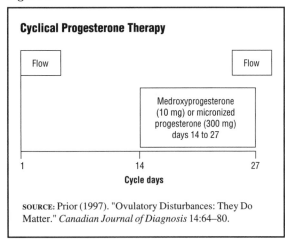

Cyclical Progesterone Therapy

Flow

Flow

Medroxyprogesterone (10 mg) or micronized progesterone (300 mg) days 14 to 27

1   14   27

Cycle days

SOURCE: Prior (1997). "Ovulatory Disturbances: They Do Matter." *Canadian Journal of Diagnosis* 14:64–80.

over sixty days. Women reporting a body mass index at age eighteen that was over twenty-four had increasing risks for oligomenorrhea with increasing weight.

Polyemnorrhea, (short cycles) are under twenty-one days in length, are common at extremes of reproductive life, and imply higher estrogen production. Short cycles are commonly abnormal in ovulatory characteristics and often have increased in flow.

DISTURBANCES OF OVULATION

Ovulatory disturbances are of two main types: low hypothalamic/pituitary stimulation, called "hypothalamic" or high pituitary stimulation called "anovulatory androgen excess." Ovulatory disturbances of either type include anovulation and cycles with ovulation but short luteal phase length. Anovulation (lack of egg release) universally causes ovarian cysts.

Hypothalamic ovulatory disturbances are common but not often detected because they occur in "regular" cycles of normal interval and flow. Hypothalamic ovulatory disturbances explain approximately 25 percent of infertility and 20 percent of prospectively documented cancellous bone loss. Seventy-five percent of normal weight, healthy premenopausal women experienced at least one cycle with ovulatory disturbance during one-year prospective monitoring, thus this may be an unrecognized cause for osteoporosis. Although not all

investigators agree, no other prospective one-year study has simultaneously and continuously documented both ovulation and bone loss.

Hypothalamic ovulatory disturbances are related to cortisol excess caused by physical or psychological stress including cognitive dietary restraint in normal weight women. Ovulatory disturbances may also be associated with menorrhagia and increased risk for anemia, endometrial cancer, breast swelling, nodularity and/or pain (fibrocystic) problems, troublesome premenstrual symptoms, and breast cancer.

Anovulatory androgen excess (commonly called "polycystic ovarian disease") occurs in approximately 5 percent of reproductive-age women. This may cause cycle or flow disturbances, acne, or unwanted male-pattern hair changes (increased facial and body hair and head hair loss). This type of anovulation may be related to insulin excess/resistance, gynecological age, and heredity. Health outcomes related to prolonged anovulatory androgen excess include increased risks of endometrial and breast cancers and probable cardiovascular disease (abnormal lipids, central obesity, increased waist/hip/ratio, and insulin resistance) but protection from osteoporosis.

OVERVIEW OF MENSTRUAL CYCLE AND OVULATORY DISTURBANCES

Cycle interval and ovulatory disturbances are common in adolescence and perimenopause. The majority are reversible (except in perimenopause). Treatment with cyclic progesterone is physiological and increases bone mineral and thus minimizes osteoporosis (see Figure 1). Population-based, prospective studies of menstrual cycles, ovulatory characteristics, and health parameters are needed.

JERILYNN C. PRIOR

(SEE ALSO: *Anorexia; Contraception; Endocrine Disruptors; Fecundity and Fertility; Nutrition; Reproduction; Sports Medicine; Women's Health*)

BIBLIOGRAPHY

Barr, S. I.; Janelle, K. C.; and Prior, J. C. (1994). "Vegetarian Versus Nonvegetarian Diets, Dietary Restraint, and Subclinical Ovulatory Disturbances: Prospective Six Month Study." *American Journal Clinical Nutrition* 60:887–894.

Coulam, C. B.; Annegers, J. F; and Kranz, J. S. (1983). "Chronic Anovulation Syndrome and Associated Neoplasia." *Obstetrics Gynecology* 61:403–407.

Hallberg, L.; Hogdahl, A. M.; Nillson, L.; and Rybo, G. (1966). "Menstrual Blood Loss: A Population Study." *Acta Obstetrics and Gynecology Scandinavia.* 45:330–351.

Landgren, B. M.; Unden, A. L.; and Diczfalusy, E. (1980). "Hormonal Profile of the Cycle in 68 Normally Menstruating Women." *Acta Endocrinology Copenhagen* 94:89–98.

Prior, J. C.; Vigna, Y. M.; Schechter, M. T.; and Burgess, A. E. (1990). "Spinal Bone Loss and Ovulatory Disturbances." *New England Journal of Medicine* 323:1221–1227.

Prior, J. C.; Vigna, Y. M.; Shulzer, M.; Hall, J. E.; and Bonen, A. (1990). "Determination of Luteal Phase Length by Quantitative Basal Temperature Methods: Validation Against the Midcycle LH Peak." *Clinical & Investigative Medicine* 45:377–392.

Ramcharan, S.; Love, E. J.; Frick, G. H.; and Goldfien, A. (1992). "The Epidemiology of Premenstrual Symptoms in a Population-Based Sample of 2,650 Urban Women: Attributable Risk and Risk Factors." *Journal of Clinical Epidemiology* 45:377–392.

Rich-Edwards, J. W.; Goldman, M. B.; Willett, W. C.; Hunter, D. J.; Stampfer, M. J.; Colditz, G. A. and Manson, J. E. (1994). "Adolescent Body Mass Index and Infertility Caused by Ovulatory Disorder." *American Journal of Obstetrics and Gynecology* 171:171–177.

Treloar, A. E.; Boyton, R. E.; Behn, B. G.; and Brown, B. W. (1967). "Variations of the Human Menstrual Cycle through Reproductive Life." *International Journal of Fertility* 9:77–126.

Vollman, R. F. (1977). *Major Problems in Obstetrics and Gynecology*, Vol. 7. Toronto: Saunders.

MENTAL HEALTH

The field of mental health has made many advances, particularly since 1980. These developments include an increased understanding of the brain's function through the study of neuroscience, the development of effective new medications and therapies, and the standardization of diagnostic codes for mental illnesses. However, many questions about mental health remain unanswered, and many people around the world are unable to benefit from the knowledge and treatments that are available.

Seven in ten Americans with a mental illness do not receive treatment. Biases against mental illness and lack of public awareness are among the obstacles that limit access to treatment and affect willingness to seek care. Fewer individuals with major psychiatric illnesses were institutionalized in the United States in the year 2000 than in 1980, but limited community resources had not yet met existing treatment needs. Over one-third of the homeless in the United States have a severe mental illness. The prevalence of dementia is rising as people are living longer, adding to the need for more resources. One of the main challenges for the field of mental health is overcoming the gap between an increasingly sophisticated understanding and treatment of mental illness and the availability of these advances to individuals and populations in need.

Mental, or psychiatric, illnesses are a major public health concern. They adversely affect functioning, economic productivity, the capacity for healthy relationships and families, physical health, and the overall quality of life. They cut across racial, ethnic, and socioeconomic lines to affect a significant proportion of communities worldwide. They tend to develop and manifest in the early adult years, often preventing individuals from leading full and productive lives. The National Comorbidity Survey of 1994 found nearly half of the individuals in its random U.S. sample had a psychiatric disorder over their lifetime, and almost 30 percent had one in the past year. The World Health Organization's *World Health Report 1998* lists mood and anxiety disorders among the leading causes of morbidity and mood disorders as the leading cause of severely limited activity. Mental disorders account for a quarter of the world's disability. Comorbidity (having more than one illness) is common and even further increases the risk of disability. Suicide is the eighth leading cause of death in the United States and the third leading cause in the fifteen- to twenty-four-year-old age group. More people die by suicide than homicide.

Dianne Hales and Robert Hales define mental health as

the capacity to think rationally and logically, and to cope with the transitions, stresses, traumas, and losses that occur in all lives, in ways that allow emotional stability and growth. In general, mentally healthy individuals value themselves, perceive reality as it is, accept its limitations and possibilities, respond to its challenges, carry out their responsibilities, establish and maintain close relationships, deal reasonably with others, pursue work that suits their talent and training, and feel a sense of fulfillment that makes the efforts of daily living worthwhile (p. 34).

A healthy pregnancy, adequate parenting, secure attachments to caretakers, regular involvement in groups, and stable intimate relationships all contribute to the development and maintenance of mental health. Mental health does not imply the absence of distress and suffering, or strict societal conformity. Mental health and illness, idiosyncratic beliefs and delusions, sadness and depression, and worry and severe anxiety lie on a continuum. An essential criterion for defining behavioral patterns or symptoms of psychological distress as a mental disorder is that they become significant enough to be functionally disabling and impose substantial increased risks ranging from an important loss of freedom to suffering pain, disability, or death.

Both genetic inheritance and environmental factors influence one's vulnerability to mental illness. Twin and family studies and genetic research have demonstrated the former, though specific genes have been difficult to identify, and there may be multiple genes involved in most psychiatric disorders. Traumatic events throughout one's lifetime, including childhood abuse or neglect, major losses, violence, military combat, and dislocation (as among the urban homeless or wartime refugees) are known to threaten mental stability. Nontraumatic stressors, including unemployment, bereavement, and relational or occupational problems, can impact mental health. Nutritional deficiencies (such as vitamin B12), infections (such as syphilis and HIV [human immunodeficiency virus]), and heavy metal poisoning (such as lead) can all cause psychiatric syndromes. Substance abuse contributes significantly to the exacerbation or even precipitation of other psychiatric illnesses and complicates their treatment. Poverty and homelessness are risk factors for many of these problems, but may also be the outcome of psychiatric illness and the inability to function independently.

Many models of mental health and illness have been proposed. Emil Kraepelin (1856–1926) contributed to the development of the precise categorization of mental illnesses, particularly in distinguishing the long-term course of psychotic and mood disorders. Sigmund Freud (1856–1939) developed the theory of psychoanalysis, through which he claimed that symptoms of psychiatric disorders, as well as many phenomena of everyday life, have unconscious meanings and sources. Erik Erikson (1902–1994) formulated a theory of human development with specific tasks and crises at different stages of the life cycle. Failure to master these stages can lead to various forms of psychopathology. Neuroscientists have demonstrated molecular models of illness, which involve genetic, developmental, functional, anatomical, and molecular abnormalities of the brain. The biopsychosocial model, proposed by George Engel in the 1970s, integrates the biological, genetic, and molecular mechanisms of illness with a psychological understanding of personality development and response to stress as well as social, cultural, and environmental influences.

The *Diagnostic and Statistical Manual of Mental Disorders* (its 4th edition, *DSM-IV*, was published in 1994) is the product of research on standardized diagnostic criteria aimed at creating a common, validated descriptive system for all mental health care providers. It is nearly universally accepted, as it classifies and describes categories of illness and aims to be neutral about controversial theories of etiology (see Table 1). The following descriptions of various mental disorders are based on *DSM-IV* criteria.

Affective disorders involve a cyclical pattern of significant mood disturbance. A major depressive episode may be precipitated by a stressful life situation but also has genetic factors. Disturbances in appetite, sleep, energy, concentration, and sexual interest are common symptoms. The majority of patients respond to treatment with antidepressant medication and/or psychotherapy. An individual who has long-term (over two years) of minor to moderate depressive symptoms may have

Table 1

Lifetime and 12-month prevalence of DSM-III-R disorders

Disorders	Lifetime prevalence (%)			12-month prevalence (%)		
	M	F	Total	M	F	Total
Affective disorders						
Major depressive episode	12.7	21.3	17.1	7.7	12.9	10.3
Manic episode	1.6	1.7	1.6	1.4	1.3	1.3
Dysthymia	4.8	8.0	6.4	2.1	3.0	2.5
Any affective disorder	14.7	23.9	19.3	8.5	14.1	11.3
Anxiety disorders						
Panic disorder	2.0	5.0	3.5	1.3	3.2	2.3
Agoraphobia without panic disorder	3.5	7.0	5.3	1.7	3.8	2.8
Social phobia	11.1	15.5	13.3	6.6	9.1	7.9
Simple phobia	6.7	15.7	11.3	4.4	13.2	8.8
Generalized anxiety disorder	3.6	6.6	5.1	2.0	4.3	3.1
Any anxiety disorder	19.2	30.5	24.9	11.8	22.6	17.2
Substance use disorders						
Alcohol abuse without dependence	12.5	6.4	9.4	3.4	1.6	2.5
Alcohol dependence	20.1	8.2	14.1	10.7	3.7	7.2
Drug abuse without dependence	5.4	3.5	4.4	1.3	0.3	0.8
Drug dependence	9.2	5.9	7.5	3.8	1.9	2.8
Any substance abuse/dependence	35.4	17.9	26.6	16.1	6.6	11.3
Other disorders						
Antisocial personality	5.8	1.2	3.5	—	—	—
Nonaffective psychosis*	0.6	0.8	0.7	0.5	0.6	0.5
Any of the disorders above	48.7	47.3	48.0	27.7	31.2	29.5

*Includes schizophrenia, schizoaffective disorder, schizophreniform disorder, delusional disorder, and atypical psychosis.

SOURCE: Kessler, R.C. et al. (1994). "Lifetime and Twelve–Month Prevalence of DSM–III–R Psychiatric Disorders in the United States: Results from the National Comorbidity Study." *Archives of General Psychiatry* 51:8–19.

dysthymia. Substance abuse, medical disorders (such as hypothyroidism), and normal life cycle events in which hormonal changes are prominent (such as the postpartum period) can all cause symptoms of depression and should be considered carefully during an assessment. An adjustment disorder is a milder disturbance of mood that may occur in response to a stressful life situation, such as a personal loss or financial crisis, and that usually resolves when the stress is relieved. About 1 percent of the general population has bipolar disorder, also called manic-depressive disorder, in which manic episodes are present as well as depressive episodes. Mania is characterized by a persistently elevated or irritable mood for at least a week, often with decreased need for sleep, rapid speech, impulsivity in spending and other behaviors, and grandiosity. In more severe manic and depressive episodes, psychotic symptoms may emerge, which can complicate treatment. Bipolar disorder is treated with mood stabilizers, such as

lithium or valproic acid, and supportive management. Antidepressant medications alone can precipitate mania in susceptible patients.

Psychotic disorders are characterized by "positive" symptoms such as hallucinations, delusions, and bizarre behaviors, as well as "negative" symptoms such as paucity of speech, poverty of ideas, blunting of affective expression, and functional deterioration. Cognitive problems such as disorganization of thought processes also occur. Schizophrenia is a chronic, disabling illness that affects almost 1 percent of the world population, independent of ethnic or cultural background. Risk factors include a family history and possibly psychosocial stressors. The precise cause is still unknown, but it is clear that certain areas of the brain and certain neurotransmitters are involved. Many of those affected are unable to maintain work or relationships and require supportive services to help them manage basic needs such as shelter and food. Treatment includes antipsychotic medication, comprehensive social services including social and occupational rehabilitation if possible, and substance abuse treatment if necessary. Newer antipsychotic medications such as clozapine, olanzapine, and risperidone have been able to treat more symptoms generally with fewer side effects, allowing many to lead more productive lives. Some patients with schizophrenic-type illness also experience prominent affective symptoms nonconcurrently and may have schizoaffective disorder. These patients often require a mood stabilizer as well as antipsychotic medication. Substance use, especially hallucinogens and stimulants (such as amphetamines and cocaine), can precipitate psychotic symptoms, and these may even endure beyond the period of substance use. Some medical conditions (such as epilepsy and delirium) and some medications (such as steroids) can also cause psychotic symptoms and should be considered in the assessment and treatment of psychosis.

Anxiety disorders are among the most prevalent psychiatric disorders in the general population, and these disorders lead to both psychological distress and increased health care utilization. Panic disorder often manifests with somatic symptoms, such as palpitations, chest pain, nausea, trembling, dizziness, and shortness of breath, and can be easily confused with a medical disorder by both patients and doctors. Patients develop persistent concerns about having further panic attacks. Some develop agoraphobia, or a fear of being in public places where their attacks may be triggered. Other phobias include simple phobia, such as fear of heights or specific animals, and social phobia, which is a marked and persistent fear of certain or all social situations, such as speaking in public or being around others in general. People with obsessive-compulsive disorder have obsessions, characterized by recurrent or persistent thoughts, impulses, or images that are experienced as intrusive and inappropriate, and/or compulsions, characterized by repetitive behaviors or mental acts often performed in response to an obsession. After one experiences a traumatic event, in which actual or threatened death or severe injury is witnessed or experienced, one may develop post-traumatic stress disorder. Intrusive recollections of the event (such as nightmares), avoidance of reminders of the event, and increased arousal (such as increased vigilance for potential threats) can all cause significant distress and impairment following a wide range of traumatic events, including an accident, military combat, torture, or rape. Generalized anxiety disorder is characterized by excessive and persistent anxiety or worry about a number of events or activities, such as work or school performance. For all anxiety disorders, specific psychopharmacologic and psychotherapeutic (such as cognitive-behavioral therapy) techniques of treatment can be effective and complementary.

Substance-use disorders are quite common and occur in all segments of society. They can lead to accidents, violent crime, and major problems in school and at work. They can cause or complicate various medical and psychiatric illnesses. Liver failure, ulcers, heart attacks, cognitive disorders, and depression are among the potential outcomes of various substances. These disorders pose major public health concerns for public safety, health costs, economic productivity, and pregnancy risks, among others. Substance abuse is defined as a maladaptive pattern of use indicated by continued use despite persistent or recurrent social, occupational, psychological, or physical problems caused or exacerbated by the use of the substance; or recurrent use in situations that could be physically hazardous (such as driving while intoxicated). With substance dependence, signs of physical dependence such as withdrawal symptoms are often present, and the person spends a great deal of time involved in substance-related activities, uses more of the substance than intended, is unable to cut down, and continues to use the substance despite social, occupational, or physical problems related to it. The first steps of treatment involve developing insight, acknowledging the problem, and wanting to change. There are various self-help groups (such as Alcoholics Anonymous), comprehensive treatment programs, psychosocial interventions, and medications that can help lead to successful recovery for the majority of those with substance-use disorders.

Childhood disorders include pervasive developmental disorders, such as autism, which occurs in four out of ten thousand people; mental retardation, which can be caused by a variety of genetic abnormalities or prenatal insults; and attention deficit–hyperactivity disorder, which can lead to significant problems in school and in social relationships. Childhood abuse and neglect are tragically quite common, with one million children affected annually in the United States alone. These can have major adverse effects on development of personality, relationships, and the ability to function in the world.

Personality disorders are usually first evident in late adolescence and are characterized by pervasive, persistent maladaptive patterns of behavior that are deeply ingrained and are not attributable to other psychiatric disorders. Biological and genetic factors, as well as developmental difficulties, are significant contributors. Other disorders described in *DSM-IV* include eating disorders, with restriction (anorexia) and/or binging and purging (bulimia) and impulse control disorders (e.g., kleptomania). Somatoform disorders cause physical symptoms with no apparent medical cause (e.g., hysterical paralysis).

Gender, race, ethnicity, and culture are important factors in determining the expression and risk of mental disorders, and these factors also impact on treatment considerations. Certain disorders are more prevalent in women, such as depression and eating disorders, and some in men, such as substance abuse. Cultural background may influence the idioms of psychological distress. For example, *nervios* describes for many Latinos a constellation of somatic, anxiety, and depressive symptoms distinct from particular *DSM-IV* diagnoses. Psychiatric disorders are the main risk factor for suicide, but rates vary significantly depending on gender, age, race, religion, marital status, and culture.

PAUL J. ROSENFIELD
STUART J. EISENDRATH

(SEE ALSO: *Community Mental Health Centers; Dementia; Depression; Schizophrenia; Stress*)

BIBLIOGRAPHY

Bromet, E. J. (1998). "Psychiatric Disorders." In *Maxcy-Rosenau-Last Public Health and Preventive Medicine,* 14th edition, ed. Robert B. Wallace. Stamford, CT: Appleton and Lange.

Diagnostic and Statistical Manual of Mental Disorders (DSM-IV) (1994), 4th edition. Washington, DC: American Psychiatric Association.

Eisendrath, S. J., and Lichtmacher, J. (1999). "Psychiatric Disorders." In *Current Medical Diagnosis and Treatment 1999,* eds. L. M. Tierney, Jr., S. J. McPhee, and M. A. Papadakis. Stamford, CT: Appleton and Lange.

Engel, G. (1980). "The Clinical Application of the Biopsychosocial Model." *American Journal of Psychiatry* 137(5):535–544.

Hales, D., and Hales, R. E. (1995). *Caring for the Mind: The Comprehensive Guide to Mental Health.* New York: Bantam Books.

Jamison, K. R. (1999). *Night Falls Fast.* New York: Alfred Knopf.

Kaplan, Harold I., and Sadock, Benjamin J., eds. (1995). *Comprehensive Textbook of Psychiatry.* 6th edition. Philadelphia: Williams and Wilkins.

Kessler, R. C.; McGonagle, K. A.; Zhao, S.; Nelson, C. B.; Hughes, M.; Eshleman, S.; Wittchen, H. U.; and Kendler, K. S. (1994). "Lifetime and Twelve Month Prevalence of DSM-III-R Psychiatric Disorders in the United States: Results from the National Comorbidity Study." *Archives of General Psychiatry* 51:8–19.

U.S. Public Health Service (1999). *The Surgeon General's Call to Action to Prevent Suicide.* Washington, DC: Author.

World Health Organization (1998). *World Health Report 1998: Life in the Twenty-first Century, A Vision for All.* Report of the Director-General. Geneva: Author.

MENTAL HEALTH CENTERS

See Community Mental Health Centers *and* Mental Health

MENTAL RETARDATION

The term "mental retardation" refers to persons with deficits in both their intellectual and adaptive (everyday) functioning. These individuals typically show IQ scores below 70, as well as difficulties in meeting the demands of everyday living, whether it be in communicating and socializing with others or attending to grooming and domestic chores. Mental retardation manifests itself in the developmental years, before age eighteen.

Anywhere from 1 to 3 percent of the population is estimated to be mentally retarded. The majority of these persons (about 85 percent), show mild levels of delay, with IQs ranging from 55 to

70. Approximately 10 percent show moderate delays, with IQs from 40 to 55. With proper supports, individuals with mild to moderate mental retardation successfully live and work in their communities, or in supervised settings such as group homes. The remainder of persons show severe to profound levels of mental retardation (IQs of 40 and below), and many of these individuals have sensory, motor, or medical problems that further complicate their care.

Mental retardation has multiple causes. Approximately 50 percent of persons with mental retardation do not have a clear-cut organic or biological cause for their delay. The low IQ of these persons is likely due to a combination of environmental and genetic factors. The other 50 percent of persons with mental retardation have a known biological etiology. These include prenatal causes such as genetic disorders or alcohol exposure in utero; perinatal causes such as premature birth; and postnatal causes such as head trauma and exposure to lead.

There are now over 750 known genetic disorders that cause mental retardation, accounting for about half of those with organic etiologies. Some of these can be screened for during pregnancy—including Down syndrome, the most common chromosomal cause of mental retardation. Other disorders include fragile X syndrome, Prader-Willi syndrome, and Williams syndrome. People with these and other syndromes often show distinctive personalities, behavioral problems, and intellectual strengths and weaknesses that can be used to guide their care.

Some organic causes of mental retardation can be prevented. As many as two in one thousand children are born with fetal alcohol syndrome, which is prevented by refraining from drinking alcohol during pregnancy. Babies born with phenylketonuria, or PKU, are placed on a special, phenylalanine-reduced diet, thereby avoiding the severe mental retardation that otherwise characterizes this disorder.

People with mental retardation are at higher risk than those in the general population for behavioral and psychiatric problems such as autism, hyperactivity, and self-injurious behaviors. Throughout the early to mid-1900s, many of these individuals, as well as those without behavioral problems, were placed in large institutions. Since the advent of deinstitutionalization in the 1960s, most children with mental retardation have been cared for by their families. To improve the quality of life for these children, the Americans with Disabilities Act and other federal legislation emphasize community inclusion and specialized services such as early intervention, special education, and school-to-work transition. Many individuals also benefit from occupational, physical, and speech-language therapies, as well as from programs that teach daily living skills. With proper support, most people with mental retardation successfully live, work, and play in their communities.

ELISABETH M. DYKENS

(SEE ALSO: *Fetal Alcohol Syndrome; Genetics and Health; Medical Genetics; Mental Health; Phenylketonuria*)

BIBLIOGRAPHY

Arc of the United States. "Information about Mental Retardation and Related Topics." Available at http://www.thearc.org.

Dykens, E. M. (2000). "Psychopathology in Children with Intellectual Disabilities." *Journal of Child Psychology and Psychiatry* 41:407–417.

Dykens, E. M.; Hodapp, R. M.; and Finucane, B. M. (2000). *Genetics and Mental Retardation Syndromes: A New Look at Behavior and Intervention.* Baltimore, MD: Paul H. Brookes.

Hodapp, R. M., and Dykens, E. M. (1996). "The Child with Mental Retardation." In *Child Psychopathology,* eds. E. J. Mash and R. A. Barkley. New York: Gilford Press.

King, B. H.; Hodapp, R. M.; and Dykens, E. M. (2000). "Mental Retardation." In *Comprehensive Textbook of Psychiatry,* 7th edition, eds. H. I. Kaplan and B. J. Sadock. New York: Williams & Wilkins.

MERCURY

Mercury (Hg) is a naturally occurring silvery metal that has been associated with adverse health effects throughout history. Elemental mercury is a liquid at room temperature, and, because of this, Aristotle named mercury "quicksilver." There are three forms of mercury: elemental mercury (Hg^0), organic mercury (e.g., methylmercury), and inorganic mercury (e.g., Hg^+, Hg^{2+}). Many different organic and inorganic mercury compounds are found in nature because of mercury's ability to form covalent or ionic bonds with other chemicals. Mercury has numerous commercial uses—including its use in the extraction of gold from ores—and is an ingredient in alkaline batteries (approximately 0.025% of battery content), mercury vapor lamps, thermostats, and mercury amalgam fillings (in the United States, 50% of a dental filling is made of mercury). Humans can be exposed to mercury compounds via the oral, inhalation, and dermal routes. The primary source of exposure to mercury compounds is attributed to the ingestion of fish and other seafood (marine mammals, crustaceans) that have bioaccumulated mercury compounds. Dental amalgams, which leach mercury, are another source.

Adverse health effects from elemental and inorganic mercury compounds have been observed, particularly in occupational settings. Health consequences commonly observed from exposure to compounds such as elemental mercury vapor and mercuric chloride include tremors, bleeding gums, abdominal pain, vomiting, and kidney damage.

Health effects from organic mercury compounds have also been well-documented, primarily because of the tragic mass poisonings from organic mercurials in locations such as Minamata, Japan, and in Iraq. These mass poisonings were primarily associated with central nervous system toxicity and death. Adverse health effects observed in poisoned individuals and their offspring included ataxia, dysarthria, impaired vision and hearing, and death. Methylmercury is particularly toxic because 95 percent of an ingested dose is absorbed into the bloodstream and can cross the blood-brain and placental barriers, causing adult and fetal neurotoxicity. One of the reasons that offspring are particularly susceptible is that methylmercury can accumulate at 30 percent higher levels in fetal red blood cells than in maternal red blood cells. Besides damaging the brain and peripheral nervous system, methylmercury may also adversely affect the adult and fetal cardiovascular systems.

Research continues to be performed on the potential neurodevelopment effects of ingesting low levels of mercury in seafood. Three particularly important, ongoing studies involve residents of New Zealand and the Seychelles and Faroe Islands who consume significant portions of seafood as part of their normal diets. Analyses performed to date on mother-offspring pairs from the Seychelles identified adverse neurodevelopmental impact in offspring attributable to maternal methylmercury exposure from seafood. Mild developmental effects were also reported among offspring of New Zealand and Faroe Island residents who ingested seafood containing relatively high levels of methylmercury. These studies are particularly pertinent to assessing potential health effects among Native Arctic populations who consume marine mammals (beluga whales, ringed seals) as part of their normal diet. An increased level of mercury has been noted in the Arctic environment since the 1970s, possibly due to anthropogenic sources such as fossil fuel combustion, or possibly from increased natural releases of mercury from geologic sources. It is hypothesized that the cold Arctic climate acts as a sink for mercury; a particularly troublesome prospect for Native Arctic populations who continue to consume mercury-laden mammals and seafood.

MARGARET H. WHITAKER
BRUCE A. FOWLER

(SEE ALSO: *Environmental Determinants of Health; Foods and Diets; Heavy Metals; Minamata Disease; Occupational Safety and Health*)

BIBLIOGRAPHY

Agency for Toxic Substances and Disease Registry (1999). *Toxicological Profile for Mercury* (Update). Washington, DC: U.S. Department of Health and Human Services.

Arctic Monitoring and Assessment Programme (1999). *Arctic Pollution Issues: A State of the Arctic Environment Report.* Available at http://www.amap.no.

National Research Council (2000). *Toxicological Effects of Methyl Mercury.* Washington, DC: Committee on the Toxicological Effects of Mercury. Board on Environmental Studies and Toxicology. Commission on Life Sciences.

Tenenbaum, D. J. (1998). "Northern Overexposure." *Environmental Health Perspective* 106(2): A64–A69.

U.S. Environmental Protection Agency (1997). *Report to Congress on Mercury*. Available at http://www.epa.gov/oar/mercury.html.

World Health Organization (1990). *Methyl Mercury,* Vol. 101. Geneva: International Programme on Chemical Safety, WHO.

—— (1990). *Inorganic Mercury,* Vol. 118. Geneva: International Programme on Chemical Safety, WHO.

MESOTHELIOMA

Mesothelioma is a rare cancer of the lining of the chest, the abdomen, or other tissues. It has become increasingly more frequent since 1900, however, paralleling the use of asbestos. Exposure to asbestos is the most common cause of this disease, with the vast majority of cases occurring following exposures that may have taken place decades earlier. Mesotheliomas can be seen ten years after first exposure, but they peak at three to four decades after exposure. The risk is lifelong, and the prognosis is extremely poor, with death often occurring within twelve months of diagnosis, no matter what the treatment. Newer, extensive surgical techniques may alter this historical experience.

All fiber types of asbestos cause this disease, although there is continuing controversy over the differential ability of the different fiber types to do so. The one other recognized cause of this disease in humans is another group of fibrous materials called zeolites. In animal studies, however, a wide variety of other fibers have been known to cause mesotheliomas.

Mesotheliomas appear as several cellular patterns and may be difficult to diagnose. Special panels of experts are available to assist with making these evaluations. The most common lesions with which these may be confused are lung cancers.

ARTHUR L. FRANK

(SEE ALSO: *Asbestos; Occupational Safety and Health*)

BIBLIOGRAPHY

Osinubi, O. Y.; Gochfeld, M.; and Kipen, H. M. (2000). "Health Effects of Asbestos and Nonasbestos Fibers." *Environmental Health Perspectives* 108(54):665–674.

Selikoff, I. J., and Lee, D. H. K. (1978). *Asbestos and Disease*. New York: Academic Press.

META-ANALYSIS

Meta-analysis is the statistical synthesis of the data from a set of comparable studies of a problem, and it yields a quantitative summary of the pooled results. It is the process of aggregating the data and results of a set of studies, preferably as many as possible that have used the same or similar methods and procedures; reanalyzing the data from all these combined studies; and thereby generating larger numbers and more stable rates and proportions for statistical analysis and significance testing than can be achieved by any single study. The process is widely used in the biomedical sciences, especially in epidemiology and in clinical trials. In these applications, meta-analysis is defined as the systematic, organized, and structured evaluation of a problem of interest. The essence of the process is the use of statistical tables or similar data from previously published peer-reviewed and independently conducted studies of a particular problem. It is most commonly used to assemble the findings from a series of randomized controlled trials, none of which on its own would necessarily have sufficient statistical power to demonstrate statistically significant findings. The aggregated results, however, are capable of generating meaningful and statistically significant results.

There are some essential prerequisites for meta-analysis to be valid. Qualitatively, all studies included in a meta-analysis must fulfill predetermined criteria. All must have used essentially the same or closely comparable methods and procedures; the populations studied must be comparable; and the data must be complete and free of biases—such as those due to selection or exclusion criteria. Quantitatively, the raw data from all studies is usually reanalyzed, partly to verify the original findings from these studies, and partly to provide a database for summative analysis of the entire set of data. All eligible studies must be included in the meta-analysis. If a conscious decision is made to exclude some, there is always a suspicion that this was done in order to achieve a desired result. If a pharmaceutical or other commercial organization conducts a meta-analysis of studies aimed at showing its product in a favorable light, then the results will be suspect unless evidence is provided of unbiased selection. One criterion for selection is prior publication in a peer-reviewed medical journal, but there are good arguments in favor of including well-conducted unpublished studies under some circumstances.

A variation of the concept is a systematic review, defined as the application of strategies that limit bias in the assembly, critical appraisal, and synthesis of all relevant studies of a specific topic. Meta-analysis may be, but is not necessarily, used as part of this process. Systematic reviews are conducted on peer-reviewed publications dealing with a particular health problem and use rigorous, standardized methods for the selection and assessment of these publications. A systematic review can be conducted on observational (case-control or cohort) studies as well as on randomized controlled trials.

JOHN M. LAST

(SEE ALSO: *Epidemiology; Observational Studies; Statistics for Public Heath*)

BIBLIOGRAPHY

Dickerson, K., and Berlin, J. A. (1992). "Meta-Analysis: State of the Science." *Epidemiologic Reviews* 14:154–176.

Petitti, D. B. (2000). *Meta-Analysis, Decision Analysis and Cost Effectiveness Analysis in Medicine,* 2nd edition. New York: Oxford University Press.

MIASMA THEORY

Miasmas are poisonous emanations, from putrefying carcasses, rotting vegetation or molds, and invisible dust particles inside dwellings. They were once believed to enter the body and cause disease. This belief dates at least from classical Greece in the fourth or fifth century B.C.E., and it persisted, alongside other theories and models for disease causation, until the middle of the nineteenth century. To some extent the belief still persists today. It was most clearly enunciated by Italian physician Giovanni Lancisi (1654–1720) in *De noxiis paludum effluviis* (*Of the poisonous effleuvia of malaria*, 1717).

The miasma theory was advanced to explain many important diseases, including tuberculosis

and malaria (from *mala aria*, meaning "bad air"). Many eminent leaders of medical opinion were convinced that the cholera epidemics of the nineteenth century were caused by miasmas, even as the evidence mounted for the germ theory, which was gathering momentum at that time. William Farr stated firmly in his annual report on vital statistics in Great Britain in 1852 that the inverse association of cholera mortality with elevation above sea level confirmed the miasma theory as its cause. Farr rejected John Snow's argument, based on evidence and logical reasoning, that cholera was caused by contaminated drinking water. Though the miasma theory soon proved to be a wrong explanation for the cause of cholera, it was partially sustained as an explanation for malaria. Some malaria control measures based on miasma theory, particularly draining swamps and marshes, are part of modern control strategies; though not, of course, because miasmas cause malaria, but because mosquito breeding sites are eliminated.

JOHN M. LAST

(SEE ALSO: *Farr, William; Snow, John; Theories of Health and Illness*)

MICROBIOLOGIST

State or local public health departments have the responsibility to protect their citizens from communicable diseases. The responsibility of a microbiologist in clinical laboratories is to identify the microorganisms that cause infectious diseases—through the application of advanced standard microbiological laboratory methods and techniques—and to record and report that information to clinicians, disease investigators, and the state health department. Maintenance and improvements of the quality of laboratory standards are maintained in compliance with the requirements of Clinical Laboratory Improvement Amendments (CLIA #88), the Occupational Safety and Health Administration (OSHA), and other regulatory agencies.

BASSAM F. HALASA

(SEE ALSO: *Clinical Laboratories Improvement Act; Occupational Safety and Health Administration*)

MICRONUTRIENT MALNUTRITION

Thirty percent of the world's population is affected by vitamin A, iron, or iodine deficiency, and almost all the world's population is folate deficient. Thus, the health of many millions of people are adversely affected by these micronutrient deficiencies.

DISEASES CAUSED BY MICRONUTRIENT DEFICIENCY

Vitamin A deficiency causes blindness and increased mortality among children. Iron deficiency causes anemia, especially in women, pregnant women, and children. This iron-deficiency anemia causes loss of IQ points in children and loss of productivity in adults. In some countries it is estimated that iron deficiency is responsible for a 3 percent decrease in gross national productivity. Iodine deficiency causes goiter and mental retardation in its severest form, and loss of IQ points at lower levels of deficiency. Folate deficiency causes anemia, especially in pregnant women; and it may additionally result in spina bifida and anencephaly, two of the most common birth defects, in offspring of folate-deficient women. Folate deficiency also appears to be a major contributor to heart attack, strokes, and colon cancer.

PREVENTING MICRONUTRIENT DEFICIENCY

The very good news is that there is technology in hand that can prevent at least 75 percent of micronutrient deficiency in the world, at a cost of about thirty-five cents (U.S.) a year.

Iodination of table salt can nearly eliminate iodine deficiency diseases. During the 1990s, concerted international efforts led to more than 75 percent of the world's population having iodine deficiency eliminated. This success was achieved because there was an understanding of the need to solve the iodine deficiency problem, the political will to solve the problem, an effective, cheap intervention available, and because strong and persistant individuals who advocated for the prevention of iodine deficiency diseases worked with industry and governments to eliminate iodine deficiency on a country-by-country basis.

Folic acid fortification of grains is a cheap and very effective way to eliminate folate deficiency. The United States has required that enriched grains contain 1.4 parts per million, an action that was followed within months by a near tripling of serum folates in the population. Fortification of wheat and corn flours around the world offer the possibility of eliminating folate deficiency for 75 percent of the world's population.

Fortification of flour with iron has also been shown to be a very effective way to increase blood-iron levels and to eliminate iron-deficiency anemia. Fortification of grains with iron can eliminate about 75 percent of the iron deficiency remaining in the world today. Fortification of infant formulas is an effective way to increase iron consumption among children.

Vitamin A is fat soluble. Sugar, margarine, milk, and edible oils can be fortified at sufficient level to lower vitamin A deficiency in a population. These foods should be fortified in countries where there is significant consumption. Research to identify even more foods to be fortified is needed to provide the technical basis to eliminate 75 percent of vitamin A deficiency. Genetically modified foods containing an increased amount of vitamin A is another promising approach to preventing vitamin A deficiency.

SUPPLEMENT STRATEGIES

Consumption of pills with vitamin A, iron, iodine, and folic acid are very effective and cost-effective ways to treat micronutrient diseases or to prevent micronutrient diseases. They are necessary where there is no widely consumed food that can be fortified, and before effective fortification of foods has been instituted in a country. Supplement strategies are also likely to be needed to complement fortification programs. People living in urban areas may be consuming foods that can be fortified, but rural people in the same country may not be consuming such foods and thus require a supplement strategy for prevention and cure. The downside of supplement programs is the difficulty in getting the population to consume supplements on a continuing basis. There has, however, been good success with once-a-year vitamin A programs and once-a-week programs for iron for women of reproductive age. Iron and folic acid supplements are also effective in preventing and treating folate- and iron-deficiency anemia of pregnancy. For many years, and without recommendations from the medical/nutritional establishment, 25 percent of American adults have regularly consumed multivitamin supplements. So it is clear that supplements can play a role in preventing and curing micronutrient malnutrition.

Eating a healthy diet is highly desirable and should be encouraged. Changing the foods eaten can make a contribution to preventing micronutrient deficiency. The problem with dietary diversity is that change is usually slow—with progress measured in years. This slowness is in sharp contrast to the instant change in consumption by fortification and supplement programs.

THE ELIMINATION OF MICRONUTRIENT DEFICIENCY

Smallpox was eradicated from the earth about two hundred years after the vaccine that provided the scientific basis for eradication was developed. It has been a little over fifty years since the polio vaccine was developed, and the elimination of polio from the world is in sight. The scientific understanding of the problem of iodine deficiency and an effective fortification strategy have existed for seventy years, and iodine deficiency may soon be obliterated. Vitamin A deficiency, iron deficiency, and folate deficiency have been known for seventy years, but only modest progress has been made to eliminate these micronutrient deficiencies. A concerted international effort could eliminate at least 75 percent of the world's population deficiencies of vitamin A, iron, and folate by 2010. The public health challenge is to create the political will to implement the effective strategies—especially fortification—to eliminate micronutrient deficiency.

GODFREY P. OAKLEY, JR.

(SEE ALSO: *Foods and Diets; Nutrition*)

BIBLIOGRAPHY

Asian Development Bank (2000). *Manila Forum 2000: Strategies to Fortify Essential Foods in Asia and the Pacific.* Proceedings of a Forum on Food Fortification Policy for Protecting Populations in Asia and the Pacific from Mineral and Vitamin Deficiencies. Manila, Philippines: Asian Development Bank; Washington, DC: International Life Sciences Institute; Ottawa, ON: Micronutrient Initiative. Publication Stock No. 090400.

National Academy of Science, Board on International Health, Food and Nutrition Board, and Institute of Medicine (1998). *Prevention of Micronutrient Deficiencies: A Toolkit for Policymakers and Public Health Workers.* Washington DC: National Academy Press. Available at http://www.nap.edu.

MIGRANT WORKERS

According to the United States Public Health Service, there are an estimated 3.5 million migrant and seasonal farmworkers in the United States—men, women, and children who work in all fifty states during peak periods of agriculture. A migrant farmworker is an individual who moves from a permanent place of residence in order to be employed in agricultural work. Seasonal farmworkers perform similar work but do not move from their primary residence for the purpose of seeking farm equipment.

Migrant farmworkers tend to be either newly arrived immigrants or individuals with limited skills or opportunities. Although American agriculture depends on the labor of these workers, employment is usually of short duration and requires frequent moves. Many men travel without their families, and most workers return during the winter to a home base, usually in Florida, Texas, California, Puerto Rico, or Mexico. Migrant farmworkers are predominantly Latino (78 percent); 2 percent are African American, 18 percent Caucasian, less than 1 percent Caribbean, and less than 1 percent Asian. Almost half have less than a ninth grade education, and many speak little or no English. Children of migrant farmworkers often change schools several times a year.

Most migrant farmworkers earn annual incomes below the poverty level and few receive benefits such as Social Security or worker's compensation. The transient nature of their work often prevents them from establishing any local residency, excluding them from benefits such as Medicaid and foot stamps. The majority of migrant farmworkers are either U.S. citizens or legal residents of the United States. Some foreign workers enter the United States under guest-worker programs when there are not enough available workers to satisfy the demand.

Farm work is considered to be second only to mining in the rating of most hazardous occupations. There is a high exposure to pesticides through topical exposure, inhalation, and ingestion, resulting in the highest rate of toxic chemical injuries of any group in the United States. Farm injuries, exposure to heat and sun, and poor sanitation in the fields are other factors that contribute to the dangers of this work. Every year nearly three hundred children die and twenty-four thousand are injured in farm work.

Housing regulations attempt to provide decent living conditions for migrant workers, but housing is often overcrowded, poorly maintained, and lacking in ventilation, bathing facilities, and safe drinking water. These conditions contribute to an increased risk of accidents, sanitation-related diseases, and infectious diseases. Several studies have shown a 40 percent positivity rate in tuberculosis testing of migrant populations. One migrant farmworker group was found to have a 5 percent incidence of HIV (human immunodeficiency virus) infection. Another study showed that 78 percent had parasitic infections.

Health care problems faced by migrant farmworkers are similar to those of other disadvantaged populations, but the factors of poverty, mobility, difficult living and working conditions, and cultural isolation put them more at risk for illness and injury. Those who work with migrant farmworkers find that, not only do common disease conditions occur more frequently, but they are often more severe because they are allowed to progress to more advanced stages before accessing care.

Unstable living and working conditions, conflicts arising from the process of acculturation, perceptions of mental illness, isolation, and discrimination all contribute to a high incidence of metal-health problems among migrant farmworkers. A 2000 study documented a 26.7 percent incidence of psychiatric disorders among a sample of male Mexican farmworkers in California. A national survey of migrant women showed that approximately 20 percent had experienced physical or sexual abuse during the previous year. These same factors make migrants more vulnerable to substance abuse, depression, and self-medication.

Migrant farmworkers themselves cite dental problems as one of their greatest health concerns. Gingivitis, dental caries, and baby bottle tooth decay are common.

In 1962, President John F. Kennedy authorized the creation of a system of health care services specifically for migrant and seasonal farmworkers. The Migrant Health Program continues to be administered as part of the Bureau of Primary Health Care within the Health Resources and Services Administration, and consists of a national network of migrant health clinics. Studies have found, however, that these services were reaching less than 15 percent of the farmworkers in the United States.

It is a challenge to provide health care to the transient migrant farmworker in the context of the traditional health care system. Migrant health centers must attempt to provide health care services that are sensitive to the unique cultural, financial, and occupational needs of farmworkers. Staff must be able to communicate in the languages of the farmworkers, and clinic services must be offered in the evening, since farmworkers will not risk a loss of wages or employment by seeking care during work hours. Transportation services are often an essential component of migrant health programs.

Migrant health programs employ outreach programs to make services more available to farmworker patients. Clinicians often travel to farmworker camps in the evenings to assess and triage health problems. Multidisciplinary care is typical—nurses, health educators, nurse practitioners, physician assistants, nurse midwives, physicians, dentists, and others collaborate to provide necessary services. Lay health advisors are often recruited from the ranks of the farmworkers population and trained in basic preventive medicine. These individuals help to reinforce preventive health concepts through teaching, triage, and referral.

Providing continuity of care is a constant focus in migrant health care programs. A farmworker may only be in one location a few weeks or months, so for services that require long-term attention, such as prenatal care or treatment of diabetes, follow-up must be carefully planned. Portable records with detailed treatment information are often given to farmworkers to present to other health care facilities as they travel. Electronic data-transfer systems have also been implemented to allow centers to communicate information such as immunization records and tuberculosis treatment.

CANDACE KUGEL
EDWARD L. ZUROWESTE

(SEE ALSO: *Community and Migrant Health Centers; Fair Labor Standards Act; Farm Injuries; Health Resources and Services Administration; Occupational Safety and Health; Rural Public Health*)

BIBLIOGRAPHY

Alderete, E.; Vega, W. A.; Kolody, B.; and Aguilar-Gaxiola, S. (2000). "Lifetime Prevalence of Risk Factors for Psychiatric Disorders among Mexican Migrant Farmworkers in California." *American Journal of Public Health* 90:608–614.

Centers for Disease Control and Prevention (1992). "Prevention and Control of Tuberculosis in Migrant Farm Workers: Recommendations of the Advisory Council for the Elimination of Tuberculosis." *Morbidity and Mortality Weekly Report* 41:1–13.

Dever, G. E. A. (1991). *Migrant Health Status: Profile of a Population with Complex Health Problems.* Austin, TX: National Migrant Resource Program, Inc.

Johnston, H. (1985). *Health for the Nation's Harvesters: A History of the Migrant Health Program in Its Economic and Social Setting.* Farmington Hills, MI: National Migrant Worker Council, Inc.

Migrant Clinicians Network (1997). *Practice-Based Research Network on Domestic Violence and Migrant Farmworkers.* Austin, TX: Migrant Clinicians Network.

Power, J. G., and Byrd, T., eds. (1998). *U.S.-Mexico Border Health: Issues for Regional and Migrant Populations.* Thousand Oaks, CA: Sage.

Rivara, F. P. (1985). "Fatal and Nonfatal Farm Injuries to Children and Adolescents in the United States." *Pediatrics* 76:567–573.

Rothenberg, D. (1998) *With These Hands: The Hidden World of Migrant Farmworkers Today.* New York: Harcourt Brace.

United States Department of Labor (1994–1995). *National Agricultural Workers Survey.* Washington, DC: Author.

MIGRATION

See Acculturation; Assimilation; *and* Immigrants, Immigration

MINAMATA DISEASE

"Minamata disease" is the term used to describe the poisoning that occurred among residents of Minamata, Japan due to the ingestion of methylmercury-containing seafood. From the 1920s through the 1960s, the Chisso Company used mercury as a catalyst in the production of acetaldehyde, a chemical intermediate with numerous uses including plastics and perfume production. The Chisso Company dumped waste methylmercury from the acetaldehyde production into Minamata Bay. The methylmercury bioaccumulated within the food chain, from plankton and other microorganisms up to fish and shellfish. This posed a significant health hazard to residents of the area who obtained much of their protein from Minamata Bay seafood.

In the early 1950s, Minamata Bay residents began to exhibit symptoms of neurological illness, such as uncontrollable trembling, loss of motor control, and partial paralysis. Children also began to be born with Minamata disease, exhibiting symptoms similar to cerebral palsy (impaired neurological development and seizures). By the late 1950s, scientists from Japan's Kumamoto University strongly suspected that methylmercury was the cause of Minamata disease.

Methylmercury concentrates in neural tissues, which explains why neurotoxicity was the major adverse effect observed in Minamata Bay. Offspring of Minamata Bay residents afflicted with Minamata disease also exhibited neurotoxicity because methylmercury can be transferred across the placenta. Between 1953 and 1960, 628 cases of illness were documented, including 78 deaths. Total cases of morbidity and mortality caused by Minamata disease from the 1950s to the year 2000 are thought to range in the thousands but the exact number is not known.

MARGARET H. WHITAKER
BRUCE A. FOWLER

(SEE ALSO: *Food-Borne Diseases; Mercury*)

BIBLIOGRAPHY

Tsubaki, T., and Irukayama, K. (1977). *Minimata Disease. Methylmercury Poisoning in Minamata and Niigata, Japan.* Amsterdam: Elsevier Scientific Publishers.

Ui, J. (1992). *Industrial Pollution in Japan*. Tokyo: United Nations University Press. Available at http://www.unu.edu/unupress/unupbooks.

World Health Organization (1990). *Methyl Mercury*. Environmental Health Criteria 101. Geneva: Author.

MINERALS

See Nutrition

MINING

Mining activities have been carried out by humans for millennia. The first book on mining, (and the health hazards associated with it), was *De re metallica* by Agricola, published in Switzerland in the sixteenth century. Mining is among the most hazardous of all occupations. Mining activities take place all over the world, and are often a major source of a country's natural wealth.

There are many types of mining operations, ranging from precious metals, such as gold, to other metals, and to minerals such as asbestos, sand, granite, and iron ore. Nonmetal mining can take many forms, including coal mining, which supplies much of the world's energy, and the mining of other materials such as clay, diamonds, semiprecious stones, and related substances.

Mining can take place on the surface of the earth or in underground settings. Depending on where in the world it is carried out, it may utilize nothing more than manual labor, or extraordinarily large and sophisticated mining equipment may be involved. Mining operations can vary in size from several people working alone (often family members) to large facilities employing hundreds of workers.

Traumatic injuries of many types are associated with mining activities. In underground mines there is the ever-present danger of explosion, foul air, water hazards, and other difficulties related to the use of mechanized equipment in confined spaces. Many injuries also take place in the transportation and processing of ore and other mined products.

Depending on the nature of the material being mined, there may also be a risk of damage to various organs. Particularly vulnerable are the lungs, with many lung diseases associated with exposures related to mining. These include the pneumoconioses, or dust diseases of the lung, which are caused by coal, silica, asbestos, kaolin, talc, and many other dusts. There is also a risk of lung cancer posed by some of these materials, and the fumes from diesel vehicles that may be used in underground mining settings also pose a threat. In many underground mining operations there is a risk of exposure to radioactive materials, especially in the form of radon gas, which can lead to high rates of lung cancer.

Although most mining-related lung disease is entirely preventable with the use of good ventilation, respirators when necessary, and other precautions, not only do traumatic injuries remain high, but long-term health effects are still quite common. The National Institute of Occupational Safety and Health (NIOSH) regularly documents these issues, and releases data regarding the respiratory problems related to mining.

Organizations involved with overseeing mining activities include NIOSH, which certifies respirators for use, and the Mining Safety and Health Administration (MSHA), which directly oversees safety practice at working mines, including oversight of dust sampling. There is still considerable medical research being done related to mining activities.

Mining activities also have a high potential for adversely affecting the general environment through air pollution, the fouling of bodies of water through runoff, or the contamination of soil with waste products.

ARTHUR L. FRANK

(SEE ALSO: *National Institute for Occupational Safety and Health; Occupational Lung Disease; Occupational Safety and Health*)

BIBLIOGRAPHY

Rosen, G. (1943). *The History of Miner's Diseases*. New York: Schumans.

MINORITY RIGHTS

Modern concepts of public health recognize health "not merely as the absence of disease or infirmity," as defined by the World Health Organization (WHO), but "a state of complete physical, mental, and social well-being" (1978). Modern public health theory further recognizes this broad characterization of health as a fundamental human right and the attainment of the highest possible level of health as an important worldwide social goal. Thus, there is an enlightened understanding that societal factors, such as the denial of human rights, clearly affect the health status of populations.

As far back as the fourth century B.C.E., Aristotle expressed this connection among health, human rights, and treatment by society. He wrote: "If we believe men have any personal rights at all as human beings, they have an absolute right to such a measure of good health as society, and society alone, is able to give them." It is clear that a society that practices or tolerates discrimination, or that otherwise fails to respect and protect the human rights of minorities and other groups, compromises the health—the physical, mental, social, and spiritual well-being—of its citizens, especially minorities and other marginalized groups subjected to discrimination.

Despite the provisions under many countries constitutions and laws and under numerous international human rights instruments (e.g., the Universal Declaration of Human Rights, the International Covenant on Economic, Social, and Cultural Rights, Convention on the Elimination of Discrimination Against Women) aimed in large part at ensuring equal rights and protection for minorities against discrimination, health disparities exist among different populations in many countries. In the United States, for example, minorities generally have shorter life spans, and they receive less, and often inferior, medical treatment. Minorities also disproportionately lack health insurance—an important means of obtaining access to health care in the United States. The rate of uninsured African Americans is more than 50 percent higher than that of whites. Although employers provide most of the private insurance for workers and their families in the United States, African-American workers and their families are much less likely to have insurance through their employers than whites. A wide gap in income also exists, with African Americans three times more likely than whites to live in poverty.

In much of the world, women experience discrimination and resulting poor health. The global AIDS (acquired immunodeficiency syndrome) epidemic highlights the interrelationship between health and the lack of women's rights. Women and girls face human rights issues in a number of social and economic spheres that increase their risk of exposure to and inadequate care for HIV/AIDS (human immunodeficiency virus/acquired immunodeficiency syndrome), resulting in higher incidence of illness and death from the disease. According to the WHO, these include lack of control by women and girls over their own sexuality and sexual relationships, resulting in coerced sex and sex abuse; poor reproductive and sexual health; inadequate or delayed access to health care and support for women with AIDS (due to family resources being devoted to caring for the man); clinical management of the disease based on research on men; cultural practices such as genital mutilation; stronger AIDS-related stigma and discrimination against women; obstacles to educational and employment opportunities for girls and women; and other similar human rights violations. Noting the intimate relationship between autonomy in decisions relating to sexuality and economic independence, WHO concludes that unless and until the scope of human rights is fully extended to economic security, women's right to safe sexuality and protection from illness and death from AIDS will not be achieved.

For public health to ensure the health of all members of society, both as a discipline and a field of practice, it must address inequality in the provision of preventative care, in access to health care, in treatment for the ill, and in all the other health functions traditionally viewed as its mission. It also must address the underlying societal conditions and determinants of health, including discrimination in education, employment, access to income, and other areas of society, and to promote policies and interventions to create favorable societal conditions that will ensure the equal treatment of all people in all realms of society.

ROSE NATHAN

(SEE ALSO: *Access to Health Services; African Americans; American Indians and Alaska Natives; Demography; Ethnicity and Health; Hispanic Cultures; Inequalities in Health; Social Class; Social Determinants*)

BIBLIOGRAPHY

Centers for Disease Control and Prevention. "Eliminating Racial and Ethnic Disparities." In *CDCFY2000 Performance Plan-XV.* Atlanta, GA: Author.

UCLA Center for Health Policy Research (2000). *Racial and Ethnic Disparities in Access to Health Insurance and Health Care.* Los Angeles, CA: UCLA.

World Health Organization (1978). *Declaration of Alma-Ata.* Geneva: Author.

—— (2000). *Women and HIV/AIDS.* Fact Sheet No. 247. June 2000. Available at http://www.who.int/inf-fs/en/fact247.html.

MOBILIZING FOR ACTION THROUGH PLANNING AND PARTNERSHIPS

To achieve optimal health, each community must use its resources wisely, taking into account its unique circumstances, and must form effective partnerships for taking strategic action. The National Association of County and City Health Officials (NACCHO), in cooperation with the Public Health Practice Program Office, Centers for Disease Control and Prevention (CDC), has developed new guidelines to assist communities in their pursuit of health. This communitywide strategic planning tool for improving health is called MAPP (Mobilizing for Action through Planning and Partnerships).

A work group comprised of local health officials, CDC representatives, community representatives, and academicians developed MAPP between 1997 and 2000. The vision for implementing MAPP is "communities achieving improved health and quality of life by mobilizing partnerships and taking strategic action."

The NACCHO work group built on the lessons learned from a previous planning tool, *Assessment Protocol for Excellence in Public Health* (APEXPH). Released in 1991, APEXPH has guided hundreds of local health departments through an internal organization capacity assessment and collaborative community health assessment process.

Communities using MAPP go beyond the concepts of APEXPH and other planning tools by focusing on the local public health system—all the entries that contribute to public health in a community. To quote the Institute of Medicine, "the

Figure 1

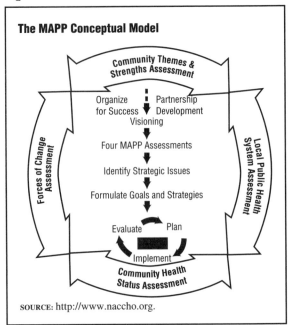

The MAPP Conceptual Model

SOURCE: http://www.naccho.org.

public health depends on the interaction of many factors; thus, the health of a community is a shared responsibility of many entities, organizations, and interests in the community, including health service delivery organizations, public health agencies, other public and private entities, and the people of a community" (Institute of Medicine Committee on Public Health, 1996).

The focus on the local health system also provides a crucial link with the National Public Health Performance Standards Program (NPHPSP) being developed by CDC, NACCHO, and other national public health organizations. The local-level instrument of the NPHPSP is an integral part of the MAPP assessment of the local public health system.

Another key characteristic of MAPP is its use of broad-based information to determine strategies needed to achieve health in the community. The MAPP process is based on proven strategic planning concepts, but it includes four unique and comprehensive assessments that collectively drive the identification of strategic issues. The four MAPP Assessments (see Figure 1) are:

- *Community themes and strengths*: identifies themes that interests and engage the community, perceptions about quality of life, and community assets.

- *Forces of change*: identifies forces that are or will be affecting the community or the local public health system.

- *Local public health system*: measures the capacity of the local public health system to conduct essential public health services.

- *Community health status*: assesses data about health status, quality of life, and risk factors in the community.

The MAPP process creates an expectation for an unprecedented union among the community organizations, agencies, groups, and individuals that, taken together, comprise the local public health system. Broad ownership ensures that the effort is sustainable, that actions build on collective wisdom, and that resources from throughout the community contribute to health improvement.

PAUL J. WIESNER
LIZA C. CORSO

(SEE ALSO: *Centers for Disease Control and Prevention; Institute of Medicine; National Association of County and City Health Officials; Public Health Practice Program Office*)

BIBLIOGRAPHY

Institute of Medicine Committee on Public Health (1996). *New Partnerships for the Future of Public Health*. Washington, DC: National Academy Press.

Mays, G. P.; Halverson, P. K.; and Miller, C. A. (1998). "Assessing the Performance of Local Public Health Systems: A Survey of State Health Agency Efforts." *Journal of Public Health Management and Practice* 4:63–77.

National Association of County and City Health Officials (1991). *Assessment Protocol for Excellence in Public Health*. Washington, DC: Author.

—— (2000). *Mobilizing for Action through Planning and Partnerships*. Washington, DC: Author.

MOLECULAR EPIDEMIOLOGY

The use of molecular techniques such as DNA typing has transformed epidemiologic investigation by making it possible to trace precisely the path taken by a specific strain of an infectious pathogen, such as the gonococcus, as it passes from one host to another. DNA/RNA typing is also an essential part of genetic epidemiology; it can help to identify cancer-prone family lineages, for example. Molecular techniques are used in cancer epidemiology to identify precancerous changes in studies of environmentally and occupationally induced cancers. In short, molecular methods are a powerful tool in many aspects of observational and analytic epidemiology.

JOHN M. LAST

(SEE ALSO: *Cancer; Contagion; Epidemiology*)

MONITORING DRUG USE

Since 1975, the *Monitoring the Future* study has provided annual data on trends in use of licit and illicit drugs among America's young people, and the reasons for those trends. The study, funded by a series of research grants from the National Institute on Drug Abuse, consists of annual surveys of nationally representative samples of eighth and tenth grade students (since 1991), and twelfth grade students (since 1975); and mail-out surveys of subsamples of previously participating twelfth grade students (since 1976). In-school questionnaires are administered by professional interviewers to about 50,000 students in approximately 420 public and private schools per year. Approximately 12,500 mail-out surveys are completed each year, following respondents through forty years of age.

PATRICK M. O'MALLEY

(SEE ALSO: *Alcohol Use and Abuse; Lifestyle; Marijuana; Smoking Behavior; Substance Abuse, Definition of; Tobacco Control*)

MONTAGU, LADY MARY WORTLEY

The celebrated eighteenth-century poet Lady Mary Wortley Montagu (1689–1762), merits a place in public health history for her early advocacy of the practice of smallpox inoculation, which was also called variation, or ingrafting. Lady Mary, who herself survived smallpox in 1716, learned of the practice in Constantinople, where her husband served as English ambassador from 1716 to 1718. While in Constantinople, she met Dr. Emanuel Timoni, who had published an account of inoculation in the Western scientific press in 1716. With Timoni's encouragement, Charles Maitland, the British surgeon brought by the Worthley family to Constantinople, successfully inoculated the Worthley's son. In a letter to Mrs. Sarah Chiswell, a London friend, Lady Mary described the ingrafting procedure, which consisted of taking dried secretions from smallpox blebs, or pustules, and either blowing them into the nostrils or injecting them into a vein or under the skin. This process produced a mild case of smallpox, which conferred lifelong immunity to natural smallpox. The process was hazardous—it occasionally caused serious disease or even death. Because smallpox was so lethal and disfiguring, however, it was considered an acceptable risk.

A severe epidemic of smallpox in London in 1721 led Lady Mary to begin a campaign in favor of inoculation that began with the inoculation of her young daughter. Shortly thereafter, royal permission was given to experimentally inoculate six condemned prisoners at Newgate Prison, all of whom survived and were pardoned. Lady Mary's strong connections with the royal family, and their adoption of inoculation among themselves, led to considerable public support for the practice, through strong opinions both for and against inoculation were widely published in the newspapers of the day.

Because it was occasionally fatal, many English physicians opposed the procedure. However, influential figures such as James Jurin (secretary of the Royal Society), John Arbuthnot, and Hans Sloane were supporters. Some historians believe that inoculation made a measurable impact on eighteenth-century mortality in England, particularly among the aristocracy, who were most likely to employ the practice. In the nineteenth century, inoculation was almost entirely supplanted by vaccination after William Jenner discovered in 1798 that immunity to smallpox could be established more safely by using material from the lesions of cows infected with cowpox or vaccinia.

NIGEL PANETH
ELLEN POLLAK

(SEE ALSO: *Jenner, Edward; Smallpox*)

BIBLIOGRAPHY

Grundy, I. (1994). *Lady Mary Wortley Montagu: Comet of the Enlightenment.* Oxford: Oxford University Press.

Lawrence, A. W., ed. (1930). *The Travel Letters of Lady Mary Wortley Montagu.* London: Jonathan Cape.

MORNING AFTER PILL

See Contraception

MORTALITY RATES

The English statistician, William Farr (1807–1883) once remarked, "Death is a fact. All else is inference." He meant that everyone dies, but though useful deductions can be made about life and death, the information is imperfect and there are traps in interpretation for the unwary. Nevertheless, facts about deaths are a reliable and consistent source of information about the health of various populations. The information can be arranged in a hierarchy of reliability, ranging from certainty (the fact of death), through near certainty (age and sex), to the place and circumstances of death. The exact cause of death is probably the least reliable piece of information for most deaths. Even among persons dying in a hospital after being diagnosed with a specific disease, autopsies sometimes shows the ante-mortem diagnosis to be wrong. When people die at home after being attended by a family doctor, the cause of death stated on the death certificate is correct only an estimated 50 to 60 percent of the time. The accuracy of death certifications is highest when death is due to a violent cause such as a traffic crash or gunshot wound, and lowest when death is sudden and there is no autopsy. The certified cause of death is often whatever happens to be most fashionable—heart attack or stroke being most in vogue in the late twentieth and early twenty-first centuries.

The aggregated data in death certificates are used to calculate mortality rates that can be manipulated in various ways to show general and specific health indicators and trends, and to make predictions about the likely future course of events. The commonly used varieties of mortality rates are: crude; age-standardized; cause-specific; infant and perinatal; maternal; and the standardized mortality ratio. Every kind of mortality rate has its uses and it's limitations.

Crude Mortality Rates. These rates reflect the number of deaths in a defined population during a specified period—usually a year—divided by the midyear population. Because of variations in age composition and other factors, crude rates are seldom useful for comparisons.

Age-Standardized Mortality Rates. Irregularities in crude rates can be reduced by making adjustments. The simplest and best way to do this is usually to calculate what the rate would be if the population concerned had the age composition of a standard population—one in which the composition is precisely known, such as that of a census year.

Cause-Specific Mortality Rates. The greatest value of mortality rates for studies of common conditions like cancer and coronary heart disease is in comparisons of cause-specific mortality rates in different populations (different regions, occupations, time periods). Such comparisons have illuminated understanding of many causal and associated factors and have prompted much detailed study of these diseases.

Infant and Perinatal Mortality Rates. The indicator of health most commonly used for comparing nations and trends over time is the infant mortality rate. This is the number of deaths in one year of infants under one year of age, divided by the number of liveborn infants. It is strongly correlated with social and economic conditions. The perinatal mortality rate is a more sensitive indicator of the standards of care for women before, during, and immediately after childbirth. The perinatal mortality rate is the number of fetal deaths between twenty-eight weeks gestation and one-week post-partum divided by the number of live births in a year multiplied by one thousand. It is considered to be a good indicator of the quality of care received by pregnant women.

Maternal Mortality Rates. This is a measure of the risk of dying from puerperal causes—causes associated with pregnancy, childbirth and the postpartum period. The World Health Organization defines this as any time up to forty-two days after termination of pregnancy, irrespective of the duration of pregnancy or its outcome in a live birth, stillbirth, miscarriage, or abortion. Maternal mortality rates are very low in the industrial nations, reflecting high standards of care during pregnancy and childbirth. In countries where women have no other recourse than induced abortion to control their fertility, almost a million women die annually of puerperal causes—a terrible loss of life that could be prevented by easier access to family planning. Cultural, political, and religious opposition inhibits these societies from addressing this appalling problem.

Standardized Mortality Ratio (SMR). This is the ratio of the number of deaths observed in a specified population to the number that would be expected if that population had the same mortality rate as a standard population. The standard population is arbitrarily chosen; it may be a recent census year or an artificial, computer-generated one. The SMR is a very useful statistic, often used to compare outcomes in two or more groups under study.

Throughout the twentieth century, death rates fell steadily everywhere in the industrial nations, reflecting improved living conditions, greater longevity, and improved control over causes of premature death. A sad exception was the experience of the nations of Eastern Europe and the former Soviet Union after the collapse of communism. In these nations, social chaos and the decay of what was once a relatively efficient pubic-health system led to lethal epidemics of diphtheria and other communicable diseases that were previously controlled by immunization programs. This experience demonstrated the necessity of maintaining effective and efficient public health services.

JOHN M. LAST

(SEE ALSO: *Infant Mortality Rate; Maternal and Child Health; Perinatology; Rates; Rates: Adjusted; Rates: Age-Adjusted; Standardization [of Rates]; Vital Statistics*)

MULTI-DRUG RESISTANCE

The proliferation of drug-resistant strains of many pathogenic organisms is an increasing public health problem. Many pathogenic organisms develop antibodies, enzymes, or other metabolic means of adaptation to drugs such as antibiotics that initially are efficacious. For example, staphylococci, gonococci, and pneumococci have all evolved an enzyme that denatures penicillin, rendering it useless. The bacillus of tuberculosis has evolved strains resistant to all the first-generation drugs developed to combat it. The malaria parasite has evolved strains that resist antimalarial drugs. Insecticides such as DDT that were initially 100 percent effective in destroying insect vectors such as the anopheline mosquito are similarly rendered inefficacious. This has happened because of widespread, often indiscriminate use of these drugs (and insecticides). Not all the exposed pathogens are killed, and those that survive selectively breed to produce resistant strains.

JOHN M. LAST

(SEE ALSO: *Antibiotics; Drug Resistance; Pathogenic Organisms*)

MULTIFACTORIAL DISEASES

The simplest way to consider the cause of a disease is to think of it as occurring when a person is exposed to a pathogenic agent. In the nineteenth century, most people got typhoid, cholera, smallpox, or plague when they were exposed to the agents that caused these diseases. Whether or not a particular person actually got these diseases was, of course, affected by the pathogenicity of the agent and the susceptibility of the person to that agent. This disease paradigm led to the well-known epidemiologic triad of host, agent, and environment. But the emphasis in those days clearly was on pathogenic agents of overwhelming pathogenicity and virulence. In 1965, a famous microbiologist, Rene Dubos, pointed out that this way of thinking about disease agents was not as useful in modern times as it once was. He said that the microbial diseases most common today arise from the activities of microorganisms that are ubiquitous in the environment. These microorganisms are much less virulent, they often persist in the body without causing obvious harm, and they cause disease only when the infected person becomes vulnerable to them. This concept caused a shift in emphasis from the virulence and pathogenicity of disease agents to those factors that strengthen or weaken people's resistance to them.

This way of thinking about microbial diseases is just as relevant when people think about diseases caused by physiochemical and behavioral factors.

Consider cigarette smoking. There is no question that cigarette smoking enormously increases the risk of many diseases, including coronary heart disease. But is smoking the cause of these diseases? Many people who smoke cigarettes do not develop heart disease. Why are some people vulnerable to the disease agent (cigarette smoking) while other people are not? There clearly are other agents involved in the cause of this disease, and those studying this, or any other disease must consider a variety of disease agents that are involved in the causal chain. Since not one of them is the single and inevitable cause of the disease, they are referred to as "risk factors" for the disease; and diseases such as coronary heart disease are referred to as "multifactorial diseases." Most diseases of concern today are multifactorial diseases.

The problem faced with multifactorial diseases in public health is how to think about interventions to prevent them. How do those concerned with the prevention of coronary heart disease, for example, develop a strategy to prevent it? A focus on cigarette smoking only ignores other risk factors such as hypertension, high serum cholesterol, obesity, and physical inactivity. An expanded prevention program on these other risk factors, however, still does not solve the problem. If a multifactorial prevention program was developed that simultaneously focused on all the risk factors for coronary heart disease, and if everyone currently involved successfully lowered their risk, new high-risk people would continue to enter the population to take their place. This is because there is another, more fundamental layer of risk factors. For example, people in lower socioeconomic levels of society are at a higher risk for cigarette smoking, hypertension, elevated serum cholesterol, and obesity than those who are better off financially. Thus, even as one reduced the risk of people already at high risk, new people will continue to enter the at-risk population.

When dealing with the prevention of multifactorial diseases, there are many risk factors operating at many different levels. Some exist at the societal level, others at the community or neighborhood level, others at the level of individual behavior, and others at the biological level.

Prevention programs for multifactorial diseases must be designed to deal with as many of these levels as possible. This requires many disciplines working together. The success that has been achieved in reducing cigarette smoking in the United States has come about because of laws restricting smoking in designated areas, increases in taxes on cigarettes, limitations on advertising, increased understanding of the biology of addiction, and the development of effective methods for helping people stop smoking. Not one of these approaches could be successful on its own. Even with this impressive achievement, however, young people continue to take up cigarette smoking at high rates. Clearly, multifactorial intervention approaches are necessary to deal with multifactorial diseases, and a continued effort is needed to expand the reach of current prevention programs. These prevention programs will become even more important as the population continues to age and as medical care delivery systems become increasingly overburdened.

S. LEONARD SYME

(SEE ALSO: *Causality, Causes, and Causal Inference; Environmental Determinants of Health; Health Promotion and Education; Prevention; Risk Assessment, Risk Management; Social Determinants; Tobacco Control*)

BIBLIOGRAPHY

Cassel, J. (1976). "The Contribution of the Social Environment to Host Resistance." *American Journal of Epidemiology* 104:107–123.

Dubos, R. (1965). *Man Adapting*. New Haven, CT: Yale University Press.

MULTIPLE CHEMICAL SENSITIVITIES

Multiple chemical sensitivities (MCS), alternatively referred to as idiopathic environmental intolerances (IEI), is a term used to distinguish persons with medically unexplained symptoms—such as fatigue, concentration problems, headaches, and respiratory symptoms—when those symptoms are attributed to and/or triggered by environmental exposures. There is no other diagnostic label that concisely describes individuals who report such symptoms. The term sometimes encompasses individuals with pathologic (medically explained) conditions who attribute their diseases to chemical exposures, although mainstream academic opinion does not support this point of view.

The most widely cited definition for MCS (Cullen, 1987) includes the following four criteria: (1) the condition is acquired following a documented environmental exposure; (2) symptoms involve more than one organ system, and predictably recur and abate in response to environmental stimuli; (3) symptoms are elicited by chemical exposures that are demonstrable, but very low; and (4) the manifestations of MCS are subjective and without clinical evidence of explanatory organ system dysfunction. A common modification of these criteria does not require that the condition be acquired at a specific instance or from a specific putative exposure, allowing it to develop more gradually.

The classification and natural history of MCS is based to a large extent on the presence or absence of a diagnosable psychiatric condition such as affective disorders and anxiety disorders. Much higher rates (50–70%) of such diagnoses are present in those who meet MCS criteria than in controls, although not necessarily higher than in those with other medically unexplained-symptom syndromes, such as chronic fatigue syndrome (CFS). Lower rates of psychiatric conditions appear to be seen in those patients who report a clear defining episode at the onset.

The exact relationship between environmental exposures and symptoms of MCS has not been defined and has been difficult to study. During attempts at clinical trials, the specific odor of the inciting agent has interfered with the usual experimental design, in which the subject should be unaware of the exposure. A clinical follow-up study suggested that exposure reduction through avoidance improved well-being, although paradoxically did not reduce levels of symptoms. To date, no studies have shown MCS to be progressive in terms of physical dysfunction or medical complications.

The extent of MCS in the general population is unknown, as no population-based studies using the MCS clinical definition have been published. However, significant amounts of various MCS correlates, such as self-reported sensitivity to chemicals (15%) and self-reported receipt of a physician diagnosis of MCS (6%) have been reported in a rigorous population-based study from California, suggesting the problem is of appreciable magnitude. The presence of MCS symptoms in those diagnosed or labeled with CFS, fibromyalgia, and Gulf War syndrome is well established. No controlled epidemiologic studies have addressed the issue of etiologic exposures, although pesticide exposures, solvent exposures, and construction-related exposures are cited in some surveys and case discussions.

Etiologic theories embrace four major categories: pathologic and toxicologic; psychophysiologic; psychiatric; and belief systems. The majority of scientific support currently is for mechanisms primarily focused in the control nervous systems, such as conditioned responses to odors or variations of panic disorders.

How best to prevent MCS is unclear, as it depends upon knowing the mechanisms by which MCS originates and is exacerbated. If exposures act primarily through psychiatric, psychophysiologic, or perceptual mechanisms, then control of exposure may not be an appropriate paradigm for prevention. On the other hand, if certain exposures clearly lead to an excess risk for such symptoms, then prevention of exposure would be beneficial.

HOWARD M. KIPEN
NANCY FIEDLER

(SEE ALSO: *Environmental Determinants of Health; Gulf War Syndrome; Risk Assessment, Risk Evaluation.*)

BIBLIOGRAPHY

Cullen, M. R. (1987). "The Worker with Multiple Chemical Sensitivities: An Overview." In *Occupational Medicine: State of the Art Reviews,* Vol. 2, ed. M. Cullen. Philadelphia, PA: Hanley and Belfus.

Kipen, H. M., and Fiedler, N. (1999). "Invited Commentary: Sensitivities to Chemicals—Context and Implications." *American Journal of Epidemiology* 150:13–16.

—— (2000). "A 37-Year-Old Mechanic with Multiple Chemical Sensitivities." *Environmental Health Perspective* 108(4):377–381.

Kreutzer, R.; Neutra, R. R.; and Lashuay, N. (1999). "Prevalence of People Reporting Sensitivities to Chemicals in a Population-Based Survey." *American Journal of Epidemiology* 150:1–12.

MULTIPLE RISK FACTOR INTERVENTION TRIALS

A risk factor is part of the chain of causation leading to a disease and is a strong and independent predictor of excess risk. The idea of a controlled experiment to intervene with people at high risk of heart attack due to multiple elevated risk factors arose in the late 1960s.

Major risk factors for coronary heart disease (CHD), high blood pressure, high blood cholesterol level, and cigarette smoking had already been established by careful observational studies. The great public health question of the day was whether dietary modification to lower blood cholesterol levels could prevent heart attacks. Medical leaders concluded that it would not be feasible to carry out a definitive trial on this question due to the cost—and because dietary intervention would inadvertently influence other lifestyle risk factors. The search began, therefore, for a feasible alternative strategy of prevention.

In theory, controlled interventions in people without manifest CHD, but who have more than one major risk factor would: (1) test the hypothesis of whether prevention of CHD, with a reduction in total mortality is at all possible; and (2) provide the best likelihood of demonstrating quickly and efficiently the possibility of a major reduction in the incidence of heart attacks.

The theory and practical aspects of the multiple risk factor intervention trials (MRFIT) were first developed by prevention strategists in the United States, Richard Remington, Jeremiah Stamler, and Henry Taylor, who submitted to the National Institutes of Health in 1969 the first MRFIT proposal, nicknamed "JUMBO" because of its complexity. Reviewers were unable to arrive at consensus on its support, but because of the urgent need to answer its fundamental questions the MRFIT idea was widely adopted.

The World Health Organization organized one model of a MRFIT in which workers at industrial sites in Belgium and Britain were randomly assigned to comparative health promotion programs. In the United States, the National Heart,

Lung, and Blood Institute designed and organized a MRFIT which randomly assigned 12,866 men, thrity-five to fifty-seven years of age, with multiple elevated risk factors to special intervention programs (SI) or to "usual care" (UC). Similar programs were also pursued in Norway and other countries.

These ambitious MRFIT projects were carried out during the 1970s, coincident with a period of mass sociocultural change in health awareness and behavior, which, in turn, was accompanied by a precipitous fall in heart attack and stroke death rates in the industrial nations of the West. With the notable exception of the successful Oslo study, where, at the outset, cholesterol and smoking levels were extremely high and health awareness lower than elsewhere, the MRFIT studies were unable to demonstrate significantly reduced multiple risk factor levels or heart attack rates, over and above favorable changes occurring in their control groups. Thus, most of the scientific community regarded the MRFIT experiments as a failure. The investigators concluded, however, that the risk factor trends and heart attack rates were moving in a favorable direction—though within study designs too weak to reach significance. Long-term follow-up of the U.S. MRFIT and the Belgian MRFIT detected lower heart attack rates among the treated groups. Moreover, ongoing observational studies of U.S. MRFIT subjects greatly increased the understanding of relationships among lifestyle interventions, risk factors, and mortality.

The concept of reducing multiple risk factors to prevent heart attack and stroke remains intact because of the overwhelming observational evidence of the causal role of such risk factors. There is continued development of effective preventive practices and public health strategies for reducing risk levels, along with ongoing surveillance of population heart attack rates. Favorable national trends in health behaviors and multiple risk factor levels were accompanied by a steady and brisk decline in coronary death rates from the 1960s until the mid-1990s, when the rate of fall diminished. This was associated with a slowing of the reduction in risk factor levels, and with a failure of health promotion to reach underserved populations among the poor, the elderly, young people, and women. Preventive strategies are now directed not only at the highest multifactor risk segments of industrial societies but to whole countries at excess risk, and to

the prevention of elevated multiple risk factors in the first place—what is termed "primordial prevention."

HENRY BLACKBURN

(SEE ALSO: *Cardiovascular Diseases; Chronic Illness; Framingham Study; Multifactorial Diseases; Noncommunicable Disease Control; Observational Studies; Risk Assessment, Risk Management*)

BIBLIOGRAPHY

Gotto, A. M. (1997). "The Multiple Risk Factor Intervention Trial (MRFIT): A Return to a Landmark Trial." *JAMA* 277:595–597.

Multiple Risk Factor Intervention Trial Research Group (1982). "Multiple Risk Factor Intervention Trial: Risk Factor Changes and Mortality Results." *JAMA* 248:1465–1477.

MULTIPLE SCLEROSIS

Multiple sclerosis (MS) is a disorder that affects primarily the myelinated white matter of the central nervous system (CNS), the brain, optic nerves, and spinal cord. There is no known cause. Myelin is the fatty sheath that insulates nerve fibers (axons). Partial or complete loss of myelin due to MS impairs nerve conduction through affected axons, producing symptoms and functional impairment referable to them. Thus, MS may produce mild to severe weakness, lack of coordination, disordered sensations, partial loss of vision, impaired control of bladder and bowel function, impaired cognition, or any combination of these effects.

Early in the course of the disorder, symptoms are often brief and transient—impaired function caused by a particular episode, or relapse, tends to improve, in what is called a "remission." Remissions may be partial or total. However, over the course of years, incomplete recovery from relapses may occur, leading to the accumulation of impaired function and producing some degree of disability in about 70 percent of affected individuals. Among those who become disabled, some do not experience improvement from the beginning. However, it is important to realize that, although it is a common cause of disability among young to middle-aged individuals, MS is very unpredictable in a particular person; it does not necessarily disable and it does not necessarily shorten life span appreciably.

The average age of occurrence of the first symptom(s) is thirty-three, but MS may show itself as early as childhood or as late as age sixty or beyond. It affects almost twice as many women as men, and primarily in men and women of predominantly or mixed Caucasian parentage. Approximately 350,000 people in the United States have MS, and it is estimated to affect about 3 million people worldwide. However, MS is rare among South and East Asians, and among blacks in Africa. These differences suggest that susceptibility to develop MS may be genetically determined. However, among identical twins where one has MS, no more than 50 percent of the unaffected twins will go on to develop MS. This lends support to the concept that an environmental trigger, perhaps a viral infection, acts in concert with the genetic setting to produce MS. Siblings and children of those with MS have a somewhat greater chance of developing MS, but no specific genetic pattern has been identified. It is likely that multiple genes are involved in conferring susceptibility.

The frequency of MS has been studied closely since the 1930s. However, despite improved diagnostic methods (and improved treatment), the incidence (number of new cases per year in the population) does not appear to have increased.

Even after many years of intensive research, the cause of MS remains elusive, and it is a challenging subject for research. The most widely accepted hypothesis at this time is that an infection triggers an autoimmune response in genetically susceptible individuals. Autoimmunity implies that the body's immune-defense system erroneously and inappropriately attacks normal tissues, in this case the myelin and/or the cell that synthesizes and supports myelin, the oligodendrocyte.

Diagnosing MS is often very challenging. To do so involves documenting the occurrence of two or more episodes of impaired function, occurring at different times, that are referable to CNS white matter, while excluding all other possible causes of the problems. The fact that MS affects primarily the CNS white matter makes it possible to visualize very accurately areas of inflammation and demyelination via magnetic resonance imaging (MRI). MRI is an invaluable aid to diagnosis, although the MRI picture alone is not sufficient to be certain of the diagnosis. MRI is also used to identify new relapses, and to quantify the number and size of past episodes. Similarly, the cerebrospinal fluid typically shows alterations that may support a diagnosis, but a diagnosis cannot be made without appropriate clinical history and neurological examination.

Even though its cause is still mysterious, treatments have been developed that have reduced the number of relapses by more than 30 percent. These agents include recombinant interferon beta (IFNß; particular brand names include Avonex, Betaseron, and Rebif) and glatiramer acetate (Copaxone), each of which is widely used. Laboratory and clinical studies of many other possible treatments are underway, which is a very hopeful indicator of more effective therapies to come in the future. In addition to these disease-modifying agents, treatment often includes the use of medications intended for purely symptomatic relief, as well as physical therapy and occupational therapy. The challenges posed by an uncertain clinical course, and by chronic disability among some individuals, makes psychological support a key part of management.

The National Multiple Sclerosis Society (http://nmss.org/), similar organizations in other countries, and the International Federation of Multiple Sclerosis Societies (http://www.who.int/ina-ngo/ngo/ngo076.htm) are excellent sources of further information about the disorder, ongoing research, and treatment.

DONALD H. SILBERBERG

(SEE ALSO: *Environmental Determinants of Health; Genes; Genetic Disorders; Genetics and Health*)

BIBLIOGRAPHY

Burks, J. S., and Johnson, K. P., eds. (2000). *Multiple Sclerosis: Diagnosis, Medical Management, and Rehabilitation.* New York: Demos.

Figure 1

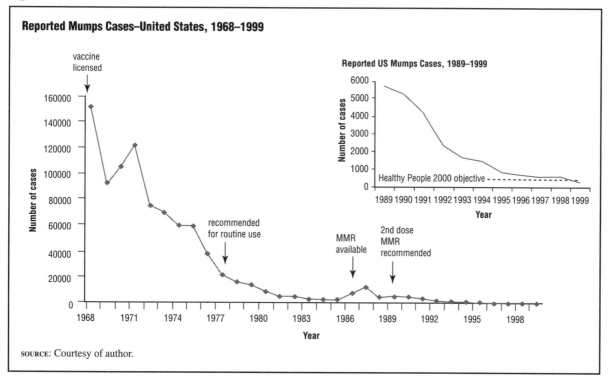

Reported Mumps Cases–United States, 1968–1999

SOURCE: Courtesy of author.

Paty, D. W., and Ebers, G. C., eds. (1998). *Multiple Sclerosis*. Philadelphia, PA: F. A. Davis.

MUMPS

Mumps is an acute infectious disease caused by a paramyxovirus. Humans are the only known natural host. Mumps disease is usually mild, characterized by fever and swelling of one or both parotid salivary glands. The parotiditis usually develops an average of sixteen to eighteen days after direct contact, through the nose or mouth, with the saliva of an infected individual. In approximately 20 to 40 percent of cases, however, mumps disease occurs asymptomatically or with an uncharacteristic presentation.

Even though mumps is regarded as a fairly benign disease in the twenty-first century, in the prevaccine era mumps caused much morbidity and mortality in the United States. In 1967, mumps accounted for over one-third of encephalitis cases and one death occurred out of approximately 20,000 mumps cases. Mumps infection during pregnancy is not associated with birth defects, but infection during the first trimester is associated with a greater occurrence of fetal death. Other conditions caused by mumps include meningitis, orchitis, mastitis, pancreatitis, neuritis, arthritis, nephritis, thryroiditis, pericarditis, and deafness.

Mumps parotiditis occurs equally among males and females. Severe mumps disease, however, such as encephalitis, has been observed to occur more frequently among boys than girls. Other gender-specific manifestations are also influenced by age. After puberty, orchitis commonly occurs among males, though sterility rarely results. Among post-pubescent females, mastitis is a common manifestation.

Mumps infection can be confirmed by isolation of the virus from throat swabs, urine, or spinal fluid. Blood tests to detect antibodies to mumps virus can be used to differentiate between a current mumps infection and a previous infection. Skin testing is not reliable.

In countries without mumps vaccination, epidemics occur every two to five years, affecting most frequently those ages five to nine. Mumps disease exhibits seasonally with more cases occurring during the winter and spring. Historically, mumps outbreaks occur in situations where individuals are grouped together, such as military camps, prisons, boarding schools, and aboard ships. In community outbreaks, school-aged children are often infected first and then infect family members at home.

The mumps virus was first identified in 1934. By 1948 a killed virus vaccine was licensed, but it was later discontinued because it did not produce long-lasting immunity. The current mumps vaccine in the United States is a live, attenuated vaccine (the Jeryl-Lynn strain) licensed in December 1967. Since introduction of the Jeryl-Lynn mumps vaccine, the reported number of mumps cases in the United States has decreased dramatically, from over 150,000 in 1968 to 387 cases in 1999 (see Figure 1).

The availability of this vaccine, the use of the combination measles, mumps, and rubella (MMR) vaccine beginning in 1986, and the two-dose recommendation in 1989 of MMR has immunized many children who would have otherwise have developed mumps disease.

LAURIE KAMIMOTO

(SEE ALSO: *Communicable Disease Control; Immunizations*)

BIBLIOGRAPHY

American Academy of Pediatrics (2000). "Mumps." In *2000 Red Book: Report of the Committee on Infectious Diseases*, 25th edition, ed. L. K. Pickering. Elk Grove Village, IL: American Academy of Pediatrics.

Baum, S. G., and Litman, N. A. (2000). "Mumps Virus." In *Principles and Practice of Infectious Diseases*, 5th edition, eds. G. L. Mandell, J. E. Bennett, and R. Dolin. Philadelphia: Churchill Livingstone.

Plotkin, S. A., and Wharton, M. (1999). "Mumps Vaccine." In *Vaccines*, 3rd edition, eds. S. A. Plotkin and W. A. Orenstein. Philadelphia, PA: W. B. Saunders.

MUNICIPAL SOLID WASTE

The estimates of North American garbage production are staggering: The average American disposes of over 3.5 kilograms of trash each day, up more than 50 percent since 1970. The health implications of solid waste include the pollutant burden contributed by various forms of waste management (including incineration, composting, etc.). The "green" approach emphasizes the three Rs: reduction, reuse, and recycling. Alternatives such as incineration and landfills are viewed as unhealthful. However, removal of hazardous materials such as mercury-containing batteries by source separation has had substantial success in reducing toxic emissions from incinerators.

There are many ways to collect garbage, and many ways to process it. Landfills and ocean dumping have long been the mainstay of solid waste management, but these are being phased out. Limitation of disposal options has resulted in long-distance transportation of garbage from urban areas to locales where it can still be disposed of.

THE WASTE STREAM

Solid waste comes from various sources. The following are estimated percentages for New York City. Municipal solid waste (residential, institutional, commercial, and industrial): 55 to 60 percent by weight; construction and demolition waste: 15 to 20 percent (hazardous materials such as asbestos should be separated); sewage sludge: 1 to 2 percent; medical waste (including potentially infectious material): 1 to 2 percent; and harbor debris: less than 1 percent. Dredge spoil can make up to 15 to 20 percent of the waste in a coastal city with a harbor. Other forms of waste that can vary by location include agricultural waste, mining waste, and hazardous waste.

Waste streams differ in the following attributes: (1) physical (e.g., compactibility, density); (2) combustion (temperature, residual ash percentage, heat content in BTUs); (3) chemical composition percentage of nitrogen, carbon, oxygen, chlorine; and concentrations of toxic polyaromatic hydrocarbons (PAHs) and metals; (4) potential for recycling various components; and (5) ease of separation.

A comprehensive waste management program must combine a variety of social, transportation, and treatment technologies. Social issues involve the acceptability of particular programs such as mandatory recycling. Components, in order of desirability, include prevention of wastes at the source; reuse, recycling, or composting; energy recovery; and putting in a landfill only those materials not amenable to other strategies. The plan should consider impacts on air quality, water quality, traffic, noise, odor, socioeconomic effects, and community acceptance.

Developing and evaluating a comprehensive waste management system requires confidence that existing health standards are adequately protective, that all components are maintained and operated according to specifications, and that monitoring and enforcement will work.

WASTE TREATMENT

There are more than thirty technological approaches to managing solid waste. One of the most common is incineration, which requires a burner and often a supplemental source of fuel. The temperature and the residence time of the waste in the burner determine the efficiency with which organic matter is converted to carbon. Noncombustible material, particularly metals, accumulate in the ash and must be removed—either to landfills or for incorporation into concrete and other construction products. As organic matter cools in the stack, unwanted products such as dioxins may also form.

Composting allows organic material to undergo biodegradation and photodegradation, resulting in simple organic molecules that can actually be beneficial to the environment.

Recycling and reuse are likely to be effective for those materials that find a ready market. In both the public and private sector, procurement practices can be controlled by fiat or by incentives to minimize waste. Consumer education programs play a large role in reducing waste, particularly in conjunction with community recycling programs. Incentives for source reduction should encourage replacement of disposables with reusable supplies and equipment.

HEALTH RISKS

Health risks involve contamination of soil and water by leachate from landfills and by emissions of toxic materials from incinerators. The latter include particulates; sulfur dioxide and oxides of nitrogen; hydrogen chloride and hydrogen fluoride; carbon monoxide; chlorinated products, including dioxins and furans; metal residues in ash; and volatile organic compounds, including acrolein and phosgene.

POLLUTION CONTROL DEVICES

Standards governing emissions can be health based, but they are often based on technological considerations including the best available control technology (BACT) and the lowest achievable emission rate (LAER). Filters (e.g., baghouses), electrostatic precipitators, scrubbers, and other devices are used to remove metals and volatile material from the stack prior to emission into the environment. Unfortunately, there are very few published data on emissions from which the efficiency of pollution control devices can be documented.

IMPLICATIONS FOR SITING

Regardless of the choice of technology, siting of a facility should take into account certain considerations. Sites should minimize proximity to residential areas, unrelated workplaces, and exposure to sensitive terrestrial and aquatic ecosystems, and they should be of adequate size to minimize exposure to surrounding communities. An adequate distance should be kept from high-rise buildings to reduce the impact on elevated receptor populations, and stack height is also an important element (higher stacks allowing material to dispose further, thereby achieving dilution). Nearby communities should be involved in the earliest stages of planning, including a clear presentation of the cost/benefit and risk/benefit considerations. An assurance of adequate maintenance and safe operation can be backed up by posting a bond with the community, allowing it to monitor a facility and even shut it down under certain circumstances.

MICHAEL GOCHFELD

(SEE ALSO: *Community Health; Hazardous Waste; Landfills, Sanitary; Mercury; Not In My Backyard [NIMBY]; Pollution*)

BIBLIOGRAPHY

Gochfeld, M. (1995). "Health Implications of Solid Waste Management." In *Environmental Medicine*, eds. S. Brooks, et al. St. Louis, MO: Mosby.

New York City Department of Sanitation (1991). *Solid Waste Management Plan: Environmental Impact.* New York: Author.

Travis, C. C., and Hattemer-Frey, H. A. (1991). *Health Effects of Municipal Waste Incineration.* Boca Raton, FL: CRC Press.

MURDER

See Homicide

MUSCULOSKELETAL DISORDERS

Musculoskeletal disorders are among the most common of human afflictions. They affect all age groups and frequently cause disability, impairments, and handicaps. They consist of a variety of different diseases that cause pain or discomfort in the bones, joints, muscles, or surrounding structures, and they can be acute or chronic, focal, or diffuse. Approximately 33 percent of U.S. adults are affected by musculoskeletal signs or symptoms, including limitation of motion or pain in a joint or extremity. In one study of Detroit residents who kept track of daily health symptoms in a diary, musculoskeletal symptoms constituted the most frequent category of health symptoms. The prevalence of musculoskeletal disorders generally increases with age, with the majority of persons aged seventy-five and over having some form of musculoskeletal disorder, especially arthritis.

Not only are musculoskeletal disorders highly prevalent, but, because of their association with aging, they are likely to become more prevalent as the population ages throughout the world. All racial groups are affected. While many of these disorders are not devastatingly disabling to affected individuals, their prevalence is so great that more mobility and other limitations are accountable to these disorders than to any other type. While much of the substantial cost of these disorders is due to the medical care and medications and other treatments required by patients, the preponderance of costs is due to work loss, which is a frequent consequence of these disorders.

Contained within the broad category of musculoskeletal disorders are a number of specific diseases and causes of pain, several of which affect a large percentage of the population. Musculoskeletal disorders range from back pain to rheumatoid arthritis and gout, and include different types of arthritis, tendinitis, and musculoskeletal pain. The most common musculoskeletal disorders are listed in Table 1, along with their point prevalence among adults in Western populations. The most prevalent disorders are low back pain, osteoarthritis, and so-called soft tissue rheumatism. Even though they afflict millions of persons around the world, several of the common musculoskeletal disorders fall into the category of moderately prevalent, including gout, a form of episodic arthritis; fibromyalgia, a disorder of diffuse muscular pain and a subtype of soft tissue rheumatism; and rheumatoid arthritis, an inflammatory systemic disorder that causes widespread joint pain.

LOW BACK PAIN

Low back pain, one of the most frequent of musculoskeletal disorders, affects up to 80 percent of people sometime in their lives, and in any given month 20 to 30 percent of adults have an episode. Generally, the pain is in the lower back on one or both sides, occasionally extending into the buttocks or thighs. In most persons the cause of back pain is unknown. It may arise from any number of pain-sensitive structures in the lumbar spinal column, including joints, ligaments, muscles, and soft tissues.

Generally, back pain is episodic, with half of the episodes remitting within a week and 90 percent going away within a month. Back pain of long duration, which occurs in only a small minority of patients, accounts for most of the societal cost of low back pain and much of the work loss and disability. Persons at high risk of low back pain include those between age twenty and forty, and those whose jobs involve physical labor—especially lifting, pushing, or pulling heavy objects, or twisting during lifting. Truck drivers are the occupational group who experience the most back pain. Another risk factor for low back pain is cigarette smoking, and poor physical fitness may also contribute to its occurrence. The high rate of back pain in particular occupations has suggested

Table 1

> **The Most Common Musculoskeletal Disorders in Adults Aged 45 Years And Older: Point Prevalence in Adult Populations in Western Europe and the U.S.**
>
> **Extremely common (prevalence > 5%)**
> Low back pain
> Osteoarthritis
> Tendinitis or bursitis
>
> **Common (prevalence 0.5-5%)**
> Gout
> Fibromyalgia
> Rheumatoid arthritis
>
> SOURCE: Felson, D. T. "Epidemiology of the Rheumatic Diseases." *Arthritis & Allied Conditions*, W. Koopman, ed. New York: Lippincott, Williams and Collens, 2000.

that altering work tasks may be a successful way to prevent episodes of back pain. Indeed, industry training programs have achieved success in lessening the rate of low back pain in some occupations.

OSTEOARTHRITIS

Osteoarthritis is the most common form of arthritis and, depending on how it is defined, affects 10 to 20 percent of all adults and a much larger percentage of the elderly.

SOFT TISSUE RHEUMATISM

Among the most common of musculoskeletal disorders are those which cause pain in muscular or tendinous areas of the extremities but not in joints. These are collectively termed "soft tissue disorders" and include a variety of localized forms of tendinitis and bursitis, as well as other more generalized pain disorders. These disorders are common causes of pain in the shoulder, elbow, hip, neck, and foot.

Muscles are attached to the bones they move by string-like structures called tendons. While soft tissue pain can often be localized to particular muscles and their attached tendons, the cause of this pain is poorly understood. For tendinitis, the cause may be related to muscle and tendon overuse. For shoulder and neck pain, overuse may be coupled with an acute or chronic injury. These disorders are often self-limited and respond to anti-inflammatory medications, but they often recur. Seven percent of the U.S. population has had an episode of shoulder pain lasting at least a month. Ten percent of the population reports neck pain of this duration. The prevalence of most of these disorders increases with age, and they are more prevalent in women than men.

Fibromyalgia is a generalized chronic disorder of diffuse muscular pain that constitutes a subtype of soft tissue rheumatism. Fibromyalgia affects up to 2 percent of women of all ages (it is much less prevalent in men) and is associated with a sleep disorder; with diffuse aching in the neck, back and extremities; and with fatigue and depressive symptoms (either as a trigger of the disorder or as a consequence of it). Treatment includes analgesic and sleep medications.

DAVID T. FELSON

(SEE ALSO: *Osteoarthritis; Rheumatoid Arthritis*)

BIBLIOGRAPHY

Felson, D. T. (2000). "Epidemiology of the Rheumatic Diseases." In *Arthritis & Allied Conditions*, ed. W. Koopman. Philadephia, PA: Lippincott, Williams & Collens.

MYOCARDIAL INFARCTION

See Coronary Artery Disease

N

NARCOTICS

See Addiction and Habituation

NATIONAL ACADEMY OF SCIENCES

The National Academy of Sciences (NAS) is a private, nonprofit, self-perpetuating society of distinguished scholars engaged in scientific and engineering research, dedicated to the furtherance of science and technology and to their use for the general welfare. Upon the authority of the charter granted to it by the Congress in 1863, the NAS has a mandate that requires it to advise the federal government on scientific and technical matters.

It carries out its work largely through committees of pro bono experts who employ an evidence-based, deliberative process to produce scientifically valid, nonpartisan reports. Studies originate in several ways: by Congress mandating that a federal executive branch agency contract with the NAS; by direct request of executive branch agencies, private foundations, or other private organizations; or as self-initiated projects when the academy determines that an important or highly sensitive issue might not be the subject of a request from an outside organization. Last, in addition to committee studies, NAS plays a unique convening role by sponsoring workshops, roundtables, symposiums, forums, and other activities that enable parties on all sides of an issue to come together and discuss problems and solutions in a neutral, unbiased setting. Dr. Bruce Alberts is the current president of the National Academy of Sciences.

Members and foreign associates of the academy are elected in recognition of their distinguished and continuing achievements in original research; election to the academy is considered one of the highest honors that can be accorded a scientist or engineer. The academy membership is comprised of approximately 1,900 members and 300 foreign associates, of whom more than 170 have won Nobel Prizes.

The academy is governed by a council comprised of twelve members. The Council is responsible to the membership for the activities undertaken by the organization and for the corporate management the National Academy of Sciences, a corporation created by an act of Congress that also includes the National Academy of Engineering (NAE), the Institute of Medicine (IOM), and the National Research Council (NRC). It has delegated the governance of the National Research Council to the NRC Governing Board, which includes members of the Councils of the NAS, NAE, and IOM.

The full text of National Academy of Sciences publications is available online at the National Academy Press web site, www.nap.edu. Additional information about the institute and its activities, as well as a list of all publications, can be found at http://www.national-academies.org.

KENNETH I. SHINE

NATIONAL AMBIENT AIR QUALITY STANDARDS

The U.S. Clean Air Act of 1970 called for the establishment of outdoor standards for those air pollutants for which adverse health effects have been shown to occur as a result of outdoor air pollution. Currently, six pollutants are regulated under this heading: ozone, sulfur dioxide, particulates, nitrogen dioxide, carbon monoxide, and lead. For each of these pollutants an ambient standard has been established by the Administrator of the U.S. Environmental Protection Agency (EPA), following a thorough review of the scientific evidence.

This review is overseen by the Clean Air Scientific Advisory Committee (CASAC), whose congressionally mandated advisory role requires it to publicly evaluate the science underlying the association between an air pollutant and its adverse effects, paying attention to the basic toxicology, animal studies, controlled human exposure studies, and the epidemiological evidence. CASAC then recommends to the EPA Administrator a pollutant level or range of levels and durations of exposure at which no adverse effects are believed to occur. The EPA Administrator then sets the standard based upon this information, including within the standard an adequate margin of safety for sensitive populations, as required by the Clean Air Act. The language of the act also requires the EPA Administrator to pay no attention to economic, social, political, or other considerations associated with the management activities required to meet the standard. These can be considered, however, when choices are made as to how to most effectively decrease air pollutant levels that exceed the ambient standard. The ability of the EPA to develop standards based on science has been recently reaffirmed by a U.S. Supreme Court decision upholding the new particulate and ozone standards.

The duration of exposure on which the National Ambient Air Quality Standards (NAAQS) are based is to a large extent dependent upon the toxicology of each particular compound: the eight- to twelve-hour equilibration period for carbon monoxide in the human body is the basis for the eight-hour carbon monoxide standard, and the recognition of the longer-term effects of ozone has been instrumental in the recent switch of the ozone standard from a one-hour to an eight-hour averaging time. An unusual but valuable aspect of the Clean Air Act is the requirement to revisit each standard every five years. This has spurred additional research and review, which has led to revision of air pollutant standards.

Management of air pollutant levels that exceed the standards is done by each state, with oversight by the EPA. This oversight includes guidance for the positioning of air pollutant monitoring equipment so as to ensure that potential hot spots are not missed. Once it is established that a state has an air pollutant measurement that exceeds the allowable standard, it is required to develop a state implementation plan that details the approach it will take to meet the standard. This is updated yearly as needed. The failure to develop and adhere to the implementation plan puts the state in jeopardy of losing federal funding, although this rarely occurs.

BERNARD D. GOLDSTEIN

(SEE ALSO: *Ambient Air Quality [Air Pollution]; Carbon Monoxide; Clean Air Act; Environmental Protection Agency; Lead; Sulfur-Containing Air Pollutants [Particulates]*)

NATIONAL ASSOCIATION OF COUNTY AND CITY HEALTH OFFICIALS

The National Association of County and City Health Officials (NACCHO) is a national organization representing local U.S. public health agencies. NACCHO's mission is to promote national policy, develop resources and programs, and support effective local public health practice and systems that protect and improve the health of people and communities.

NACCHO was established in 1994 with the merging of the U.S. Conference of Local Health Officials and the National Association of County Health Officials. Both of the two predecessor organizations were founded in the 1960s. NACCHO's members are local public health agencies, also called local health departments, in the United States. NACCHO serves the 3,000 local health departments in the country; over 1,100 local health departments, serving 75 percent of the U.S. population, are active, dues-paying members of NACCHO.

The organization's headquarters are in Washington, D.C., where the work of the organization is organized by a staff of about fifty. Local health departments are represented on NACCHO's thirty-two-member board of directors by local health officials (usually the chief executive) elected by the membership. Over three hundred local health officials serve on a variety of NACCHO advisory committees and national workgroups addressing a wide variety of public health issues.

NACCHO provides a number of services, ranging from professional meetings for local health officials to the development of tools to enhance local practice, and from public advocacy of national policies of importance to local practitioners to timely research on topics of relevance. NACCHO works closely with a number of federal partners, including the Health Resources and Services Administration (HRSA), the Centers for Disease Control and Prevention (CDC), the Agency for Toxic Substances and Disease Registry (ATSDR), the Environmental Protection Agency (EPA), and the National Highway Traffic Safety Administration (NHTSA). NACCHO receives a significant portion of its operating revenues through the development of tools and services funded by these federal partners to benefit local public health practice. Examples include community assessment tools (APEX*PH*, PACE-EH), work on public health capacity issues (workforce development, accreditation, performance standards, information technology), and a variety of projects in key practice areas (tobacco use prevention, clean indoor air, brownfields, maternal and child health, food safety, safe communities, hepatitis-C prevention, rural health, and bioterrorism preparedness). NACCHO generates reports and provides training in many of these areas.

NACCHO also serves as the National Program Office for the W.K. Kellogg Foundation's Turning Point project. This project provides technical support and resources to forty-one community partnerships located in fourteen states around the county. The partnerships are working through collaborative partnerships to transform and strengthen their local public health systems to better protect and improve the health of their communities.

THOMAS L. MILNE

(SEE ALSO: *Association of State and Territorial Health Officials; Community Health; Mobilizing for Action through Planning and Partnerships*)

NATIONAL ASSOCIATION OF LOCAL BOARDS OF HEALTH

The idea for a national organization serving the interests of local boards of health was conceived at the 1991 American Public Health Association (APHA) meeting in Atlanta, Georgia. At that time, representatives of six state associations of local boards of health (Georgia, Illinois, Massachusetts, North Carolina, Ohio, and Utah) and the Washington State Board of Health recommended the formation of a national organization of local boards of health.

During 1992, a steering committee developed bylaws and processed the appropriate applications to create a non-profit organization known as the National Association of Local Boards of Health (NALBOH). At the 1992 APHA meeting, bylaws were ratified and the first officers and Board of Trustees were elected. NALBOH:

- Represents the interest of all local boards of health.

- Establishes and maintains communication nationally with state associations of boards of health, local boards of health, public health organizations, agencies, and elected officials.

- Promotes, identifies, or provides public health information, education and training for local board of health members, designed to improve their effectiveness in establishing sound public health policy.

NALBOH maintains a database on 3,178 local boards of health. A national survey conducted by the Centers for Disease Control and Prevention and NALBOH profiled the boards' makeup, responsibilities, and needs. To meet information and educational needs, NALBOH publishes (and distributes) a quarterly, *Newsbrief*, to all boards of health. An educational conference, designed to address the needs of board of health members, is held annually. In addition, specific topical programs and materials have been developed. Topics have included "Making Effective Public Health Policy" and leadership presentations. Guides on Tobacco Control Authority, Environmental Health, Establishing a Local Board of Health and Developing a State Association of Local Boards of Health have been prepared.

In cooperation with other national health organizations and agencies, NALBOH participates in the development of national public health policies and performance standards relevant to local boards of health.

The membership of NALBOH consists of local boards of health, tribal boards of health, state boards of health, state associations of boards of health, and individuals who share the concept of citizen boards of health.

NALBOH is governed by an Executive Board consisting of 13 members: President, President Elect, Past President, Secretary, Treasurer, seven Regional Trustees, and two State Affiliate Trustees. The Executive Board is elected by the Institutional and Affiliate members at the NALBOH Annual Education Conference.

An Executive Director and full-time staff is maintained at the NALBOH Administrative office in Bowling Green, Ohio. A Director of Liaison and Governmental Relations is housed in Washington, D.C.

NED E. BAKER

NATIONAL ASTHMA EDUCATION AND PREVENTION PROGRAM

The National Asthma Education and Prevention Program (NAEPP) was established in March 1989 by the National Heart, Lung, and Blood Institute, a component of the U.S. National Institutes of Health. Its objectives are threefold: (1) to raise awareness among patients, health professionals, and the public that asthma is a serious chronic disease; (2) to ensure that symptoms of asthma are recognized by patients, families, and the public, and that appropriate diagnosis is made by health professionals; and (3) to ensure effective control of asthma by encouraging a partnership among patients, physicians, and other health professionals, using modern treatment and education programs.

Asthma ranks among the most common chronic conditions in the United States, affecting about 17 million persons of all ages, races, and ethnic groups. This chronic inflammatory disease of the airways is characterized by recurrent episodes of breathlessness, wheezing, coughing, and constriction in the chest. Asthma can range in severity from mild to life-threatening. It is one of the leading illness-related causes of school absenteeism, accounting for over 10 million missed school days annually, and it is the leading work-related lung disease.

Interest in asthma as an important cause of morbidity and mortality was not new in 1989 when the NAEPP was launched. The National Institutes of Health had, in fact, supported research on asthma for many years. What was new was scientific evidence that chronic airway inflammation is the underlying mechanism that leads to asthma—a finding that suggested an entirely different approach to treatment—and the demonstration by behavioral scientists that health education programs based on a sharing of responsibility by patients and their families with a physician can be very effective in promoting optimal management of asthma.

In establishing the NAEPP, the National Heart, Lung, and Blood Institute built upon its considerable experience with other health-education programs (e.g., the National High Blood Pressure Education Program, begun in 1972, and the National Cholesterol Education Program, begun in 1985). It was clear that addressing the problem of asthma would require coordinated, multidisciplinary efforts among research scientists, health care providers, public health personnel, and patient advocates. The NAEPP was developed under the auspices of a coordinating committee with representatives from thirty-six major medical associations, voluntary health organizations, and federal agencies with an interest in asthma. The committee continues to provide input on program strategies and materials development, and its participating organizations are directly involved in implementation of many activities.

In 1991, the NAEPP published its *Expert Panel Report: Guidelines for the Diagnosis and Management of Asthma*. This landmark document set the stage for nationwide improvement in clinical management of asthma. It changed common perceptions about asthma and its treatment by emphasizing the role of inflammation in disease development, noting the importance of objective monitoring of lung function, and stressing the need to establish partnerships between patients and health care providers through patient education. More than 300,000 copies were distributed to physicians, health professionals, and medical schools. To promote broad use by health professionals involved in asthma care, strategically targeted companion documents were developed for nurses, emergency department personnel, pharmacists, and school personnel.

The *Expert Panel Report* also stimulated new research that so significantly increased knowledge about effective approaches to asthma care that a second expert panel was convened in 1995. Its report, *Expert Panel Report 2: Guidelines for the Diagnosis and Management of Asthma*, published in 1997, remains the most accurate, up-to-date source of information for clinicians on asthma diagnosis and management.

The guidelines developed by the NAEPP translate research findings into recommendations for patient care. There is now substantial scientific evidence that the guidelines, when followed, lead to a significant reduction in the frequency and severity of asthma attacks, and the majority of patients can live fully active lives. Outreach and education programs, especially targeted to high-risk populations at the community level, are an essential part of the NAEPP effort to ensure full utilization of the guidelines. Interventions to facilitate access to medical care and appropriate financial support for medication, monitoring aids, and environmental control measures are critical for reducing the burden of asthma. These needs are being actively addressed through a partnership with community-based asthma coalitions.

CLAUDE LENFANT
SUZANNE HURD

(SEE ALSO: *Asthma; National Institutes of Health*)

NATIONAL CENTER FOR HEALTH STATISTICS

The National Center for Health Statistics (NCHS), the United States federal government's principal vital and health statistics agency, is organizationally part of the U.S. Department of Health and Human Services' Centers for Disease Control and Prevention (CDC). Created in 1960 by the merger of the National Office of Vital Statistics and the National Health Survey, the agency monitors the nation's health.

NCHS systems develop a wide variety of information (including data) on health status, lifestyle, and exposure to unhealthy influences, the onset and diagnosis of illness and disability, and the use of health care. These data are important to policymakers in government, to medical researchers, and to others in the health community.

The agency's principal data systems include the National Vital Statistics System, the National Health Interview Survey, the National Health and Nutrition Examination Survey, the multiple component National Health Care Survey, the National Survey of Family Growth, the Longitudinal Studies of Aging, and the National Immunization Survey, among others. The agency has also developed surveys for collecting health-related data on a state and regional basis.

The Public Health Service Act affords NCHS specific legislative authority to protect the confidentiality of its information. In addition, the act mandates NCHS to undertake and support research, demonstrations, and evaluations regarding its activities, and to provide technical assistance to state and local jurisdictions.

To meet its data needs, NCHS works closely with other federal agencies, state and local governments, researchers in biomedical and public health institutions, as well as researchers in the private sector.

EDWARD J. SONDIK

(SEE ALSO: *National Health Surveys; Vital Statistics*)

NATIONAL DEATH INDEX

The National Death Index (NDI) was implemented in 1982 to facilitate retrospective and prospective studies in medical and health research by reducing the time, expense, and effort involved in ascertaining information about deaths, either for an entire study population or just for those subjects who could not be contacted. The NDI is a national, computerized index of death record information compiled from computer files submitted to the National Center for Health Statistics (NCHS) by each state's vital statistics office. The NDI contains records on virtually all deaths in the United States since 1979. About 2.4 million death records are added to the file each year.

A researcher or investigator desiring access to NDI data must submit an official application form. (The NDI is not accessible to organizations or the general public for legal, administrative, or genealogy purposes.) Once the application is approved, the investigator is instructed to submit a computer file containing identifying information on each study subject. This file is to be prepared in a specified format and then mailed to NCHS on diskette or CD-ROM. Investigators are strongly encouraged to compile as many of the NDI data items as possible: first and last name, middle initial, father's surname, Social Security number, date of birth, state of birth, state of residence, sex, race, marital status, and age at death (if known). NCHS searches this information against records in the NDI database and sends the investigator a report showing which records generated one or more possible matches with NDI records. The NDI also provides the state of death and the death certificate number for each possible match. It is the investigator's responsibility to assess the match results and to determine which are true matches based on the data items that agree or disagree. The investigator may then contact state vital statistics offices for copies of the relevant death certificates to confirm the matches or obtain information such as the cause of death.

Beginning in 1997, the NCHS obtained authorization from each state vital statistics office to enhance the NDI service by also releasing the cause of death codes for close matches. This new service is called NDI Plus. The codes are derived from the World Health Organization's *International Classification of Diseases* for both the underlying and multiple causes of death.

The NDI has been used for a variety of studies, including occupational health studies where workers exposed to hazardous chemicals or low-level radiation are tracked over time. It has been used for tracking participants in cohort studies of health problems and clinical trials of new treatments; for tracking subjects of cancer registries to determine outcomes; and for the U.S. National Longitudinal Mortality Study, where a sample of over 2 million persons drawn from Census Bureau surveys are tracked over time.

ROBERT BILGRAD

(SEE ALSO: *Mortality Rates; Vital Statistics*)

BIBLIOGRAPHY

Acquavella, J. F.; Donaleski, D.; and Hanis, N. M. (1986). "An Analysis of Mortality Follow-up through the National Death Index for a Cohort of Refinary and Petrochemical Workers." *American Journal of Industrial Medicine* September:181–187.

Boyle, C. A., and Decoufle, T. (1990). "National Sources of Vital Status Information: Extent of Coverage and Possible Selectivity in Reporting." *American Journal of Epidemiology* 131(1):160–168.

Calle, E. E., and Terrell, D. D. (1993). "Utility of the National Death Index for Ascertainment of Mortality among Cancer Prevention Study II Participants." *American Journal of Epidemiology* 137(2):235–241.

Edlavitch, S. A.; Feinleib, M.; and Anello, C. (1985). "A Potential Use of the National Death Index for Postmarketing Surveillance." *Journal of the American Medical Association* 253(9):1292–1295.

National Center for Health Statistics (1997). *National Death Index User's Manual.* Washington, DC: NCHS.

Patterson, B. H., and Bilgrad, R. (1986). "Use of the National Death Index in Cancer Studies." *Journal of the National Cancer Institute* 77(4):877–881.

Sathiakumar, N.; Delzell, E.; and Abdalla, O. (1998). "Using the National Death Index to Obtain Underlying Cause of Death Codes." *Journal of Occupational and Environmental Medicine* 40(9):808–873.

NATIONAL DISEASE AND THERAPEUTIC INDEX

The National Disease and Therapeutic Index (NDTI) is a commercial data resource maintained by IMS Health, in Plymouth Meeting, Pennsylvania. This resource was developed in 1958 to provide representative data on the population for whom drugs are prescribed, as well as the prescribers, in the United States. Analogous data resources are maintained by this company in many other countries.

The basic data is gathered in an ongoing fashion from a panel of 3,700 physicians selected to represent a statistical sample of practicing physicians. Since a large proportion of practitioners are primary-care providers (e.g., general practitioners or internal medicine specialists), these groups are well sampled. Smaller specialty groups, such as ear, nose, and throat physicians, are sparsely represented.

Each panel physician records data every quarter for a two-day period, using a special duplicate prescription form for all drugs prescribed. When a prescription is written, not only is the usual information (drug name, amount, dosing instructions and duration) written, but also the indication for the drug, the patient's gender and age, the site of prescription (hospital, clinic, etc.), other drugs the patient is taking, other diagnoses, and some physical exam and laboratory data. This data, excluding patient identification, is provided to the company for inclusion in the database.

This NDTI database provides an ongoing national estimate of the pharmaceutical prescribing practices in the United States. This data is expressed as "mentions" of a pharmaceutical, since the information on pharmaceuticals is mentioned in both the actual prescription as well as concomitant therapy. Accordingly, this information does not provide a precise estimate of the frequency of prescribing any product due to the nature of the methodology. Frequency data (e.g., number of prescriptions dispensed per quarter) is available in other databases that sample very large numbers of dispensed prescriptions at retail pharmacies. Nonetheless, because of the careful sampling of practitioners, the actual numbers of mentions are extrapolated to provide approximate national estimates of the characteristics of patients *exposed* to specific drug products and other products they are using.

This data includes information primarily on prescription pharmaceutical products, although there is some information on over-the-counter concomitant therapy. There is little information on other therapies or herbal drugs used by patients. Due to the sample, this data resource's information is most reliable in describing therapies in relatively common use by primary care physicians. It is more limited for use in describing prescription or patient characteristics typical of specialty practices such as urology or plastic surgery.

NDTI data is most often used by pharmaceutical manufacturer's marketing departments. Post-marketing surveillance and drug safety groups both within and outside the pharmaceutical industry also use this data to estimate the characteristics of populations for both epidemiological studies and for developing exposure denominators for pharmaceutical benefit and risk assessment.

JUDITH K. JONES

(SEE ALSO: *Personal Health Services; Pharmaceutical Industry*)

NATIONAL ENVIRONMENTAL POLICY ACT OF 1969

By the 1960s it had become clear that human activities were producing profound effects on the natural environment. The National Environmental Policy Act of 1969 (NEPA) was the first comprehensive environmental law enacted in the United States, and it established a broad national framework to:

- Encourage productive and enjoyable between man and his environment.

- Promote efforts which will prevent or eliminate damage to the environment and biosphere and stimulate the health and welfare of man.

- Enrich the understanding of the ecological systems and natural resources important to the nation.

- Establish a Council on Environmental Quality.

Specifically, NEPA requires that agencies assess the environmental impacts of significant activities such as the construction of airports, buildings, military complexes, and highways; parkland purchases; and other proposed federal activities. Environmental Assessments (EAs) and Environmental Impact Statements (EISs), which are assessments of the likelihood of impacts from alternative courses of action, are required from all federal agencies and are the most visible NEPA requirements.

The Council on Environmental Quality (CEQ) is based in the Executive Office of the President, and the chair of the CEQ reports to the president. The president must file an Environmental Quality Report to Congress each year. The CEQ has the job of assisting the president with preparation of this report, along with a number of responsibilities related to gathering information and developing national policies on the environment.

Soon after its establishment, the CEQ played a major in the establishment of the Environmental Protection Agency (EPA), in 1970, and since that time it has continued to be the voice for the environment within the White House. The CEQ serves as a forum for the settlement of disputes about environmental policy within the federal government where various cabinet agencies and White House offices come together to resolve issues over major policies. While the administrator of the EPA and the secretary of the interior are the most visible public figures with environmental responsibility within the federal government, the director of CEQ often serves in an advisory capacity to the president of the United States.

Perhaps one of the most important consequences of NEPA was to require that every federal agency incorporate environmental considerations into decision making. This began a process of incorporating environmental information into the work of agencies that had no prior environmental expertise and made protecting the environment and natural resources an objective of all federal agencies. As a result, most U.S. agencies have an expert staff to assess the environmental consequences of their actions.

The NEPA also served as a precedent that influenced environmental legislation in the fifty states and in other countries. The notion of an environmental impact assessment for significant activities has been incorporated into numerous other legislative efforts—often with other requirements, such as public hearings and approval processes. This in turn has increased the involvement of stakeholders in environmental decisions in many parts of the world.

LYNN R. GOLDMAN

(SEE ALSO: *Environmental Impact Statement; Environmental Protection Agency; Pollution*)

NATIONAL HEALTH INSURANCE

Proposals for a national health insurance system were heard as early as 1912, when President Theodore Roosevelt's Progressive Party platform (following the example of Germany and other European nations) called for "the protection of home life against the hazards of sickness, irregular employment and old age through the adoption of a system of social insurance adapted to American use." Shortly thereafter, the American Association for Labor Legislation (AALL) formed a Committee on Social Insurance comprising prominent members of the American Medical Association (AMA) and others. The committee recommended a compulsory plan covering the majority of workers.

Efforts to enact the AALL plan at the state level failed, largely due to opposition from organized medicine and other conservative elements that considered it a harbinger of radical social change. The AMA initially called the plan the "inauguration of a great social movement" (1917), but rapidly changed course and consistently opposed mandatory health insurance since that time. In 1920 the AMA House of Delegates resolved to oppose "any plan embodying the system of compulsory insurance which provides for medical service to be rendered contributors or their dependents provided, controlled or regulated by any state or the federal government." The labor leader Samuel Gompers joined in opposition, apparently fearing that benefits gained through legislation rather than negotiation would be vulnerable to later repeal or limitation.

In 1927 President Calvin Coolidge appointed a Committee on the Cost of Medical Care, funded by a consortia of foundations, led by Carnegie and

Millbank. The committee documented the severe and widespread problems Americans faced in obtaining and paying for medical care. The Committee called for care provided through group practice, paid for by insurance or taxation. The AMA attacked the plan a "socialism and communism—inciting to revolution." The stock market crash and onset of the Great Depression in 1929 vastly increased the number of Americans who could not afford basic medical care.

Franklin D. Roosevelt campaigned for the presidency in 1934 on a platform that promised aggressive government action to relieve the massive social and economic dislocations created by the Great Depression. Health insurance was included in a long list of problems facing the nation. Shortly after election, he named a cabinet-level Committee on Economic Security to look into "all forms of social insurance." Health insurance was included in a long list of problems facing the nation. However, the AMA's unrelenting opposition to any public health insurance again frustrated action. The President's advisors reasoned that organized medicine could hold the entire Social Security bill hostage. They recommended that, instead of including a health component, the President offer a study of health insurance options. The Social Security Act passed in 1935 with no mention of health care, but authorizing the study of actions the government might take to assure the economic security of older citizens. Subsequent Social Security Board reports called for health insurance, hospital construction grants, grants to states for indigent care, and health insurance programs. These recommendations formed the basis of the Murray-Wagner-Dingell bill.

President Harry S. Truman endorsed the Murray-Wagner-Dingell bill in 1945 and asked Congress to enact compulsory health insurance funded by payroll deductions. AMA opposition killed the bill. After Truman's upset victory in 1948, the AMA voted a special assessment of members to "resist the enslavement of the medical profession." Truman failed to win legislation, but did develop a plan to provide sixty days of free hospital care for aged Social Security beneficiaries. This idea later became the core of insurance benefits under Medicare.

The 1960 Democratic Party Platform endorsed medical care benefits for the aged under Social Security. Shortly after taking office, President John F. Kennedy made health insurance his priority domestic issue in the New Frontier. AMA reaction was rapid and predictable. Insurance companies joined in opposition. However, public response to Kennedy's 1962 rally in Madison Square Garden made it clear that health insurance had popular support. Kennedy was assassinated before Congress seriously considered his proposal. The political climate created by the Kennedy assassination was masterfully exploited by President Lyndon B. Johnson. Johnson's overwhelming defeat of Barry Goldwater in 1964 and the simultaneous election a large Democratic majority in Congress set the stage for enactment of the Great Society programs, starting with Medicare. Johnson made health insurance his top legislative priority. On July 28, 1965, Medicare and Medicaid became law, providing Social Security–based coverage for hospital and physician services to the aged, and a program of matching federal grants to states for coverage of physician, hospital and nursing home services for the poor. In a symbolic gesture, Johnson signed the bill in Independence, Missouri, joined by former President Truman.

Medicare and Medicaid rapidly changed the structure of health care in the United States. Millions of aged and poor, received services for which physicians and hospitals were fully reimbursed. This new revenue stream supported modernization of the nation's hospitals and creation of technology intensive academic medical centers. Federal involvement in the medical system also desegregated hospitals and other institutional providers. Rapid growth in national health expenditures followed—more than doubling within five years, a pattern that continued for the next twenty-five years. The pressures of this growth on public programs and privately held insurance created an unlikely alliance of interests for enactment of health insurance to expand coverage and contain costs.

In 1969 Walter Reuther, president of the United Auto Workers, formed a Committee of 100 for National Health Insurance, an alliance of labor unions and liberals activists. Reuther launched a national effort to develop and enact comprehensive health insurance. Senator Edward M. Kennedy became the leading Congressional supporter of the resulting Health Security Plan, launching his continuing role as the most consistent Congressional advocate for comprehensive national health insurance. Public and Congressional support for national health insurance legislation strengthened. President Richard M. Nixon declared his support and submitted an administration bill. For a short time in the early 1970s, a cross-party political consensus emerged that might have proved strong enough to achieve legislative action. However, the liberal-labor coalition fell apart over Kennedy's efforts to compromise with the administration and moderates in Congress. Shortly thereafter, the Watergate scandal and Nixon's resignation effectively closed the window.

President Jimmy Carter's election in 1976 reopened the debate. The Carter administration developed a plan—Health Security—that combined requirements for employers to offer health insurance to their employees with an expansion of the Medicare and Medicaid programs. Health costs were to be contained through high patient out-of-pocket spending requirements. Senator Kennedy and Representative Henry Waxman advanced their own bill—Health Care for All Americans Act— that combined a national health budget with insurance plans offered to all employers and individuals through a consortia of companies. With the Democrats in disarray, and historic opposition by organized medicine, business, the insurance industry, and conservative Republicans, any possibility of legislative action was doomed. In the aftermath of this failure, there were modest expansions of Medicaid coverage for pregnant women and children, and the introduction of new Medicare reimbursement methods for hospitals, a largely futile effort to contain hospital costs.

In the Ronald Reagan and George Bush administrations (1981–1993) the focus of health policy was largely on cost containment rather than expanding coverage. However, additional modest expansions of Medicaid emerged from the Democratic Congress. During this period the number of uninsured Americans continued to grow. Importantly, during the 1990–1991 recession, large numbers of middle class Americans lost jobs and insurance coverage, fueling new political support for health care reform.

President Bill Clinton made health reform the centerpiece of his presidential campaign, and after his 1992 election designated his wife, Hillary Rodham Clinton, to lead Administration efforts to design and enact a national health insurance bill.

On September 22, 1993, Clinton addressed a joint session of Congress to describe the plan, historically named "Health Security." The Clinton plan combined familiar elements of previous health insurance proposals with complex and novel ideas for cost containment and management of insurance competition. The core concept would have mandated employer purchased coverage through "accountable" provider plans contracting with state-regulated consumer alliances. Public funds would subsidize low-wage employers, the self-employed and near-poor. The alliances would manage competition to assure access and risk pooling. Congress was initially friendly to the plan, but its complexity, inept management of the political process by the administration, and well financed, vociferous opposition by insurance companies health plans and organized medicine combined to defeat the Clinton effort. The after-effects of the health care reform debacle helped elect the conservative 1994 Republican Congress. These developments created a political climate in which Teddy Roosevelt's goal of a national system to assure access to a health insurance for all Americans could not be achieved, and unleashed a market-driven reform of health care delivery, dramatically changing the practice of medicine. At the end of 1999, an estimated 44 million Americans remained uninsured.

SUSANNE A. STOIBER

(SEE ALSO: *Health Care Financing; Medicaid; Medicare; Poverty and Health; Uninsurance*)

NATIONAL HEALTH SURVEYS

The United States is unique in having several national health surveys. Other countries have good surveys, but for the most part they are not national and one must assume that, for example, the southeast part of a country is like the northwest. Because the United States has national surveys, we know whether the southeast is, or is not, like the northwest. That provides us a great advantage in formulating policy for a country as large and diverse as the United States. For this article, four national surveys and one state-based survey have been selected to illustrate the kinds of impact each can have. The basis for this choice was that each of the surveys has a unique design feature that makes its impact different from the others, each is household based, each covers the total noninstitutionalized population, and each is old enough to have had a demonstrable impact.

NATIONAL HEALTH INTERVIEW SURVEY

The oldest of the population-based surveys is the National Health Interview Survey (NHIS), conducted by the National Center for Health Statistics (NCHS) at the Centers for Disease Control and Prevention (CDC). The National Health Survey Act was signed into law by President Eisenhower on July 4, 1956; and the NHIS went into the field precisely one year later. It's unique design feature is that it is a continuing survey, with each weeks' sample capable of producing national estimates. This design immediately proved its worth. When the flu epidemic hit in the fall of 1957, the NHIS was able to produce weekly estimates of the number of incident cases—the first time immediate data on cases, not deaths, were available. A few years later, the NHIS data were critical in formulating the new Medicare and Medicaid programs. Estimates of the conditions of the people covered and the costs of those programs were still not precise, but they were far better than they would have been without the NHIS.

The original intent of the NHIS was to estimate the incidence of acute conditions, the prevalence of chronic ones, and the use of medical care. Over time, supplemental questionnaires were added to the base questionnaire and some of those supplements have contributed the main impact of the NHIS. The Child Health Supplements, the Supplement on Aging, the Supplement on Disability, and the Cancer Supplements have all been used by their sponsoring agencies to monitor their missions and implement new programs.

By the late 1970s, the CDC had shifted its focus to the prevention, rather than the cure, of disease. In 1979, *Healthy People: The Surgeon General's Report on Health Promotion and Disease Prevention* appeared. This was followed, in 1980, by another report, *Promoting Health/Preventing Disease: Objectives for the Nation*. That report outlined 226 health goals (*Healthy People 2010* contains 467 goals). Progress toward these goals was to be assessed by data. Most of the data, especially in that first decade, came from the NHIS. Even in *Healthy People 2010*, the NHIS provided data for more goals (73) than any other data source. Again the unique survey design of the NHIS served well; it was the only survey that was repeated every year and that had a core of unchanging questions that could be used to monitor change.

A second design feature of the NHIS is that while the base questionnaire changes relatively little, there are supplemental modules that enable the survey to be used to answer immediate and important policy questions. Some of these modules have also been used as the basis for longitudinal studies such as the Longitudinal Study of Aging.

NATIONAL HEALTH AND NUTRITION EXAMINATION SURVEY

Even when the NHIS was first in the field, its designers knew that respondents can report only what they know and what they are willing to report, and that there was a need for data based on objective standardized physical examinations. Yet the only physical data on the health of the American people came from the draft examinations, which were far from standardized. Therefore, the National Health and Nutrition Examination Survey (NHANES) was created with the unique feature that mobile examination centers were moved around the country so that the examinations and their environments were constant; the only thing allowed to vary was the people being examined. NHANES has had an impact on both policy and practice. The growth charts (which have recently been modified) have influenced well-baby care all over the world. Charting blood-lead levels over time and across population groups resulted in Environmental Protection Agency changing the schedule for removing lead from gasoline from a gradual phaseout to removing the lead at once. The standardized measures over time have enabled the National Heart Lung and Blood Institute to monitor the levels of blood pressure and cholesterol in the United States population. The availability of "normal" measures of many elements of human physiology have revised the textbook standards that, before NHANES, were dependent on such populations as twenty prisoners in a state prison.

During their early years, these two surveys were conducted by the U.S. Bureau of the Census (the NHIS still is), which was reluctant to ask sensitive questions because of the possible impact on the decennial census. Yet the need for data on the so-called sensitive topics was increasing and had to be met.

NATIONAL HOUSEHOLD STUDY ON DRUG ABUSE

In 1971 and 1972, the National Commission on Marijuana and Drug Abuse sponsored the first two studies of what is now the National Household Survey on Drug Abuse (NHSDA) sponsored by the Substance Abuse and Mental Health Services Administration. The NHSDA added two unique features. First, it was, and is, a completely anonymous survey. Second, adolescents were both oversampled and responded for themselves. Recently, it has added another feature; it is the only nationally administered survey designed to produce estimates for each state. Like the NHIS, it is a repeated cross-sectional survey, making it very useful in tracking short-term changes. In addition to informing policy, the NHSDA has changed policy. The NHSDA data showing that most users of illicit drugs are employed led to many workplace initiatives such as Executive Order 12564, that established a drug-free federal workplace in 1986. The substantial increase in use of illicit drugs by youths in the early 1990s along with data showing the relationship between marijuana use and use of harder drugs led to a major emphasis on preventive activities.

MEDICAL EXPENDITURE PANEL SURVEY

One of the interesting aspects of the legislation enabling the NHIS was that it encouraged research in survey methods. Partly because of that research it became increasingly obvious that respondents did not recall all of the medical care they or their families had received in the past year. A better method was needed to provide good estimates of the costs of medical care. For that reason a new survey was born in 1977 at the University of Chicago, a survey that is now the Medical Expenditure Panel Study (MEPS) sponsored by the Agency for Healthcare Research and Quality. The MEPS added two new dimensions to the basic household survey. The first was that instead of asking people to remember all their medical care for the past year, people were interviewed several times so that they had a shorter recall period. The second was that instead of expecting people to remember precisely what their medical insurance covered, or what was done at each medical visit, an insurance component and a medical provider component were conducted to obtain that information from the insurance or medical provider. That is, the MEPS is four surveys in one: a household component, a medical-provider component, an insurance component, and a nursing-home component. The nursing-home component adds another unique feature, all of these surveys are of the civilian noninstitutionalized population. Having the nursing-home component at least makes inclusion of the older population, the people who are most likely to use medical services, complete.

The MEPS impact on policy has always been great and has increased as issues such as the cost of medical care and the proportion of the uninsured population have grown as policy issues. One of the early discoveries from the MEPS was that the proportion of the population uninsured *at some time* during the year was much greater than the proportion uninsured at any one time. That led to a complete reassessment of the uninsured population of the United States. Recent contributions to policy have been estimating the number of children who are eligible for, but not enrolled in, Medicaid; estimating the potential number of children eligible for the State Children's' Health Insurance Program (SCHIP); examining racial and ethnic disparities in medical insurance coverage over the past decade; examining whether medical insurance is an impediment to job mobility; and the potential for participation in medical savings accounts.

There are other population surveys of selected segments of the population. The National Survey of Family Growth, up to now a survey of women of child-bearing age but soon to include men, has informed the government on many aspects of population policy, including the characteristics of people who adopt children. The Health and Retirement Survey, a collaborative project between the National Institute of Aging and the Survey Research Center at the University of Michigan, is a survey of men and women approaching retirement age designed to study the health and economic predictors of their retirement decisions. The Survey of Income and Program Participation, conducted by the U.S. Bureau of the Census, is a longitudinal survey designed to understands people's movement into and out of public programs.

These are all surveys in which the interviewer goes to the individual's home to conduct the interview. Such surveys are expensive. As the cost of conducting household interviews increased, interest in telephone surveys also increased. New techniques for overcoming problems such as multiple telephones in a single household, and techniques for scheduling calls were developed, and telephone surveys are now more widely used than personal interview surveys. They have some disadvantages for health research because the people who are least likely to have telephones are poor people—and they are also most likely to be sick or to have problems accessing medical care. However, used wisely, they can enable data collection that would not be financially possible with household surveys.

BEHAVIORAL RISK FACTOR SURVEILLANCE SYSTEM

One example of a telephone survey is the Behavioral Risk Factor Surveillance System (BRFSS). It is also a repeated cross-sectional survey like the NHIS and the NHSDA, but unlike them it is a system of state surveys that are coordinated by the National Center for Chronic Disease Prevention and Health Promotion at the CDC. The decision as to what questions will be on the next year's questionnaire is made at an annual conference attended by the state coordinators and CDC staff. There is a core of questions asked in all states, optional questions on selected topics that are asked in many states, and space for questions of major interest to that state or, sometimes, a group of neighboring states. The impact on national policy is to provide evidence of the sometimes remarkable differences among the states in important policies, such as smoking. The impact in states that actually use the data is that the states for the first time have data that are relevant to their own state policies. Many states are now using the data for substate areas, such as health planning areas.

These surveys have been in existence for more than a decade because they have proved their worth. Each fills a niche and has a rather fixed formal structure. Yet each has flexibility built into it so that in addition to fulfilling their primary purpose, they can be used to respond to immediate as well as long-term questions.

MARY GRACE KOVAR

(SEE ALSO: *Behavioral Risk Factor Surveillance System; Health Goals; Healthy People 2010; National Center for Health Statistics; Survey Research Methods; Surveys*)

NATIONAL HEALTH SYSTEMS

In every country there is a "national health system," the characteristics of which are determined by historical departments, the country's economic level, and the policies of its government. To some extent in all countries, there is a free market in which private health services to individuals are bought and sold. At the same time, governments intervene in this market to attempt to assure appropriate health services to part or all of the population.

The structure of a national health system has five principle components: resource production, organization of programs, economic support, management, and delivery of services. Within each of these components, there are various activities and functions. These are indicated in Figure 1.

The extent to which governments intervene in the free market of private health services permits a national health system to be classified along a scale that varies from low to high intervention. If we pose four steps in the scaling, they range from national health systems that are (1) very entrepreneurial to (2) welfare-oriented to (3) universal and comprehensive to (4) socialist. This scaling may apply to health systems in countries of different economic levels. If we scale economic levels in three steps, there results a matrix of 12 cells. This is shown, with illustrative countries indicated in each cell in Table 1.

In the twentieth century there was a tendency of national health systems throughout the world to evolve from column 1 to column 2 and from column 2 to column 3. Column 3 (universal and comprehensive health systems) is the most enduring, and systems in column 4 (socialist systems)

Figure 1

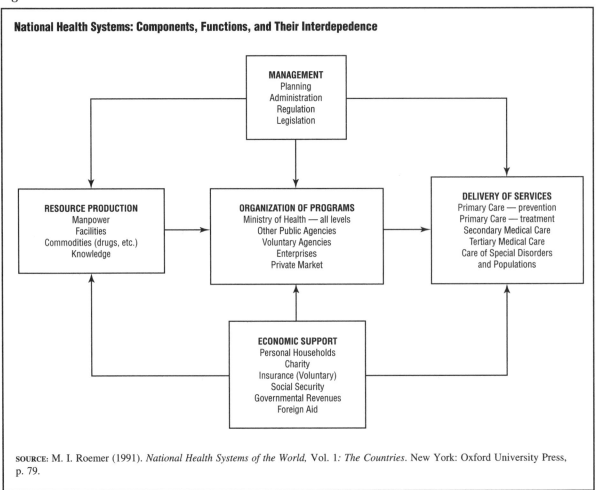

National Health Systems: Components, Functions, and Their Interdepedence

SOURCE: M. I. Roemer (1991). *National Health Systems of the World,* Vol. 1: *The Countries.* New York: Oxford University Press, p. 79.

tend to move in the other direction toward column 3. These trends mean that national health systems are achieving increasing equity for the populations they serve, without involving the complete control by government, implicit in the socialist health systems. The trends are also associated with an improvement in health status in virtually every country, as reflected by an extension of life expectancy at birth.

Trends in life expectancy at birth have shown improvement throughout the world. Considering the 30-year period from the mid-1950s to the mid-1980s, the trends in major world regions are shown in Table 2. Perhaps the most interesting feature of these data is that the improvement in all industrialized countries (from 65.7 to 72.3 years) was by 10.5 percent, while the improvement in all developing countries (from 41.0 to 57.6 years) was by 40.4 percent. In spite of the greater relative progress in the developing countries, of course, the advantages of life in the industrialized countries are still considerable.

These trends are due to actions in both the private and public sectors of national economies. Over recent decades the share of gross national product (GNP) devoted to the health system has increased in all countries. In the United States, for example, it rose from 5.3 percent of GNP in 1960 to 11.2 percent in 1987. In Honduras the share of GNP devoted to the health system rose from 5.1 percent in 1970 to 6.0 in 1976.

The proportion of health expenditures derived from governmental sources has also been increasing over the years. In the United States, for

Table 1

National Health Systems: Types Classified by Country's Economic Level and System's Health Policies, around 1986

Economic Level of Countries (GNP per capita)	Health System Policies (Market Intervention)			
	Entrepreneurial	Welfare-Oriented	Comprehensive-Universal	Socialist
High	USA	Germany	Britain	Poland
Medium	Philippines	Peru	Israel	Cuba
Low	Ghana	India	Tanzania	China

SOURCE: M. I. Roemer (1991). *National Health Systems of the World*, Vol. 1: *The Countries.* New York: Oxford University Press, p. 97.

Table 2

Life Expectancy at Birth in Major World Regions, 1950–1985

Region	Life Expectancy in Years	
	1950–1955	1980–1985
Africa	38.0	49.9
South Asia	38.8	54.4
East Asia	42.7	68.4
United States	73.0	75.0
Latin America	51.2	64.5
All Developing Countries	41.0	57.6
All Industrialized Countries	65.7	72.3
World Total	**45.9**	**59.6**

SOURCE: United Nations, Department of International Economic and Social Affairs (1989). *World Population Prospects 1988* (Population Studies No. 106). New York: U.N., pp. 166–189.

example, this share rose from 24.5 percent in 1960 to 41.1 percent in 1987. In Japan, governmental sources of health system expenditures were 60.0 percent in 1960, rising to 73.5 percent in 1987. Among developing countries the equivalent trend cannot be reported due to lack of data. A somewhat comparable trend can be noted in the proportion of central government budgets derived from public (compared with private) sources. In Uruguay, for example, this increased from 1.6 percent in 1972 to 4.8 percent in 1986, while in Bolivia over the same span of years it declined from 6.3 to 1.4 percent. Percentages, of course, can be deceptive; actual health spending for health in Bolivia continued at about the same level while the denominator of total government expenditure was rising.

The long-term meaning of these various trends suggests an improvement in health service equity throughout the world. Health care has been of rising importance in national economies, which is reflected by increasing shares of such expenditures being derived from governmental sources. This has led to gradual improvement of the health status of populations worldwide.

MILTON I. ROEMER

(SEE ALSO: *Barefoot Doctors; Inequalities in Health; International Development of Public Health; International Health; United States Agency for International Development [USAID]*)

BIBLIOGRAPHY

Roemer, M. I. (1991). *National Health Systems of the World,* Vol. 1: *The Countries.* New York: Oxford University Press.

—— (1993). *National Health Systems of the World,* Vol. 2: *The Issues.* New York: Oxford University Press.

United Nations, Department of International Economic and Social Affairs (1989). *World Population Prospects 1988* (Population Studies No. 106). New York: U.N.

U.S. Public Health Service, Office of Disease Prevention and Health Promotion (1988). *Disease Prevention/ Health Promotion: The Facts.* Palo Alto, CA: USPHS.

NATIONAL HIGH BLOOD PRESSURE EDUCATION PROGRAM

The National High Blood Pressure Education Program (NHBPEP) was established in 1972 by the National Institute of Health to translate research results on the health hazards of high blood pressure into clinical and public health practice. Before 1900, high blood pressure, or hypertension, was not generally recognized as a health problem. Only when a practical method of clinical blood pressure measurement emerged in the early 1900s were associations made between hypertension and subsequent morbidity and mortality. Those associations were confirmed by actuarial statistics, correlating blood pressure levels of life insurance policy holders with subsequent death rates. The associations were also confirmed by observation studies such as the National Heart, Lung, and Blood Institute's Framingham Heart Study, which routinely collected information regarding the health status of an entire community. These data showed that as blood pressure rose, deaths from stroke, heart disease, and all causes began to increase. The higher the blood pressure, the greater the chance of dying from a heart attack or stroke.

The first controlled clinical trial to test the efficacy of blood-pressure–lowering drugs was designed to occur during a five-year period. The results were so successful that the study was stopped at eighteen months. Those receiving blood-pressure–lowering drugs had fewer cardiovascular events than those taking a placebo. Lowering blood pressure saved lives.

The goal of the NHBPEP is to reduce death and disability through programs of professional, patient, and public education. The aim is to raise public awareness about hypertension, to urge hypertensive patients to follow their doctor's advice, and to have clinicians use the available scientific information. The strategies include developing and disseminating educational materials and programs that are grounded in a strong science base and developing partnerships among the program participants. Throughout its history, the NHBPEP has worked to mobilize and coordinate the resources of organizations. The NHBPEP is a network of federal agencies, voluntary and professional organizations, all state health departments, and numerous community-based programs. At the hub of the program is the NHBPEP Coordinating committee, composed of representatives from thirty-eight national professional, public, and voluntary health organizations and seven federal agencies. The program follows a consensus-building process to identify major issues of concern among the participants and to develop program activities. Representatives from the member organizations work together to provide guidance to the program and each other, as well as to develop and promote activities to their own constituencies. This multidisciplinary committee also defines national priorities, examines critical issues, explores future opportunities, sponsors national activities, and promotes collaboration among the program partners.

The Coordinating Committee agencies encompass a wide distribution network, supporting a mass media campaign and distribution of educational materials and documents. Among their publications are posters, public service announcements, patient education brochures, and clinical guidelines. Additional activities include designing public health interventions to address the excessive stroke mortality in the Southeast United States; publishing reports describing best treatment practices to control hypertension; conducting demonstration projects at the work site and in urban and rural settings; developing reports and intervention programs regarding hypertension among special populations or situations (e.g., African Americans, hypertensive patients with renal disease or diabetes, children and older Americans); and promoting population strategies for the primary prevention of hypertension.

The effectiveness of the NHBPEP can be measured in several ways. In 1972, the year the program began, less than one-fourth of Americans knew of the relationship between hypertension and stroke and heart disease. By 1990, nearly 90 percent of the public knew of that relationship. In 1971, only 51 percent of Americans with hypertension were aware of their condition, only 39 percent were being treated, and only 16 percent had achieved satisfactory control. Two decades later, the corresponding figures were 84, 73, and 55 percent respectively. Since the inception of the NHBPEP, death rates for strokes decreased by nearly 60 percent and heart disease by nearly 50 percent. These improvements are real, are seen in both genders, and in African Americans and whites. The story of efforts to detect, control, and prevent hypertension is one of the great public health successes of the second half of the twentieth century.

EDWARD J. ROCCELLA

(SEE ALSO: *Blood Pressure; Framingham Study; National Institutes of Health; Stroke*)

BIBLIOGRAPHY

Chairman, Sheps S. (1997). "The Sixth Report of the Joint National Committee on Prevention, Detection, Evaluation, and Treatment of High Blood Pressure." *Archives of Internal Medicine* 157 (November 24):2413–2446.

The Society of Actuaries and Association of Life Insurance Medical Directors of America (1979). *Blood Pressure Study 1979.* Chicago.

Veterans Administration Cooperative Study Group on Antihypertensive Agents (1967). "Effects of Treatment on Morbidity in Hypertension I: Results in Patients with Diastolic Blood Pressures Averaging 115 through 129 mmHg." *Journal of the American Medical Association* 202:1028–1034.

—— (1970). "Effects of Treatment on Morbidity in Hypertension: II. Results in Patients with Diastolic Blood Pressure Averaging 90 through 114 mmHg." *Journal of the American Medical Association* 213:1143–1152.

NATIONAL INSTITUTE FOR OCCUPATIONAL SAFETY AND HEALTH

The National Institute for Occupational Safety and Health (NIOSH) is the primary federal agency conducting research on the safety and health of the workplace. NIOSH is part of the Centers for Disease Control and Prevention in the U.S. Department of Health and Human Services. The Institute was established in 1971 by the Occupational Safety and Health Act (OSH Act) of 1970 to provide research, information, education, and training in the field of occupational safety and health. To conduct its programs, NIOSH draws from several public health disciplines, including industrial hygiene, epidemiology, nursing, engineering, medicine, statistics, psychology, the social sciences, and communication.

NIOSH develops and promotes the use of national and state-based surveillance systems to identify, quantify, and track injuries and illnesses. Epidemiological analyses of these databases help identify unsafe or unhealthy workplace conditions. NIOSH also supports laboratory and field research to further identify, assess, and control occupational hazards and exposures and the diseases and injuries they cause. The research is conducted both intramurally by NIOSH personnel and extramurally through research grants and cooperative agreements. In 1996, NIOSH and more than five hundred other organizations and individuals enhanced these collaborations by establishing the National Occupational Research Agenda (NORA) to guide occupational safety and health research on a broader scale. NORA provides a framework of priorities for both intramural and extramural research programs.

In addition to identifying risks, NIOSH develops and evaluates prevention measures such as control technology, personal protective equipment, and work practices. NIOSH assesses potential health problems at worksites upon the request of employers, employees, and other government entities. These evaluations often identify new occupational health problems and provide the industry-wide expertise needed to target prevention initiatives.

NIOSH uses the knowledge gained from research, surveillance, and prevention efforts to deliver critical information to workers, employers, the public, and the public health community. The institute produces and disseminates various informational materials, including policy and criteria documents, technical and surveillance reports, and educational documents. NIOSH also evaluates the effectiveness of worker training programs to ensure that the messages of workplace safety and health are effective for individual workers.

As directed by the OSH Act, NIOSH works to maintain adequate numbers of occupational safety and health professionals and researchers by establishing, strengthening, and expanding graduate and undergraduate educational programs and special training grants.

For further information contact NIOSH at 1–800-35-NIOSH (1–800-356–4674) or visit the NIOSH web site, http://www.cdc.gov/niosh.

JULIE M. BRADLEY

(SEE ALSO: *Occupational Disease; Occupational Safety and Health; Occupational Safety and Health Administration*)

BIBLIOGRAPHY

Rosenstock, L., and Cullen, M. R. (1994). *Textbook of Clinical Occupational and Environmental Medicine.* Philadelphia, PA: W. B. Saunders.

U.S. Department of Health and Human Services, Public Health Services, National Institute for Occupational Safety and Health (2000). *Worker Health Chartbook, 2000.* Cincinnati, OH: National Institute for Safety and Health.

NATIONAL INSTITUTE OF ENVIRONMENTAL HEALTH SCIENCES

The National Institute of Environmental Health Sciences (NIEHS) was founded in 1969. Its mission is to reduce the burden of disease caused by environmental factors through defining how environmental exposures affect human health and how individuals differ in their susceptibility to exposures. The focus of NIEHS is on disease prevention rather than on treatment, which tends to characterize the mission of the other Institutes within the National Institutes of Health.

NIEHS has its headquarters and intramural laboratories in North Carolina, in close proximity to research laboratories of the Environmental Protection Agency. The NIEHS extramural program funds individual competitive research grants and a variety of research centers throughout the United States. These include generalized Centers of Excellence as well as research centers focused on hazardous waste and on children's health and the environment. In recent years the NIEHS has extended its grants and centers program beyond basic laboratory science to a broader range of public health disciplines and activities, including K–12 programs, community outreach activities, and international environmental health. NIEHS also administers the National Toxicology Program (NTP) which, in concert with other federal agencies, evaluates the hazards of chemicals.

BERNARD D. GOLDSTEIN

(SEE ALSO: *Environmental Determinants of Health; Environmental Impact Statement; Environmental Protection Agency; Exposure Assessment; National Institutes of Health; Toxic Substances Control Act; Toxicology*)

NATIONAL INSTITUTE ON AGING

The National Institute on Aging (NIA), one of twenty-five institutes and centers of the U.S. National Institutes of Health, was established in 1974 to support biomedical, behavioral, and social research on aging processes and the diseases, problems, and needs of older people. The mission of the NIA is to improve the health and well-being of older Americans. In addition to providing support for research and research training through the award of grants, the NIA offers free information to the public through the National Institute on Aging Information Center (NIAIC), the Alzheimer's Disease Education and Referral (ADEAR) Center, and through various publications, including *Age Pages*, which is a collection of fact sheets on different topics, and numerous informational booklets.

JEAN S. KUTNER

(SEE ALSO: *AARP; Alzheimer's Disease; Medicare*)

NATIONAL INSTITUTE ON DRUG ABUSE

The National Institute on Drug Abuse (NIDA) was established by Congress in 1974, and it became part of the National Institutes of Health of the U.S. Department of Health and Human Services in October 1992. NIDA's mission is to lead the nation in bringing the power of science to bear on drug abuse and addiction. This charge has two critical components: The first is the strategic support and conduct of research across a broad range of disciplines. The second is to ensure the rapid and effective dissemination and use of the results of that research to improve drug abuse and addiction prevention, treatment, and policy.

Recent scientific advances have improved our understanding of the nature of drug abuse and addiction. The majority of these advances, which have implications for how to best prevent and treat addiction, have been supported by NIDA. NIDA supports over 85 percent of the world's research on the health aspects of drug abuse and addiction, and NIDA-supported science addresses essential questions about drug abuse, ranging from the molecule to managed care, and from DNA to community outreach research.

NIDA is seizing upon opportunities and technologies to further an understanding of how drug abuse affects the brain and behavior, and is working to ensure the rapid and effective transfer of scientific data to policymakers, health care practitioners, and to the general public. The scientific knowledge that is generated through NIDA research contributes to improving overall health in the United States.

NIDA has explored the biomedical and behavioral foundations of drug abuse, ranging from its causes and consequences to its prevention and treatment. Among the many and diverse accomplishments, NIDA-supported research has:

- Identified the molecular sites in the brain where opiates, cocaine, PCP, and THC (the active ingredient in marijuana) have their initial effect. These discoveries, together with computer-aided drug design, are paving the way for development of new medications to break the cycle of addiction.

- Used molecular genetic technologies to clone the genes for the major receptors for virtually every abusable drug, thus providing scientists with the tools necessary to study how drugs of abuse exert their many behavioral effects.

- Supported the development and evaluation of three medications—LAAM, naltrexone, and buprenorphine—for the treatment of opiate addiction.

- Defined nicotine addiction and the scientific basis for therapy using nicotine gum and skin patches.

- Measured the positive impact of community drug-prevention strategies that involve the media, schools, families, neighborhoods, and the workplace.

- Demonstrated that successful drug abuse treatment reduces criminality as well as relapse to addiction.

- Pioneered community-based research on AIDS (acquired immunodeficiency syndrome) prevention efforts that showed that drug users can change AIDS risk behaviors, and thus reduce their susceptibility to HIV (human immunodeficiency virus) infection and AIDS.

- Demonstrated that participation in methadone treatment significantly reduces HIV seroconversion rates and decreases high-risk behaviors.

- Supported the development and evaluation of pharmacologic treatment for newborns withdrawing from exposure to narcotics.

- Used advanced imaging techniques to identify the specific brain circuits that are involved in craving, euphoria, and other sequelae of drug addiction. These findings will provide the foundation for the development of new, targeted medications to block individual aspects of drugs.

- Demonstrated that prenatal exposure to cigarettes and marijuana have long-term effects on cognitive performance.

The results of these and other achievements through NIDA-funded research provide a scientific foundation for helping to solve the medical, social, and public health problems of drug abuse and addiction. More information about NIDA can be found at www.drugabuse.gov.

LUCINDA L. MINER

(SEE ALSO: *Addiction and Habituation; Cocaine and Crack Cocaine; Drug Abuse Resistance Education [DARE]; Marijuana; Substance Abuse, Definition of*)

NATIONAL INSTITUTES OF HEALTH

The National Institutes of Health (NIH) is the principal federal agency that supports and conducts biomedical research on the prevention and treatment of disease. It is the center of biomedical research in the United States and the foremost medical research enterprise in the world, with a budget in 2001 of $20.3 billion. An agency of the U.S. Public Health Service, it is a part of the U.S. Department of Health and Human Services. There are twenty-seven institutes and centers that comprise the National Institutes of Health, and the research supported by these institutes ranges from basic molecular and genomic biology to translational and applied studies involving individuals and large populations. Training for careers in biomedical research is also an important part of the NIH mission, as is the dissemination of information from this research to the public, to health providers, and to scientists.

HISTORY OF NIH

The history of NIH reflects an interweaving of the disciplines of public health, medicine, and basic biology, with a changing emphasis among these areas as health science progressed. The NIH had its origins in the Laboratory of Hygiene, which was created in 1887 to research cholera and other infectious diseases. The laboratory was an outgrowth of the Marine Hospital Service created in 1798 and, in turn, became the Public Health Service in 1912. Early activities focused on infectious and communicable diseases brought to the United States on incoming ships, and on the prevention of epidemics of yellow fever and cholera. In 1914, Dr. Joseph Goldberger described his findings that pellagra was a nutritional deficiency disease, rather than an infectious disease, and could be prevented by appropriate diet. This discovery marked a shift from infectious disease investigation. Research on the importance of nutrition in disease causation was fostered by this discovery, and the essential nature of vitamins in health followed.

The modern era of NIH began in 1930 with the redesignation of the Hygienic Laboratory as the National Institute of Health. In 1935, 45 acres of land in Bethesda, Maryland, were donated for the use of the National Institute of Health. Additional gifts of land were made and the buildings and grounds on the current site and were dedicated in 1940.

The National Cancer Institute Act was passed in 1938, and the first awards for research fellowships were made the following year. Laboratories at NIH were important in improving prevention and medical care during World War II. The contributions of science to the war effort provided a compelling rationale for the remarkable investment in biomedical research that followed during the second half of the twentieth century.

The Public Health Service Act of 1944 provided the legislative authority for post–World War II research programs and made the National Cancer Institute a part of NIH. In 1948, the National Heart Institute was authorized, and the name of NIH officially became the National *Institutes* of Health. The research emphasis shifted to investigation of basic biology and biochemistry and the disorders of biology that lead to disease. Prevention and treatment of diseases have been based largely on understanding the fundamental alterations in biology following World War II. Support for research conducted at colleges and universities also increased with an expanding budget. Other institutes and centers have been authorized and totaled twenty-seven in 2001. A clinical center on the Bethesda campus was dedicated in 1953 as the principal on-campus or intramural resource for clinical research. This facility combines patient facilities (inpatient and outpatient) with laboratories to foster integration of research from patient to laboratory.

During the second half of the twentieth century, the breadth and complexity of biomedical research activities conducted at NIH and supported at non-NIH sites increased. From 1950 onward, research emphasis shifted to chronic diseases, which had assumed epidemic proportions in the United States and other industrialized countries. Basic levels of molecular biology and genomics were increasingly probed. This led to an important benchmark at the turn of the millennium—the publication of the human genome map. Information on the inherited susceptibility and the interplay between genetic and environmental factors will eventually provide insights that will be translated into practical research.

Studies of large populations, like the Framingham Heart Study, have also been initiated by NIH to delineate risks for disease. Similarly, large interventional trials have tested effective means of preventing and managing these risks. These investigations were an outgrowth of an improved understanding of disease causation and the need to extend these findings to patients and populations. The growth of knowledge has been exponential, and the investment in biomedical research has produced a remarkable return to the public in improved health and increased longevity. Political support for the NIH budget has been consistent and bipartisan, reflecting broad public-interest support and confidence in the benefits of health research.

SUPPORT OF RESEARCH

Research activities are conducted in the laboratories of NIH by intramural scientists and are further supported through extramural grants and contracts at 2,570 academic and research facilities in the United States and worldwide. The NIH laboratories and clinical facilities are located principally in Bethesda, Maryland, with additional laboratories located elsewhere in Maryland and in Montana. Intramural research accounts for only about 10 percent of the budget of NIH. The overwhelming majority of funds thus support research being conducted at extramural sites. These extramural research studies are supported by grants and contracts awarded to nonfederal scientists working in universities, medical schools, hospitals, and research institutions. In 2000, there were over 37,000 grants and contracts supporting research and over 16,000 grants supporting research training.

Both intramural and extramural research undergoes rigorous scientific review before being funded, and oversight continues during the course of the work. Investigators who want to conduct research prepare an application describing the proposed work. This application can be initiated by the investigator, or it can be submitted in response to an NIH-initiated solicitation. Grants and contracts to non-NIH institutions and scientists are awarded after review and evaluation by panels of scientists expert in the particular research area for which support is requested. These proposals are reviewed and scored for scientific merit and relevance.

The initial scientific review by scientific peers is followed with review by an advisory council of senior scientists representing the institute or center involved, and this council is charged with overseeing the development of a balanced portfolio of sponsored research. The grants and contracts are funded by the institutes and centers from funds appropriated to them by Congress. This review by panels of nongovernmental scientific peers (the peer-review system) has been fundamental to the evaluation and support of meritorious research and to sound investment of public funds in research. The process of peer review is now used by many other governmental and nongovernmental organizations in the United States and internationally. The researchers report on progress during the conduct of the project and, importantly, report their results in journals and meetings, making the findings available to other investigators and to the public.

ORGANIZATION AND SCOPE OF NIH RESEARCH

The NIH supports and conducts research at all levels of scientific inquiry, from molecular biology through clinical research on individuals, to the study of large groups and communities. Support for training is provided at the levels of predoctoral, postdoctoral, and established investigators. Training is supported for all levels of scientific study. The institutes and centers typically support research and research training related to a specific condition (e.g., cancer, heart disease) or phase of life (e.g., child health and human development, aging) or for cross-cutting issues (e.g., health disparities, complementary and alternative medicine). Some centers are engaged in scientific review or support of research resources.

The development of the institutes has followed the evolution of public and Congressional interest in diseases and health issues. There is now a belief that research should be the foundation for health policy, medical care, and public health action. The orientation by condition or phase of life has derived from public and Congressional advocacy related to medical and public health issues. One strength of this organizational structure is the integration of basic scientists with clinical researchers in the investigation of diseases.

This vertical integration allows scientists to unite basic biology with clinical and public health science and to promote a translation of scientific advances to human clinical studies. This integration occurs in both intramural and extramural research programs, and both clinical and public health applications benefit from this orientation. Clinical research flourishes with the integration of basic research, and this has influenced medical training and specialty emphasis. Each institute or center supports the full spectrum of research, with a few exceptions.

The vertical organizational structure of the NIH requires special efforts to integrate research across the institutes at each scientific level—a horizontal integration. The commonalities of basic biologic mechanisms compel collaboration among scientists who might be studying, for example, the biology mechanisms involved in cancer or heart disease. Similarly, there are joint risks for conditions such as cancer and heart disease and this requires collaborative study of the risks to exposed populations. During the 1990s, the institutes emphasized cross-institute and trans-NIH research to afford an integration of populational research across institutes. To foster this integration, several programmatic offices within the Office of the NIH Director have been developed. The Office of Disease Prevention and the Office of Behavioral and Social Sciences Research are examples. These offices work with the institutes to develop crosscutting research in the areas of prevention and behavioral research, respectively, and to coordinate activities with other federal agencies and the private sector.

Examples of the vertical and horizontal integrations illustrate how this structure advances knowledge. The mapping of the human genome and discovery of specific genes related to particular diseases afford an opportunity to identify individuals at risk for disease and to develop approaches that might modify this risk and prevent disease. Importantly, the interplay between genetic and environmental risk can be determined and appropriate interventions developed. Variations of BRCA-1 and BRCA-2 genes were found in studies of families having a high risk of breast cancer, for example. Subsequent population studies have disclosed the prevalence and penetrance of these genes in more general populations and have provided realistic estimates of when to screen for the genetic variation. The abnormality encoded by these genes is being investigated and could lead to behavioral interventions to modify the risk of breast cancer.

Prevention research exemplifies cross-institute collaboration. Several personal and environmental risks affect development of more than one disease, and there may be beneficial as well as adverse effects. The use of hormonal replacement by menopausal women can have beneficial effects on cardiovascular disease, osteoporosis, and mental acuity, in addition to the aesthetic effects for which they are commonly taken. However, this therapy also poses risks for breast cancer and cancer of the uterus. To quantify the benefits and risks of hormonal replacement therapy for this range of clinical conditions, a large clinical trial is in progress utilizing the scientific expertise of several institutes and dependant on scientists at academic institutions with a range of specialty expertise in the conditions being studied. The planning, conduct, and monitoring of this large trial has required the participation of epidemiologists, biostatisticians, clinical trialists, and community organizers.

A description of the institutes and offices, their missions, and recent accomplishments are available at the NIH web site at http://www.nih. gov/. A list of all currently funded grants and contracts is available at http://www-commons.cit. nih.gov/crisp/, including an abstract describing the research project or program. A special web site containing all NIH-supported clinical trials is available at http://clinicaltrials.gov/. This site provides information to patients and referring physicians regarding available clinical trials.

WILLIAM R. HARLAN

(SEE ALSO: *Centers for Disease Control and Prevention; Healthy People 2010*)

BIBLIOGRAPHY

Mullan, F. (1989). *Plagues and Politics: The Story of the United States Public Health Service.* New York: Basic Books.

National Institutes of Health. *NIH Almanac.* Washington, DC: U.S. Department of Health and Human Services. Published annually. Available online at http://www.nih.gov/about/almanac/index.html.

Shorter, E. (1987). *The Health Century.* New York: Doubleday.

Swain, D. C. (1962). "The Rise of a Research Empire: NIH, 1930–1950." *Science* 138:1233–1237.

NATURAL DISASTERS

Natural disasters occur when forces of nature damage the environment and manmade structures. If people live in the area, natural disasters can cause a great deal of human suffering. As a result of disasters, people may be injured or killed, or may lose their homes and possessions. The impact is so great that the affected community often must depend on outside help in order to cope with the results (Noji, Gunn and William).

Examples of natural forces that can cause widespread human suffering include earthquakes, tornadoes, hurricanes, floods, volcanic eruptions, wilderness fires, and extreme hot or cold temperatures. Between 1975 and 1996, natural disasters worldwide cost 3 million lives and affected at least 800 million others (Noji). In the United States, damage caused by natural hazards costs close to one billion dollars per week.

PUBLIC HEALTH EFFECTS OF NATURAL DISASTERS

The physical force of a disaster can directly cause injury and death to the population, and each type of disaster can result in its own combination of physical injuries. In earthquakes, buildings and the objects inside them can fall, injuring those who live or work there. Floods can result in drowning, and wildfires can cause burns and illness from smoke inhalation. In addition to the direct injury and death caused by the disaster's force, there can be other serious adverse effects on the well being of those living in the area.

The large numbers of people who are suddenly ill or injured can exceed the capacity of the local health care system to care for them. In addition to the burden of increased numbers of patients, the system itself can become a victim of the disaster. Hospitals may be damaged, roads blocked, and personnel may be unable to perform their duties. The loss of these resources occurs at a time when they are most critically needed.

The disaster also can hamper the ability to provide routine, non-emergency health services. Many people may be unable to obtain care and medications for their ongoing health problems. The disruption of these routine services can result in an increase in illness and death in segments of the population that might not have been directly affected by the disaster.

Much has been written about the mental health aspects of natural disasters. The popular images of a community paralyzed by the shock of the disaster, panicking or looting, are unfounded. Actually, people tend to come together following a natural disaster. Survivors offer immediate assistance to those who are injured or trapped in earthquake damaged buildings, help with sandbagging efforts in floods, offer shelter and assistance to those made homeless, and volunteer goods or money to those in need. However, living in a disaster area can be highly stressful. Staying in damaged buildings, relocating to shelters, dealing with the death or injuries of loved ones, as well as the prolonged time and energy involved in recovering from the affects of the disaster can result in feelings of anxiety and depression. While these might be normal responses to stress and unpleasant events, the degree to which a disaster can disrupt daily living may contribute to an increase in these feelings.

ENVIRONMENTAL HEALTH AND POPULATION DISPLACEMENT

Certain disasters can interfere with the functioning of water and sewage systems as well as the provision of gas and electricity. The loss of these everyday services can increase the risk for sickness even in uninjured people. For example, drinking unclean water or eating inadequately stored or prepared food can cause serious intestinal illness.

The most serious consequences of natural disasters are related to mass population displacements. Many people cannot stay in their homes because the buildings are so badly damaged that they are structurally unsafe. Others refuse to stay in otherwise stable buildings because they fear that they might collapse. While this often occurs following violent storms, it is particularly the case after earthquakes, when potentially damaging aftershocks commonly occur. In many cases, those displaced by disasters find shelter in the homes of people they know, while others must go to shelters staffed by disaster relief authorities such as Red Cross/Red Crescent Societies and government agencies.

Placing large numbers of people in crowded shelters poses a risk for additional health problems. It can be difficult to provide so many people with clean drinking water, sufficient waste disposal, and safe, nutritious food. This temporary living situation can also increase the chances for outbreaks of certain diseases. It is important to remember that only those diseases that are found in the affected community during predisaster times pose a danger to displaced populations after a disaster occurs. For example, it would be unlikely for those living in a shelter following a flood in the upper Midwest portion of the United States to experience an outbreak of malaria (as malaria does not exist in that part of the world), but poor sanitary services could contribute to an outbreak of conditions such as infectious diarrhea or some forms of respiratory illness. In addition, an occasional outbreak of more serious illnesses that might occasionally appear in the community during nondisaster times, such as meningitis or measles, would be a more significant health risk in shelters.

When large numbers of people gather in unsheltered settings, such as parks or open fields, there is an even greater risk of illness. This is because these areas often do not have enough sanitary services. Clean drinking water may have to be trucked into the area, and prompt attention must be directed to providing facilities to handle human waste. The ability to receive, safely store, and prepare food is also a concern for the health of the displaced population. Flies, mosquitoes, and rodents that might be carrying diseases that can cause illness in humans add to the risk of living in an unsheltered setting.

NEEDS ASSESSMENTS AND SURVEILLANCE

The impact of a disaster on the public's health poses special problems for public health professionals. They must monitor the health needs of the disaster-affected population and work to ensure that emergency managers take actions to meet those needs. They also need to maintain the everyday public health programs that were in place before the disaster occurred. These challenges can be addressed in several ways.

Rapid assessment surveys can be conducted of those living in areas most impacted by the disaster. Often, aerial views of the disaster area can indicate damage to key facilities (hospitals, utility stations, major roads), residential structures, and the assembly of large numbers of people in unsheltered settings. Teams of public health, engineering, social service, and medical personnel can then go to those areas that appear most damaged and begin a survey of the people living there. The affected area is divided into smaller areas, called clusters. The teams interview a representative sample of seven people from each of thirty different clusters in the high-impact disaster area. Using a standard set of questions, they gather information about the number of injuries, deaths, houses without running water, functioning toilets, electricity, heat, and those with ongoing medical conditions (Malilay).

With the information gathered from the assessment surveys, disaster health managers can draw conclusions about which segments of the affected community are at greatest need for emergency efforts. Once the decision is made to direct resources to the most seriously affected areas, another rapid assessment may be performed to determine the effectiveness of those efforts.

Other information about the number and types of injured may be obtained from medical facilities. It is important to distinguish between patients who were injured or made ill as a result of the disaster from those who happened to seek medical attention for conditions not related to the disaster. This requires a working knowledge of the injury and illness patterns that are associated with different natural disasters. Definitions of which types of conditions will be attributed directly to the disaster or its consequences also are needed.

Computer models are being developed that can combine views of buildings, transportation ways (highways, railroads, airports, and harbors), utilities, and medical facilities with local hazards of varying severity. These models, currently being tested for earthquakes, allow emergency managers and health planners to predict the extent of damage and injuries if a hazard occurs in their community. Once these models are refined and validated, they may prove valuable to emergency response and public health planners.

As the global population continues to grow and more people live in hazard-prone areas, there will be an increase in the number and severity of mass population emergencies. Public health personnel have a key role in natural disaster preparation and response. Before a disaster occurs, they need to have systems in place to identify and track diseases. They must also understand the basic health issues of water and food safety, sanitation, and environmental hazards.

Public health practitioners routinely provide comprehensive programs of health education and preventive care that put them in close contact with those living in the community. They can use their professional skills to develop and evaluate programs for community disaster preparedness before a disaster strikes. After the disaster, they have the ability to help assess its affects on the local population. By adapting their knowledge and skills to these large-scale emergencies, public health professionals can have a significant impact on reducing the negative health affects of disasters.

STEVEN J. ROTTMAN
KIMBERLEY SHOAF

(SEE ALSO: *Famine; Refugee Communities; War*)

BIBLIOGRAPHY

Gunn, S., and William, A. (1990). *Multilingual Dictionary of Disaster Medicine and International Relief.* London: Kluwer Academic.

Malilay, J.; Flanders, W. D.; and Brogan, D. (1996). "A Modified Cluster-Sampling Method for Post-Disaster Rapid Assessment of Needs." *Bulletin of the World Health Organization* 74(4):399–405.

Noji, Eric K. (1997). *The Public Health Consequences of Disasters.* New York: Oxford University Press.

NEEDLE EXCHANGE PROGRAM

Illicit intravenous drug users (IVDUs) commonly share injection needles, transmitting blood-borne infections—notably HIV and hepatitis B and C—in the process. Needle exchange programs provide clean, sterile needles to drug users, with no questions asked. As infected IVDUs often infect others, this is considered a better approach to a serious public health problem than moralizing and admonitions to desist from using illicit intravenous drugs, though these programs have forced opposition in many quarters.

Some have suggested that a better approach would be to legalize illicit drugs and provide them under license to those who are addicted, while simultaneously providing substance abuse programs aimed at rehabilitation. In the long run this might eliminate the problem and destroy the financial base of the hugely lucrative illicit drug trade, though, in the United Stated at least, political pressure to be "tough on crime" keeps such an approach from being considered.

JOHN M. LAST

(SEE ALSO: *Blood-Borne Diseases; Drug Abuse Resistance Education [DARE]; Politics of Public Health; Public Health and the Law; Substance Abuse*)

NEEDLESTICK

"Needlestick" is a slang term for a puncture wound made by a contaminated hypodermic needle, especially one that may convey HIV infection to health workers such as nurses or physicians. Although this is a rare mode of transmission of HIV or other serious infection, the risk is real: about three or four out of every thousand episodes of needlestick in Europe and North America have led to confirmed HIV infection. The risk is reduced by education, which must begin with junior staff when they are first in contact with patients, and with rigorous attention to sterile procedures, including universal precautions.

JOHN M. LAST

(SEE ALSO: *Communicable Disease Control; HIV/AIDS; Universal Precautions*)

NEIGHBORHOOD HEALTH CENTERS

Neighborhood health centers (NHCs) comprise a wide array of organizations, typically nonprofit or public entities that provide services in medically underserved areas. NHCs typically exist where economic, geographic, or cultural barriers limit access to primary health care for a substantial portion of the population. The clinics seek to tailor services to the needs of the community or special populations they serve. They do this by building a community-based primary care infrastructure and by striving to provide family-oriented, culturally competent primary care, often linked to social services. The NHCs attempt to provide accessible and dignified health services to low-income persons and others with barriers to receiving care. The centers are often created by community groups, physicians, churches, and/or hospitals. Well over fifteen million of the nation's neediest people receive primary health care through NHCs.

Many types of NHCs exist, the largest being a network of approximately 700 Community and Migrant Health Centers with over 3,000 delivery sites, funded by the Health Resources and Services Administration of the U.S. Department of Health and Human Services (USDHHS). These sites are located in federally designated Medically Underserved Areas. There are also free clinics available throughout the country. The number of free clinics grew from approximately 130 in 1992 to over 300 in 1998, according to the Free Clinic Foundation of America. Free clinics are staffed predominantly by volunteers. Significant numbers of faith-based clinics, hospital owned or affiliated clinics, clinics operated under the direction of city governments also exist, as well as some free-standing unaffiliated clinics.

Many NHCs target their service to all ages and attempt to provide comprehensive services, which can include some or all of the following: outpatient medical, dental, supplementary and/or subsidiary hospital follow-up, mental health, substance abuse, and WIC nutrition. Some even provide transportation to connect those in need with the service providers. Other NHCs target their services to specific populations, such as women, children, ethnic groups, the homeless, the elderly, residents of public housing, schools, persons with special needs (e.g. HIV positive), or runaway children.

NHCs are financed in many different ways. Support comes from government (city, county, state, or federal support or grants), foundations, philanthropy, volunteers, churches, hospitals, health plans, individual contributors, community-action organizations, and others. Most NHCs charge fees, typically using a sliding fee scale based upon an individual's income. Not all organizations charge, however. Free clinics provide services at little or no charge, relying heavily on volunteers and nonpatient financial support.

RICK WILK

(SEE ALSO: *Access to Health Services; Community and Migrant Health Centers; Community Mental Health Centers; Community Organization; Primary Care; Social Medicine; Social Work; United States Department of Health and Human Services [USDHHS]*)

BIBLIOGRAPHY

Hawkins, D., and Rosenblum, S. (1997). "The Challenges Facing Health Centers in a Changing Health Care System." *Access to Community Health Care: A National State Data Book*. Washington, DC: National Association of Community Health Centers, Inc.

Siegal, S. (1998). "Access to Primary Health Care: Tracking the States." *Health Policy Tracking Services Series*. Washington, DC: National Conference of State Legislators.

NEWBORN SCREENING

Newborn screening is an organized process of identifying medical conditions in newborn babies that, if untreated, can cause developmental delays, serious illness, or even death. Generally, these conditions cause no symptoms in the first days of life. Screening programs have therefore been developed to identify and treat babies with these conditions before permanent damage occurs. In the United States, these programs are usually mandated by state public health laws.

In 1964, phenylketonuria (PKU) became the first disorder subject to generalized newborn screening. Phenylketonuria causes mental retardation due to the baby's inability to metabolize the amino acid phenylalanine, which then accumulates in the blood. It can be successfully treated with a diet low in phenylalanine. PKU is diagnosed through a blood sample. Since 1964, technological advances allow screening for many more diseases on the same blood sample, including adrenal hyperplasia, biotinidase deficiency, blood sample, including cystic fibrosis, galactosemia, homogystinuria, hypothyroidism, maple syrup urine disease, and sickle cell disease. Abnormal results are reported to the baby's doctor with recommendations for further confirmatory testing and treatment.

Screening for hearing impairment was implemented in the 1970s. Initially, only known risk factors, such as a family history, prompted a hearing test. In the 1990s, universal newborn hearing screening began to be implemented in the United States and in Europe. Children with moderate to severe hearing impairment benefit by diagnosis and treatment early in life to maximize speech and language development.

JOHN H. VOLLMAN

(SEE ALSO: *Child Health Services; Hearing Disorders; Maternal and Child Health; Screening; and articles on specified diseases mentioned herein*)

BIBLIOGRAPHY

Erbe, R. W., and Levy, H. L. (1997). "Neonatal Screening." In *Emery and Rimoin's Principles and Practice of Medical Genetics*. New York: Churchill Livingstone.

National Institutes of Health (1993). "Early Identification of Hearing Impairment in Infants and Young Children." *NIH Consensus Statement* 11(1):1–24. Washington, DC: Author.

NIGHTINGALE, FLORENCE

Florence Nightingale was born in Florence, Italy, on May 12, 1820. The daughter of upper-class British parents, Nightingale pursued a career in nursing, despite family objections, believing it to be God's will. In 1851 she received her initial training in Kaiserworth at a hospital run by an order of Protestant Deaconesses. Two years later she gained further experience as the superintendent at the Hospital for Invalid Gentlewomen in London, England.

After reading a series of correspondence from the *London Times* in 1854 on the plight of wounded soldiers fighting in the Crimea, Nightingale asked the British secretary of war to secure her entrance into the military hospitals at Scutari, Turkey. He not only granted her permission but designated her the head of an official delegation of nurses. Nightingale worked for the next two years to improve the sanitary conditions of army hospitals and to reorganize their administration. The *Times* immortalized her as the "Lady with the Lamp" because she ministered to the soldiers throughout the night.

Upon her return to England, Nightingale conducted an exhaustive study of the health of the British Army and created a plan for reform that she compiled into a five-hundred-page report entitled *Notes on Matters Affecting the Health, Efficiency, and Hospital Administration of the British Army* (1858). In 1859 she published *Notes on Hospitals*, which was followed in 1860 by *Notes on Nursing: What It Is and What It Is Not*. That same year she established a nursing school at St. Thomas's Hospital in London.

Nightingale wanted to make nursing a respectable profession and believed that nurses should be trained in science. She also advocated strict discipline, an attention to cleanliness, and felt that nurses should possess an innate empathy for their patients. Although Nightingale became an invalid following her stay in the Crimea, she remained an influential leader in public health policies related to hospital administration until her death on August 13, 1910.

JENNIFER KOSLOW

(SEE ALSO: *History of Public Health; Leadership; Nurse*)

BIBLIOGRAPHY

Baly, M. E. (1986). *Florence Nightingale and the Nursing Legacy*. London: Croom Helm.

Bullough, V.; Bullough, B.; and Stanton, M. P., eds. (1990). *Florence Nightingale and Her Era: A Collection of New Scholarship*. New York: Garland.

Small, H. (1948). *Florence Nightingale: Avenging Angel*. London: Constable.

NO-FAULT LEGISLATION

See Legislation and Regulation

NOISE

Sound is an essential form of human communication. However, unwanted sounds, or noise, can lead to a variety of medical problems, including deafness and elevated blood pressure; there is also evidence for an increased pulse rate. There is some evidence suggesting that environmental noise may affect the learning ability of children.

Sound waves are generated by vibrations moving through the air, and they are perceived through a complex interaction of vibrations hitting the inner ear. External vibrations are translated, through bones, into additional vibrations, which are then picked up by hair-like structures in the inner ear. These vibrations are further translated into neurologic signals, which are registered in the brain and received as intelligible information.

Noise can be normal sounds that get in the way of being able to perceive wanted sounds. Sound is measured in units called decibels, and the human ear is well-designed to perceive and interpret sounds at low decibel levels and across a wide spectrum of vibration. Sounds that are too loud, however, can damage the ability of the ear to make sense of what is perceived. A graphic measurement of what one can hear is called an audiogram, and hearing loss can be traced on audiograms. There is some hearing loss that is considered normal with aging, called presbycusis. Additional hearing loss and other physiological damage, may result from excessive loud noise.

There is some controversy as to what level of sound is too high, particularly in workplaces. It is thought that the maximal tolerable noise level for an eight-hour workplace exposure is about seventy-five decibels. The current allowable standard is eighty-five decibels. The standard was decreased from the previous ninety decibel level after a hard-fought battle to try and prevent a significant number of cases of hearing loss. At eighty-five decibels, hearing protection and noise monitoring becomes mandatory. There are several ways that noise can be reduced, either through changes in noise-making equipment itself, or by providing personal protective equipment to individuals who must work in noisy environments. The two basic types of personal protection are earplugs and earmuffs. Earmuffs, which can be put on and taken off more easily, are useful where the noise may be intermittent, such as at airports. Earplugs are more practical for people who spend considerable continuous periods of time in noisy environments.

In addition to noisy workplace environments, there are certain general environments where noise may be a particular problem. Among these are subway systems, where passengers may be intermittently exposed to high noise levels, and in communities located near airports. Over time there has been a considerable effort to diminish the noise around airports, both through the use of quieter engines and through changes in flight paths. In some extreme situations, homes have been bought and people moved out of flight paths near airports to help reduce the risk and annoyance associated with such noise.

ARTHUR L. FRANK

(SEE ALSO: *Hearing Disorders; Hearing Protection; Occupational Safety and Health*)

BIBLIOGRAPHY

Moller, A. G. (1992). "Noise as a Health Hazard." In *Public Health and Preventive Medicine,* 13th edition, eds. J. M. Last and R. M. Wallace. Norwalk, CT: Appleton and Lange.

NOMOGRAM

A nomogram is a chart that displays values of three related variables in vertical columns in such a way that when a ruler is placed across values in any two columns, the corresponding value of the variables in the third column can be read directly from the chart. A common application is a display of heights, weights, and body-mass index—the latter being mathematically computed from height and weight and, in practice, can be read from the nomogram chart to derive the value for individual patients or clients in a doctor's office.

JOHN M. LAST

(SEE ALSO: *Health Measurement Scales*)

NONCOMMUNICABLE DISEASE CONTROL

Noncommunicable diseases are usually thought of as chronic conditions that do not result from an acute infectious process. These conditions cause death, dysfunction, or impairment in the quality of life, and they usually develop over relatively long periods—at first without causing symptoms; but after disease manifestations develop, there may be a protracted period of impaired health. Generally, these conditions or diseases result from prolonged exposure to causative agents, many associated with personal behaviors and environmental factors. The major noncommunicable diseases are listed in Tables 1 and 2. Noncommunicable diseases also include injuries, which have an acute onset, but may be followed by prolonged convalescence and impaired function, as well as chronic mental diseases.

Noncommunicable diseases are the leading cause of functionary impairment and death worldwide. These conditions have been the leading cause of death in the United States and other high-income countries over the last fifty years, and they are emerging as a leading cause of death in low- to middle-income countries. Table 1 depicts the leading causes of death worldwide showing that noncommunicable diseases and injuries account for

Table 1

Causes of Death Worldwide: Estimates for 1999
(in thousands)

Total Deaths	55,965	
Communicable Diseases	17,380	(31%)
Non-Communicable Diseases	33,484	(59.8%)
Injuries	5,101	(9.1%)
Cardiovascular Diseases	16,970	(30.3%)
Cancers	7,065	(12.6%)
Respiratory Diseases	3,575	(6.4%)
Digestive Diseases	2,409	(3.7%)
Neuropsychiatric Disorders	911	(1.6%)
Genitourinary Diseases	900	(1.6%)

SOURCE: Adapted from The World Health Report 2000: Health Systems: improving performance. Geneva: World Health Organization, 2000.

Table 2

Burden of Disease Worldwide: Estimates for 1999
(in thousands)

	Disability-Adjusted Life Years	
Total DALYS	1,438,154	
Communicable Diseases	615,105	(42.8%)
Non-Communicable Diseases	621,742	(43.2%)
Injuries	201,307	(13.9%)
Cardiovascular Diseases	157,185	(10.9)
Neuropsychiatric Disorders	158,721	(11.0)
Cancers	84,500	(5.9)
Respiratory Diseases	70,017	(4.9)
Congenital Abnormalities	36,557	(2.5)

SOURCE: Adapted from The World Health Report 2000: Health Systems: improving performance. Geneva: World Health Organization, 2000.

over two-thirds of deaths. In addition, these diseases cause pain, disability, loss of income, disruption of family stability, and an impaired quality of life.

Disability-adjusted life years (DALYs) constitutes one means of assessing the effect of disease, as shown in Table 2. (DALYs are a measure accounting for years of life spent with diminished function resulting from health conditions of varying severity.) Over the past century, dynamic changes have occurred in the worldwide prevalence of noncommunicable diseases, and even more rapid transitions are expected in the twenty-first century. These changes have been driven by social, economic, and public health progress, and the strategies for change have been illuminated by research.

ASCENDENCY OF NONCOMMUNICABLE DISEASES

In 1900, the average life expectancy worldwide was about forty-seven years, and there were few differences among different countries. The leading causes of death in the United States and worldwide were communicable diseases and nutritionally related conditions (see Tables 1 and 2). Infant and childhood mortality was high because of infections and poor nutrition—the short average life span mainly reflected high mortality in the early years of life. During the first half of the twentieth

century, the high-income, industrialized countries of the world made major advances against infectious and childhood diseases through improved public health measures, nutrition, vaccines, and, to a lesser degree, antibiotics. Childhood mortality declined in these countries, survival to middle and late adult life increased, and noncommunicable diseases emerged in the middle of the twentieth century as the major threat to health. This "epidemiologic transition" from communicable to noncommunicable diseases as the major threats to health did not begin in low- and middle-income countries (LMICs) until the last half of the twentieth century. In many countries with rapidly developing economies, such as Malaysia and Korea, the transition was rapid in the latter half of the century. The public health experience of high-income countries was applied successfully by these countries. Currently, many middle-income countries have health profiles that resemble those of high-income countries. But this epidemiologic transition to noncommunicable disease not only differs across countries but has been interrupted by recent events.

Unfortunately, the trend in many countries have been impacted by a new epidemic plague—HIV/AIDS (human immunodeficiency virus/acquired immunodeficiency syndrome). Many countries in Africa and southern Asia have high infection rates for HIV, and the disease principally affects young adults and newborn infants in these areas. From 1980 onward, the rapid transmission of this fatal disease has not been preventable except by behavioral change; there is no vaccine for prevention, and affordable treatment has not been available in low-income countries. This leaves many countries with a double burden of health problems—a new epidemic of infectious disease and unresolved infectious conditions, as well as a growing set of noncommunicable diseases.

The state of the epidemiologic transition varies around the world, reflecting the social, cultural, economic, and health resource factors in various countries. The health status of the nations of the world is reported by the World Health Organization, and models have been developed to predict future disease patterns by region and country. These models are based on observed trends in disease prevalence (frequency) for countries and regions of the world. The book *Global Burden of Disease*, edited by Christopher Murray and Allen Lopez provides a prediction of health status in 2020. Rather than taking cause of death and age at death as the principal measures of health, Murray and Lopez have combined measures of morbidity (impaired health) and mortality to assess health status (see Table 2).

According to estimates of the burden of disease, high-income countries in 1990 experienced a preponderance of noncommunicable disease compared to the burden worldwide, as measured by disability-adjusted life years (DALYS), a measure that portrays years of life lost due to disabling conditions, and thus represents the impact of these conditions. Worldwide in 1990, infectious diseases and perinatal conditions top the list. However, by the year 2020 the worldwide burden is projected to shift to noncommunicable diseases, as indicated in the right column. There is an important dimension not obvious from these tables. High-income countries contain 15 percent of the world's population but account for only 8 percent of the disease burden. Comparisons of high-income countries and LMICs indicate that noncommunicable diseases rates were similar across the two levels of economic income in 1990. A major burden of noncommunicable disease does exist in LMICs, but is overwhelmed by the burden of communicable diseases. If the communicable diseases are controlled successfully, there will be a new worldwide "epidemic" of noncommunicable disease.

Already, many middle-income countries that are managing the epidemic of HIV/AIDS are experiencing increased survival to middle adult life and increasing rates of chronic disease and injuries. This change in disease patterns is useful to the health planner who needs to evaluate resource needs, and to the economist who links health, productivity, and economic development as an argument to allocate resources to health services.

There was an alarming rise in chronic diseases and injuries in high-income countries (the United States, Canada, Australia, European nations, and Japan) during the middle of the twentieth century. This increase was especially striking for ischemic heart disease, which became the leading cause of death in these countries in the 1950s and 1960s. This disease results from the formation of plaques containing cholesterol and blood clots in the arteries that supply oxygen and nutrients to the heart muscle. The concerns about this epidemic prompted studies that explored the causes and prevention of the plaques and resultant disease. From 1960 to the present there has been a striking decline in ischemic heart disease deaths in the high-income countries, representing another epidemiologic transition to prevention and management of chronic diseases and increasing survival. Life expectancy has increased in these countries, principally from adding to the years of life after the age of fifty. Somewhat later, in the 1990s, cancer deaths began to decline. This "postindustrialization" improvement in health and survival has important implications beyond the increased life expectancy for these countries. First, noncommunicable diseases can be controlled with prevention and treatment when the modifiable environmental causes are identified and controlled and effective health services are available. Second, research studies can identify the risks and the means to modify them. This information can be applied to individuals and to groups to improve health. Third, the lessons learned from high-income countries might be applied to low income countries to stanch the anticipated epidemic of noncommunicable diseases.

CAUSES AND PREVENTION

Modifiable Causes. The causes of noncommunicable diseases are often divided into modifiable

Table 3

Burden of Diseases (1999)
(Measured in Disability-Adjusted Life Years)

High Income Countries 1999	Worldwide 1999	Worldwide 2020 (Projected)
Ischemic Heart Disease	Lower Respiratory Infection	**Ischemic Heart Disease**
Unipolar Major Depression	Perinatal Conditions	**Unipolar Major Depression**
Cerebrovascular Disease	Diarrheal Diseases	**Motor Vehicle Accidents**
Cancer	HIV/AIDS	**Cerebrovascular Disease**
Motor Vehicle Accidents	**Unipolar Major Depression**	**Chronic Obstructive Pulmonary Disease**
Chronic Obstructive Pulmonary Disease	**Cerebrovascular Disease**	Tuberculosis
Perinatal Conditions	Malaria	Lower Respiratory Infections
Lower Respiratory Infections	**Motor Vehicle Accidents**	War
	Chronic Obstructive Pulmonary Disease	

SOURCE: Adapted from *World Health Report,* WHO, 2000 ([1]) and The Global Burden of Disease ([2]).
[1] The Global Burden of Disease edited by Murray, C. J. L. and Lopez, A. D. World Health Organization.
[2] The World Health Report 2000: Health Systems: Improving Performance.

and nonmodifiable factors, although these distinctions are blurring with greater knowledge. Chronic diseases result from genetic, behavioral, and environmental factors and the interactions between them. These factors, generally termed "risk factors," produce molecular and structural changes in organs and tissues but produce few if any early symptoms or signs of disease. After relatively long periods of time, usually decades, disease manifestations and impairment of health result. Risk factors place an individual at a greater likelihood of developing disease, but do not predict disease with absolute certainty. For most chronic diseases, several risk factors contribute.

At the population level, a high prevalence of risk factors can put populations or communities at greater risk and result in more disease. Risk factors for future disease development and early structural changes may be found during the "silent" period before disease becomes manifest.

The prevention of noncommunicable diseases entails a definition of the risk factors and application of interventions to favorably alter risk before overt symptoms or signs develop. At an even earlier level, it may be possible to prevent the development of risk factors through changes in the environment and personal health behaviors. Primary prevention of chronic disease is therefore an important goal, as morbidity and mortality may be averted or forestalled, and promotion of health, or "primordial prevention," is perhaps the foremost goal. Prevention research seeks to identify risks

and to test interventions that modify risk and thereby prevent disease. Chronic diseases result from multiple factors that often interact in an additive or multiplicative fashion to increase risk, but there are also factors that can obviate or decrease disease risk. Because most chronic diseases take years to develop, with overt manifestations occurring in middle to late adult life, there is considerable potential for early identification and modification of risk in childhood, adolescence, and early adulthood.

Injuries include trauma from unintentional causes, such as vehicular and occupational injuries, as well as intentional injuries, such as interpersonal violence and self-inflicted trauma. With increased industrialization and the growth of vehicular traffic, injuries are a major cause of death and DALYs (see Tables 1 and 2), and the estimated worldwide burden in 2020 suggests an even greater increase (see Table 3). Homicides, suicides, and wars are also regrettably important sources of injury-related mortality and morbidity.

The prevention of vehicular injuries has focused on improved vehicular engineering for safety, better road design and traffic regulation, and improved driver training and enforcement of impaired driver laws. Occupational hazards are addressed with regulations related to the workplace. Homicidal actions, either individual or national, continue to pose a threat, particularly with the development of weapons that pose a threat to noncombatants. The principal casualties of wars continue to be civilian populations, and the advent of chemical and biological weapons increase further the potential for mass civilian deaths, even in the absence of declared national wars.

Nonmodifiable Causes. A major nonmodifiable individual risk for disease is genetic susceptibility. This has a very important influence on disease development, but does not confer an absolute certainty that a disease will occur. In the overwhelming majority of diseases, inherited susceptibility interacts either adversely or beneficially with environmental exposures and personal behaviors to alter molecular or metabolic processes that increase the likelihood of disease development—or to mitigate such changes if the susceptibilities or the exposures are beneficial. For example, smoking and tobacco use are risks for cancer—the risk of smokers getting lung cancer is ten to forty times that of nonsmokers. However, not all smokers will develop lung cancer at the same exposure levels, as measured by number of cigarettes smoked and the duration of smoking. There is an individual difference in susceptibility, attributable in part to genetic differences or to environmental exposures to substances such as asbestos, which increases the risk further.

The delineation of the human genome will accelerate the description of genetic susceptibilities to disease and clarify the interactions between genetic differences and environmental risks. However, discovery of the individual genetic susceptibility will only provide an alert that an increased risk exists. There is no current safe means of changing the genetic makeup of individuals, and multiple changes might be required. Nevertheless, it might be possible in the future to identify those genetically at risk and have them avoid certain environmental exposures, thereby decreasing the risk for disease. The current preventive strategy, however, is to identify and eliminate or minimize damaging exposures and not to seek out and change the genetic component.

In some instances, a single gene abnormality will predominate over environmental influences. For example, familial hypercholesterolemia is a disorder resulting from a single abnormal gene that results in blood cholesterol levels two to four times above normal, depending on whether one or two alleles are inherited. Ischemic heart disease

develops in middle or early adult life. The usual modifiers of blood cholesterol levels, diet and physical activity, have little influence on cholesterol levels or disease development. The genetic risk overwhelms the environmental influences. However, the use of potent new drugs that decrease internal cholesterol synthesis in the body can lower blood cholesterol and the risk for heart disease. However, for the overwhelming majority of people, and for the majority of chronic diseases, alteration of personal and environmental exposures are the most important strategy.

Age represents a nonmodifiable factor in development of chronic disease. The mechanism is assumed to be the cumulative, long-term exposure to factors that alter function and structure, including DNA. However, increasing genetic information suggests that there are individual differences in genetic-environmental damage related to exposure.

GENERAL ENVIRONMENTAL EXPOSURES

Environmental exposures can be categorized into general environmental exposures and personal environmental exposures (see Table 4). The general environment encompasses the social, cultural, and public health aspects of life over which individuals can exert little or no personal control. For example, the quality of air and of drinking water or the exposures in the workplace environment are managed or regulated by public health or industrial organizations. If toxic exposures exist, the only personal option would be to change location or employment, but this is often not feasible. The public generally depends on public health organizations to monitor and manage the ambient environment and to make and enforce regulations in the public interest. Through public action, however, individuals can express preferences if the health risks are known.

Vehicular accidents and injuries result from increased traffic and speed of traffic, but public regulation of vehicular design, highway engineering, and regulation of driver behavior represent social policy changes that can decrease fatalities and injuries. Occupational exposures to silica, asbestos, and heavy metals can lead to lung disease, cancer, and death, and regulation and monitoring

Table 4

Modifiable Risk Factors for Non-Communicable Diseases

General Environmental Exposures

Physical environment:
    ambient air quality
    water quality
    occupational and work site
    food safety and availability

Social environment:
    income
    cognitive education
    cultural education
    access to health services
    availability of public health and community services

Personal Environmental Exposures

Smoking (and tobacco use)

Nutrition and Obesity
    dietary intake
    micronutrient adequacy
    caloric balance

Physical Activity

Alcohol/Drug Abuse

Genetic endowment
    monogenetic
    gene-environment interactions

SOURCE: Adapted from U.S. Department of Health and Human Services. Healthy People 2010: Understanding and Improving Health, 2nd ed. Washington, DC: U.S. GPO, November 2000.

---

of the workplace can minimize or eliminate the risk. Environmental aspects can also facilitate healthful behaviors. The community environment can be made more conducive to personal behaviors that decrease the risk of chronic disease. For example, provision of safe and pleasant community venues for walking or other physical activity can help individuals to develop and maintain personal commitments to increasing physical activity. Similarly, the availability of fresh fruits and vegetables at reasonable prices in local markets can foster healthful purchases and eating behaviors.

Other social and environmental characteristics can have a major influence on health, particularly that of populations. Throughout the world, groups with higher personal income and greater education have better health, less disease, and live longer. This observation was substantiated throughout the twentieth century and remains a fundamental factor for both communicable and noncommunicable diseases. The reasons for health disparities by income are not completely understood, but include access to health services, knowledge about and resources to act on health-promoting behaviors, and homes and workplaces that have less hazardous exposures. Differences in health status among countries can be explained in part by differences in per capita income, but there are exceptions—some countries that have low income levels have relatively good health status (e.g., Chile, China, and Sri Lanka). Attention to public health measures and availability of basic health services in low-income countries may account for some of the favorable differences. Within a country like the United States, which has a high prevalence of chronic disease, this income and educational gradient is also present. Three times as many people in low-income families report activity limitations as those in high-income families, and individuals in high-income families can expect to live three years longer than those in low-income families.

Disparities in health across racial and ethnic groups are not fully explained, but require study because of the major differences that exist and the need to address risks in groups with the poorest health. Important elements in such disparities include social, economic, and educational factors, as well as access to care, and the affordability of care. These factors tend to be confounding and have made it difficult to sort out the quantitative contribution of each. Some countries have provided more equitable distribution of public health and personal health care despite overall limitations in financial resources. These investments have been associated with improved health for the entire country. Considerable speculation has focused on the role of genetic differences across populations and groups as an explanation of health differences. However, this seems less important than environmental differences, as evidenced by the many instances of rapid change in disease patterns within a generation. This could not be explained by changes in the genetic pool.

PERSONAL ENVIRONMENTAL FACTORS

Personal environmental factors include behavioral choices that are made every day, though many behaviors are habitual. These personal behaviors are extraordinarily important and have been termed the underlying or true causes of chronic disease. They are outlined in Table 4. Use of tobacco, particularly smoking, is the number one preventable cause of death and disability. It directly contributes to ischemic heart disease, stroke, chronic lung disease, and several common cancers, especially lung cancer. These are the leading causes of death in industrialized countries and will be the leading causes worldwide during the coming century. Even exposure of nonsmokers to second-hand smoking increases risk. The prohibition of smoking in public places is an example of a public health regulation that decreases the risk for nonsmokers.

Dietary intake, which includes both the quantity and quality of foods, is highly important in the development of chronic diseases. An intake of calories in excess of what is expended during daily activity leads to obesity and an increased risk of diabetes, high blood pressure, heart disease, and some cancers. Increased physical activity can offset some excess caloric intake and may have additional healthful benefits as well. Since much of the industrialized world now has a predominance of inexpensive, calorically dense food and too little requirement for physical activity, it is not surprising that an epidemic of obesity, and the corresponding increased risk for disease, has occurred. As low-income countries move toward economic development and industrialization, there are similar pressures toward high caloric intake and decreased physical activity. Dietary patterns have important influences aside from the caloric content. Fruits and vegetables and whole grain products have beneficial effects on health, as does a limitation of fat intake to no more than 30 percent of calories.

Other personal behaviors and circumstances contribute to noncommunicable disease development. Alcohol use has both adverse and beneficial effects. Nonpregnant individuals and groups consuming small amounts of alcohol (about one drink per day) experience less ischemic heart disease. However, large amounts (about four or more drinks per day) contribute to chronic liver disease, depression and suicide, and injuries, especially motor vehicular injuries. Any alcohol use during pregnancy carries a risk for impaired fetal development.

Illicit drugs are addictive and impair social and occupational functioning and are associated with impaired mental health, notably depression. Both alcohol and illicit drugs can have long-term effects on intellect.

There is evidence that behavioral risk factors are influenced by the availability and affordability of tobacco, foods, and alcohol. When people immigrate to an industrialized country from an area where chronic diseases are less common, their pattern of disease changes to resemble the resident country over several decades of exposure. There has been no genetic change, but the risk factors and disease patterns change as the lifestyle changes. The influence of the new environment is especially marked in younger individuals. While genetic susceptibility is important, the factors of environment and personal behavior are robust, modifiable, and when changed effectively, can reduce disease.

RESEARCH

The determination that many attributes and behaviors carry risk for disease development has resulted from large observational studies. Groups and populations with varying personal behaviors and degrees of exposure have been studied for the development of disease, and this has allowed quantitative assessments of risk for the multiple factors associated with disease. The risk for disease is generally proportional to the level of the risk factors. The identification of these risks has provided a basis for studies to determine the effects of change. Numerous interventions to modify risk have been tested in clinical trials and community comparison studies. These provide a scientific basis for effective preventive measures that can modify risk factors and decrease disease and subsequent mortality. There is good evidence that lowering blood pressure and blood cholesterol, stopping smoking, and increasing physical activity can decrease deaths from ischemic heart disease and stroke. The majority of studies to identify and modify risk factors have been conducted in high-income countries where the resources for research are concentrated. As noncommunicable diseases increase in lesser developed countries there is a critical need to utilize findings from these studies and to conduct research that relates to indigenous exposures and cultures of LMICs. While many of the major risk factors are likely to be operative worldwide, there are new and perhaps unique risk factors and novel genetic-environmental interactions to be elucidated. The modification of behavioral risks will be dependent on understanding and integrating cultural aspects into lifestyle changes.

The profile of risk factors is constantly evolving, and in some instances there are infectious or communicable factors. Recent research indicates that infectious organisms, viruses, or bacteria may be resident as chronic infections and can initiate or contribute to the development of chronic disease. For example, the principal cause of peptic ulcer of the stomach or duodenum was long thought to be increased gastric acidity from stress and poor dietary habits. But, studies have clearly demonstrated that *Helicobacter pylori*, a fairly ubiquitous bacterium causing no acute symptomatology, can infect the stomach and cause peptic ulcer, and perhaps gastric cancer. Antibiotic treatment can eliminate peptic ulcer, and this affords evidence for its causative role. Similarly, human papilloma virus (HPV) is present in the early stages of cancer of the cervix. This association has led the testing of a vaccine to eliminate the infection and possibly prevent the development of cervical cancer. Chlamydia has been found in the atherosclerotic plaques of some persons with heart disease, though the role of the organism is unclear. Studies to eliminate the infection may provide insights that would serve to prevent and treat the condition.

Chronic conditions tend to result from the action of multiple factors, genetic and environmental, that increase the risk of disease. As research broadens the understanding of the multiple risks for disease, it would be expected that risk factors might have quantitatively different effects in different countries and cultures and expand the opportunities for intervention and prevention.

After considering these risk factors at the individual and community level, it is instructive to ask whether national changes in risk factors predict countrywide changes in noncommunicable disease. Observations of disease changes indicate that there is an approximate correlation between changes in risk factors and increases or decreases

in the relevant chronic diseases. A striking example is the emergence of chronic diseases in LMICs undergoing social changes associated with adoption of harmful behaviors. Smoking and obesity are becoming more common in countries undergoing rapid economic development, and these countries are experiencing the same epidemic of chronic diseases as the industrialized nations. The rates of heart disease, stroke, and diabetes have increased rapidly from 1950 to 1980 in rapidly industrializing countries. As is true with migrant groups undergoing change in risk and disease, environmental factors are critical. However, genetic propensity for particular disease expression may differ across populations and across countries. Subcontinental Indians who migrate to high-income countries and develop obesity have higher rates of diabetes and heart disease than non-migrating, native-born with the same levels of obesity. Two explanations have been offered. The first is that there is a greater genetic susceptibility in this population, but it is not expressed until the sufficient environment—excess calories—is available. The second is that in utero and early life experiences, especially food deprivation, change the expression of the genes as a means of promoting survival. A thrifty gene would conserve energy and store fat for survival in times of deprivation, but would be detrimental to health in times of plenty. Because developing countries are making the transition from relative privation to adequacy or excess, this becomes an important consideration in determining modifiable causes of chronic diseases.

A LOOK AHEAD

The experience of high-income countries indicates that noncommunicable diseases can be prevented and managed with declines in death and disability. This "postindustrial" epidemiologic transition is based on the development and application of scientific information. Risk factors predict disease and their modification through public health and personal health measures can change disease patterns in individuals, groups, and populations. Technological development can assist this change through the development of vaccines, medicines, and foods. However, personal behaviors and public health policies will always be important. These innovations can be transported throughout the world, but at a financial cost and with the need to assure cultural integrity. Cost, education, and cultural diversity will be barriers to be surmounted worldwide. Further investigation of risk will include appreciation of gene-environment interactions and exploration of new exposures. The improvement of health for all will depend on this progress.

WILLIAM R. HARLAN
LINDA C. HARLAN

(SEE ALSO: *Access to Health Services; Aging of Population; Alcohol Use and Abuse; Behavior, Health-Related; Blood Pressure; Causes of Death; Chronic Illness; Communicable Diseases; Environmental Determinants of Health; Epidemiologic Transition; Genetics and Health; Global Burden of Disease; Health Promotion and Education; Homicide; Inequalities in Health; International Health; Life Expectancy and Life Tables; Mental Health; Occupational Disease; Physical Activity; Primary Prevention; Race and Ethnicity; Risk Assessment, Risk Management; Smoking Behavior; Social Determinants; Substance Abuse, Definition of; Suicide; Violence; World Health Organization*)

BIBLIOGRAPHY

Murray, C. J. L., and Lopez, A. D. *The Global Burden of Disease.* Geneva: World Health Organization.

World Health Organization (2000). *World Health Report 2000–Health Systems: Improving Performance.* Geneva: Author.

NONGOVERNMENTAL ORGANIZATIONS, INTERNATIONAL

See International Nongovernmental Organizations

NONGOVERNMENTAL ORGANIZATIONS, UNITED STATES

Societies and their institutions are commonly divided into three sectors: public or governmental, for-profit or corporate, and nonprofit or independent. This number is sometimes reduced to two—public and private. The public sector includes governmental institutions, while the private includes both for-profit and nonprofit organizations. Institutions within the nonprofit or independent sector are often referred to as nongovernmental organizations (NGOs). This term is somewhat misleading, since it suggests a broader scope—that is, everything outside the governmental sector—than is usually intended. In general, the term refers only to nonprofits and does not include any organizations in the corporate sector.

Broadly speaking, NGOs include charitable organizations such as hospitals, museums, and orchestras; voluntary health agencies such as the American Cancer Society and American Heart Association; foundations or grant-making institutions such as the Robert Wood Johnson Foundation and the Carnegie Endowment for International Peace; social welfare organizations such as the National Association for the Advancement of Colored People and the National Center for Tobacco-Free Kids; and professional and trade organizations such as chambers of commerce and business leagues. Certain types of NGOs are also called voluntary organizations, development agencies, civil society organizations, membership organizations, mutual aid societies, advocacy organizations, and grassroots organizations.

NGOs are committed to addressing social needs and improving the human condition. In addition to this broad mandate, many NGOs share a number of other characteristics. They recruit and engage volunteers for many of their activities and are usually led by volunteer boards; they place mission before profits; and they engage in activities, such as grassroots advocacy campaigns, that would be difficult or impossible for other organizations. By focusing on a specific mission and drawing on the passionate support of local communities and loyal volunteers, NGOs are able to address issues that organizations in other sectors cannot or will not. Perhaps most important, NGOs enjoy a unique independence in their service to the public. Unlike organizations in the public sector, which are often subject to constant political pressure and regulation, and those in the corporate sector, which are beholden to their owners and shareholders, NGOs are accountable primarily to the public's trust.

With the rise of the modern nation state, social development has increasingly been viewed as the responsibility of government. The growth of social democracies and the welfare state during the twentieth century clearly reflects this belief. However, despite massive investment in social programs, governments have never been able to address fully the many needs of their citizens, nor are these needs often met by the corporate sector. NGOs have emerged in large part to bridge the gap between what governments and corporations can do and what society needs or expects.

The unique history and culture of the United States has played an important role in the growth of NGOs and their precursors, which include a range of disparate associations from volunteer fire departments, church groups, and missions to public and voluntary associations. Alexis de Tocqueville, the nineteenth-century French observer of American democracy and customs, was one of the first to comment on the unusual inclination of Americans to volunteer for community-based efforts. What he saw in America was the embodiment of modern longing for a fresh beginning and a fair start for all amid infinite possibilities. Everything American seemed limitless: its space, its resources, its energy, its pioneering spirit. These Americans are curious, he said. There is present an unusual neighbor-helping-neighbor philosophy. No sooner would someone's barn burn down than the entire community would pitch in to raise a new one. This, he said, was uniquely American. It is only since the 1850s, however, that NGOs in the modern sense have emerged and have begun to influence U.S. society on a broad scale. By the year 2000, the nonprofit sector within the United States included more than a million organizations, about 6 percent of all organizations in the country. Together these organizations allocated and dispensed more than $500 billion a year and employed one in fifteen Americans.

Present-day NGOs are often legal corporations with full-time staffs and governing boards and in the United States are categorized by the Internal Revenue Service as 501 (c)(3)s, (c)(4)s, and (c)(6)s. Their organizational structures are more formal and complex, and their operations are more strategic and businesslike. In fact, although NGOs are commonly defined in opposition to government and for-profit organizations, they frequently display characteristics of both. Many NGOs receive support from the government and for-profit corporations, and they often work in collaboration with these groups, each bringing their particular competencies to bear on a common issue. Such collaborations, especially those with the corporate sector, have often led to an increased professionalism and efficiency in NGOs. In fact, many choose to refer to themselves as not-for-profits, rather that nonprofits, indicating that although they are not in the business of making a profit, they are by no means averse to raising more funds for their work. Of course, unlike for-profit corporations, which distribute earnings and dividends to their shareholders, NGOs roll their surplus revenues into ongoing activities or hold them in reserve to cover future needs.

An important subset of NGOs is involved directly in public health issues and education. International NGOs, such as CARE, Oxfam, and Doctors without Borders, often focus on economic development and disaster relief, seeking to address crisis situations and broad infrastructural issues in order to improve the overall health and well-being of a community. Domestic NGOs provide similar services to low-income areas in the United States in addition to deploying resources and manpower during natural disasters. NGOs that focus on educational and occupational issues may indirectly address public health issues by empowering individuals with new skills and competencies, thereby improving their overall standard of living.

Voluntary health agencies (VHAs) are more directly involved in public health issues, often focusing on a particular disease or risk factor. They were among the earliest nongovernmental organizations established in the United States, with several dating back to the beginning of the twentieth century. Some of the larger and more well known VHAs are the American Cancer Society, the American Heart Association, the March of Dimes, the Planned Parenthood Federation of America, the National Easter Seal Society, the American Lung Association, and the Arthritis Foundation. VHAs are involved in a wide variety of activities including research, advocacy, public education, and patient services. Through experience and recruitment, they have acquired broad expertise in the practice of public health and have become critical to the pursuit and achievement of certain public health principles, such as universal access to health care.

Although it does not focus on a single disease or risk factor, the American Red Cross is viewed by some as an early prototype for the modern voluntary health agency. In October 1863, the International Red Cross and Red Crescent Movement was created in Geneva, Switzerland, to provide nonpartisan care to the wounded and sick in times of war. The American Association of the Red Cross was founded shortly thereafter in 1881. Initially, the organization was led by its president, Clara Barton, and an executive board comprised of eleven members. Shortly after its founding, the Red Cross was called into action to provide aid to the victims of a string of disasters, including war, fires, floods, famine, and hurricanes. To do so, the organization sought out volunteer support and public contributions. Since then, volunteer involvement has been an essential element of its organizational structure. As the organization expanded throughout the country, it began to establish local chapters, creating a model for local involvement that is still used today. Each chapter is responsible for local activities, subject to the policies and regulations of the national organization, and local revenues are generally shared with the parent organization. Over the next two decades, the Red Cross quickly established its place in society, and as the organization entered the twentieth century, its humanitarian efforts were well known and respected among the general public.

The model established by the Red Cross was soon duplicated by a number of other groups established to combat leading causes of death. In 1892, Lawrence F. Flick, a former field hand and tuberculosis patient, founded the Pennsylvania Society for the Prevention of Tuberculosis, the first American association of lay and medical professionals dedicated to the conquest of a single disease. In 1904, a national association was established, which quickly developed wide public support. Americans joined the association by the thousands, boosting the number of local affiliates from 23 in 1904 to 431 in 1910. With their support, the association helped accelerate the decline in mortality from tuberculosis through a variety of public health education efforts. The association also developed an early and innovative fundraising campaign, the Christmas seals program. Over the years, the control of tuberculosis has been so successful that the association has refocused its efforts and is now known as the American Lung Association.

The American Cancer Society was another pioneer in the voluntary health movement. In 1913, fifteen prominent physicians and business leaders gathered in New York City to found the American Society for the Control of Cancer (ASCC). Their mission was to disseminate knowledge concerning the symptoms, treatments, and the prevention of cancer; to investigate conditions under which cancer is found; and to compile statistics in regard thereto. The society soon began to establish chapters throughout the country. For many years, however, the majority of its members were concentrated on the East Coast, and consequently, much of its work was focused there. Then, in 1936, Marjorie G. Illig, an ASCC field representative and chair of the General Federation of Women's Clubs Committee on Public Health, established the Women's Field Army, one of the most successful volunteer recruitment structures ever created. Members of the Field Army donned khaki uniforms, complete with insignia of rank and achievement, and went out into the streets to raise money and help educate the public. Clarence Little, the ASCC's managing director at the time, wrote that, "In 1935 there were fifteen thousand people active in cancer control throughout the United States. At the close of 1938, there were ten times that number." In 1945, the ASCC was reorganized as the American Cancer Society. A year later, New York philanthropist Mary Lasker helped raise over $4 million dollars for the society, $1 million of which was used to establish and fund the Society's research program. In the year 2000, the American Cancer Society was the largest voluntary health agency in the world, with over 18 million volunteers and donors, a staff of eight thousand, and $600 million dollars in annual revenue.

No history of voluntary health agencies would be complete without mentioning the National Foundation for Infantile Paralysis (March of Dimes). In 1938, the foundation began collecting dimes to fund polio research. Seventeen years later, on April 12, 1955, the Salk vaccine became available to the public. Without the foundation's support, this achievement might have been delayed for many years. Indeed, in some ways, the story of the foundation exemplifies the power and possibility of the independent sector: polio was vanquished in large part through the voluntary actions of everyday Americans.

During this period, the foundation was led by Basil O'Connor, a Wall Street lawyer. O'Connor not only directed one of the most successful public health campaigns in history but also reinvigorated the voluntary health movement by applying modern marketing techniques to fundraising and simultaneously inspiring a legion of devoted volunteers to his cause. O'Connor's March of Dimes campaign was enormously successful. In 1938, O'Connor enlisted some of the nation's shrewdest advertising and public relations experts to help develop and implement the inaugural campaign. For weeks, the public was inundated with polio information. Hundreds of thousands of dollars in free advertising was devoted to the cause, and celebrities from Edgar Guest to Walt Disney to Shirley Temple donated their time. The campaign culminated with an on-air appeal from Eddie Cantor, Jack Benny, Bing Crosby, and others, urging listeners to send their dimes to the White House. The public response was enormous. Nearly $2 million was raised during that first campaign and future efforts proved equally successful. Although far more people were affected by cancer and heart disease than polio in 1938, O'Connor was able to capture the public's attention, propelling the National Infantile Paralysis to the forefront of the voluntary health movement.

Since these first organizations came into prominence, many more NGOs have been established. Some are small organizations with only a handful of staff and volunteers. Others operate on a global scale. Whatever the case, NGOs continue to play a critical role in U.S. society. In the future, success will lead to obsolescence for some NGOs, but others will evolve to address unresolved issues and emerging threats, improving the health and well-being of the public.

JOHN R. SEFFRIN

(SEE ALSO: *American Cancer Society; American Heart Association; American Lung Association; American Medical Association; American Public Health Association; Official U.S. Health Agencies*)

BIBLIOGRAPHY

Carter, R. (1992). *The Gentle Legions.* New Brunswick, NJ: Transition.

Fernando, J. L., and Heston, A. W., eds. (1997). "Introduction: NGOs Between States, Markets, and Civil Society." *Annals of the American Academy of Political and Social Science* 554:46–65.

Green, A., and Matthias, A. (1997). *Non-Governmental Organizations and Health in Developing Countries.* New York: St. Martin's Press.

NONIONIZING RADIATION

Nonionizing radiation, in contrast to ionizing radiation, is electromagnetic radiation that does not have sufficient energy to remove electrons from an atom or molecules to form an ion (or charged particle) during a collision. Instead, it imparts energy to other particles, which typically results in heating. Nonionizing radiation includes frequencies of the electromagnetic spectrum ranging from 1 hertz (Hz) up to 3×10^{10} Hz (300 gigahertz) and its wavelengths range from 10^9 meters down to 10^{-7} meters. As the frequency of a wave decreases and the wavelength increases, the energy decreases. Included within this category of nonionizing radiation are—in order of decreasing energy: the lower frequency portion of ultraviolet (UV) radiation, visible light, infrared radiation (IR), microwave radiation, radio frequency radiation, and extremely low frequency (ELF) radiation.

Some types of nonionizing radiation have both beneficial and harmful effects on human health. For example, exposure to UV radiation facilitates the synthesis of vitamin D in the human body, and vitamin D plays an important role in intestinal calcium absorption. Lack of vitamin D can result in lead overdosing, kidney damage, and elevated serum cholesterol levels. UV is also used as an antimicrobial agent—it can penetrate food packaging and sterilize the contents—and it is used in tanning beds and salons. On the other hand, acute UV exposure can cause eye and skin damage in humans, and long-term exposure has been found to cause elastosis (loss of skin elasticity) and skin cancer in humans. The sun is the major source of UV radiation.

Lasers, one type of nonionizing radiation device that operates at below UV frequencies, are used for a variety of important scientific and industrial processes, but inappropriate exposures can cause severe injuries in humans. Infrared radiation, which can be used in home electrical appliances, welding, furnaces, and foundries, can cause skin and eye damage through excessive heating.

Lower-frequency nonionizing radiation, such as microwave, radio frequency, and ELF radiation, have many beneficial uses—such as tracking radar, weather radar, microwave ovens, radio navigation, satellite communication, broadcast radio and television, and a variety of other communications devices including two-way radios and cellular phones. Acute effects from direct exposure to high levels of this type of radiation can include severe burns, electric shocks, and even death. The human health effects of chronic exposure to these types of radiation are less clear. The higher frequencies in this range, such as microwaves, may cause adverse heating effects. The majority of studies, which have focused on exposure to ELF radiation, have examined cancer, adverse reproductive outcomes, neurodegenerative diseases, and cardiac abnormalities. However, difficulties in conducting these studies, including defining and measuring the biologically relevant exposure and variation in subjects' responses, have left substantial uncertainty.

The most effective means of preventing exposure to most types of nonionizing radiation is to maintain a safe distance from the source. Other means of preventing or limiting exposure, such as using shields, are far more difficult and costly, particularly as the size of the source increases. Unlike ionizing radiation, nonionizing radiation penetrates through most materials relatively unchanged. Special metallic grids can be designed to exclude radiation of particular frequencies, but this is not currently practical, physically, for handheld devices such as cellular phones and two-way radios, and is very onerous for large-scale implementation, such as around houses or buildings.

DANIEL WARTENBERG

(SEE ALSO: *Electromagnetic Fields; Radiation, Ionizing*)

BIBLIOGRAPHY

Ducatman, A. M., and Haes, D. L., Jr. (1994). "Nonionizing Radiation." In *Textbook of Clinical Occupational and Environmental Medicine*, eds. L. Rosenstock and M. R. Cullen. Philadelphia, PA: W. B. Saunders Company.

Michaelson, S. M. (1975). *Fundamentals and Applied Aspects of Nonionizing Radiation*. New York: Plenum.

Wilkening, G. M. (1991). "Nonionizing Radiation." In *Patty's Industrial Hygiene and Toxicology*, eds. G. D. Clayton and F. E. Clayton. New York: Wiley.

NONMALEFICENCE

The term "nonmaleficence" derives from the ancient maxim *primum non nocere*, which, translated from the Latin, means "first, do no harm." Professionals in the health sciences, and in public health practice in particular, have a tradition of utilitarian approaches, meaning that the greatest good should be accomplished through any public health action. Obligations not to harm others (e.g., through theft, disablement, or killing) are clearly distinct from, and usually more stringent than, obligations to help others (e.g., by providing benefits, protecting interests, and promoting welfare). For example, the obligation not to injure others is a societal expectation, whereas the act of rescuing someone in danger is generally considered a heroic act.

In public health research and practice, professionals intervene through asking people to participate in research by, for instance, answering questions, submitting themselves to vaccination or screening programs, through issuing health advisories, or through legislation. Under the utilitarian theory of ethics that serves as the foundation for public health, the duty not to cause harm through any intervention is interpreted to mean that any given intervention must result in more good than harm on a population basis. In medical practice, what the physician does for a patient should have a greater chance of benefiting than harming the patient. Both applications of the duty not to harm are supported by rigorous risk-benefit analyses, often based on studies of effects of animals (e.g., toxicological research of new drugs). They are enforced through regulations under administrative law designed to protect the public health interest, as well as through codes of professional practice.

A common public health concern involving the principle of doing no harm involves product safety. Harms can arise when manufactured products are used by consumers. The crucial question is whether or not adequate knowledge existed before the product went to market about the potential for harms to occur. If the manufacturer did not take precautions (e.g., adequate product testing) to ensure safety, the duty to cause no harm would have been breached because, with due care, harm could have been prevented. The breach would be real regardless of whether or not harm was intended.

The actions of individuals can also be contrary to the principle of nonmaleficence. For example, the leading cause of death in North America among people aged eighteen to thirty-four is accidental injury. The majority of these injuries involve motor vehicles. If a driver should fail to obey the speed limit or drive while intoxicated, he or she is placing other drivers in a dangerous situation. While there is no specific intent to harm, reasonable care was not taken to avoid harm. Breach of the obligation to cause no harm in the absence of a specific intent to harm is called "negligence" and may be treated as such under the law.

COLIN L. SOSKOLNE
LEE E. SIESWERDA

(SEE ALSO: *Beneficence; Codes of Conduct and Ethics Guidelines; Ethics of Public Health*)

BIBLIOGRAPHY

Beauchamp, T. L., and Childress, J. F. (1994). *Principles of Biomedical Ethics,* 4th edition. New York: Oxford University Press.

NORM

The terms "norm" and "normal" generally refer to what is customary or usual, or sometimes to what is desirable. In a technical sense, "norm" applies to standards or criteria, and may be applied to either a measurable variable, such as height or weight, or to a way of behaving. In medicine and in public health, "normal" has several meanings: it can mean healthy, or in a more precise sense it may mean that the value of a variable such as temperature or blood pressure is within generally accepted limits applicable to healthy people. In statistics, a *normal distribution* is defined as a continuous frequency distribution of infinite range in which values are symmetrically distributed about a central mean.

JOHN M. LAST

(SEE ALSO: *Assessment of Health Status; Health; Statistics for Public Health*)

Figure 1

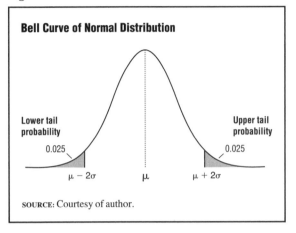

SOURCE: Courtesy of author.

NORMAL DISTRIBUTIONS

In studies of public health, information is frequently collected for variables that can be measured on a continuous scale in nature. Examples of such variables include age, weight, and blood pressure. The shape of the distribution associated with these variables is useful to describe the frequency of values across different ranges. More specifically, distributions allow for the probability of obtaining a specific value of a variable to be calculated, while providing estimates of the average, and range, of possible values. The normal distribution is the most widely used distribution to describe continuous variables. It is also frequently referred to as the *Gaussian* distribution, after the well-known German mathematician Karl Friedrich Gauss (1777–1855).

Normal distributions are a family of distributions characterized by the same general shape. These distributions are symmetrical, with the measured values of the variable more concentrated in the middle than in the tails. They are frequently referred to as "bell-shaped." The area under the curve of a normal distribution represents the sum of the probabilities of obtaining every possible value for a variable. In other words, the total area under a normal curve is equal to one. The shape of the normal distribution represents specified mathematically in terms of only two parameters: the mean (μ), and the standard deviation (σ). The standard deviation specifies the amount of dispersion around the mean, whereas the mean is the average value across sampled values of the variable. It is a characteristic of normal distribution that 95 percent of the possible values for a variable lie within ±2 standard deviations. This is illustrated in Figure 1.

Several biological variables are normally distributed (e.g., blood pressure, serum cholesterol, height, and weight). The normal curve can be used to estimate probabilities associated with these variables. For example, in a population where the birth weight of infants is normally distributed with a mean of 7.2 pounds and a standard deviation of 2.1 pounds, one might wish to find the probability a randomly chosen infant will have a birth weight of less than 3 pounds. Such information might help in planning for future obstetric services.

Since the normal distribution can have an infinite number of possible values for its mean and standard deviation, it is impossible to calculate the area for each and every curve. Instead, probabilities are calculated for a single curve where the mean is zero and the standard deviation is one. This curve is referred to as a standard normal distribution (Z). A random variable (X) that is normally distributed with mean (μ) and standard deviation (σ) can be easily transformed to the standard normal distribution by the formula $Z = (X-\mu)/\sigma$.

The normal distribution is important to statistical work because most hypothesis tests that are used assume that the random variable being considered has an underlying normal distribution. Fortunately, these tests work very well even if the distribution of the variable is only approximately normal. Examples of such tests include those based on the t, F, or chi-square statistics. If the variable is not normal, alternative nonparametric tests should be considered; however, such tests are inconvenient because they typically are less powerful and flexible in terms of types of conclusions that can be drawn. Alternatively, mathematical theory (e.g., the central limit theorem) has proven that normal distribution–based hypothesis testing can be performed if a large enough number of samples are taken. This latter option is based on an important principle that is largely responsible for the popularity of tests based on the normal function—that if the size of the samples is large enough, the shape of the sampling distribution approaches normal shape even if the distribution of the variable in question is not normal.

PAUL J. VILLENEUVE

(SEE ALSO: *Chi-Square Test; Sampling; Statistics for Public Health*)

NOSOCOMIAL INFECTIONS

A nosocomial, or hospital-acquired, infection is a new infection that develops in a patient during hospitalization. It is usually defined as an infection that is identified at least forty-eight to seventy-two hours following admission, so infections incubating, but not clinically apparent, at admission are excluded. With recent changes in health care delivery, the concept of "nosocomial infections" has sometimes been expanded to include other "health care–associated infections," including infections acquired in institutions other than acute-care facilities (e.g. nursing homes); infections acquired during hospitalization but not identified until after discharge; and infections acquired through outpatient care such as day surgery, dialysis, or home parenteral therapy.

Early studies reported at least 5 percent of patients became infected during hospitalization. With the increased use of invasive procedures, at least 8 percent of patients now acquire nosocomial infections.

The most frequent types of infection are urinary-tract infection, surgical-wound infection, pneumonia, and bloodstream infection (see Table 1). These infections follow interventions necessary for patient care, but which impair normal defenses. At least 80 percent of nosocomial urinary infections are attributable to the use of an indwelling urethral catheter. Surgical-wound infection follows interference with the skin barrier, and is associated with the intensity of bacterial contamination of the wound at surgery. Nosocomial pneumonia occurs most frequently in intensive-care-unit patients with endotracheal intubation on mechanical ventilation—the endotracheal tube bypasses normal defenses of the upper airway. Finally, primary nosocomial bloodstream infection occurs virtually only with the use of indwelling central vascular catheters, and correlates directly with the duration of catheterization.

Table 1

Frequency of most common nosocomial infections

Infection Site	Incidence	
	All patients	Device-related
Urinary tract infection	2.34/100 admissions	5.3-10.5/1,000 catheter days
Surgical site infection	4.6-8.2/1,000 discharges	2.1-7.1% of wounds
Pneumonia	0.5-1.0/100 admissions	9-47% ventilated patients 1-3%/ventilator day
Central vascular line	—	1.4% of central catheters 1.7/1,000 catheter days

SOURCE: Mayhall, ed.

The clinical status of the patient is important in the development of infection. Many hospitalized patients, such as leukemia patients or transplant patients, have profoundly impaired immunity due to both their disease and therapy. These patients are highly susceptible to infection, frequently with organisms that do not cause infection in normal persons. Patients with neurologic problems may have swallowing difficulties due to aspiration of bacteria from the mouth or stomach, which can lead to pneumonia. Patients who have received antimicrobials may develop nosocomial infectious diarrhea caused by *Clostridium difficile*.

The hospital environment may also contribute to infections. Repeated outbreaks of Legionnaire's disease caused by organisms in a hospital's potable water or in air conditioning cooling towers have occurred. Increases in *Aspergillus* spores in the air during hospital construction cause fungal pneumonia in some immunocompromised patients, with a mortality rate of over 50 percent. Bacterial contamination of sterile intravenous fluids or equipment has repeatedly caused outbreaks of nosocomial infections. Finally, patients may acquire tuberculosis or chicken pox from other patients.

NATURE AND DIMENSION OF PUBLIC HEALTH PROBLEM

The high frequency of nosocomial infections places a substantial burden on individual patients and on the health care system. There is increased morbidity, including delayed wound healing, delayed rehabilitation, increased exposure to antimicrobial therapy and its potential adverse effects, and prolonged hospitalization. The average prolongation of stay is 3.8 days for urinary infection, 7.4 days for surgical-site infection, 5.9 days for pneumonia, and 7 to 24 days for primary bloodstream infection. Some infections, such as infection occurring in a hip or knee replacement, result in prolonged or even permanent disability and require repeated rehospitalization and reoperation. Nosocomial infections also cause mortality. The case-fatality rate for patients with ventilator-associated pneumonia is 42 percent, with an attributable mortality of 15 to 30 percent. For nosocomial bloodstream infection, the case fatality rate is 14 percent, with an estimated attributable mortality of 19 percent.

Nosocomial infections are costly. The direct costs of hospital-acquired infections in the United States is estimated to be $4.5 billion per year. In England, the cost for one health unit is estimated to be 3.6 million pounds per year. Prolongation of stay necessitated by nosocomial infection limits access of other patients to hospital resources, and contributes to overcrowding on wards and in emergency departments.

Nosocomial infections also contribute to the emergence and dissemination of antimicrobial-resistant organisms. Antimicrobial use for treatment or prevention of infections facilitates the emergence of resistant organisms. Patients with infection with antimicrobial-resistant organisms are then a source of infection for other hospitalized patients. Some bacteria, such as methicillin-resistant *Staphylococcus aureus*, may subsequently spread to the community.

CONTROL AND PREVENTION

Prevention of nosocomial infections requires a systematic, multidisciplinary approach. This is usually achieved under the leadership of an institutional infection-control program. The principle activities of such a program include surveillance, outbreak management, policy development, expert advice, and education. An optimal program may decrease the incidence of nosocomial infections by 30 to 50 percent.

Surveillance of nosocomial infections, by itself, may decrease the incidence. When each surgeon is provided with their own wound-infection rates and with other surgeons' rates for comparison, the institutional surgical-wound infection rate decreases. Outbreak control includes early identification of potential outbreaks, as well as evaluation and intervention if an outbreak is identified. Continuing education of hospital staff about the importance of, and their role in, preventing nosocomial infections is necessary. The infection-control program also provides expert consultation to other hospital programs such as occupational health, clinical microbiology, and pharmacy.

Institutional policies and practices must be developed and adhered to. In particular, optimal handwashing and glove use must be facilitated and reinforced, as transmission of organisms between patients occurs primarily on the hands of staff members. Isolation guidelines to identify and segregate patients who have an increased risk of transmitting infection to other patients or staff are also essential. Other important policies include: for urinary infection, the use and care of the indwelling catheter; and for surgical wound infection, optimal surgical technique including preoperative preparation and prophylactic antimicrobials. Many national or local standards and regulations will also prevent nosocomial infection, and institutions must be in compliance. These regulations cover hospital construction, municipal water supply, laundry management, food handling, waste disposal, sterilization and other reprocessing procedures, as well as standards for pharmacy and microbiology laboratory practice.

An effective infection-control program requires dedicated staff with appropriate training and sufficient resources. The number of personnel is determined by the size and complexity of the facility. Infection-control practitioners, usually from a nursing background, are responsible for program activity. In larger hospitals, program leadership is provided by a physician with training in epidemiology and infection control. Smaller facilities may obtain such expertise by contractual arrangement with outside experts. Oversight of the infection-control program is usually provided by a multidisciplinary infection-control committee. The program director, however, should report directly to senior hospital management to ensure optimal program effectiveness.

LINDSAY E. NICOLLE

(SEE ALSO: *Antisepsis and Sterilization; Barrier Nursing; Contagion; Hospital Administration*)

BIBLIOGRAPHY

Centers for Disease Control and Prevention (1999). "Guidelines for Prevention of Surgical Site Infection." *Infection Control and Hospital Epidemiology* 20:247–278.

Health Canada Laboratory Centre for Disease Control (1998). "Handwashing, Cleaning, Disinfection, and Sterilization in Health Care." *Canadian Communicable Disease Report* 24S8(Supp.).

—— (1999). "Routine Practices and Additional Precautions for Preventing Transmission of Infection in Health Care." *Canadian Communicable Disease Report* 25S4(Supp.).

Mayhall, C. G., ed. (1999). *Hospital Epidemiology and Infection Control*, 2nd edition. Philadelphia, PA: Lippincott Williams and Wilkins.

Scheckler, W. E.; Brumhall, D.; Buck, A. S.; Farr, B. M.; Friedman, C.; Garibaldi, R. A.; Gross, P. A.; Harris, J. A.; Hierholzer, W. J., Jr.; Martone, W. J.; McDonald, L. L.; Solomon, S. L. (1998). "Requirements for Infrastructure and Essential Activities of Infection Control and Epidemiology in Hospitals: A Consensus Panel Report." *Infection Control and Hospital Epidemiology* 19:114–124.

Shlaes, D. M.; Gerding, D. N.; John, J. F.; Craig, W. A.; Bornstein, D. L.; Duncan, R. A.; Eckman, M. R.; Farrer, W. E.; Greene, W. H.; Lorian, V.; Levy, S.; McGowan, J. E.; Paul, S. M.; Ruskin, J.; Tenover, F. C.; and Watanakunakorn, C. (1997). "Society for Healthcare Epidemiology of America and Infectious Diseases Society of America Joint Committee on the Prevention of Antimicrobial Resistance: Guidelines for the Prevention of Antimicrobial Resistance in Hospitals." *Infection Control and Hospital Epidemiology* 18:275–291.

NOT IN MY BACKYARD (NIMBY)

The so-called NIMBY (not in my backyard) syndrome reflects the propensity of local citizens and officials to insist on siting unwanted but necessary facilities anywhere but in their own community. The term has gained currency in relation to the siting of facilities that have a potential for adverse impacts on the environment, such as municipal waste incinerators and hazardous waste facilities. But it is equally applicable to the siting of prisons, methadone clinics, and psychiatric halfway houses—all of which are often subject to intense local opposition. For all of these examples, the best approach to the problem is that of primary prevention, which would lessen the need for such facilities. Success in siting an unwanted but needed facility requires that authorities fully involve the public with openness and integrity in all aspects of the planning process.

BERNARD D. GOLDSTEIN

(SEE ALSO: *Community Health; Nuclear Waste; Nuisance Abatement*)

BIBLIOGRAPHY

Chess, C. (2000). "Evaluating Environmental Public Participation: Methodological Questions." *Journal of Environmental Planning and Management* 43(6):769–784.

NOTIFIABLE DISEASES

The collection of relevant data pertaining to disease occurrence, when collated, analyzed, and reported, leads to a public health action. This is known as Public Health Surveillance. Without a resultant action, the information gathered is archival and not satisfying a public health function. Disease control and prevention activities cannot be effectively and efficiently accomplished without analyzing occurrence data, which helps direct the development of these activities. The initial data may not be adequate for accomplishing the subsequent public health action and thus additional data may need to be collected or a research project initiated. All of our efforts in disease control and prevention work are predicated by having meaningful disease notification.

Disease reporting was initially developed more than 150 years ago in Great Britain when occurrence data related to epidemic diseases such as cholera and plague were collected. It was the accumulation of data concerning the occurrence of cholera deaths in London in the 1840s that led to epidemiological studies by John Snow that portrayed the natural history of cholera in London

from which control and prevention measures were offered and eventually accepted. Subsequently, more specific mechanisms of obtaining disease occurrence data were developed; and in the United States in the early 1900s, laws were passed that initiated the development of the disease reporting system. Through the years, this system has become more sophisticated both in the United States and throughout the world. No part of the world is truly isolated, and thus it is recognized that worldwide disease reporting is important if diseases are to be controlled and prevented. Each country will have its own arrangements for developing surveillance data according to its own needs and resources. The World Health Organization (WHO) maintains worldwide coverage of selected diseases and solicits the reporting of other diseases on a voluntary basis. By international law, plague, cholera, and yellow fever are reportable to WHO. Data on these diseases are summarized in a weekly epidemiologic report prepared and distributed by the WHO.

There are multiple uses of disease notification data. A major use is that of providing information concerning the natural history of disease. For example, data for malaria in the United States from 1920 to 1999 depicts a gradual decrease in incidence, apparently due to control measures, but with a number of sporadic increases, reflecting, for example, returning members of the armed forces or immigrants from malarious areas of the world. The system also may be used to portray changes in the occurrence of a disease. Another use is to monitor the effectiveness of control and prevention measures, such as the decreasing incidence of measles reflecting the nation's vaccination program. Another use of the data is to assist in the detection of a national epidemic that may not be apparent when looking at data from a single state. When data are accumulated from several states, however, the occurrence of an epidemic may become apparent. This is exemplified by the data for the epidemic of salmonellosis in 1984 in the Midwest caused by contaminated milk. The Centers for Disease Control and Prevention (CDC) has developed guidelines, including threshold values, which assist in identifying the occurrence of a disease epidemic. Disease notification data may also be useful in suggesting the need for research, including field investigations in order to explain unusual features of disease occurrence.

Within the Untied States, each state has its own laws concerning what diseases are reportable and how they should be reported to the state health department. The number of diseases reportable within the states varies from thirty-five to 120. These state laws include penalties for not reporting reportable diseases; however, there is no information available concerning whether any health care practitioners have been charged with not reporting a reportable disease.

The CDC is the agency within the United States Public Health Service that is charged with the responsibility for maintaining the notifiable disease system for the United States. The diseases that are reportable from states to CDC are decided upon by agreement between the states and CDC, though this is a voluntary reporting system. The diseases to be reported to CDC are discussed at an annual meeting. As of January 2000, sixty diseases were reportable. In some states, the laws do not include all nationally notifiable diseases. The National Notifiable Diseases Surveillance System (NNDSS) asks for the number of cases of each disease that have been reported within the state on a weekly basis. However, there are supplemental CDC reporting systems for many of these diseases for which the states are asked to fill out a more specific reporting from that calls particularly for data that allows for the determination of potential risk factors. Routine reporting through the NNDSS from the states to CDC is accomplished by computer, whereas the supplemental systems have specific forms that are filled out and forwarded to CDC.

Public health surveillance may either be passive or active. Passive surveillance is the form of surveillance that is most commonly utilized throughout the world and consists of the routine reporting of a disease being initiated by the health care provider. Occasionally a specific request for reporting a disease is made by a public health agency, initiated because an acute outbreak of disease requires rapid accumulation of information in order to consider effective control and prevention measures. Usually such reporting is maintained only for a limited period of time. Also, a group of health care practitioners may be specifically requested to report a disease or diseases. This group may be proportionately representative of the entire group of health care providers, or they may be a selected sample in order to get more quantitative

reporting. If the reporters are randomly selected on the basis of population density, the resulting data may be extrapolated to the entire population. Disease reporting may also be directed toward a specific population among whom a particular disease has a higher incidence than in the general population.

Reporting is usually the responsibility of the health care provider who makes the diagnosis of a patient's illness. However, a surrogate may be used; for example, in a hospital a ward clerk may be designated to initiate the report. Reporting may also be the responsibility of the laboratory in which the etiologic agent is identified, which allows more specific reporting of certain diseases such as gastrointestinal diseases.

The most common reporting system is morbidity reporting, where each case of a reportable disease is reported. Mortality reporting may also be used, such as with influenza. The weekly occurrence of deaths due to "Influenza and Pneumonia" are used to portray the occurrence of influenza. Reporting may also be accomplished by noting absenteeism in schools or large industrial establishments, or by the utilization of pharmaceuticals purchased in pharmacies. Reporting within states is usually accomplished on a weekly basis using reporting forms, postcards, fax machines, or computers.

The sensitivity of reporting varies, but for the common diseases it is low, maybe as low as 5 percent. However, if the methods of reporting, case definitions, and the reporters do not change, then the data will still adequately represent the trend of the disease occurrence for control and prevention purposes. Sensitivity can be increased by offering a reward (such as financial) for reporting a confirmed case of a disease. Such an award system was very important in the worldwide smallpox eradication program in the 1960s and 1970s.

At regular intervals the accumulated data concerning notifiable diseases should be analyzed by time, place, and person to the level permitted by the details reported. Once analyzed, a report should be prepared providing quantitative information concerning the occurrence of disease, as well as information concerning recommended control and prevention measures. Field investigations can also be reported. CDC prepares the *Morbidity and Mortality Weekly Report* (MMWR), which is available through the CDC's web site. Additionally, the MMWR may be obtained in hard copy from the Government Printing Office or the Massachusetts Medical Society. CDC also prepares an annual summary of all of the data for the preceding year, which are compared to the data accumulated over the past thirty to forty years. Disease-specific reports are published by CDC at regular intervals and may also be obtained through the CDC web site or from the above two agencies.

The reporting of data analyses back to the health care providers is important so they are encouraged to continue reporting. Not only is this important for continuity, but is also allows them to be updated on disease occurrence, on current method and prevention, and on the success of implementation of these measures.

Disease reporting systems should be evaluated at regular intervals to assure that they are functioning as planned. Important attributes to consider in evaluating such effectiveness include sensitivity, specificity, predictive value positive, representativeness, flexibility, simplicity, acceptability, and timeliness. Sensitivity refers to whether all true cases of the particular disease have been reported. Specificity refers to noncases not being reported as cases. Predictive value positive is the proportion of reported cases that truly are cases. A flexible system can adapt to changes in disease occurrence, or in changes in the reporting system, and still continue to function. Simplicity indicates a minimum of effort on the part of those involved in reporting or maintaining the system, and acceptability that reporting is acceptable to the health care providers who are asked to report. Timeliness refers to the fact that the data reported can be used in a timely manner for the control and prevention of that disease. Representativeness means that the cases reported does represent the occurrence of the disease, as it is occurring at the time of reporting. Another important consideration is cost-effectiveness, that is, whether the disease reporting for a particular disease saves money compared to not maintaining reporting for that disease.

The practice of disease notification is becoming more sophisticated not only in the United States but throughout the world. The use of computers is making reporting quicker and more accurate, and it supports more sophisticated analysis of the data. Improving laboratory support by means of more rapid and detailed identification of etiologic agents has also increased the effectiveness disease reporting.

In the future, health care practitioners, after seeing a patient, will be able to record the history, physical examination, and laboratory findings on a computer that will be programmed to automatically report the reportable data to the local health department, form which it will automatically be reported to the state health department. This will release the health care provider from having to make a special effort to file a report and improve the timing, accuracy, and sensitivity of reporting.

PHILIP S. BRACHMAN

(SEE ALSO: *Information Systems; Surveillance*)

BIBLIOGRAPHY

Brachman, P. S. (1998). "Surveillance." In *Bacterial Infections of Humans–Epidemiology and Control*, 3rd edition, eds. A. S. Evans and P. S. Brachman. New York: Plenum Publishing Corporation.

Langmuir, A. D. (1963). "The Surveillance of Communicable Diseases of National Importance." *New England Journal of Medicine* 268:182–192.

Thacker, S. B., and Berkelman, R. C. (1988). "Public Health Surveillance in the United States." *Epidemiologic Reviews* 10:164–190.

Thacker, S. B., and Stroup, D. F. (1998). "Public Health Surveillance." *Applied Epidemiology: Theory to Practice*, eds. R. C. Brownson and D. B. Petitti. Oxford: Oxford University Press.

NUCLEAR POWER

The use of nuclear power to generate electricity began in the late 1950s. At the close of the twentieth century, nuclear power was supplying about 20 percent of the electricity generated in the United States and about 16 percent worldwide.

Nuclear power has been the most controversial of all energy sources. Public concerns about reactor safety and environmental issues were especially heightened by the 1979 accident at Three Mile Island in Pennsylvania and the much more serious accident in 1986 at Chernobyl in Ukraine. Construction of new nuclear power plants has slowed considerably since then, and some industrialized countries may abandon this energy source. Concerns about disposal of spent nuclear fuel have also affected public confidence in nuclear power. Although many scientists believe that spent fuel and other highly radioactive wastes can be disposed of safely in a geologic repository located far below ground, disposal sites for these wastes have not been approved, and the need to store spent fuel until disposal facilities are available raises safety and environmental concerns. The public also has not supported development of new disposal facilities for low-level radioactive wastes generated at nuclear power plants and in many other commercial activities. Other factors contributing to public concerns have included environmental problems at sites operated under nuclear weapons programs and fears that plutonium produced at nuclear power plants could be diverted for use in nuclear weapons.

Public concerns about safety and environmental issues have been exacerbated by financial risks in the nuclear power industry, including the high cost of constructing and operating nuclear power plants, potentially high costs of decommissioning nuclear facilities, and costs for storage and disposal of spent fuel and other nuclear wastes. Nuclear power may not remain competitive with other energy sources unless these costs are reduced.

Proponents of nuclear power emphasize its significant benefits. Past accidents notwithstanding, the nuclear power industry has an enviable safety record in those industrialized countries that require extensive reactor safety systems. Uranium used in nuclear fuel is abundant, which reduces dependence on foreign energy supplies and preserves oil and natural gas for essential uses. Nuclear reactors produce the greatest amount of energy per amount of fuel of any nonrenewable energy source, and the environmental damage from use of nuclear power is less than with other major energy sources, especially coal. Perhaps most importantly, the use of nuclear power in place of coal, oil, and natural gas greatly reduces emissions of carbon dioxide, which is believed to be a factor in global warming, and other hazardous air pollutants.

Given these benefits, many energy experts believe that nuclear power is an important energy source for the future. A major challenge will be to address public concerns about safety and environmental issues. The keys to meeting this challenge may include resolving concerns about nuclear waste disposal, siting of new reactors in remote areas, developing smaller reactors that incorporate passive safety systems, and using standard power plant designs to lower construction and operating costs.

DAVID C. KOCHER

(SEE ALSO: *Chernobyl; Energy; Not In My Backyard [NIMBY]; Nuclear Waste; Risk Assessment, Risk Management; Three Mile Island*)

BIBLIOGRAPHY

Cohen, B. L. (1990). *The Nuclear Energy Option: An Alternative for the 90s.* New York: Plenum Press.

Gofman, J. W., and Tamplin, A. R. (1971). *Poisoned Power: The Case Against Nuclear Power Plants.* Emmaus, PA: Rodale Press.

Jungk, R. (1979). *The New Tyranny: How Nuclear Power Enslaves Us.* New York: Grosset & Dunlap, Inc.

Rhodes, R. (1993). *Nuclear Renewal: Common Sense about Energy.* New York: Whittle Books.

NUCLEAR WASTE

Nuclear waste has many sources that are grouped into two broad categories. The first category is nuclear fuel-cycle waste, which consists of any waste arising from the separation and processing of uranium to fabricate nuclear fuel, from nuclear reactors used for any purpose, and from any subsequent uses of radioactive materials contained in nuclear fuel or produced in a reactor. Uses of nuclear reactors include generation of electricity; production of plutonium for use in nuclear weapons; production of radioisotopes for use in medicine, industry, or commerce; and research and development. The different types of nuclear fuel-cycle waste include the following:

- High-level radioactive waste arises mainly when spent nuclear fuel from a reactor is chemically reprocessed to remove plutonium for use in nuclear weapons. This highly hazardous waste contains high concentrations of radioactive fission products, such as strontium-90, iodine-131, and cesium-137, and long-lived radionuclides heavier than uranium, such as plutonium and americium.

- Spent nuclear fuel, which resembles high-level waste, is waste if it is not chemically reprocessed. Spent fuel from nuclear power reactors in the United States is not reprocessed at the present time, but reprocessing is carried out in other countries.

- Transuranic waste arises mainly when plutonium removed from spent fuel is used in fabricating nuclear weapons. This waste mostly contains plutonium and other heavy radionuclides, such as americium, in lower concentrations than in high-level waste or spent fuel, although there are exceptions.

- Mill tailings are the very large volumes of residues containing naturally occurring radionuclides that arise mainly when uranium is chemically separated from ores for use in nuclear fuel. The radiation hazard of mill tailings is due mainly to the elevated levels of radium and high emanation rates of radon gas.

- Low-level radioactive waste includes any nuclear fuel-cycle waste other than high-level waste, spent fuel, transuranic waste, and mill tailings. Low-level waste arises in many activities, including operations at nuclear facilities; uses of reactor-produced radioisotopes in medicine, industry, or commerce; cleanup of radioactively contaminated sites; and research and development. Most low-level waste contains relatively low concentrations of radionuclides, but some wastes can be as hazardous as high-level waste or spent fuel.

The second broad category includes any nuclear waste other than the nuclear fuel-cycle wastes described above. Nuclear waste in this category thus includes naturally occurring or accelerator-produced radioactive material (NARM). Waste containing naturally occurring radioactive material, such as potassium-40, uranium, thorium, or radium, does not include mill tailings. Important wastes of this type include spent radium sources, waste from removal of radionuclides from drinking water, residues from processing of various ores or minerals and other industrial activities, coal ash from electricity generation, and phosphate waste from fertilizer production. Accelerator-produced waste includes accelerator targets any waste arising in the production of medical radioisotopes in accelerators (such as cyclotrons), and subsequent uses of these radioisotopes. Accelerator-produced waste contains mainly short-lived radionuclides and often resembles low-level radioactive waste. In general, NARM waste, especially waste containing naturally occurring radioactive material, has received less attention than nuclear fuel-cycle waste.

DAVID C. KOCHER

(SEE ALSO: *Not In My Backyard [NIMBY]; Nuclear Power; Risk Assessment, Risk Management*)

BIBLIOGRAPHY

League of Women Voters Education Fund (1993). *The Nuclear Waste Primer: A Handbook for Citizens,* revised edition. New York: Lyons & Burford.

NUISANCE ABATEMENT

Before there were statutes and regulations dealing with public health, some protections were afforded by common law—the body of law developed through the case-by-case adjudication of disputes. The ancient protections against nuisances are common law rules that were originally intended for protection of private property rights and that, incidentally, benefitted public health.

A "nuisance" (also called a "private nuisance") is a condition or activity that unreasonably interferes with the use and enjoyment of private property. Examples of nuisances that affect public health include toxic chemicals leaching from a nearby mine into a landowner's well water; excessive noise; smoke or other air pollutants; and even hordes of flies from a neighbor's manure pile. A nuisance is usually ongoing; a one-time or brief occurrence would not usually be a substantial enough interference with property rights to constitute a nuisance. (This does not mean there is no remedy for harm caused by a one-time occurrence, such as a chemical explosion.)

A landowner may file a court action seeking redress from the responsible party for a nuisance. One remedy is damages (i.e., money) to compensate for harm resulting from the nuisance. Courts can also grant injunctive relief, such as ordering the responsible party to abate the nuisance. A court can also enjoin (bar) an anticipated activity that has a high likelihood of causing a nuisance, such as building an incinerator in a residential area.

Injunctive relief can be intrusive and onerous, and therefore it is granted only if justified in light of all the relevant circumstances, including the respective harms and benefits to each party, where the fault lies, and the existence of alternative remedies. For example, if homeowners sue to enjoin construction of a factory in their neighborhood, the court would weigh such factors as the health effects and decreased property values likely to be suffered by the residents, as well as the feasibility and cost to the company of locating the project elsewhere. If homeowners seek injunctive relief due to pollution from an existing factory, the cost on the defendant's side of the equation is likely to be much greater, and thus harder to overcome, especially if relief would require shutting down the factory.

The cause of action for nuisance discussed above is sometimes called private nuisance, to distinguish it from public nuisance. Whereas a private nuisance is an invasion of private property rights, a public nuisance is an interference with a right held in common by the public. The common law rules against public nuisance were developed, in part, for the protection of the public health and safety. Pollution of a river that interferes with the public's right to swim or fish is an example of a public nuisance. A governmental entity, or any individual affected by a public nuisance, can sue in court for abatement of the nuisance or other relief.

Today, there are other avenues available to accomplish goals that once relied solely on the common law. Federal and state environmental statutes, such as the Clean Water Act and the Clean Air Act, provide protections against public nuisances that harm the environment and public health. Much like the common law rule against public nuisances, many of these statutes can be enforced in court not only by governments, but also by affected citizens. Although invoked less frequently nowadays, the old common law protections against private and public nuisance are still generally recognized and available if needed.

RUSSELLYN S. CARRUTH

(SEE ALSO: *Clean Air Act; Clean Water Act; Public Health and the Law; Regulatory Authority; Toxic Torts*)

BIBLIOGRAPHY

Bonine, J. E., and McGarity, T. O. (1992). *The Law of Environmental Protection,* 2nd edition. Eagan, MN: West Publishing Co.

Boston, W., and Madden, M. S. (1994). *Law of Environmental and Toxic Torts.* Eagan, MN: West Publishing Co.

Findley, R. W., and Farber, D. A. (1996). *Environmental Law in a Nutshell.* Eagan, MN: West Publishing Co.

NURSE

Nurses in public health settings work with community leaders, health and social-service agencies, high-risk groups, families, and individuals to identify and resolve unmet environmental, social, and health needs. Their role is to provide education about lifestyle and behavior choices that can help prevent illness and foster good health. public health nurses work in clinics, homes, schools, and other community locations. *The Future of Public Health,* published by the Institute of Medicine in 1988, initiated debate among public health nurse leaders and started a trend away from care of individuals in clinics toward an increased involvement with community groups such as healthy connections networks. This trend is expected to continue in the twenty-first century.

JUDITH CAZZOLI

(SEE ALSO: *Behavior, Health-Related; Behavioral Change; Future of Public Health; Public Health Nursing*)

BIBLIOGRAPHY

Public Health Nursing Section of the American Public Health Association (1990). *The Definition and Role of Public Health Nursing in the Delivery of Health Care.* Washington, DC: APHA.

NURSING HOMES

Nursing homes are residential health care facilities that provide nursing care and supervision twenty-four hours per day. In addition to skilled nursing services, physical, occupational, and speech therapy are usually offered. These therapies are designed to enable residents to recover and improve functional ability lost as a result of disease or injury. In addition, residents may receive social services and engage in recreational activities designed to improve physical and mental health. Residents also receive assistance with activities of daily living such as eating, dressing, walking, toileting, transferring between a bed and chair, and bathing. Typically, a nursing-home resident will need help in three or more of these activities of daily living.

Nursing homes form part of the continuum-of-care options available for persons with chronic or long-term health care needs. This continuum ranges from independent home care to care within intensive-care units of hospitals. Not all nursing homes are the same. Some nursing homes provide basic services, called "custodial services." Others, called "subacute" facilities provide highly skilled and technologically complex services that resemble medical units in hospitals. Many provide a mix of services.

LENGTH OF STAY

The average length of time that a person spends in a nursing home varies by the type of facility and the services rendered. For example, a person who resides in a nursing home in which he or she receives largely custodial services is likely to be there as long as several years. In fact, such a person will not usually return to an independent or community living environment. However, a person in a subacute facility is generally there only a matter of weeks. Such a person often receives intensive nursing or rehabilitation services and returns home or goes to an independent community environment.

Nursing-home residents generally have long-term health care needs that have resulted from one or more chronic illnesses, disabilities, or injuries. These conditions are rarely completely cured. Such conditions include, but are not limited to, strokes, fractured hips, arthritis, and mental confusion. These conditions often place a substantial burden on the health and economic status of individuals, affecting their quality of life and contributing to the decline of the person's overall ability to live independently.

REGULATION

The nursing-home industry is the second most regulated industry in the United States, second only to the nuclear industry. Nursing homes are required to be licensed by state health departments. They are inspected at least annually to determine compliance with approximately 150 different state and federal regulations, and results of these inspections are available to the public. In addition, nursing homes are regularly inspected or reviewed by other state and local organizations including, but not limited to, fire marshals, sanitarians, and patient-advocate organizations. The Joint Commission on Accreditation of Healthcare Organizations (JCAHO) may accredit nursing homes that voluntarily meet certain health and safety requirements.

FINANCING

There are four basic ways to pay for nursing-home care. These include private funds, insurance, Medicare and managed-care plans, and Medicaid. In general, people pay for approximately 25 percent of nursing-home care from their own personal financial resources. Basic room and board in a nursing home averages approximately $46,000 per year. Because of the costs, long-term care insurance is on the rise, and the extent of coverage varies greatly depending upon the insurance carrier and the individual policy. The American Association of Retired Persons (AARP) provides an analysis of the major insurance companies and their types of coverage. This information can be easily accessed through the Association's web site. Medicare and Medicaid are important governmental programs that provide coverage for nursing-home care.

Medicare. Medicare is a federal medical-insurance program that generally provides coverage to persons who are sixty-five years of age or older, persons of any age with permanent kidney failure, or those receiving Social Security benefits. Medicare coverage for nursing-home care is limited. Nursing homes that receive reimbursement from the federal Medicare program must be certified. All, or only part, of a facility may be designated as Medicare certified. A nursing home must meet the federal conditions of participation in order to be certified and maintain certification. During the annual state inspection or survey, compliance with the conditions of participation is assessed.

As of January 1, 2001, a person who is admitted to a skilled nursing facility within thirty days of a three-day hospital stay, and who is receiving care for the condition for which he or she was in the hospital, may receive up to one hundred days of either total or partial coverage from Medicare. The hundred days of coverage are not automatic. In order to qualify for Medicare benefits, the person must receive daily skilled nursing care or therapy services, and be certified for those services by a group of professionals, known as a utilization review committee, who reviews the case. If the person meets all of these requirements, he or she will receive coverage as follows:

- Full coverage for a semi-private room, meals, nursing care, rehabilitation therapy, drugs prescribed by the physician, medical supplies and equipment for the first twenty days

- Partial coverage for up to an additional eighty days if the physician and the reviewing professionals certify continued need for skilled services

Government statistics show that patients receive an average of twenty-four days of coverage under Medicare.

Medicaid. Medicaid is a program of health insurance for eligible low-income persons. Both the federal and state governments fund Medicaid. The program was not initially established to provide long-term coverage for persons in nursing homes; however, it has become the primary method of payment for low-income individuals in these facilities. While it varies from state to state, Medicaid pays for approximately 65 to 75 percent of nursing-home care. In order to receive payment from Medicaid, nursing homes must also be certified.

Individuals applying for Medicaid must do so through the county office of the U.S. Department of Human Services in their state. Medicaid applicants must meet both financial and medical eligibility criteria. In order to meet the financial criteria, an individual's assets must be less than $2,000; or $3,000 for a couple in the nursing home at the same time. Assets include cash, real and personal property (excluding the primary residence), cars, stocks, bonds, and the cash value of life-insurance policies, investments, and trusts—if the trust provides for the person's care.

Many people have too many assets at the time of admission to a nursing home to qualify for Medicaid. They must typically "spend down" their assets to meet the financial eligibility requirement. In the past, these spend-down requirements have often left the community-living spouse destitute. As a result, more liberal laws now provide for the financial protection of such spouses. As of January 2001, most states allow the spouse of a nursing-home resident to retain half of the couple's assets and the family home and furnishings, so long as these assets don't exceed a state established minimum. These laws are subject to review both at the state and federal level.

MARIA R. SCHIMER

(SEE ALSO: *Aging of Population; Geriatrics; Gerontology; Medicaid; Medicare*)

BIBLIOGRAPHY

American Geriatrics Society (1993). "Regulation and Quality of Care Standards in Nursing Facilities." *Journal of the American Geriatrics Society* 48(1): 1519–1520.

Besdine, R. W.; Rubenstein, L. W.; and Snyder, L., eds. (1996). *Medical Care of the Nursing Home Resident: What Physicians Need to Know*. Philadelphia, PA: American College of Physicians.

—— (1997). *Unrealized Prevention Opportunities: Reducing the Health and Economic Burden of Chronic Disease*. Atlanta, GA: Author.

Franklin, M. B. (2000). "Paying Today for Tomorrow's Care." *Kiplinger's Personal Finance Magazine* 54(1):114–116.

Hoffman, E. (2000). "Nursing Homes Don't Have to Break You." *Business Week* (November 20):169–170.

Schick, F. L., and Scick, R., eds. (1994). *Statistical Handbook on Aging Americans*. Phoenix, AZ: Onyx Press.

U.S. Department of Health and Human Services (1994). *National Health Interview Survey on Disability (Phase 1)*. Hyattsville, MD: Author.

NUTRITION

Few subjects are more important to public health than food. One of the major ways in which humans interact with their environment is through our food. The science of nutrition has developed through the study of the components of foods that are required to sustain life and to maintain health. Improper diet can cause disease if important nutrients are missing from the diet, and inappropriate dietary practices can increase the risk of certain diseases.

Essential nutrients are substances that must be in the human diet to support life. These essential nutrients include vitamins, inorganic elements, essential amino acids, essential fatty acids, and a source of energy, and water. A lack of a nutrient or an insufficient amount of a nutrient can result in a deficiency disease that can be life threatening in extreme cases. The essential nutrients are widely distributed in foods and most people can obtain sufficient amounts of them if they consume a varied diet.

ELEMENTS OF HUMAN NUTRITION

Energy. Most of the food consumed is used by the body to supply energy. The body is able to digest and absorb into the blood stream components of carbohydrates, fats, and protein that can be metabolized by the body to release energy. Energy is used to maintain body temperature, support metabolic processes, and to support physical activity. People are generally in a state of energy balance, that is, they consume as much energy as they use to support their bodies and daily living. They tend to gain weight if they are in positive energy balance, or lose weight if they take in less than they expend. Most excess energy is stored by the body as fat. Energy needs are usually expressed in kilocalories, but in much of the world's scientific literature, energy expenditure is expressed in joules or kilojoules (1 kilocalorie equals 4.184 kilojoules).

The energy expended by the body when at rest is quite constant between individuals and can be

Table 1

Energy Expenditure during Selected Activities

Activity	Kcal expended per hour[1]
Walking, 2 to 2.5 miles per hour (mph)	185–255
Walking, 5 mph	555
Jogging 5.5 mph	655
Tennis	400
Aerobic exercise	275
Cross country skiing	600

[1]These values represent above resting metabolic rate for a 70 kg person.

SOURCE: Powers, S. K., and E. T. Howley, eds. (2000). *Exercise Physiology*, 4th ed., New York: McGraw-Hill.

estimated quite closely by prediction equations that take into account age, sex, and body weight. The resting metabolic weight of a 70-kilogram (154-lb.) man, for example, is estimated to be 1750 kilocalories per day, and for a 58-kilogram (128-lb.) woman, 1350 kilocalories per day. The total daily energy needs are related to the amount of physical activity expended in the course of everyday life. A person whose life style involves light amounts of activity may have a total energy expenditure of about one and one-half times their resting metabolic rate, while a person who is engaged in very intense physical activity may expend over twice as much energy as their resting metabolic rate in the course of twenty-four hours. Exercise can increase the metabolic rate considerably, depending on the type and duration of the activity. The amount of energy expended by certain types of physical activity is shown in Table 1.

Protein. The principal structural components of body soft tissues are proteins, which are made by the body from amino acids. The amino acids along with the nucleic acids are the principle nitrogen-containing components of the body and of most foods. The enzymes that regulate most body processes are also proteins. The body can synthesize many of the amino acids needed for protein syntheses, but some amino acids must be obtained from the proteins in the diet. The dietary essential amino acids for humans are threonine, valine, leucine, isoleucine, methionine, lysine, histidine, and tryptophan. Two others can only be formed from essential amino acids: tryosine from phenylalanine, and cystine from methionine. Human dietary protein requirements are quite modest. An adult man of average weight is estimated to need about sixty-three grams of protein per day, while an average woman is estimated to need about fifty grams. The protein must supply the essential amino acids required by humans and sufficient total nitrogen to allow syntheses of the other amino acids required for protein synthesis.

Fats. Fats are synthesized from carbohydrates, but the body is unable to make certain fatty acids, which are components of fats. These essential fatty acids, notably linoleic and linolenic acid, must be supplied by dietary fats. Fats that are solid at room temperature, such as butter or lard, usually contain high amounts of saturated fatty acids such as palmitic or stearic acid. Fats that are liquid at room temperature such as vegetable oils are higher in unsaturated fatty acids, which include oleic acid as well as the linoleic and linolenic acid. Fat is the most concentrated source of energy available to humans, supplying about nine kilocalories per gram of dietary fat, compared to four kilocalories per gram of carbohydrate and protein. Fat is also the principal storage form of energy in the body.

Vitamins. Vitamins are a diverse group of dietary essentials that have important functions in the body. The vitamins known to be required by humans are listed in Table 2. Many of them are components of co-enzymes, molecules that are required for some enzymes to carry out certain metabolic processes. Others, such as vitamin E and vitamin C, act as antioxidants, protecting body components from damage from oxygen needed by the body for metabolism. Some are more like hormones, such as vitamin D, which regulates the absorption of calcium from the intestine and the formation of bones. Vitamin D can actually be formed by the action of ultraviolet light from the sun on vitamin D precursors found in the skin, but since this synthesis may not be sufficient at times, humans need a dietary source of vitamin D. Vitamin A is a component of visual pigments in the eye that respond to light stimuli and are essential for sight.

A deficiency of a vitamin may result in a characteristic deficiency disease related to the body function affected by the lack of the vitamin. Vitamin D deficiency can cause soft bones in children, a condition called rickets; vitamin A deficiency

Table 2

Vitamins and Inorganic Elements Required in Human Diets to Support Life and Maintain Health

Vitamins	Inorganic Elements
Vitamin A (retinol, retinal, retinoic acid)	Calcium
	Phosphorus
Vitamin C (ascorbic acid)	Potassium
Vitamin D (D_3 cholecalciferol, D_2 ergocalciferol)	Sodium
	Chlorine
Vitamin K (menaquinones, phylloquinone)	Magnesium
	Iron
Vitamin E (tocopherols)	Iodine
Vitamin B_6 (pyridoxine)	Zinc
Vitamin B_{12}	Selenium
Biotin	Copper
Riboflavin	Manganese
Niacin	Chromium
Folacin	Fluorine
Thiamin	Molybdenum
Choline[1]	Boron

[1]Choline can be synthesized by the body but recent evidence suggests that dietary choline may be needed at some stages of the life cycle.

In addition to these elements, substantial evidence indicates that arsenic, nickel, silicon, and vanadium have important physiological functions that may make them nutritional essentials. They are required in very small amounts and a dietary deficiency has not been convincingly described.

SOURCE: Powers, S. K., and E. T. Howley, eds. (2000). *Exercise Physiology*, 4th ed., New York: McGraw-Hill.

may cause night blindness and even blindness in its more severe form. Many of the vitamins have multiple functions in the body, and deficiency diseases can be severely debilitating in severe cases. Vitamins are required in very small amounts by the body. Only a few micrograms of vitamin B_{12} is required each day, while vitamin C requirements may be from sixty to one hundred milligrams per day.

Inorganic elements. Humans also require several inorganic elements as components of the diet. The inorganic elements known to be required by humans are listed in Table 2. These elements may have a structural function, such as calcium and phosphorus, which are needed for bone synthesis, or they may have a catalytic function similar to some of the vitamins. They are required for the action of many enzymes in the body. Sodium and potassium are essential for fluid balance. Iodine is an essential component of thyroxin, the hormone produced by the thyroid gland. Some of the inorganic elements are required in extremely small quantities, only micrograms per day, while other elements may be needed in higher amounts. Soils vary in their content of some of the trace elements, and plants grown in some areas may be deficient in an essential element. This has been true for iodine, where a deficiency is still observed in many areas of the world, and selenium, where geographically based human deficiency disease has been observed.

NUTRITION RECOMMENDATIONS

In the United States, the National Academy of Sciences, through the National Research Council and The Institute of Medicine, has convened expert groups since 1941 to establish nutrition recommendations to be used by individuals and institutions for planning nutritionally adequate diets. These groups have established recommended dietary allowances (RDAs) as the daily dietary intake level for a specific nutrient that is sufficient to meet the nutritional requirements of nearly all (97–98 percent) individuals in the life stage and gender group specified. In the most recent recommendations, dietary reference intakes (DRIs) have been specified that have attempted to estimate average nutrient requirements, RDAs, and an upper limit of safe nutrient intake. Where data are not sufficient to set a precise RDA, new recommendations called adequate intake (AI) define a recommendation for some nutrients.

The RDAs and AIs are used to plan diets for groups in hospitals, the military, large institutions, to set standards for government food programs such as school lunches, to establish nutritional labeling, and for counseling individuals. Similar dietary recommendations have been made by expert groups convened in many countries and also by international organizations such as the World Health Organization and the Food and Agricultural Organization of the United Nations. These recommendations are periodically revised to include information from most recent research findings. The latest recommendations for dietary reference intakes can be obtained in the United States from the National Academy Press, 2101 Constitution Avenue, NW, Washington, D.C. 20418.

Recommendations have been established for most nutrients where sufficient research data are available to make reliable estimates. The nutrient recommendations are given for different age groups and are differentiated by sexes because of different nutritional needs at different stages of life. Infants and young children who are growing rapidly have different nutrient needs compared to adults. Women who are menstruating need more iron to replace blood lost in the menstruation compared to postmenopausal women or men. Similarly, there are special needs for pregnant and lactating women. There is increasing evidence accumulating about the needs of the elderly, and nutrition recommendations now include a category for individuals over seventy years of age.

Recent revisions of nutrition recommendations have taken into account public health concerns about osteoporosis, a condition in which bone mineral is lost and older individuals become more vulnerable to bone fractures. New recommendations stress the importance of maintaining a high level (1200 mg/day) of calcium intake by both men and women over fifty years of age in an attempt to reduce loss of bone mineral. Similarly, recommendations for folic acid intake have also been revised to stress the importance of sufficient folic acid consumption by women who may become pregnant. Insufficient folic acid has been associated with a higher incidence of birth defects. The concern for adequate intake of folic acid led to the fortification of enriched grain products with folic acid in the United States beginning in 1998.

Nutrient recommendations also take into consideration the efficiency by which nutrients are digested and absorbed from foods. The form in which iron is ingested has a major influence on how much food iron is absorbed into the body. Iron in animal products is well absorbed because it is found as a component of hemoglobin or muscle pigments, while iron in plants, found as inorganic salts, is poorly absorbed. Some components of plants, such as phytic acid and tannins, also interfere with iron absorption. Therefore, dietary recommendations for iron intake must consider the availability of iron in the foods being consumed.

PUBLIC HEALTH ISSUES

In the early part of the twentieth century, nutritional disorders were common. Pellagra, a disease caused by a deficiency of nicotinic acid, was widespread in the southern United States. Rickets, from vitamin D deficiency, was common, and goiters from iodine deficiency were widespread. Iron-deficiency anemia and riboflavin deficiency were frequently observed. In parts of Asia, beriberi, a disease caused by thiamin deficiency, was a public health problem. The discovery and characterization of the vitamins made it possible to produce them in large amounts, and the enrichment of grain products with niacin, riboflavin, thiamine, and iron largely eliminated B-vitamin deficiencies in the United States as a public health problem. Similarly, the addition of vitamins A and D to milk provided protection from deficiency of the nutrients. The use of iodized salt essentially eliminated goiter from the U.S. population.

Unfortunately, nutritional deficiencies have not been eliminated from much of the world even today. A combination of poor diet, poor sanitation, and lack of safe water leading to frequent intestinal infections, causes more than 200 million of the world's children to be shorter and weigh less than children in good environments at the same age. These malnourished children are often born underweight from mothers who are also underweight and of poor nutritional status. Measures of the degree of malnutrition that are frequently used include a comparison of a child's weight for age, height for age, and weight for height with norms established by similar measurements on a well-nourished population of children. A usual convention classifies a child whose weight for age is more than two standard deviations below the standard as malnourished, and those three standard deviations below the standard are usually considered severely malnourished. The most vulnerable time for growth faltering in children is the period from six months of age to two years, when breast feeding stops and weaning foods are introduced. A combination of poor weaning foods, exposure to contaminated water, and poor sanitation that results in frequent bouts of diarrhea and the occurrence of other childhood diseases contributes to the poor growth of children after weaning.

The United Nations estimates that more than two-hundred million of the world's children are stunted, with the largest numbers being found in South Asia and in Africa. Similarly, about 4 percent of the world's population is considered at risk for iodine deficiency disorders including *goiter*,

cretinism, and *mental retardation.* Vitamin A deficiency is estimated to affect about 3.3 million children in the world. Iron deficiency anemia is also the most prevalent nutritional deficiency in the world. Over 90 percent of those effected live in developing countries. The United Nations has estimated that severe anemia is a contributing factor to 50 percent of maternal deaths in developing countries.

Nutritional deficiencies are common in the refugees displaced by wars and natural disasters. Assistance is provided by the United Nations High Commissioner for Refugees to more than 26 million people world wide, and there are other internally displaced people in the world that may number as many as 31 million. The difficulty of providing food for these displaced groups puts them at risk for nutritional deficiencies.

Nutritional deficiencies are rare in most industrialized nations in Europe, Asia, and the Americas, and among the higher income groups of the developing world. The public health issues related to nutrition in these nations are concerned with over–consumption of energy, inadequate levels of activity, and improper food choices. Dietary practices are known to be risk factors for severe chronic diseases, including hypertension, atherosclerotic cardiovascular disease, and several types of cancers. The amount and type of fats seem to influence the risk of atherosclerotic cardiovascular diseases and to risk of certain forms of cancer. The consumption of saturated fatty acids and trans fatty acids found in certain hydrogenated cooking fats increases the levels of serum total cholesterol and cholesterol associated with serum low density lipoproteins (LDL) and thus increases the risk of artheriosclerosis and coronary heart disease. Diets high in fruits, vegetables, legumes, and cereal products are associated with a lower occurrence of coronary heart disease and certain cancers.

Genetic variations occur among individuals in their response to food. Variations in various blood lipoprotein components can effect an individual's response to dietary fat and cholesterol, and risk of coronary heart disease. There appears to be a genetic component to susceptibility to obesity. As more information is known about the human genome, it may be possible to predict more accurately individual risks for disease, and the dietary factors that may modify this risk.

Obesity. Dietary patterns that are characterized by the consumption of energy-rich, high-fat foods are considered to be factors contributing to obesity, particularly when the high intake of energy is not accompanied by appropriate physical activity. Obesity in adults is defined by reference to the body mass index (BMI), a relationship that takes into account both height and body weight. The BMI is calculated as weight in kilograms/height in meters squared. In pounds and inches it is calculated by weight (pounds)/height (inches)^2 × 704.5. A person with a body mass index between 20 to 25 is considered in the normal range, while a body mass index of 25 to 30 is considered overweight, and over 30 is considered obese.

The prevalence of obesity in the United States has increased markedly in recent years. The prevalence of overweight children ages six to eleven in surveys conducted in the early 1970s was 6.5 percent of males and 4.9 percent for females. By 1988–1994, the prevalence of overweight in this age grouping had increased to 11.4 percent and 9.9 percent for males and females respectively. On the basis of surveys carried out between the years 1988 and 1994, more than 50 percent of American adults were considered overweight on the basis of having a BMI greater than 25. In further surveys, 17.9 percent of U.S. adults were considered obese in 1988, compared with 12 percent in 1991. The increasing prevalence of obesity is of considerable public health concern as excess weight is associated with greater risk of mortality, non-insulin dependent Type II diabetes mellitus, hypertension, stroke, osteo-arthritis, and some cancers. The annual number of deaths attributed to obesity in the United States has been estimated at more than 280,000 persons.

The control of obesity is difficult, and weight reduction is difficult to maintain. The most effective weight loss schemes seem to be those that reduce weight slowly, from one-half to one pound per week, and that involve both reduction in energy intake and an increase in physical activity. For overweight individuals, a reduced intake of from 300 to 500 kilocalories per day should result in a loss of one-half to one pound per week, while severely obese individuals may need to reduce energy intake by 500 to 1000 kilocalories per day to achieve a one to two pound per week weight loss.

Table 3

Dietary Guidelines for Americans

Aim for fitness
- Aim for a healthy weight
- Be physically active each day

Build a Healthy Base
- Let the Pyramid guide your food choices
- Choose a variety of grains daily, especially whole grains
- Choose a variety of fruits and vegetables
- Keep food safe to eat

Choose sensibly
- Choose a diet that is low in saturated fat and cholesterol and moderate in total fat
- Choose beverages and foods to moderate your intake of sugar
- Choose and prepare foods with less salt

SOURCE: From the United States Department of Agriculture/Department of Human Services: Dietary Guidelines for Americans 2000.

Dietary guidelines. The concern for appropriate food choices have led many countries to issue dietary guidelines that provide advice that goes beyond the recommendations for individual nutrients covered by the recommended dietary allowances. The year 2000 dietary guidelines for Americans are shown in Table 3. These are issued by the U.S. Department of Agriculture and the U.S. Department of Health and Human Services and are revised about every five years. This publication represents the only official dietary advice to consumers by the U.S. Government. The full text of the bulletin provides more detailed advice on food choices. Many countries have published similar dietary guidelines to guide food choices to reduce the dietary risk factors associated with chronic disease.

To give advice to consumers regarding appropriate food choices to implement dietary guidelines, food guides have been developed. One of the most popular representations of a food guide is the dietary pyramid that has been published by the U.S. Department of Agriculture and the Department of Human Services. This food guide illustrates the importance of building a healthy diet on a base of cereal-based foods supplemented liberally with fruits and vegetables. Foods high in protein and fat should be consumed sparingly. The pyramid provides the number of recommended daily servings of the food groups.

Food supplies. The world population is projected to increase about 25 percent from the year 2000 to 2020, to about seven and one-half billion people. Most of this increase is projected to be in developing countries located in the tropical zones of the earth. The population of Asia is projected to increase by 800 million, and the population of Africa is projected to double. The International Food Policy Research Institute (IFPRI) has projected that food production will be able to increase such that the world per capita food available will supply about 2,900 kilocalories per person per day in the year 2020, compared to 2,700 kilocalories in 1993. The equitable distribution of food supplies will remain a major problem. The daily food available in sub-Saharan Africa is projected to supply only about 2,300 kilocalories per capita in the year 2020, barely sufficient to support a productive life. IFPRI estimates that one out of every four of the world's children will be malnourished in the year 2020. To achieve the projected increase in food supplies, continued improvements in crop yields will be necessary.

In contrast to the limited food supplies in many developing nations, developed countries are projected to have a food supply that will provide 3,470 kilocalories per capita per day in the year 2020. The U.S. Department of Agriculture indicates that the available food in the United States in 1994 provided 3,800 kilocalories per capita. This food supply provided annually 193 pounds of red meat, poultry, and fish, 585 pounds of dairy products, 194 pounds of cereal products, 151 pounds of fresh, canned, or dried fruits, 208 pounds of fresh, canned, frozen, dried, or fried vegetables and pulses, and 147 pounds of sugar. These figures represent food availability and do not represent actual consumption or account for wastes and losses in marketing and food preparation. Even with the variety of food available, consumers in the United States do not generally meet the dietary guidelines and food guide recommendations. For example, in food consumption surveys, only 38 percent of those surveyed reported consuming the recommended number of servings per day of cereals, 41 percent of the servings of vegetables (heavily weighted toward potatoes and starchy vegetables), and 23 percent of the servings of fruits. The reported diets provided 33 percent of the energy from fats and 11 percent from saturated fats. Food choices by consumers appear to depend on a variety of factors, such as cost, food preferences, convenience of preparation, and cultural norms, in addition to perception as to effects on health.

Food safety. In addition to providing nutrients, food can also potentially be a source of harm to a consumer. Hazards associated with food include microbiological pathogens, naturally occurring toxins, allergens, intentional and unintentional additives, modified food components, agricultural chemicals, environmental contaminants, and animal drug residues. It has been estimated that more than 80 million cases of food-borne illness occur annually in the United States, resulting in more than 9,000 deaths, primarily from microbiological contamination. The transformation of a safe food into a potentially dangerous one can occur anywhere in a food system that consists of producers, shippers, processors, wholesalers, retailers, and consumers.

An effective food safety system requires regulation, surveillance, consumer education, and continued research to detect and prevent food-borne illnesses. The increase in world trade in food also involves international dimensions in food safety issues. Import regulations dealing with food safety may also have the effect of restricting access to markets, and food safety becomes an issue in world trade.

The United States has a complex system of food-safety regulation. The Food and Drug Administration (FDA) is responsible for domestic and imported foods in interstate commerce except for poultry and meat products. The FDA has responsibility for standards for food labeling, inspects food-processing plants, and regulates food animal drugs and feed additives and all food additives. The Food Safety and Inspection Service (FSIS) of the U.S. Department of Agriculture (USDA) inspects meat and poultry products to ensure they are safe and correctly marked, labeled, and packaged. The Environmental Protection Agency (EPA) licenses pesticide products and establishes tolerances for pesticide residues in food products and animal feeds. The Centers for Disease Control and Prevention (CDC) are responsible for surveillance of illnesses associated with food consumption in association with the FDA and the USDA. These agencies also collaborate with state and local public health agencies that are concerned with food safety.

The consumption and preparation of food also has great social and cultural significance, contributing to the daily enjoyment of life. Public health concerns about dietary practices often must compete with these values as an individual makes food choices. This makes the issues associated with food and nutrition more complex than the medical and public health issues discussed here.

MALDEN C. NESHEIM

(SEE ALSO: *Blood Lipids; Energy; Foods and Diets; Nutrition in Health Departments*)

BIBLIOGRAPHY

Institute of Medicine, Food and Nutrition Board (1989). *Diet and Health: Implications for Reducing Chronic Disease.* Washington, DC: National Academy Press.

—— (1997). *Dietary Reference Intakes for Calcium, Phosphorous, Magnesium, Vitamin D, and Fluoride.* Washington, DC: National Academy Press.

—— (1997). *Dietary Reference Intakes: Thiamin, Riboflavin, Niacin, Vitamin B$_6$, Folate, Vitamin B$_{12}$, Pantothenic Acid, Biotin, and Choline.* Washington, DC: National Academy Press.

Institute of Medicine, National Research Council (1998). *Ensuring Safe Food.* Washington, DC: National Academy Press.

Mokdad, H. H.; Serdula, M. K.; Dietz, W. H.; Bowman, B. A.; Marks, J. S.; and Koplan, J. P. (1999). "The Spread of the Obesity Epidemic in the United States 1991–1998." *Journal of the American Medical Association* 282:1519–1522.

Must, A.; Spadano, J.; Coakley, A.; Field, E.; Colditz, G.; and Dietz, W. H. (1999). "The Disease Burden Associated with Overweight and Obesity." *Journal of American Medical Association* 282:1523–1529.

National Research Council, Food and Nutrition Board (1989). *Recommended Dietary Allowances,* 10th edition. Washington, DC: National Academy Press.

Pandya-Lorch, R.; Andersen, P. P.; and Rosegrant, M. (1997). *The World Food Situation: Recent Developments, Emerging Issues, and Long Term Prospects.* Washington, DC: International Food Policy Research Institute.

Shils, M. E.; Olson, J. A.; and Shike, M. (1994). *Modern Nutrition in Health and Disease,* Vols. 1 and 2, 8th edition. Philadelphia, PA: Lea and Febiger.

—— (1999). *Modern Nutrition in Health and Disease,* 9th edition. Baltimore, MD: Williams and Wilkins.

Stipanuk, M. (2000). *Biochemical and Physiological Aspects of Human Nutrition.* Philadelphia, PA: W. B. Saunders Company.

Sub-Committee on Nutrition (ACCI/SCN) United Nations Administrative Committee on Coordination (1997). *Third Report on the World Nutrition Situation.* Geneva: World Health Organization.

Triano, R. P., and Flegal, K. M. (1998). "Overweight Children and Adolescents: Description, Epidemiology, and Demographics." *Pediatrics* 101:497–503.

United Kingdom Department of Health (1991). *Dietary Reference Values for Food Energy and Nutrients for the United Kingdom: Report of the Panel on Dietary Reference Values of the Committee on Medical Aspects of Food Policy.* London: HMSO.

United States Department of Agriculture and the United States Department of Health and Human Services (2000). *Nutrition and Your Health: Dietary Guidelines for Americans.* Home and Garden Bulletin no. 232, 5th edition. Washington, DC: United States Government Printing Office.

U.S. Department of Agriculture (1992). *The Food Guide Pyramid.* Home and Garden Bulletin no. 252. Washington, DC: Human Nutrition Information Service.

World Health Organization (1985). *Energy and Protein Requirements: Report of a Joint FAO/WHO/UNU Expert Consultation.* WHO Technical Report Series 724. Geneva: Author.

NUTRITION IN HEALTH DEPARTMENTS

The purpose of a nutrition program in a health department is to promote the nutritional health of the residents living under the health department's jurisdiction. A public health nutritionist with a master's or doctoral degree in nutrition or a related field is trained to direct the program. The program may include providing medical nutrition therapy for chronic diseases such as diabetes, promoting wellness through advice on healthful food patterns, and assessing the nutritional status of children with special needs in their homes. The nutritionist also targets programs to nutritionally at-risk populations such as pregnant women, infants, children, and the elderly.

MARY ANN McGUCKIN

(SEE ALSO: *Eating Disorders; Foods and Diets; Nutrition;*)

BIBLIOGRAPHY

Dodds, J. M., and Kaufmann, M., eds. (1991). *Personnel in Public Health Nutrition for the 1990's.* Washington, DC: The Public Health Foundation.

Owen, A. L.; Splett, P. L.; and Owen, G. (1999). *Nutrition in the Community: The Art and Science of Delivering Services,* 4th edition. Boston: WCB/McGraw Hill.

NUTRITIONAL DISORDERS

See Nutrition

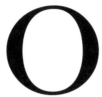

OBESITY

See Nutrition *and* Physical Activity

OBJECTIVES

See Health Goals *and* Healthy People 2010

OBSERVATIONAL STUDIES

An observational study is a study in which inferences are drawn or hypotheses tested through observational methods. Two common varieties are the descriptive study, where events are simply observed and described as they take their natural course, and the analytic epidemiologic study, which does not include any intervention or experimentation; examples include the case-control study and the cohort study. As human experimentation is fraught with ethical problems and often not feasible, many important epidemiologic discoveries have had to rely entirely on observational studies.

JOHN M. LAST

(SEE ALSO: *Case-Control Study; Cohort Study; Cross-Sectional Study; Descriptive Study; Epidemiology*)

OCCUPATIONAL DISEASE

The term "occupational disease" refers to those illnesses caused by exposures at the workplace.

They should be separated, conceptually, from injuries that may also may occur at workplaces due to a variety of hazards.

In 2001, some 137 million Americans were working, either full-time or part-time, out of a total population of some 280 million. Women make up 46 percent of the workforce.

Occupational diseases may occur in varying time frames, from the instantaneous development of illness following exposure to toxic chemicals to decades between onset of exposure and the development of disease, as occurs with many occupationally related cancers. Many time frames in between these extremes may be seen as well. Examples of varying time frames include instantaneous reactions to exposure to chemicals such as chlorine or ammonia gas; a delay of some six to twelve hours with fumes of aerosolized zinc, as occurs when welding on galvanized steel; a delay of weeks to months with lead poisoning; a delay of decades with occupational carcinogens; and even the finding of congenital malformations in children whose parents may have been exposed to hazardous materials.

Although not all occupational exposures that cause illness lead to death, considerable numbers of deaths each year are associated with workplace exposures. While it is relatively easy to count deaths due to occupational injuries, it is much more difficult for delayed illnesses. For injuries, the most recent available data indicates that more than 6,200 fatal occupational injuries occur in the

United States each year, with more than 40 percent associated with transportation, and most of these related to motor-vehicle fatalities. Homicides are the second leading cause of death in the workplace, accounting for some 14 percent of the total. The leading causes of death from injuries vary by sex, with motor vehicles accounting for the greatest number of deaths in men, and homicides in women. Workers older than sixty-five have the highest rates of occupational-injury deaths. Also, smaller workplaces (those with less than ten workers) have the highest fatality rate. Many large companies invest in occupational safety and health programs and do ongoing workplace assessments. Companies with strong programs are known to have lower injury rates.

As noted above, deaths from occupational illness for most diseases are hard to enumerate. The only diseases for which reasonably good data exists are the pneumoconioses, such as asbestosis, coal-workers pneumoconiosis, and silicosis. For many other diseases, such as those from chemical exposure, various occupational cancers, and other problems, individual fatalities are difficult to recognize and record.

In the years for which data was available in the year 2000, almost 430,000 nonfatal occupational illnesses were recorded annually in the United States, with approximately 60 percent of these occurring in the manufacturing sector. The rate was almost fifty cases per 10,000 full-time workers. However, it should be recognized that many workplace-related illnesses go unreported, in part because they are unrecognized, and in part because of record keeping that is not optimal.

Among the occupational diseases most commonly reported, those relating to repeated trauma, such as carpal tunnel syndrome, tendonitis, and noise–induced hearing loss, accounted for more than 60 percent. Carpal tunnel syndrome alone accounted for almost 30,000 cases with days away from work. For those cases of carpal tunnel syndrome with workplace absence, half needed twenty-five or more days away from work. Skin diseases represented about 13 percent (58,000 cases) of work related illnesses. Dermatitis, or inflammation of the skin, resulted in more than 6,500 cases that required time away from work.

It is well recognized that these types of injuries are underreported, but a better sense can be gotten from the seven states that have an active SENSOR (Sentinel Event Notification System for Occupational Risks) program in place for some diseases. No state looks at all diseases in this way, but those that collect data concentrate upon silicosis, occupational asthma, and adult lead poisoning.

There are insufficient numbers of occupational physicians properly trained to care for the hundreds of thousands of cases of occupational disease. Only about 10,000 of some 800,000 American doctors practice in the field of occupational medicine, and only a small percentage of these have had training leading to certification as specialists in this field. Most occupational diseases are treated by primary-care physicians, and, unfortunately, many of them have had little or no training in occupational disease.

There are two government agencies that have a special role in evaluating occupational disease. The National Institute for Occupational Safety and Health (NIOSH) of the U.S. Department of Health and Human Services has the responsibility for research and prevention activities with regards to workers' health. NIOSH advises as to allowable levels of exposure, based upon scientific review. Within the Department of Labor is the Occupational Safety and Health Administration (OSHA), which has the responsibility of actually setting and enforcing workplace regulations. One of the difficulties that OSHA faces is an insufficient number of inspectors to evaluate what actually goes on at most workplaces; given the number of inspectors in the United States at the present time, it would take more than two decades for all workplaces to be inspected even once. OSHA's resources focus on fatalities. In addition to government agencies, there are a variety of voluntary groups, such as the American Conference of Governmental Industrial Hygienists and the National Safety Foundation, that make recommendations for safe and healthful practices in the workplace.

ARTHUR L. FRANK

(SEE ALSO: *Asbestos; Carpal Tunnel Syndrome, Cumulative Trauma; Environmental Determinants of Health; Ergonomics; Farm Injuries; Mining; National Institute for Occupational Safety and*

Health; Occupational Lung Disease; Occupational Safety and Health; Occupational Safety and Health Administration)

BIBLIOGRAPHY

National Institute for Occupational Safety and Health (2000). *Worker Chartbook, 2000.* Washington, DC: NIOSH.

OCCUPATIONAL LUNG DISEASE

The lungs are one of the body's organs most in contact with the surrounding environment. Thousands of breaths are taken each day, and if there are hazardous substances in the air many types of disease may develop.

Among the occupational lung problems are asthma and the closely related hypersensitivity pneumonias; irritant and toxic gases, some of which may prove rapidly fatal; cancer-causing agents; inorganic dusts, such as cement, which cause acute bronchitis; organic dusts that produce a variety of problems, such as byssinosis, which is caused by cotton dust; and the pneumoconioses, or chronic dust-caused diseases of the lung.

Most, if not all, of these problems are entirely preventable. For some, such as byssinosis, there is now better recognition and response, leading to the development of fewer new cases. Similarly, stricter regulations over time have reduced the incidence of some of the pneumoconioses, but others continue to be significant health problems, including silicosis in certain groups of silica-exposed workers, such as sandblasters. With lower levels of exposure to asbestos the risk of asbestos has been diminishing, but the cancer-associated risks continue.

A wide variety of substances in many workplace settings can give rise to asthmatic and allergic phenomena. These include such diverse illnesses as baker's asthma from exposure to flour dust; asthmatic responses to animals among those who regularly handle them, such as veterinarians or research scientists; and sensitization to plastics, such as occurs in meat wrapper's asthma or in those who solder wires that are coated with teflon. A wide variety of organic materials can lead to hypersensitivity pneumonias. These include "tea picker's lung" and "coffee grinder's lung."

If any gas replaces enough oxygen at a worksite, a worker may die from simple asphyxiation due to the lack of oxygen. More frequently, however, other effects occur such as the acute and chronic damage to the lung caused by oxides of nitrogen that occur in agricultural silos or damage from acute exposure to chlorine, ammonia, and other chemicals widely used in chemical production facilities. Harmful levels of carbon monoxide can occur from vehicle exhaust in confined spaces or from furnaces or space heaters not working properly. Phosgene can develop from mixing together household-cleaning chemicals.

For the pneumoconioses, first described in the eighteenth century, these scarring diseases of the lung can lead to severe pulmonary distress over time. Among the materials that can cause a pneumoconiosis are asbestos, coal dust, silica, talc, kaolin, mica, flint, and certain metal dusts such as tin, which causes stannosis. Some materials also have carcinogenic potential (such as asbestos and silica). In addition, many of these occupational lung hazards have interactive effects when combined with cigarette smoke.

ARTHUR L. FRANK

(SEE ALSO: *Asbestos; Asthma; Chronic Respiratory Diseases; Lung Cancer; Mining; Occupational Disease; Occupational Safety and Health*)

BIBLIOGRAPHY

National Institute of Occupational Safety and Health (1986). *Occupational Respiratory Disease.* Washington, DC: U.S. Department of Health and Human Services.

OCCUPATIONAL SAFETY AND HEALTH

THE HISTORY OF WORK

As long as humans have existed they have had to work. Initially, there was a need to hunt to catch food and have materials to make clothing. Generally, males would do the hunting and women would do the processing of the materials. Food would be preserved by drying, salting, or other methods for use over time; clothing would be made; and shelter would be fashioned from the hides of animals. When societies became more complex and humans changed into settled creatures, agriculture became a dominant force in their existence. As crops became cultivated and animals domesticated, there was still a need for essentially year-round labor, with both cultivation and processing activities being divided among the males and females of families, and this would generally include children as well. Only as societies became more complex did nonagricultural activities become possible, such as work from artisans fashioning useful household products, religious goods, and goods used for war or hunting. Eventually, societies were able to sustain other artisans who pursued writing, music, and visual arts such as painting.

Throughout recorded history, there have been references to work under a variety of conditions. The Old Testament includes rules about safe practices with regards to agriculture and how to treat workers. The Greeks and Romans used slaves, generally those captured in battle, to do both domestic work and to work in especially hazardous conditions, such as in mining. The writings of the ancients even discuss some early preventive measures, such as using inflated pig bladders to breathe into to avoid dusty atmospheres.

The first written discussions specifically directed toward matters of occupational safety and health were those of Paracelsus, in the fifteenth century. In the early eighteenth century, Bernadino Ramazzini wrote the first text on occupational medicine, *De morbis artificium diatriba*, and he is generally regarded as the "father of occupational medicine." Ramazzini wrote about the health hazards for dozens of occupations ranging from ditch diggers to tailors, from religious activities to those quite secular. In the United States, in the early twentieth century, Dr. Alice Hamilton became the first woman physician appointed to a faculty position at Harvard University, where she worked at the School of Public Health promoting safe and healthful work practices in the United States. She has been recognized as the leader of the occupational medicine movement in the United States, which came relatively late compared with that in Europe.

Except for hunting, agriculture is the most longstanding work activity. Even today, some 70 percent of the world's working population is engaged in agriculture. In sharp contrast, less than 2 percent of Americans continue to be engaged in agriculture; however, these small numbers, utilizing modern equipment, can feed and help clothe much of the rest of the population of the United States, and much of the world. By contrast, much of the agricultural work done in the rest of the world is still tied to direct human labor, sometimes assisted by animals, and somewhat more rarely by modern equipment. Farming continues to be an occupation associated with great risk.

Beginning in earnest in the eighteenth century, the Industrial Revolution of Europe led to large numbers of individuals settling in cities and working in factories. As more and more people worked in factories, and the hazards of factory work became known, regulations came into place regarding who could work, and under what conditions. Initially, there were no restrictions on ages or hours of work, but gradually child-labor laws, laws regulating the work of women, and mandated maximum hours of work were put in place. Today, in the United States, laws such as the Fair Labor Standards Act control child labor, to some extent.

GOVERNMENT REGULATIONS

Until about 1970, there were few federal regulations in the United States with regard to workplace safety and health issues. Each state had its own set of laws with regards to what were considered fair labor practices for workers, as well as a workers' compensation system for individuals that were injured. There was state-by-state enforcement of such regulations. In 1970, laws were passed establishing two government agencies: the National Institute for Occupational Safety and Health (NIOSH) within the U.S. Department of Health and Human Services (USDHHS), which was mandated to undertake research and prevention activities related to work; and the Occupational Safety and Health Administration (OSHA) within the Department of Labor, which was mandated to set national standards for workplace safety and health and to enforce such standards. Workers' compensation, however, has been left on a state-by-state basis, despite efforts toward federal standardization. Compared with Europe, workers' compensation legislation came much later in America, and is more varied.

Other regulations have to do with such issues as workplace drug testing and how such testing must be done. The Americans with Disabilities Act prohibits discrimination for those with handicaps and also requires that certain accommodations be made in the workplace for those who develop disabilities. There are no international standards that are universally utilized with regards to workplace safety and health, but such standards do exist for manufacturing production and quality-control issues regarding manufactured goods. One federal law specifically compensates for coalworker's pneumoconiosis, which is caused by the inhalation of coal dust.

The oversight of occupational safety and health is delegated to OSHA, but other agencies regulate what can leave workplaces by way of emissions (the Environmental Protection Agency), or as products (the Food and Drug Administration or the Consumer Product Safety Commission).

NIOSH once maintained a list of the "top ten" issues considered the most serious in the area of occupational safety and health. Included were occupational cancers, occupational lung disease, skin disorders, and similar problems. In 1996 a major overhaul of this approach was undertaken, and currently the governing construct for research carried out by NIOSH is the National Occupational Research Agenda, or NORA. Replacing the traditional top-ten list are twenty-one areas covering basic toxicology, human interactions in the workplace, emerging technologies, and psychological aspects of work in ways that are much more comprehensive than what had existed previously. It also evaluates combinations of exposures in the workplace, since workers are rarely exposed only to one material at a time, and it includes issues such as workplace organization to see how this impacts on occupational safety and health.

In regulating workplace-related issues, one must note the interactions with normal life events and exposures; and care must be taken to fully understand what is truly workplace-related, what is not, and where and when workplace exposures may have some role in the development of injuries or illnesses. Common life events such as stress, smoking, drug use, and other factors such as noise may interact with what goes on in the workplace.

Substance abuse is another serious workplace issue. There are rules regarding the testing of employees, either at the time of hire and/or during their employment. Certain federal regulations mandate that specific workers, like those in transportation, are required to be tested if there is an accident. Special certification is required as one aspect of drug-testing activities.

Those best equipped to understand occupationally related problems are physicians trained in occupational medicine, a branch of the field of preventive medicine, but in which there are few specialists. Although there are approximately 800,000 physicians in the United States, only about 10,000 practice occupational medicine on a full-time or part-time basis, and of these, only about 20 percent have ever had formal training and certification as specialists in occupational medicine. Most occupational medicine is practiced by primary-care physicians who generally have little training in this field. Medical schools spend virtually no time, if any, on occupational medicine. NIOSH provides some small level of funding to train occupational physicians as well as occupational health nurses, safety specialists, and other related health personnel.

OCCUPATIONAL INJURIES

As the term "occupational safety and health" implies, there are two aspects to this field. One is the area of safety, which seeks to make workplaces safe for workers so that they do not suffer injuries. Poorly designed or laid-out workplaces or equipment may pose a serious hazard to workers, and more than 400,000 injuries occur at work each year. Separate from the concept of safety is that of occupational health, where the goal is to prevent the occurrence of illnesses among workers because of exposures at their place of work.

With regards to safety issues, the greatest number of injuries seen at work, most of which are preventable, involve hearing loss, musculoskeletal disorders, and cumulative trauma problems such as carpal tunnel syndrome.

Equipment-related injuries are a major source of difficulty, and motor-vehicle injuries, specifically, make up the largest number of fatalities related to the workplace. In addition, there are always thousands of cases of broken bones, materials getting into the eyes, burns, and similar injuries that occur each year. The nature of these problems will vary by work sector, age, gender, and other factors, but hundreds of thousands of individuals suffer from workplace-related injuries each year. Many of the injured go on to have a permanent disability that may threaten their livelihoods.

Other workers are at risk due to exposure to fumes and gases. Damage to lungs, or even death, can occur when entering confined spaces where oxygen may be reduced. This includes such diverse settings as grain silos, manure pits, or oil storage tanks. Vehicle exhausts are also known to cause harm or death.

A variety of professionals specialize in issues of occupational safety. For example, certified industrial hygienists are the most experienced at assessing workplaces and monitoring workers to see what kinds of exposures are actually taking place. With regard to safety issues, certified safety professionals constitute a group well qualified to assess safety at workplaces and to put in place safety programs for workers. Other occupational safety professionals include engineers who can make assessments in the workplace. Along with industrial hygienists, they can address such issues as ventilation or other protective measures.

As noted above, these are specialists in the field of occupational medicine who are best equipped to recognize and deal with the medical aspects of these problems. The specialty of occupational medicine requires college, medical school, and a minimum three-year period of specialized training. Among the areas that an occupational disease specialist must study are toxicology, epidemiology, organization of the workplace, regulations that control workplace exposures, as well as the diagnosis, treatment, and prevention of occupational problems.

OCCUPATIONAL DISEASES

Occupational diseases are illnesses that occur because of workplace exposures. Each organ system can have its own set of problems due to a wide variety of exposures.

Skin. The largest organ of the body is the skin, and a considerable number of diseases occur because of exposures of the skin to various agents. These diseases include dermatitis, sensitizations, interactions with drug or chemical exposures, and other difficulties. The skin may also be the route of

entry of foreign matter into the body, such as occurs with many chemicals and some viruses, such as HIV (human immunodeficiency virus), which may enter through an accidental inoculation by needlesticks or vials of tainted blood breaking. Some chemicals dry out the skin and make it more likely that other substances may get in. There are barrier creams available to protect the skin, and protective clothing may be used to prevent skin burns, such as when welding.

Lungs. Another large organ of the body frequently affected by workplace exposures is the lungs. The lungs are directly connected to the outside, and materials taken into the lungs may potentially cause local, or even systemic, disease. Protecting the lungs are a variety of biological process that attempt to block or eliminate foreign substances. These include the hairs in the nasal passages; the mucociliary escalator that exists at the top of the respiratory tract; and macrophages, special cells found in the lungs and elsewhere in the body that gobble up foreign materials. Even though defenses efficiently protect the lungs, many types of occupational lung diseases can develop. Among the most important is occupational asthma, which involves asthma-like symptoms triggered by exposures at the workplace to chemicals, animal hair, or other factors. In addition, a wide variety of dusts causes diseases in the lung, characterized by scarring due to the formation of collagen, the major component of connective tissue. The pneumoconioses can result from exposure to materials such as asbestos, coal dust, silica, talc, or man-made materials such as fibrous glass products. Other substances can enter the lungs and cause disease, including a variety of heavy metals, and a wide variety of substances with the capacity to produce lung cancer and related disorders.

Cardiovascular System. A number of substances are known to cause heart disease. For example, cobalt salts will cause a cardiomyopathy—a weakening of the heart muscle and its ability to pump blood. Other materials can cause changes in the electrical pattern of the heart, known as arrhythmias. Some materials, such as carbon disulfide, a material used in the manufacture of nylon, can cause premature blockage of the arteries in the heart.

Reproductive Organs. The reproductive organs of both men and women can be affected by workplace exposures. Among women, the problem is rarely one of sterility, but of difficulty in becoming pregnant, or having pregnancies characterized by birth defects. Some materials are thought to have estrogenic-like properties that block the normal reproductive cycle.

In men, exposure to lead or to some pesticides, such as dibromochloropropane, can lead to reduced fertility. Some men even become sterile following exposure to certain materials in the workplace. There are still significant questions of whether alterations in the male gene pattern from workplace exposures can be passed on to offspring.

Urinary Tract. Different exposures can cause disease in the various parts of the urinary tract, which consists of the kidney, the ureter (which carries materials from the kidney to the bladder), and the bladder. For example, a number of materials cause malfunction of the kidney, such as exposure to certain solvents that may damage the kidneys sufficiently so that dialysis is required to cleanse the blood of materials that are normally filtered out through the kidney. Certain occupations or exposures may lead to kidney cancer, such as working with printing inks.

Similarly, the bladder can be affected. Certain chemicals, such as beta-naphthalamine or benzidine-based clothing dyes, may cause bladder cancer. Cancer may also result from parasitic diseases, such as schistosomiasis, which may occur due to the parasites entering the body or agricultural workers.

Nervous System. A variety of substances can do damage to the nervous system—some acutely, and some over time. Certain pesticides can have acute, and sometimes lethal, affects on the nervous system, while other exposures may take weeks, months, or years to develop into disease. Manganese found in welding rods can lead to the development of a clinical picture that looks very much like Parkinson's disease. Lead can also damage the nervous system, leading to drooping wrists and ankles. Hearing loss, due to damage to nerves in the ear, is a major workplace problem.

Hematologic System. The blood-forming organs can also be affected by exposures in the workplace. Some substances cause anemia, such as lead and arsine, and some solvents can completely shut off blood production. Certain agents, such as

benzene and ionizing radiation, can produce leukemias.

Liver. A number of agents are known to damage the liver. Most significant are a wide variety of solvents, many of whose use has been curtailed over time. These solvents can produce both acute and chronic disruptions of the cellular architecture of the liver, as well as its function. Some of these agents are used directly, like carbon tetrachloride in dry cleaning, while other are made into other products such as rocket fuel, pesticides, munitions, and paints.

Infectious Agents. A wide variety of infectious agents are also relevant to the workplace. Health care personnel, for example, are at an especially high risk of developing tuberculosis, various forms of viral hepatitis, and HIV/AIDS (acquired immunodeficiency snydrome). The handling of animals or animal hides can produce a wide range of problems, including anthrax and allergic asthma.

Musculoskeletal System. Another set of problems being seen more frequently in the workplace affect the musculoskeletal system. Many muscles and joints in the body can be involved, including the shoulder, elbow, wrist, hip, knee, and ankle. Back injuries are a major problem; prevention approaches include learning proper lifting techniques, use of assist devices, and exercise. A field of study called "ergonomics" specifically evaluates the relationship between persons and machines, and looks to develop tools or methods of working that can minimize injury. Should injuries occur, a variety of professionals may become involved in caring for the patient, including physicians, physical therapists, occupational therapists, and other rehabilitative specialists.

OCCUPATIONAL CANCERS

One special concern is the development of a variety of cancers due to workplace exposures. Cancers can be caused by exposure to a wide range of substances from organic chemicals, metals, certain dusts and fibers, and to physical agents such as radiation.

Many organ systems in the body can be affected. Some substances are only known to produce one type of cancer, whereas some can produce many types of cancers in many organs of the body. For example, asbestos produces a wide range of cancers, including lung cancer; mesothelioma, a rare cancer affecting the lining of the lung, or the pleura; various gastrointestinal-tract cancers, including those of the stomach, colon, and rectum; kidney cancer, and cancer of the oropharynx. Radiation, in various forms, can initiate leukemias, lung cancer, and other cancers, depending on the nature of the source material and the dose. Arsenic, a metal, can cause skin cancer, lung cancer, and an otherwise rare cancer known as a hemangiosarcoma (cancer of the lining of blood vessels). Some fifty or more materials are known or highly suspected of producing a cancer in humans, and many others are still under study.

According to the concept of "sentinel cancers," exposure to certain materials may signal special problems in the workplace. For example, mesotheliomas are almost always tied to asbestos exposure, and hemangiosarcomas result from thorotrast, vinyl chloride, or arsenic.

Some basic principles apply to occupational exposures that can lead to cancer. Not everyone exposed to a particular carcinogenic substance will develop cancer, but the risk is elevated, often many times. The risk of developing a cancer is closely tied to the dose received. The "dose-response" concept means that as the dose goes higher, the risk also increases. This concept applies to many aspects of occupational toxicology, not just cancer.

There is also the phenomenon of latency. For human cancers tied to workplace exposures, the malignancy often appears after ten years, although some are more rapid, such as radiation-induced cancers or leukemias related to benzene. After twenty years, the rate of cancer development often increases, and many risks last over an entire lifetime even if exposure extended for a relatively brief period or stopped many years before.

Some materials, acting together, produce far more cancer that the substances do acting separately. This is called the "synergistic" or the "multiple factor" effect. The first described synergistic effect was that asbestos and cigarette smoking lead to far more lung cancer than either cause alone. Radiation and cigarette smoking have a similar combined effect.

ORGANIZATIONS INVOLVED IN OCCUPATIONAL SAFETY AND HEALTH

A wide variety of organizations, in addition to governmental agencies, are involved in issues of workplace safety and health. In the United States, organizations that have an interest in this field are the American Public Health Association, the American College of Occupational and Environmental Medicine, the American College of Preventive Medicine, and the Society of Occupational and Environmental Health.

On the international level, a variety of organizations are concerned with these issues. These include the World Health Organization, the International Labor Office, and the Collegium Ramazzini.

All these groups are concerned about the development of injuries and diseases in workers, and they also have a major focus on the prevention of these problems.

Other groups active in the protection of workers include various labor organizations, such as individual labor unions and some overarching groups such as the AFL-CIO. Worker health protection makes up a large part of their mandate. These groups examine, among other issues, the transfers of hazardous exposures around the world. It is unfortunately still true that hazardous materials that are banned for use in the United States can, in some cases, continue to be manufactured in the United States for export to other countries. Among these chemicals are dibromochloropropane and DDT, with often tragic consequences associated with their use. Similarly, using certain materials that are highly hazardous and known to cause disease, such as asbestos, are now almost eliminated in the United States but are exported for manufacture and use elsewhere around the world. More than twenty countries have now banned the use of asbestos inside their country, and there is a growing worldwide movement to eliminate the use of this material since safer substitutes can be found.

What is dismaying is that as workplaces in the United States and other major industrialized countries become safer over time, the knowledge about the hazards and the measures to control hazards are not being exported to developing countries along with the hazardous materials. As the world becomes more globalized, the hazards faced by workers become the same all over the globe. It needs to be recognized on a international level that almost all occupational injury and disease are entirely preventable.

ARTHUR L. FRANK

(SEE ALSO: *Asbestos; Benzene; Ergonomics; Fair Labor Standards Act; Hamilton, Alice; HIV/AIDS; Lead; National Institute for Occupational Safety and Health; Occupational Disease; Occupational Safety and Health Administration; Pesticides; Ramazzini, Bernardino; Risk Assessment, Risk Management; Toxicology*)

BIBLIOGRAPHY

National Institute of Occupational Safety and Health (1994). *National Occupational Research Agenda Update*. Washington, DC: U.S. Department of Health and Human Services.

—— (2000). *Worker Health Chartbook, 2000*. Washington, DC: Department of Health and Human Services.

Rom, W. (1998). *Environmental and Occupational Medicine*, 3rd edition. Philadelphia, PA: Lippencott-Raven.

Weeks, J. L.; Levy, B. S.; and Wagner, G. R. (1991). *Preventing Occupational Disease and Injury*. Washington, DC: American Public Health Association.

OCCUPATIONAL SAFETY AND HEALTH ADMINISTRATION

The mission of the Occupational Safety and Health Administration (OSHA) is to assure that every U.S. worker goes home whole and healthy every day. Toward that end, the agency sets and enforces workplace safety and health standards, encourages voluntary compliance through consultation and partnerships, and promotes safety training and education for workers and employers. Since Congress passed the Occupational Safety and Health Act of 1970 (OSH Act), which created OSHA as an agency within the U.S. Department of Labor, workplace fatalities have been cut in half and occupational injury and illness rates have declined 40 percent. At the same time, U.S. employment has nearly doubled.

Under the OSH Act, employers are responsible for providing a safe and healthful work environment in line with standards set by OSHA.

Protecting workers against workplace hazards requires every employer and every worker to make safety and health a top priority. OSHA's charge is to offer leadership and encouragement to workers and employers in carrying out this responsibility. OSHA has a staff of about 2,250, including about 1,250 inspectors in 67 field offices. Sharing the responsibility for oversight of workplace safety and health are twenty-five states that run their own OSHA programs with about 2,800 employees, including about 1,250 inspectors.

Early OSHA standards focused primarily on safety and establishing precise safety requirements, such as the specific height for guardrails on stairs. Newer standards take a performance or program approach, identifying a safety or health objective and providing a framework for employers to use in achieving that goal. OSHA standards cover the gamut of workplace safety and health issues, including machine guarding, fall protection, chemical-hazard communication, and protection against blood-borne pathogens such as HIV (human immunodeficiency virus) and hepatitis B.

OSHA's enforcement program has changed dramatically over the years. The agency has continually attempted to target its resources toward the most hazardous worksites, as well as respond to worker complaints and investigate fatal accidents. Initially, OSHA focused on sites in industries with high injury rates. More recently, OSHA has obtained site-specific injury and illness data and has been able to concentrate on individual sites with poor safety and health records. The agency conducts about 35,000 inspections each year; states running their own OSHA programs inspect an additional 55,000 workplaces. To foster voluntary compliance with OSHA standards and assist employers in setting up ongoing safety and health programs, OSHA offers free consultations and seeks to establish partnerships with individual workplaces and with trade groups and unions.

The OSHA consultation program, designed for smaller employers, provides free assistance to employers who request help with safety and health programs and specific problems. Employers agree in advance to correct serious hazards identified by the consultant. The consultation program is administered by state authorities and is completely separate from the enforcement effort. OSHA's premier partnership is the Voluntary Protection

Programs (VPP). Individual workplaces that meet criteria for excellence in safety and health may apply to the agency for VPP recognition. VPP sites serve as models for their industries and their communities, and they average 50 percent fewer injuries than their non-VPP counterparts. The OSHA Strategic Partnership Program (OSPP) is open to sites with a similar commitment but varying levels of achievement. It includes both national and regional partnerships. These partnerships combine the resources of OSHA, trade groups, and unions to develop successful strategies for preventing injuries and illnesses and measure the results.

To further assist employers and workers, OSHA maintains an extensive web site (http://www.osha.gov) that includes the agency's standards, publications, training materials, interactive software covering specific standards and hazards, small business information, an online complaint filing system for workers, and links to many other sources of information on job safety and health. The agency also offers safety and health training at its Chicago-area training institute and through twelve educational centers located at community colleges and universities around the country. OSHA is developing satellite-delivered and web-based training programs to make its training available to a wider audience. Through its New Directions grants, OSHA encourages nonprofit organizations such as unions and trade associations to develop additional training materials and offer training courses.

Improving work environments is a long-term proposition that requires daily diligence and on-going commitment in the face of competing priorities for time, energy, and resources. OSHA's mandate is to aid employers and employees to make this commitment and continually pursue excellence in job safety and health.

OCCUPATIONAL SAFETY AND HEALTH ADMINISTRATION

(SEE ALSO: *National Institute for Occupational Safety and Health; Occupational Safety and Health; Occupational Safety and Health Administration*)

BIBLIOGRAPHY

Occupational Safety and Health Administration. *All About OSHA*. (OSHA 2056). Available at http://www.osha.gov.

OCEAN DUMPING

Pollution of the open seas by human activities has become a serious problem. Ocean dumping is the dumping or placing of materials in designated places in the ocean, often on the continental shelf. A wide range of materials is involved, including garbage, construction and demolition debris, sewage sludge, dredge material, and waste chemicals. In some cases, ocean dumping is regulated and controlled, while some dumping occurs haphazardly by ships and tankers at sea, or illegally within coastal waters. Incineration at sea of organic wastes, with subsequent dumping, has been allowed as a viable disposal process, both in the United States and in Europe.

An important, but little recognized source of ocean dumping is the elimination of bilge water from tankers carrying oil and other products. Bilge water can contain a number of toxic chemicals, as well as biological agents that can affect marine ecosystems and marine organisms, some of which are subsequently consumed by humans. Dumping of radioactive wastes and soil from contaminated nuclear defense sites has periodically been suggested as a viable disposal method, and canisters of nerve gas have been disposed of at sea. In addition to permitted ocean dumping, there is always the possibility of collisions, groundings, and accidents that result in de facto ocean dumping, often of materials not otherwise allowed.

At one time, drums containing hazardous waste were dumped, but the disintegration of canisters caused sufficient concern to halt this process. Some of the drums containing hazardous chemicals were dumped in shallow seas, such as the North Sea, that are intensely fished, creating a potential risk to humans from the consumption of contaminated fish and shellfish.

A number of U.S. federal laws apply to at-sea incineration, including the Resource Conservation and Recovery Act, Toxic Substances Control Act, Water Pollution Prevention and Control Act, Air Pollution Prevention and Control Act, Dangerous Cargo Act, Ports and Waterways Safety Act, Deep Water Ports Act, and the Ocean Dumping Act. Most states also have a number of laws and regulations to control operations.

There are three main direct public health risks from ocean dumping: (1) occupational accidents, injuries, and exposures; (2) exposure of the public to hazardous or toxic materials washed up on beaches; and (3) human consumption of marine organisms that have been contaminated by ocean disposal. Periodically, medical and other wastes from both legal and illegal dumping have washed up on beaches, resulting in exposure to beachgoers and, in some cases, the closure of beaches until the wastes could be removed. Consumption of fish and shellfish contaminated from radioactive wastes may pose a serious problem worldwide because of nuclear waste dumping in the oceans.

One of the main sources of toxic chemicals off the Atlantic coast of the United States has been ocean-dumped municipal sewage sludge. In addition to biologic agents, sludge contains toxic residues. These same areas are fished heavily, both commercially and recreationally. From a public health perspective, pregnant women, women about to become pregnant, and young children are most at risk from the consumption of contaminated fish and shellfish.

JOANNA BURGER

(SEE ALSO: *Ambient Water Quality; Medical Waste; Municipal Solid Waste; Oil Spills; Sewage System; Wastewater Treatment; Water Quality*)

BIBLIOGRAPHY

Goyal, S. M.; Adams, W. N.; O'Malley, M. L.; and Lear, D. W. (1984). "Human Pathogenic Viruses at Sewage Sludge Disposal Sites in the Mid-Atlantic Region." *Applied Environmental Microbiology* 48:758–763.

Kennish, M. J. (1991). *Ecology of Estuaries: Anthropogenic Effects.* Boca Raton, FL: CRC Press.

Lipton, J., and Gillett, J. W. (1991). "Uncertainty in Ocean-Dumping Health Risks: Influence of Bioconcentration, Commercial Fish Landings and Seafood Consumption." *Environmental Toxicology and Chemistry* 10:967–976.

Nielsen, S. P.; Iosipe, M.; and Strand, P. (1997). "Collective Dose to Man from Dumping of Radioactive Waste in the Seas." *Science of the Total Environment* 202:136–146.

ODDS RATIO

The odds ratio (OR) provides a measure of the strength of relationship between two variables,

Table 1

Frequencies in a 2 x 2 Table.

	OUTCOME +ve	OUTCOME −ve
Exposure (outcome positive)	a	b
Exposure (outcome negative)	c	d

SOURCE: Courtesy of author.

most commonly an exposure and a dichotomous outcome. It is most commonly used in a case-control study where it is defined as "the ratio of the odds of being exposed in the group with the outcome to the odds of being exposed in the group without the outcome." In the standard 2x2 epidemiological table, this ratio can be expressed as the "cross-product" (ad/bc), as seen in Table 1.

This concept can be extended to a situation with multiple levels of exposure (e.g., low, moderate, or high exposure to an environmental containment). One exposure level is assigned as the "reference" level. For each of the remaining exposure levels, one divides the odds of that exposure level in the outcome positive group (compared with the reference level) by the odds of that exposure level in the outcome negative group.

The OR ranges in value from 0 to infinity. Values close to 1.0 indicate no relationship between the exposure and the outcome. Values less than 1.0 suggest a protective effect, while values greater than 1.0 suggest a causative or adverse effect of exposure.

The OR is closely connected to logistic regression. This analytic method models the natural logarithm of the OR as a linear function of the predictor variables. It is a powerful and very common method for the analysis of epidemiological studies.

The OR is one of the most common measures encountered in observational epidemiology. The value of the OR for case-control research was first

Table 2

Frequencies of Erysipelas by Obesity

	erysipelas	No erysipelas
Obese	68	97
Non-obese	61	197

SOURCE: Courtesy of author.

recognized by Jerome Cornfield in 1951. His work provided the theoretical base for the application of the case-control approach to studying disease etiology. The OR estimates the incidence-density ratio or the cumulative incidence ratio that would have been observed if it had been feasible to perform a cohort study rather than a case-control study. Depending on the method used to obtain control subjects, the OR either is identical to one of the incidence ratios or is close to them if the disease is rare. Some epidemiologists modify the term to reflect the type of study being done (e.g., prevalence odds ratio, exposure odds ratio, or disease odds ratio).

Although mainly used for the analysis of case-control studies, the odds ratio can also be applied in cross-sectional and cohort studies. It also plays a major role in certain approaches to the meta-analysis of randomized clinical trials (e.g., the Peto method).

An example of the use of the odds ratio can be found in a paper published by A. Dupuy et al. This paper studied 129 patients with erysipelas of the leg and a control group of 294 people without erysipelas of the leg. Obesity was considered as a risk factor. Analysis of the data produced the 2x2 table shown in Table 2.

This gives an OR of $(68 \times 197)/(61 \times 97)$ or 2.3. That is, people with erysipelas are 2.3 times more likely to be obese than people without erysipelas. This supports the suggestion that obesity increases the risk of developing erysipelas.

GEORGE WELLS

(SEE ALSO: *Case-Control Study; Epidemiology; Statistics for Public Health*)

BIBLIOGRAPHY

Dupuy, A.; Benchikhi, H.; Roujeau, J. C.; Bernard, P.; Vaillant, L.; Chosidow, O.; Sassolas, B.; Guillaume, J. C.; Grob, J. J.; and Bastuji-Garin, S. (1999). "Risk Factors for Erysipelas of the Leg (Cellulitis): Case-Control Study." *British Medical Journal* 318:1591–1594.

OFFICE ON SMOKING AND HEALTH

Federal legislative acts since 1965 have accorded regulatory responsibility to the administrative branch of the U.S. government in relation to tobacco advertising, labeling, public education, and reporting to Congress on tobacco sales, marketing practices, and ingredients. These responsibilities were assigned to the Office of Smoking and Health when it was created within the Office of the Assistant Secretary of Health in 1978. The office's authority was transferred to the Centers for Disease Control and Prevention (CDC) in 1986 and placed within the National Center for Chronic Disease Control and Health Promotion in 1988.

The mission of the office is to lead and coordinate strategic efforts aimed at preventing tobacco use among youths, promoting smoking cessation among youth and young adults, protecting nonsmokers from environmental tobacco smoke, and eliminating health disparities associated with tobacco. These goals are accomplished through efforts to expand the science of tobacco control, build capacity in states and organizations to conduct tobacco-control programs, communicate information to constituents and to the public, facilitate action with and among partners, and provide technical assistance to the global community.

LAWRENCE W. GREEN

(SEE ALSO: *Environmental Tobacco Smoke; Smoking Cessation; Tobacco Control*)

OFFICIAL U.S. HEALTH AGENCIES

The role of the U.S. government in health policies and programs has its roots in the Constitution. This role is made clear by Lawrence A. Gostin:

The Constitutional design reveals a plain intent to vest power in government at every level to protect community health and safety. By its very first sentences, the Constitution provides sole legislative or policy making authority in the Congress, and the first enumerated legislative power is to provide for the common defense and general welfare of the United States. The legislative role is to enact laws necessary to safeguard the population from harms and promote health (e.g., food and drug purity, occupational health and safety, and a healthy environment) (Gostin 2000, p. 2838).

The powers granted to the federal government to regulate interstate commerce, to tax, and to spend have been the most important powers used to protect and promote the health of the population. It was not until the policies advocated by President Franklin Roosevelt in the 1930s, including Social Security, that the welfare clause was used to expand the federal role in domestic social programs. The Medicare program enacted in 1965 to finance hospitals and physicians' services for the elderly and disabled and the Medicare Program—a joint federal-state program to finance health care to certain categories of the poor—was based on the authorities granted in the original Social Security Act of 1935, which represented a fundamental shift in the role of the federal government.

While the Department of Health and Human Services is the lead federal agency on health, the United States government has health functions in over forty different departments and agencies, including the Departments of Agriculture, Veteran's Affairs, Commerce, Defense, Education, Energy, Health and Human Services, Housing and Urban Development, Interior, Justice, State, Transportation, and Treasury, as well as such independent agencies as the Consumer Product Safety Commission, the Environmental Protection Agency, the Nuclear Regulatory Commission, the National Science Foundation, and the United States International Development Corporation, which includes the U.S. Agency for International Development. (For a detailed description of the various federal department, agencies and commissions that carry out federal health functions see: G.T. Kurian, ed. [1998]. *A Historical Guide to* *the U.S. Government.* New York: Oxford University Press.)

Policies affecting public health begin with the legislative branch, which consists of the two houses of Congress (the Senate and the House of Representatives). Both the Senate and the House of Representatives affect how or if policies affecting health and environmental programs become law. Congress often determines which federal department or agency will implement these policies. Congress also plays a primary role in the funding of the federal government's public health functions. No money can be spent by a federal department or agency unless appropriated by Congress.

The states play a central role in promoting and protecting the population's health. The states have what are described as reserved powers that permit them to exercise all the powers inherent in government that are neither granted to the federal government nor prohibited to the states by the Constitution. Critical to the states' role in public health are police powers—Gostin defines police power as:

The inherent authority of the state (and, through delegation, local government) to enact laws and promulgate regulations to protect, preserve, and promote the health, safety, morals, and general welfare of the people. To achieve these communal benefits, the state retains the power to restrict, within federal and state constitutional limits, personal interests in liberty, autonomy, privacy, as well as economic interests in freedom or contract as uses of property (Gostin 2000, p. 2980).

The role assigned to the states has made the relationship of the federal government and the states in domestic social programs, including public health, critical to achieving domestic policy objectives. These roles have evolved, particularly since the expansion of the federal role during Roosevelt's New Deal in the 1930s. Federalism, which describes this relationship, traces its roots to the Latin word for covenant. To describe the formation of political society by mutually consenting individuals, the related word "compact" had been used by philosopher John Locke almost one hundred years before the ratification of the U.S. Constitution. In the United States, the ultimate arbiter of the role of the federal government and the states is the Supreme Court. Many courts, including the court as of the year 2000 have been strong defenders of the states' rights against federal domination. Other courts (e.g., the Warren Court) have defined a stronger federal role (e.g., civil rights, women's reproductive rights).

State health agencies and local departments of health are increasingly structured within the framework of federal categorical grant in aid programs for public health, environmental health, and medical care. The multiple departments and agencies at the federal level that fund public health programs are often reflected in the organization of the programs at the state and local level.

THE SIX CORE FUNCTIONS

The role of the U.S. government in protecting and promoting the health of the population is broad and complex, but can be described within six broad functions: (1) policy-making, (2) financing, (3) public health protection (e.g., standard setting and regulation), (4) collecting and disseminating information, (5) capacity building for population health, including research and training, and (6) direct management of health services. The interactions of the three branches of the federal government with each other and with the state governments are critical to the performance of each function. This article, however, focuses on the executive branch of the federal government. The policy-making involves Congress, the president, cabinet secretaries, and their key staffs. The judicial branch may play a key role (e.g., abortion, civil rights, environmental health, federal-state roles). Financing depends first and foremost on the authorization for and appropriation of funds by Congress. After these funds are appropriated there is control by the Office of Management and Budget in the White House, with the actual distribution of funds by the departments and agencies (e.g., Health Care Financing Administration). All the other activities are primarily carried out by departments and agencies, with oversight by the White House and Congress.

All of the six basic functions must be effectively performed at the federal level for an effective federal health function. When working in a coordinated fashion, these independent functions create a synergy that supports a population-based

approach to health. The current priorities and the organization of federal health programs, however, reveal a confusion about the federal health mission and how to organize to achieve it. In terms of expenditures, the highest priorities are financing medical care for individuals and biomedical research. Public health priorities have been reflected in multiple-disease focused, categorical public health programs that are more often treatment than prevention oriented.

An alternative priority for federal health action would be to set as a goal the 1988 definition of the mission of public health by the Institute of Medicine's Committee for the Study of the Future of Public Health:

> *The Committee defines the mission of Public Health as fulfilling society's interest in assuring the conditions in which people can be healthy. Its aim is to generate organized community efforts to address the public interest in health by applying scientific and technical knowledge to prevent disease and promote health. The mission of public health is addressed by private organizations and individuals as well as by public agencies. But the governmental public health agency has a unique function: to see to it that the vital elements are in place and that the mission is adequately addressed (IOM 1988, p. 5).*

Little emphasis has been placed on this public health mission and on capacity building for population health, or on collecting and disseminating information on the health of the population, particularly at the state and local level.

Policy-making. Health policy-making is a critical function of the federal government. It involves creating and using an evidence base, informed by social values, so that decision makers can shape legislation, regulation, and programs to achieve the agenda of national leaders. This involves interaction of executive and legislative branches, influenced by a variety of stakeholders in the nongovernment sector, and often tempered by action by the judicial branch.

Policies are reflected in the legislation authorizing particular programs, and in the appropriation of funds by Congress for particular purposes that do not require a special legislation (e.g., *Healthy People 2010*).

The judicial branch can affect federal public policy and its public health functions by modifying the legal basis for public health initiatives in decisions rendered by federal courts, including and the U.S. Supreme Court. While Congress must enact the laws that establish federal public health policies and appropriate the funds to implement these laws, the judicial branch can influence public policy in the United States by interpreting policies in relation to the Constitution and federal laws. For instance, the Supreme Court, under Chief Justice Earl Warren, made decisions of fundamental importance in two areas directly related to the public's health: civil and reproductive rights. More recently the Rehnquist court has limited the interpretation of the commerce clause by the Congress.

Depending on the priority placed by the president in health issues, many public health and environmental health policy proposals develop in the White House, including the Office of Management and Budget (OMB), as well as by cabinet departments, independent agencies (e.g., EPA), and commissions (e.g., Consumer Product Safety Commission). Within the executive branch, health-policy direction comes from the Executive Office of the President, particularly the Office of Management and Budget, the Council on Environmental Quality, and the Domestic Policy Council (directed by a special assistant to the president).

The U.S. Department of Health and Human Services (USDHHS) plays a major role in initiating, shaping, and ultimately implementing and monitoring the effects of legislation passed by Congress and signed by the president. It does this in coordination with the Executive Office of the President, particularly the Office of Management and Budget (OMB), Congress, state governments, regulated industries, providers, beneficiaries, and other interest groups. The position of Secretary of Health and Human Services has the widest responsibilities over the public health programs at the federal level, but this role is limited because of this wide dispersion of federal public health and medical care programs. The organization and management of USDHHS was changed substantially in 1994, when the Social Security Administration (the core of the department from 1953 to 1994) was removed from USDHHS by Congress and established as an independent agency. In 1995 the secretary assumed direct authority over the eight agencies of the U.S. Public Health Service (PHS), designating them as operating divisions reporting to the secretary. The assistant secretary for health thus became a staff officer not a line manager. Another factor affecting the secretary's role was the enactment of welfare reform in 1996, which eliminated federal welfare programs that had operated for over sixty years and transferred the policy and program decisions to the states—with federal financial support but little policy direction. The decreased role of welfare policy increased the relative importance of the health policy and program role of the secretary.

The secretary delegates responsibility to the components of USDHHS. The Center for Medicine and Medical Services (CMMS), the Administration on Aging (AOA), the Agency for Children and Families (ACF), and the operating divisions of the U.S. Public Health Service (i.e., the National Institutes of Health [NIH], the Centers for Disease Control and Prevention [CDC], the Agency for Toxic Substances and Disease Registry [ATSDR], the Health Resources and Services Administration {HRDA], the Substance Abuse and Mental Health Services Administration [SAMHSA], the Indian Health Service [HIS], and the Agency for Healthcare Research and Quality [AHRQ]). The secretary's role as the country's chief public health official goes beyond the administration of federal programs, because the secretary serves as the president's principal health advisor.

Financing. The federal government plays a very large role in the financing of health care. In Medicare, the federal government directly finances the health care of the elderly, but Medicare only covers about 50 percent of the cost of health care for the elderly (e.g., it does not cover prescription drugs). The federal government also provides a large subsidy for state Medicaid programs, providing 50 to 80 percent of their funds. Federal employees have their purchasing of health insurance subsidized by the federal government, as do the dependents of military personnel.

Medicare, Medicaid, and the State Child Health Insurance Programs (SCHIP) are administered by the Centers for Medicare and Medicaid Service (CMMS). Through these programs, CMMS provides health insurance directly or indirectly to over 74 million Americans. To run these programs,

CMMS has a relatively small staff to implement policy through regulations and oversee the performance of the insurance companies that administer Medicare Part A (hospital insurance) and Part B (medical insurance) and pay the providers for services rendered. These are called fiscal "intermediaries" (Part A) and "carries" (Part B). The CMMS also oversees the state agencies that administer Medicaid and SCHIP. It is also the responsibility of CMMS to combat fraud and abuse in the Medicare and Medicaid programs. Additional responsibilities for CMMS include setting national policies for paying health care providers, conducting research on the effectiveness of health care services, and the enforcement of the policies related to the quality of health care services. The regulation of clinical laboratories performing tests on patients paid by Medicare also falls under the jurisdiction of CMMS with advice from CDC.

Public Health Protection. Public health protection is the most classic of the public health functions performed by the federal and state governments. Governments at all levels use their health status and disease surveillance capacity to assess health risks and use their standard-setting and regulatory powers to protect the public from these risks.

Based on the scientific evidence available through risk assessments, standard setting and regulation at the federal level involves four broad areas: (1) provider certification (e.g., for clinical laboratories through the Clinical Laboratory Improvement Act and certification of providers such as hospitals who meet the standards of the Joint Commission on Accreditation of Healthcare Organizations and thus qualify for Medicare payment); (2) purchaser and insurance certification (e.g., through collaboration with states to establish criteria for financial viability of health plans and health insurance entities that permit them to operate in the market place); (3) standard setting (e.g., for age appropriate clinical preventive services, immunization schedules, clean water, air quality, and workplace safety, as well as health care quality standards set by HCFA for providers of health care to receive Medicare funding); and (4) regulations (e.g., for the safety and quality of foods; the safety and efficacy of prescription drugs, biologics such as blood products and vaccines, medical devices, and cosmetics; highway safety; occupational health and safety; air and water pollution control; pesticides; radiation; toxic wastes; and consumer products.)

Financing agencies, such as HCFA (which administers Medicare and Medicaid), also implement regulations to assure compliance with the intent of Congress with respect to the administration of programs. Types of regulatory measures include command and control regulations, performance standards, and guidance documents. An example of the regulatory power the federal government has is the power to issue a health provider and/or purchaser/insurer certification; as in 1966, when hospitals had to be certified that they were in compliance with the Civil Rights Act of 1964 (e.g., that they barred segregation) in order to receive Medicare payments. Over 3,000 hospitals had to desegregate prior to the implementation of Medicare on July 1, 1966, in order for them to receive Medicare payments.

The basis for standard setting in regulating remains grounded in science; the research base is largely generated by DHHS agencies. These regulations are reviewed by USDHHS and OMB before they become final.

The principal federal regulatory agencies are the Food and Drug Administration (drugs, biologics, medical devices, cosmetics), the Department of Agriculture (meat, poultry, and eggs), the Department of Energy (radiation-related environmental management, civilian radioactive waste management), the Department of Labor (occupational health and safety), the Department of Transportation (auto and highway safety), the Department of Treasury (alcohol, tobacco, and firearms), as well as the Centers for Disease Control and Prevention and HCFA (clinical laboratories, health care providers), the Environmental Protection Agency (air and water pollution control), the Consumer Product Safety Commission and the Nuclear Power Regulatory Commission.

Collecting and Disseminating Information. The federal government is responsible for the collection and dissemination of information relating to public health and the health care delivery systems. This part of the assessment function is critically important to public health practice and risk assessment. The U.S. Census carries the most basic of the federal data collection responsibilities.

The National Center for Health Statistics (NCHS) in HHS is the primary agency collecting and reporting health information. Data gathering for public health purposes is a shared responsibility with state and local governments. The collection and dissemination of information includes at least six functions: (1) reporting requirements for federal grant-in-aid funded programs; (2) disaster surveillance; (3) national vital and health statistics; (4) population surveys (e.g., Health Information Survey, National Health and Nutrition Examination Survey); (5) health care cost, delivery, and utilization information; and (6) research findings. The federal government presents information about the health of the nation through its annual publication *Health, United States*. It also publishes many other reports. Particularly important surveys conducted by the NCHS are the Health Interview Survey and the National Health and Nutrition Examination Survey (NHANES). The Agency for Healthcare Research and Quality (AHRQ) conducts the National Medical Care Expenditure Survey, while the Health Care Financing Administration (HCFA) conducts the Medicare Beneficiary Survey and it also collects and disseminates information on national health expenditures.

In the future, the development of the National Health Information Infrastructure will be critical to enhancing the capacity for collaboration among the federal, state, and local governments. The proliferation of categorical public health programs (there are more than 200) at the federal level has made coordination and collaboration more complex and more difficult at all levels of government.

Capacity Building for Population Health. Capacity building for population health must assure the ability of federal agencies to effectively discharge their responsibilities to promote and protect the health of the population. It must also assure that other levels of government, which share responsibilities for health, have the resources—human, financial, and organizational—to carry out their responsibilities, whether delegated to them by the federal government or those for which they have primary responsibility.

The major federal investments in capacity building have supported biomedical research, human resource development, and capital development of facilities (e.g. hospitals) for personal health care

services and biomedical research, mirroring the federal health policies that support the financing of health care and biomedical research.

The research and training function is dominated by the support of biomedical research (basic and clinical) by the National Institutes of Health. Located in Bethesda, Maryland, the National Institutes of Health (NIH) comprises twenty-seven separate institutes and centers, including the National Institute of Environmental Health Sciences, located in North Carolina. The NIH approached $20 billion dollars in 2001. The mission of NIH is to help fund work in its own laboratories and in universities, hospitals, private research institutions, and private industry to uncover new knowledge that can potentially improve the quality of medical care and the understanding of disease processes. While part of the PHS, the research at NIH is focused primarily on basic biomedical and clinical research, with little emphasis on the health of the population (e.g., determinants of health) or prevention. The NIH also supports research training, but in a more modest scale than in the past.

The largest support for health professions training consists of Medicare's funding of graduate medical education (GME). Funding for GME provides direct salary support of residents in training in hospitals caring for Medicare patients (called direct medical education payments) and payment to teaching hospitals for the higher costs of treating Medicare patients in teaching hospitals (indirect medical education payments). The GME payments dwarf the funding for health-profession training funding by the Health Resources and Services Administration or other operating divisions within USDHHS.

Health-services research is supported very modestly, and far below what is needed. Public health research and training is a third category that receives only limited support by the USDHHS, particularly through CDC and HRSA.

There never has been a systematic or adequate federal investment in public health infrastructure (e.g., public health laboratories), broad-based information systems for disease surveillance or environmental risk, population health, water quality, food safety) and population health education and work force training. Compared to the billions spent by Medicare to support graduate medical education, the federal government spends less than $5 million annually for public health training.

Collaboration among agencies (departments within the federal government) to promote population health requires managerial capacity building, particularly information systems to meet the needs of various collaborating agencies that go beyond the limited data systems that serve primarily to assure program accountability. This is often made more difficult because Congress sometimes places increased demands on agencies (e.g., FDA, HCFA) but reduces their budgets for the administrative support required to meet their expanded responsibilities.

Federal-state relations are a particularly important area for capacity building. The federal government is already using intermediaries, including state and local governments, for much of what it does.

Direct Management of Health Services. The Department of Defense, including the Army, Navy, and Air Force, the Indian Health Service of the U.S. Department of Health and Human Services, the Department of Veteran Affairs carry out the direct management of public health and medical services. The U.S. Public Health Service also provides commissioned officers to provide medical care to prisoners in federal prisons and to members of the Coast Guard. The medical care previously provided to merchant seamen through a system of public health service hospitals and clinics was eliminated during the Reagan administration.

JO IVEY BOUFFORD
PHILIP R. LEE
BRIAN PUSKAS
ANNE M. PORZIG

(SEE ALSO: *Environmental Protection Agency; Health Resources and Services Administration; Medicaid; Medicare; Nongovernmental Organizations, United States; Police Powers; Policy for Public Health; U.S. Consumer Product Safety Commission; United States Public Health Services [USPHS]*)

BIBLIOGRAPHY

Gostin, L. O. (2000). "Public Health Law in a New Century, Part 1: Law as a Tool to Advance the Community's Health." *Journal of American Medical Association* 283:2838.

—— (2000). "Public Health Law in a New Century, Part 2: Powers and Limits of Public Health." *Journal of American Medical Association* 283:2980.

Institute of Medicine, Committee for the Study of the Future of Public Health (1988). *The Future of Public Health.* Washington, DC: National Academy Press.

Kincaid, J. (2001). "Introduction: Federalism Values and Health Values." *SciPolicy Journal* 1(1):1–17.

OIL SPILLS

Oil is one of the world's main sources of energy, but because it is unevenly distributed it must be transported by ship across oceans and by pipelines across land. This results in accidents when transferring oil to vessels, when transporting oil, and when pipelines break, as well as when drilling for oil. While massive and catastrophic oil spills receive most of the attention, smaller and chronic oil spills and seeps occur regularly. These spills contaminate coasts and estuaries, and they can cause human health problems.

Oil is a mixture of hydrocarbon compounds, which are the decayed remains of marine animals and plants that lived in shallow inland seas, died, and drifted to the bottom. For the past 600 million years, under intense pressure and temperatures, these remains changed into the complicated hydrocarbons called petroleum. Crude oil is a mixture of gas, naphtha, kerosene, light gas, and residuals, which have different health effects.

Overall production of petroleum products rose from about 500 million tons in 1950 to over 2,500 million tons by the mid-1990s, resulting in massive transport and associated oil spills. By far the greatest oil reserves are in the Middle East, and major transportation routes emanate from there. The number of oil spills, both major and minor, has been increasing with the increasing rate of oil transport and the aging of oil tankers, as well as an increase in the size of oil tankers. Oil accounts for over half the tonnage of all sea cargo.

Since the 1960s there have been about twenty oil spills of more than 20 million gallons. Major oil spills have occurred off the coast of Mexico, the Middle East, off South Africa, in the North Pacific, and in Alaska, as well as in the pipeline in Usink,

Russia. The largest oil spill to date resulted from the Gulf War in 1991, when over 240 million gallons of oil poured into the Persian Gulf, most of it deliberately. The next largest oil spill, from the Ixtox-1 well off Mexico, involved a blowout of 140 million gallons.

The largest spills do not necessarily receive the most media coverage, either because of their location, the lack of human health or ecological effects, the lack of documentation of these effects, or a lack of media interest. For example the 1980 Nowruz field spill in Arabia (80 million gallons) and the 1992 Fergana Valley spill in Uzbekistan (80 million gallons) barely received any attention. In contrast, two smaller spills received enormous media attention: the oil tanker *Amoco Cadiz* released 68.7 million gallons off the coast of France in 1978, and the tanker *Exxon Valdez* spilled 11 million gallons into Prince William Sound in Alaska in 1989.

Short-term public health impacts from oil spills include accidents suffered by those on damaged tankers or those involved in the cleanup, and illnesses caused by toxic fumes or by eating contaminated fish or shellfish. However, there are other less obvious public health impacts, including losses and disruptions of commercial and recreational fisheries, seaweed harvesting, boating, and a variety of other uses of affected water. There are also emotional, aesthetic, and economic losses, such as when Native Americans and others are denied subsistence or recreational uses. In both the case of the *Exxon Valdez* and the *Amoco Cadiz* there were permanent changes to the social and cultural communities residing in the region, which had permanent public health consequences, including chronic psychological stress.

JOANNA BURGER

(SEE ALSO: *Ambient Water Quality; Ocean Dumping; Pollution*)

BIBLIOGRAPHY

Burger, J. (1997). *Oil Spills.* New Brunswick, NJ: Rutgers University Press.

Cahill, R. A. (1990). *Disasters at Sea: Titanic to Exxon Valdez.* San Antonio, TX: Nautical Books.

Cutter Information Corporation (1995). *International Oil Spill Statistics.* Arlington, MA: Cutter Information.

Picot, J. C., and Gill, D. A. (1996). "The Exxon Valdez Oil Spill and Chronic Psychological Stress." In *Proceedings of the Exxon Valdez Oil Spill Symposium,* eds. F. Rice, R. Spies, D. Wolfe, and B. Wright. Bethesda, MD: American Fisheries Society.

OLD AGE

See Gerontology

ONCHOCERCIASIS

Onchocerciasis, or river blindness, is a filarial infection caused by the parasitic nematode, *Onchocerca volvulus,* carried by black flies of the genus *Simulium.* It is estimated that 17.7 million people are infected with *O. volvulus,* with 95 percent of those infected found in Africa. The infection is also found in areas of Central and South America and in the Arabian peninsula. Onchocerciasis is a significant cause of blindness in endemic countries. Of those people currently infected, approximately 270,000 are blind and a further 500,000 have severe visual impairment.

Simulium spp. are biting flies that are active during the day, breeding in fast flowing, well-oxygenated waters. Infection prevalence is highest in areas adjacent to such rivers, hence the term "river blindness." Transmission occurs when an infected fly takes a blood meal from a human and injects *O. volvulus* larvae (called microfilariae) into the host. The microfilariae develop into adult worms over the next one to two years. When mature, the adult worms produce new microfilariae that migrate throughout the skin of the host. A female adult worm may live for as long as ten years and will produce 1,300 to 1,900 microfilariae per day. These new microfilariae can be taken up by a biting fly, and thus the cycle of infection is completed.

Adult worms seldom cause any symptoms except as subcutaneous nodules around bony prominences. As microfilariae migrate throughout the body the following symptoms occur: severe itching, rashes, depigmentation of the skin, especially of the lower limbs ("leopard skin"); and destruction of skin elasticity, resulting in loose, hanging folds ("hanging groin"). The most devastating effect of onchocerciasis results when micrifilariae enter the eye, leading to visual impairment and eventually to blindness. These clinical manifestations are predominantly due to the body's inflammatory response to dead or dying microfilariae and vary depending on the number of worms.

Diagnosis is made by microscopic examination of skin snips for microfilariae. Adult worms may be found in subcutaneous nodules. There are several immunodiagnostic tests that have been developed for antigen detection with varying sensitivities and specificities. A small dose of diethylcarbamazine (DEC) when given to a patient (the "Mazzotti test") results in death of microfilariae and intense itching. This reaction is an indirect, sensitive method for diagnosing very light infections.

Treatment is with a single dose of ivermectin. As this drug kills only microfilariae, and not adult worms, treatment must be repeated every six to twelve months until the adult worms die of old age. Although DEC is also an effective treatment, it tends to induce more severe side effects than does ivermectin. Visible nodules can be removed to decrease the number of adult worms.

In 1974, the World Health Organization established the Onchocerciasis Control Program (OCP) to try to eliminate the Simulium fly by spraying the river systems in West Africa. With the discovery of ivermectin, a second strategy was added to the OCP. Populations in affected regions are given an annual dose of ivermectin to decrease the effects of the infection and to reduce further spreading by eliminating microfilariae. It is estimated that since the initiation of the program, 300,000 cases of blindness have been prevented. However, in large areas of Africa onchocerciasis continues to cause significant morbidity and mortality.

MARTHA FULFORD
JAY KEYSTONE

(SEE ALSO: *Vector-Borne Diseases*)

BIBLIOGRAPHY

Burnham, G. (1998). "Onchocerciasis." *The Lancet* 351:1341–1346.

Hall, L. R., and Pearlman, E. (1999). "Pathogenesis of Onchocercal Keratitis (River Blindness)." *Clinical Microbiology Reviews* 12(3):445–453.

Molyneux, D. H., and Morel, C. (1998). "Onchocerciasis and Chagas' Disease Control: The Evolution of Control via Applied Research through Changing Development Scenarios." *British Medical Bulletin* 54(2):327–339.

Ottesen, E. A. (1993). "Filarial Infections." *Infectious Disease Clinics of North America* 7(3):619–633.

World Health Organization (2000). *Onchocerciasis (River Blindness)*. Fact Sheet No. 95. Geneva: Author.

ONE-HIT MODEL

The one-hit model of carcinogenesis is a dose-response model based on the assumption that only one genetic change is required to transform a normal cell into a cancer cell, and that any dose of a carcinogen presents a risk of cancer. Only at zero dose is there zero risk. In theory at least, even a single molecule of a carcinogen could turn a normal cell cancerous. The probability of the transformation of a normal cell into a cancer cell, according to the one-hit model, follows a Poisson probability distribution.

The one-hit model is generally recognized to be an overly simplistic representation of the biological process of carcinogenesis. Carcinogenesis is a multistep process, with several genetic changes required to produce a tumor cell. Furthermore, it is highly unlikely that a single molecule of a substance would be biologically capable of causing cancer. Carcinogens have an effective threshold for their activity because of the body's ability to detoxify chemicals, repair cell damage, and otherwise protect itself. However, for regulatory purposes, exposure to a single molecule of a carcinogen is sometimes equated with a single effective dose. That is an assumption of the one-hit process in forming regulatory policy that is health protective because it is likely to over-estimate the probability that a substance will produce cancer.

GAIL CHARNLEY

(SEE ALSO: *Cancer; Carcinogen; Carcinogenesis; Genetics and Health; Risk Assessment, Risk Management; Toxicology*)

OPHTHALMIA NEONATORUM

Ophthalmia neonatorum is a form of conjunctivitis that occurs in the first few (usually four) weeks of life. Causative infectious agents can be present in the birth canal. An infant is exposed during the birth process, and symptoms develop a few days later. Most of the serious infections leading to corneal damage are caused by *Neisseria gonorrhoeae*, but *Chlamydia trachomatis* is also a common cause of infection. Many other microorganisms have also been implicated. Prophylactic agents instilled in the eyes shortly after birth have greatly reduced the incidence in many industrialized areas, but ophthalmia neonatorum remains an important cause of blindness elsewhere.

MODENA WILSON

(SEE ALSO: *Child Health Services; Chlamydia; Gonorrhea; Newborn Screening*)

BIBLIOGRAPHY

Feigin, R. D., and Cherry, J. D., eds. (1998). *Textbook of Pediatric Infectious Diseases,* 4th edition. Philadelphia, PA: W. B. Saunders.

OPIUM

See Addiction and Habituation

ORAL CANCER

Oral cancer is a malignant growth involving the tongue, floor, palate, interior lining of the cheeks or lips, or other parts of the mouth or pharynx. Most oral cancers are squamous cell carcinomas. It is the most common cancer in parts of Southeast Asia and India; in the United States it ranked seventh, most common among blacks and twelfth among whites. Incidence and mortality rates increase with age, though in the United States they have been decreasing among whites and increasing among nonwhites. Tongue cancer incidence and mortality have been increasing since 1970 among the young in the United States. Tobacco and alcohol are major risk factors for oral cancer; used together, they increase the effects of each other.

JOHN C. GREENE

(SEE ALSO: *Alcohol Use and Abuse; Cancer; Oral Health; Tobacco Control*)

BIBLIOGRAPHY

Schottenfeld, D., and Fraumeni, J. F., Jr., eds. (1996). *Cancer Epidemiology and Prevention,* 2nd edition. New York: Oxford University Press.

ORAL HEALTH

In twenty-first century America, a healthy smile is considered necessary for social mobility and acceptance, interpersonal relations, employability, and a good self-image.

Poor oral health may lead to pain and infection, absence from school or work, poor nutrition, poor general health, an inability to speak or eat properly, and even early death. Studies done in the late 1990s showed that poor oral health may also lead to low birth-weight babies, heart disease, and stroke. It is clear that oral diseases play a significant role in compromising health potential. Up until the late 1990s, when the new HIV medications became available, over 90 percent of persons with AIDS had HIV-related oral diseases.

MAJOR ORAL DISEASES

There are many different types of oral diseases, but they are generally differentiated as being of hard tissue or soft tissue origin. Hard-tissue oral diseases are those of the teeth, supporting bone, and jaw; whereas soft tissue diseases affect the tissues in and around the mouth, including the tongue, lips, cheek, gums, salivary glands, and roof and floor of the mouth. Some oral diseases may result in both hard and soft tissue disorders or conditions such as cleft palate or oral-facial injuries. The major oral diseases and conditions are:

- Dental caries (tooth decay, cavities)

- Periodontal disease (gum disease)

- Malocclusion (crooked teeth)

- Edentulism (complete tooth loss)

- Oral cancer

- Craniofacial birth defects such as cleft lip and cleft palate

- Soft tissue lesions

- Oral-facial injuries

- Temporomandibular dysfunction (TMD)

The prevalence of oral diseases varies due to differences in the host, agent, and environment. Some diseases have higher rates in certain population groups due to personal habits such as a sugar-heavy diet or poor oral hygiene. Others may occur more frequently in individuals who put themselves at risk for injury by not wearing seatbelts or by playing contact sports without using proper mouth and head protection. Environmental and cultural factors may also affect the rates of oral diseases. For example, persons who live in a community in which the water supply is fluoridated would have much less tooth decay than those who live in a nonfluoridated community. Certain cultures, especially in developing countries, have diets almost completely devoid of refined foods that have high sugar content, and therefore have much less tooth decay compared to the average American. A 1997 report by the U.S. Department of Agriculture found that Americans consume an average of about 154 pounds of sugars a year (or 53 teaspoons a day) most of it in processed foods, drinks, and sweets. This was a 28 percent increase in added sugar or sweeteners since 1982. Tooth decay may be viewed as a disease of civilization.

A NEGLECTED EPIDEMIC

Oral diseases have been called a "neglected epidemic" because, while they affect almost the total population, oral health is not integrated into most health policies or programs. This is especially true in the United States, where, in the year 2000, there were 125 million Americans without dental insurance. In addition, many people who have dental insurance are underinsured. Under such conditions, people who are knowledgeable about oral health and have the resources to pay for it are much more likely to receive regular dental care than are the poorer members of society. This situation has resulted in major disparities in oral health status in the United States. Low-income children between ages two and five have almost five times more untreated dental disease than high-income children, and people without health insurance have four times the unmet dental needs of those with private insurance.

Vulnerable or high-risk population groups like children, the poor, the developmentally disabled, the homeless, homebound and elderly persons, persons with HIV/AIDS (human immunodeficiency virus/acquired immunodeficiency syndrome), and ethnic and cultural minorities are at greater risk for oral diseases, primarily because they do not have access to preventive services or treatment. In 2000, the first ever Surgeon General's report on oral health stressed the importance of oral health as part of total health as well as the need to reduce oral health disparities in the United States.

Although there has been much progress in the improvement of oral health, both nationally and internationally, oral diseases are still epidemic in the United States and many other countries. The nation's dental bill in the year 2000 was about $60.2 billion, or 4.6 percent of total health expenditures in the United States. In 1970, dental care accounted for 6.4 percent of total health expenditures. This 28 percent decrease is primarily due to the higher costs of hospitals and medical care.

PREVENTION

Prevention of dental disease may occur at the individual or community level. Prevention of disease at the community or population level is one of the foundations of public health practice. There are three levels of prevention. Primary prevention is aimed at preventing a disease before it occurs, through programs such as community water fluoridation, school dental sealant programs, and health education. Secondary prevention keeps an existing disease from becoming worse, and includes dental screenings for children and early detection of oral cancer in adults. Tertiary prevention consists of treatment to limit a disability or to help rehabilitate an individual after a disease has progressed beyond the secondary level. Examples of tertiary prevention include complex dental fillings, root canal treatment, and false teeth.

HEALTHY PEOPLE 2010

The United States has developed national health objectives with a focus on prevention. These objectives are renewed every ten years. This effort began with the 1979 report from the Surgeon General, *Healthy People*, and is spearheaded by the Office of Disease Prevention and Health Promotion of the U.S. Department of Health and Human Services. The purpose of these national health objectives is to provide direction for the country in preventing major health problems in the United States. Each set of national health objectives, including the Healthy People 2010 objectives, contain components on oral health (see Table 1).

PUBLIC HEALTH DENTISTS

Of the nine recognized dental specialties, only dental public health has the potential to make a population-based impact on communities such as schools, neighborhoods, cities, states, or nations or on groups of individuals such as homeless children or persons with HIV. Dental public health is "the science and art of preventing and controlling dental disease and promoting dental health through organized community efforts. It is the form of dental practice which serves the community as a patient rather than the individual. It is concerned with the dental health education of the public, with applied dental research, and with the administration of group dental care programs as well as the prevention and control of dental diseases on a community basis" (*Journal of Public Health Dentistry*, 46 no. 1). Most states in the United States have a dentist trained in public health in their state health department. The same is true in some major cities. The U.S. Department of Health and Human Services also has dentists trained in public health who work in administrative and policy-making roles.

A public health dentist is primarily involved with the three core functions of public health as defined by the Institute of Medicine: assessment, policy development, and assurance. Dental public health assessment might involve a statewide survey to determine the amount of tooth decay by age group, or a questionnaire to determine the barriers to dental care for the low-income elderly. Policy development could involve efforts to have preventive services included in a dental Medicaid program or to have a state dental practice act allow dental hygienists to work under general supervision in public schools. The assurance function might take the form of a program to provide dental care to homeless children, or to provide some other service that no one else is providing.

As of 2000, only 136 dentists out of 150,000 practicing dentists were board certified in dental public health by the American Board of Dental Public Health, and only about 1,500 dentists were working primarily in this field. Although the number of public health dentists is small, they are trained to work with a variety of health professionals and community groups to improve oral health. This would include, but not be limited to, public health dental hygienists, health educators, epidemiologists, nutritionists, nurses, academicians, researchers, and other health and human services personnel.

There are ten major areas of competencies that a dentist must attain to become board certified in dental public health. These ten competencies are: program planning; population-based prevention; developing, managing, and evaluating programs; needs assessment; communication; advocacy; study design; and critiquing the literature. Public health dentists can be contacted through the oral health program of local or state health departments, or through one of the ten regional offices of the U.S. Department of Health and Human Services.

TOOTH DECAY

Tooth decay, or dental caries, is the most common oral disease in the United States, if not the most common of all diseases. It is the primary cause of tooth loss; and may be considered a lifelong disease—18 percent of children aged 2 to 4 have had tooth decay in their primary teeth and 52 percent of those aged 6 to 8 have had tooth decay in their primary or permanent teeth; 78 percent of 17-year-olds have had tooth decay in their permanent teeth, with an average of seven affected tooth

Table 1

Oral Health Objectives in Healthy People 2010

Chapter 21 – Oral Health

1. Reduce the proportion of children and adolescents who have dental caries experience in their primary or permanent teeth.
2. Reduce the proportion of children, adolescents, and adults with untreated dental decay.
3. Increase the proportion of adults who have never had a permanent tooth extracted because of dental caries or periodontal disease.
4. Reduce the proportion of older adults who have had all their natural teeth extracted.
5. Reduce periodontal disease.
6. Increase the proportion of oral and pharyngeal cancers detected at the earliest stage.
7. Increase the proportion of adults who, in the past 12 months, report having had an examination to detect oral and pharyngeal cancer.
8. Increase the proportion of children who have received dental sealant on their molar teeth.
9. Increase the proportion of the U.S. population served by community water systems with optimally fluoridated water.
10. Increase the proportion of children and adults who use the oral health care system each year.
11. Increase the proportion of long-term care residents who use the oral health care system each year.
12. Increase the proportion of children and adolescents under age 19 years at or below 200 percent of the Federal poverty level who received any preventive dental service during the past year.
13. (Developmental) Increase the proportion of school-based health centers with an oral health component.
14. Increase the proportion of local health departments and community-based health centers, including community, migrant and homeless health centers, that have an oral health component.
15. Increase the number of States and the District of Columbia that have a system for recording and referring infants and children with cleft lips, cleft palates, and other craniofacial anomalies to craniofacial anomaly rehabilitative teams.
16. Increase the number of States and the District of Columbia that have an oral and craniofacial health surveillance system.
17. (Developmental) Increase the number of Tribal, State (including the District of Columbia), and local health agencies that serve jurisdictions of 250,000 or more person that have in place an effective public dental health program directed by a dental professional with public health training.

Other Chapters

1-8   In the health professions (including dentistry, developmental), allied and associated health profession fields, and the nursing field, increase the proportion of all degrees awarded to members of underrepresented racial and ethnic groups.

3-6   Reduce the oropharyngeal cancer death rate.

5-15 Increase the proportion of persons with diabetes who have at least an annual dental examination.

SOURCE: *Healthy People 2010: Oral Health.* Washington, D.C.: US Department of Health and Human Services; January, 2000. Conference Edition, Volume II; Ch. 21.

---

surfaces; 99 percent of adults aged 40 to 44 have had tooth decay in their permanent teeth, with an average of forty-five affected tooth surfaces; and 60 percent of persons over age 75 years of age have had tooth decay on the exposed roots of three of their teeth.

Tooth decay is an infectious disease. The percentage of people with this disease increases with age, and the severity of the disease once it occurs depends on whether or not one has had adequate fluoridation and dental treatment. Tooth decay is not self-limiting unless it is exposed to fluoride just as it is beginning and the demineralized tooth structure can remineralize. Demineralization is the dissolving of minerals such as calcium, carbonate, and phosphate in the tooth structure. Remineralization is enhanced by fluoride. Once tooth decay progresses beyond the tooth's ability to remineralize, mechanical intervention is needed

by a dentist, who removes the decayed portion of the tooth and puts in a filling. When tooth decay is not treated it may result in an acute or chronic infection and severe pain, ultimately resulting in an abscess and/or cellulitis, which will then need to be treated with antibiotics, root canal treatment, or removal of the tooth. In the United States, more teeth are lost due to tooth decay than to any other disease.

Causes of Tooth Decay. Bacteria that produce tooth decay can be transferred from a mother to a child, even at an early age. When these bacteria have repeated contact with sugars or sticky sweets, they create an acid that demineralizes the surface or enamel of a susceptible tooth, eventually causing a cavity or tooth decay. The more access to sugars the bacteria have, the greater the likelihood of tooth decay occurring. Sticky sweets are more decay-producing than other types of sugary foods because they stay in the mouth longer. The bacterial mass that resides on the teeth is called dental plaque. Plaque may also, however, contain the minerals from demineralization, which may be available for remineralization.

Prevention of Tooth Decay. Tooth decay may be prevented on the individual level and at the community level. At the individual level, good oral hygiene—brushing with a fluoride toothpaste, sealants, and regular dental checkups—is of primary importance. Avoidance of excessive amounts of sugar and sweets, can also help prevent tooth decay. During the second half of the twentieth century, fluoride became an important tool in decay prevention. When fluoride is ingested, it goes through the body and becomes part of the tooth, resulting in a stronger tooth that is more resistant to tooth decay. When fluoride is placed on the teeth, it affects the tooth and plaque directly, preventing tooth decay. Fluoride is therefore added both to toothpaste and to community water supplies (see Figure 1).

Community water fluoridation consists of the adjustment of the fluoride level of a central water supply to a level that is optimal for oral health. The recommended level of fluoride for fluoridation in the United States varies from 0.7 to 1.2 parts per million, depending on a community's mean maximum daily air temperature over a five-year period. At the recommended level, the fluoride in water is odorless, colorless, and tasteless. In 1992, when the last national data was available, about 145 million Americans, or 62 percent of the population, were using fluoridated public-water supplies (see Figure 1).

Effective community prevention programs for tooth decay are considered in terms of effectiveness, cost, and practicality. Fluoridation is the most cost-effective. Fluoridation is considered one of the ten most significant public health measures of the twentieth century. Unfortunately, it has also been one of the more misunderstood public health measures, with some people at different times making claims such as it caused mongolism, pollution, sterility, or cancer. None of these allegations has ever been demonstrated by scientific studies. Most reputable national health organizations, such as the American Academy of Pediatrics, the American Dental Association, the American Medical Association, the American Public Health Association, and most other national health organizations, have supported or endorsed fluoridation for years. Salt fluoridation, which is not used in the United States, has been used as an alternative to water fluoridation in countries where central water supplies are not readily available.

Early Childhood Caries. The threat of tooth decay begins with the first appearance of teeth in a baby's mouth. The first teeth to appear are usually the two lower front teeth, which appear at about six months of age. All twenty primary, or baby, teeth usually erupt by two years of age. The permanent teeth begin erupting at six years of age, and with the eruption of the third molars (wisdom teeth), usually between eighteen and twenty-one years of age, all thirty-two permanent teeth are in place.

Early childhood caries (ECC) may be due to several factors, including the introduction of decay-producing bacteria into the child's mouth—usually transmitted from the mother or caused by poor feeding practices, various medical conditions, poor oral hygiene, and chronic malnutrition, which may also affect tooth development. ECC, also known as baby bottle tooth decay, or nursing tooth decay, occurs in the primary teeth of infants as young as nine months of age. When an infant sleeps with a baby bottle containing milk, infant formula, or sweetened liquids, there is a prolonged source of food for the decay-producing bacteria in the child's mouth. Among American Indians, as many as 53 percent of infants have this disease, and in inner city populations as many as 11 percent are affected. When early childhood caries is not treated and the disease is allowed to progress, severe pain or infection may result.

Root Surface Caries. This type of tooth decay usually occurs in older persons whose gums have receded exposing the roots of their teeth. As people retain their teeth for longer periods of time, this type of tooth decay becomes more frequent. Over 60 percent of seventy-five-year-olds who have teeth have root caries.

GUM (PERIODONTAL) DISEASE

Gum disease is the second most common reason for the loss of teeth. There are two major types of

Figure 1

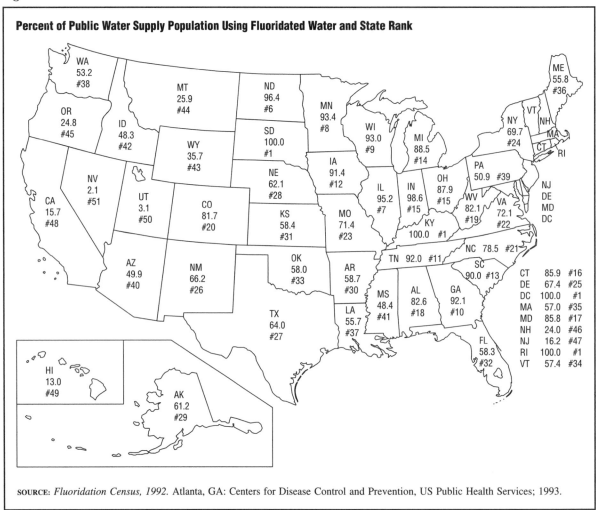

Percent of Public Water Supply Population Using Fluoridated Water and State Rank

CT	85.9	#16
DE	67.4	#25
DC	100.0	#1
MA	57.0	#35
MD	85.8	#17
NH	24.0	#46
NJ	16.2	#47
RI	100.0	#1
VT	57.4	#34

SOURCE: *Fluoridation Census, 1992.* Atlanta, GA: Centers for Disease Control and Prevention, US Public Health Services; 1993.

gum disease: gingivitis, which is an inflammation or infection of the gums, and periodontitis, which is an inflammation or infection of the gums and the surrounding bone. Gingivitis may occur in adolescents or adults and is often self-healing once the area is properly cleaned. However, poor oral hygiene, stress, lack of sleep, or poor nutrition can all aggravate the condition and lead to an acute case of gingivitis, which can be very painful.

Gingivitis may lead to periodontitis in susceptible individuals who have risk factors such as bacterial plaque, calculus (calcified deposits around teeth), smoking, or systemic diseases. Periodontitis usually increases in severity with age. It is not self-healing and requires mechanical intervention such as a deep scaling or surgery by a dentist. About 48

percent of adults aged thirty-five to forty-four have gingivitis, and 22 percent have destructive periodontal disease. Dentists who specialize in treating gum diseases are called periodontists.

The best way to prevent gum disease is with proper oral hygiene. This includes brushing the teeth properly with a fluoride toothpaste after breakfast and before going to bed, utilizing dental floss appropriately, and visiting a dentist or hygienist on a periodic basis for a professional cleaning. A combination of personal and professional prevention is very important, as there are no population-based preventive measures for gum disease. Good health habits, including proper nutrition and avoidance of tobacco products, is also important.

MALOCCLUSION

The permanent teeth may not erupt in their proper alignment, resulting in malocclusion, or crooked teeth. In its most severe form, called handicapping malocclusion, this condition can affect an individual's chewing ability. The main causes of malocclusion are a lack of space for the permanent teeth to erupt properly and the premature loss of the baby teeth, which usually guide the permanent teeth to their proper location, may also be a factor.

To prevent malocclusion due to premature loss of the primary teeth, space maintainers may be used to guide the teeth into proper alignment. Dentists who specialize in treating malocclusions are called orthodontists.

ORAL-FACIAL INJURIES

Most oral-facial injuries occur as a result of falls, automobile accidents, and sports. About 25 percent of Americans aged six to fifty have injured their upper or lower front teeth. Falls at work or at play are difficult to control. Some of them may be prevented, however, by self-discipline and by environmental controls such as railings, good lighting, smooth walkways, and proper injury-prevention education.

Oral and facial injuries are a frequent result of automobile accidents. Seatbelts, airbags, and safe driving techniques can greatly reduce the injuries. Sports-related oral-facial injuries may be prevented by wearing protective mouthguards and helmets. In competitive high school sports such as football, ice hockey, lacrosse, and soccer, mouthguards are required by many states. A school-based mouthguard program, in which a dentist fits each student athlete with a custom mouthguard, greatly improves the chances that the athletes will use the devices, which can otherwise be uncomfortable and inhibit breathing and talking.

ORAL CANCER

Oral and pharyngeal cancers occur primarily in individuals over fifty-five years of age, especially in those who smoke and drink heavily. About 30,000 Americans are diagnosed with oral cancer each year, and about 8,000 die from this disease. The earlier oral cancer is detected, the better it can be controlled. Only 7 percent of adults over the age of forty, however, have reported having an examination for oral cancer. Individuals who use spit tobacco beginning at an early age may have a greater risk for developing oral cancer and gum disease. Baseball players have traditionally used spit tobacco, luring younger children to also use it. According to the National Cancer Institute, over 15 percent of high school boys use spit tobacco. Marijuana use has also been linked to oral cancer. The incidence of oral cancer is two times greater in developing countries than in industrialized nations.

The best way to prevent oral cancer is not to smoke or to use spit tobacco, and, if one drinks, to drink in moderation. Adults, including those wearing dentures or false teeth, should have regular dental examinations that include an oral cancer screening. In 1994, the National Collegiate Athletic Association (NCAA) banned the use of spit tobacco and other tobacco products by student athletes and coaches during games and practices. Spit tobacco has also been banned in minor league baseball, and its use has been significantly reduced among major league players. Diets high in vitamin C, vegetables, and fruits may decrease the risk of oral cancer. A workshop to develop a national strategy to prevent and control oral cancer recommended a multifaceted approach that includes public advocacy, collaboration, public and professional education, and evaluation.

MOUTH ODOR

Mouth odors may be caused by poor oral hygiene or the foods that one eats. Mouth odors also occur when people have not eaten or had liquids for extended periods of time, such as in the morning upon waking. During sleep, there is a decrease in the flow of saliva, allowing bacteria to grow. Certain medications may also cause a condition known as xerostomia, or "dry mouth," which can lead to an increase in tooth decay over time. Over five hundred drugs and medicines list dry mouth as a potential side effect.

Proper oral hygiene and choice of foods can decrease or prevent mouth odors. In addition, sometimes bacteria accumulate on the tongue and brushing or scraping the back of the tongue periodically can help. Regular eating and drinking habits are also helpful. Dry mouth cannot be prevented, though water, ice chips, or sugarless gum may provide some relief.

CRANIOFACIAL DEFECTS

Approximately one to two in 1,000 children are born with a cleft lip or a cleft palate—two of the more common craniofacial defects. A cleft lip occurs when the lips of the developing fetus are not complete, resulting in a split in the child's lip. This usually occurs in the upper lip. A cleft palate is similar—the bone in the roof of the mouth is not fused properly and has an opening in it. Individuals born with cleft lips or palates should have corrective surgery and receive appropriate adjunctive therapy as needed, depending on the severity of the cleft.

There is no known way to prevent a cleft lip or palate. Proper prenatal care and food consumption during pregnancy may be important. Alcohol and tobacco consumption during pregnancy have been shown to increase the likelihood of cleft lip, so these substances should not be used by pregnant women.

TEMPOROMANDIBULAR DISORDERS

Temporomandibular (jaw) disorders (TMDs) are a group of conditions that affects the jaw joint. The lower jaw acts like a hinge with the upper jaw, and when the hinge joint is traumatized it may affect one's bite, cause pain in the chewing muscles, or cause pain or clicking in the joint located in front of the ears. This disorder affects twice as many women as men. Treatment varies depending on the severity of the problem. In many cases, the disorder dissipates by itself. This group of disorders is also referred to as myofacial pain-dysfunction syndrome of TMJ syndrome.

There is no simple way to prevent temporamandibular disorders. Avoiding trauma to the jaw or mouth may be helpful, and protective mouthguards should be used for contact sports.

MYRON ALLUKIAN, JR.

(SEE ALSO: *American Association of Public Health Dentistry; Baby Bottle Tooth Decay; Caries Prevention; Community Dental Preventive Programs; Community Water Fluoridation; Dental Fluorosis; Dental Sealants; Gingivitis; Healthy People 2010; Oral Cancer; Plaque*)

BIBLIOGRAPHY

Allukian, M. (1996). "Oral Diseases: The Neglected Epidemic." In *Principles of Public Health Practice,* eds. F. D. Scutchfield and C. W. Keck. Albany, NY: Delmar Publishers.

Beck, J. D.; Offenbacher, S.; Williams, R.; Gibbs, P.; and Garcia, R. (1998). "Periodontitis: A Risk Factor for Coronary Heart Disease?" *Annals of Periodontology* 3:127–141.

Dasanayake, A. P. (1998). "Poor Periodontal Health of the Pregnant Woman as a Risk Factor for Low Birth Weight." *Annals of Periodontology* 3:206–211.

Davenport, E. S., et al. (1998). "The East London Study of Maternal Chronic Periodontal Disease and Preterm Low Birth Weight Infants: Study Design and Prevalence Data." *Annals of Periodontology* 3:213–221.

Dental Health Foundation (1997). *The Oral Health of California's Children: A Neglected Epidemic.* San Rafael, CA: DHF.

DiAngelis, A. J., and Bakland, L. K. (1998). "Traumatic Dental Injuries: Current Treatment Concepts." *Journal of the American Dental Association* 129:1401–1414.

Genco, R. J. (1998). "Periodontal Disease and Risk for Myocardial Infarction and Cardiovascular Disease." *Cardiovascular Reviews and Reports* 19:34–40.

Greenlee, R. T.; Murray, T.; Bolden, S.; and Wingo, P. A. (2000). "Cancer Statistics, 2000." *CA–A Cancer Journal for Clinicians* 50(1):7–33.

Health Care Financing Administration. *National Health Care Expenditures.* Available at http://www.hcfa.gov/stats/stats.htm.

Horowitz, A. M., and Nourjah, P. A. (1996). "Patterns of Screening Oral Cancer among U.S. Adults." *Journal of Public Health Dentistry* 56:331–335.

Institute of Medicine (1998). *The Future of Public Health.* Washington, DC: National Academy Press.

Ismail, A. I. (1998). "Prevention of Early Childhood Caries." *Community Dental Oral Epidemiology* Supp. 1:49–61.

Kelly, M., and Bruerd, B. (1987). "The Prevalence of Nursing Bottle Decay among Two Native America Populations." *Journal of Public Health Dentistry* 47:94–97.

Klatell, J. Kaplan, A.; and Williams, G. (1991). *The Mount Sinai Medical Center Family Guide to Dental Health.* New York: Macmillan.

Lorente, C.; Cordier, S.; Goujard, J. et al. (2000). "Tobacco and Alcohol Use During Pregnancy and Risk of Oral Clefts." *American Journal of Public Health* 90(3):415–419.

Mueller, C. D.; Schur, C. L.; and Paramore, C. (1998). "Access to Dental Care in the United States." *Journal of the American Dental Association* 129:429–437.

Offenbacher, S., et al. (1995). "Periodontal Infection as a Possible Factor for Preterm Low Birth Weight." *Annals of Periodontology* 67(suppl. 10):1103–1113.

Palmer, C. (1994). "NCAA Forbids Tobacco Usage." *ADA News* 25:4.

Parker-Pope, T. (2000) "A Common Side Effect, Dry Mouth, Can Cause Serious Tooth Decay." *Wall Street Journal* (March 11).

Putnam, J. J., and Allshouse, J. E. (1999). *Food Consumption, Prices, and Expenditures, 1970–1997.* An Economic Research Service Report, Statistical Bulletin No. 965. Washington, DC: U.S. Department of Agriculture.

Ring, M. E. (1993). *Dentistry, An Illustrated History.* New York: Abradale Press.

Rosenberg, M. (1996). "Clinical Assessment of Bad Breath: Current Concepts." *Journal of the American Dental Association* 127:475–482.

Seow, W. K. (1998). "Biological Measures of Early Childhood Caries." *Community Dental Oral Epidemics* Supp. 1:8–27.

Slavkin, H. C. (1999). "Does the Mouth Put the Heart at Risk?" *Journal of the American Dental Association* 130:109–113.

"Ten Great Public Health Achievements—United States, 1900–1999" (1999). *Morbidity and Mortality Weekly Report* 48(12):241–243.

Vargas, C. M.; Crall, J.; and Schneider, D. (1998). "Sociodemographic Distribution of Pediatric Dental Caries: NHANES III, 1988–1994." *Journal of the American Dental Association* 129:1229–1238.

Weinert, M.; Grimes, R. M.; and Lynch, D. P (1996). "Oral Manifestations of HIV Infection." *Annals of Internal Medicine* 125(6):485–496.

Winn, D. M., et al. (1996). "Coronal and Root Caries in the Dentition of Adults in the United States, 1988–1991." *Journal of Dental Research* 75(Special Issue):642–651.

World Cancer Research Fund (1997). *Food, Nutrition, and the Prevention of Cancer: A Global Perspective.* Washington, DC: American Institute for Cancer Research.

Zhang, Z. F.; Morgenstern, H.; Spitz, M. R. et al. (1998). "Marijuana Use and Increased Risk of Squamous Cell Carcinoma of the Head and Neck." *Cancer Epidemiology, Biomarkers & Prevention* 8:1071–1078.

ORGANOCHLORINES

Organochlorines constitute a large class of chemical compounds that have been in the channels of trade since the late 1800s. These compounds are lipid soluble, rapidly absorbed from most routes of exposure, and cross the blood-brain barrier. Their chemistry ranges from simple monochloromethane to the polychlorinated ethylenes and ethanes. Several alkyl-chlorocompounds and polyhalogenated compounds also exist. Many anesthetic gases are polyhalogenated alkanes, as are some of the freons and fire retardants.

The discussion here will be limited to the chlorinated short-chain alkanes and alkenes. The chloromethanes range from monochloromethane through tetrachloromethane. Monochloromethane and dichloromethane are industrial compounds that have been used in foods, drugs, and solvents. Trichloromethane is chloroform, an anesthetic gas that was discovered in the mid–nineteenth century. It is still used as a solvent, and up until very recently it was found in over-the-counter cough medicines, lozenges, and mouthwashes. Tetrachloromethane is carbon tetrachloride, a solvent used for many years in the dry cleaning industry and for personal use as a fabric cleaner. It was discovered at the same time and in the same laboratory as chloroform.

The toxicity of chloroform and carbon tetrachloride has been well studied. These compounds are highly toxic to the liver and kidney, though chloroform has a greater toxicity to the kidney while carbon tetrachloride has a much greater toxicity to the liver. These compounds are toxic to their target organs regardless of the route of exposure. Chloroform is positive in the rodent bioassay for carcinogenicity. Carbon tetrachloride is so toxic that long-term bioassays are difficult to conduct.

The chloroethanes are interesting compounds. Biologically they are relatively inert compared to carbon tetrachloride and chloroform. As long as there is one nonsubstituted site on one carbon the chemical is rapidly metabolized and excreted as ethanol. However, hexachlorethane exhibits some of the same toxicity as chloroform.

The more interesting compounds are the chlorethylenes. The double-bonded carbons render these compounds much more biologically active. Monochloroethylene is vinyl chloride. This compound has anesthetic properties, is used as a polymer precursor in plastic manufacturing, and is highly reactive. In rodent bioassays and in humans, vinyl chloride induces a relatively rare type of hemangiosarcoma, among other tumors. Vinyl chloride is one of those rare carcinogens that induces virtually identical cancers in animals and humans. In addition, vinyl chloride exhibits some mutagenic activity. Dichlorethylenes are much different in their structure and toxicity. Vinylidene chloride and 1,2-cisdichloroethylene appear to be more toxic than the transisomer, but their toxicity, mutagenicity, and carcinogenicity are much less than the potency of vinyl chloride, if they possess those properties at all.

Trichloroethylene (1,1,2-trichlorethylene [TCE]) was once widely used for several clinical and industrial application. TCE was a diluent in anesthetics until the 1970s. It was thought to be the agent that led to nausea and vomiting after gaseous anesthesia. TCE, an excellent degreasing agent and industrial solvent, was also used as a decaffeinating agent in coffees until banned by the regulatory agencies. There is a great deal of controversy over the potency of TCE as a toxicant. However, the compound exhibits enough water solubility to present a hazard in many drinking water supplies. TCE is mutagenic in several in vitro bacterial assays and is carcinogenic in some bioassays.

The next chemical in the series is tetrachloroethylene (perchloroethylene, PERC, or PCE). PERC is very lipid soluble but is also found in some water supplies. It was widely used as a dry cleaning agent and a degreaser for metal finishing. For many years PERC and TCE were used as a drug for the treatment of gut-dwelling parasites. These chemicals are not of the same class as the aromatic chlorinated compounds, but they are found as air pollutants and water pollutants throughout the world. Their use in foods and drugs in the United States and elsewhere has been curtailed. The danger of these compounds is the broad possibility for exposure. Industrial hygiene practices have limited exposure in the workplace, but exposure in the home and on the street is measurable. These are excellent solvents that remain in use in the channels of trade.

MICHAEL GALLO

(SEE ALSO: *Carcinogenesis; Persistent Organic Pollutants [POPs]; Tetrachloroethylene; Toxicology*)

OSTEOARTHRITIS

Osteoarthritis, which is also called degenerative arthritis or degenerative joint disease, is primarily a disease that results from the breakdown and loss of cartilage in joints (e.g., knees, hips, wrists). Cartilage, a connective tissue that covers the surfaces of articular joints, is essential for proper joint function because it allows the ends of bones to slide over one another smoothly. Osteoarthritis results from both mechanical (e.g., trauma to joints) and biological (metabolic) events that interfere with the maintenance of healthy cartilage. Eventually, cartilage may be lost, causing the bones in the joint to rub together, and bony spurs may form.

SIGNS, SYMPTOMS, AND DIAGNOSIS

Osteoarthritis is characterized by joint pain, tenderness, swelling, and limitation in joint movement. The joints most often affected are the joints of the fingers, the base of the thumb, the hips, the knees, the neck (cervical spine), and the lower back (lumbar spine). Unlike some types of arthritis that affect multiple organ systems, any inflammation associated with osteoarthritis is limited to the joints. Pain after joint use that subsides with resting the joint is a classical sign of osteoarthritis. As osteoarthritis worsens, pain may occur at rest or at night. Health care providers diagnose osteoarthritis based on a history of joint symptoms, physical examination, and radiographic (X-ray) changes. X-ray changes may include joint-space narrowing, changes in the bones, and the presence of bony spurs.

In addition to the physical symptoms, osteoarthritis also impacts psychological, social, and economic well-being. Psychological effects include stress, depression, anger, feelings of helplessness, and anxiety. The social impacts may include decreased community involvement and lack of understanding by family, friends, and coworkers. The economic status of people with arthritis and their families is also affected. The financial burden of health care and days lost from work may seriously impact the financial well-being of persons with arthritis and their families.

Age is a major demographic risk factor for the development of osteoarthritis. Although aging does not cause osteoarthritis, the prevalence of osteoarthritis increases with age. Almost half of people over the age of sixty-five have arthritis—mostly osteoarthritis. Osteoarthritis is also more common among women than among men. In addition to age, risk factors for osteoarthritis include joint injury and being overweight (especially for knee and hip osteoarthritis). Reduction of weight has been shown to reduce the risk of symptomatic osteoarthritis in overweight people.

THE BURDEN OF OSTEOARTHRITIS

Osteoarthritis is the most common form of the more than one hundred conditions that are considered arthritis and other rheumatic conditions. In 1998, these conditions affected 43 million Americans, and they are among the most common chronic diseases. Arthritis is also a leading cause of disability—it limits activities for 7 million Americans. The costs of arthritis are enormous. In 1992, the costs of medical treatment and lost wages were estimated at $65 billion. The cost of osteoarthritis alone may currently exceed $15.5 billion.

Osteoarthritis affects as many people as all of the other types of arthritis combined. Almost 22 million Americans have osteoarthritis—almost one of every twelve people in the United States. Prevalence estimates of osteoarthritis will differ by how the data are collected or how the diagnosis is made. For example, people who have pain due to osteoarthritis may not show X-ray changes, and those with X-ray changes consistent with osteoarthritis may not have symptoms. The prevalence of osteoarthritis is high and will get even higher as the number of older Americans increases. In 2020, an estimated 60 million Americans will have arthritis—osteoarthritis alone is likely to affect over 30 million people. Osteoarthritis is a major

cause of disability. Sixty to 80 percent of people with osteoarthritis are limited in their activities because of the disease.

OSTEOARTHRITIS TREATMENT AND CONTROL

There is no known cure for osteoarthritis, yet there are effective treatment and control strategies. Management of osteoarthritis is directed toward reducing pain, minimizing or preventing disability, and improving quality of life. Achieving these goals not only requires good clinical care, but also depends on the active involvement of the person with osteoarthritis in self-management strategies and proactive efforts by the public health system.

Clinical Care. The American College of Rheumatology (ACR) has published guidelines on the medical management of osteoarthritis of the hip and knee that outline the key components of appropriate management. The guidelines list therapeutic strategies, including medications, rehabilitation therapies, and surgery. Medical management of osteoarthritis primarily focuses on prescribing appropriate medications and recommending self-management strategies or making referrals to rehabilitation, self-management, or surgical services.

Medication recommendations for osteoarthritis are evolving. Nonsteroidal anti-inflammatory drugs (NSAID) were, until recently, the primary medication treatment for osteoarthritis. However, due to concerns about the gastrointestinal toxicity of NSAIDs, the 1995 ACR medical-management guidelines concluded that the first-line medication for symptomatic osteoarthritis should be acetaminophen. NSAIDs were recommended for those individuals who do not get sufficient pain relief from acetaminophen. In 1998, a new form of NSAID, called COX-2 Inhibitors, was released. COX-2 medications are similar to other NSAIDs in their effect on pain and joint inflammation, but they have significantly fewer gastrointestinal side effects. Physicians now vary in whether they initiate treatment for osteoarthritis with acetaminophen, another NSAID, or a COX-2 medication.

Other treatments are also used. For example, symptomatic knee osteoarthritis may benefit from an injection of cortisone into the joint. The role of other treatments, such as glucosamine, chondroitin, and injections of hyaluronan are under investigation.

Rehabilitation services, such as physical and occupational therapy, are also important in the management of osteoarthritis. Therapists may prescribe therapeutic exercise to increase joint range of motion, muscle strength, and aerobic conditioning; they make teach strategies to reduce fatigue and stress on joints; and they may recommend environmental or task modification and assistive devices to make it easier to perform daily activities. Rehabilitation services may also be used after joint surgery.

Persons with severe symptomatic osteoarthritis, marked by pain and declining function, may benefit from total joint replacement. Both total hip and knee replacement have substantially reduced pain and improved function in the vast majority of individuals who have received them.

Self-Management Strategies. The ACR guidelines for medical management of osteoarthritis recommend specific self-management strategies as well as clinical interventions. The guidelines specify self-management education, exercise and aerobic conditioning, and weight control as integral to optimal health outcomes in osteoarthritis.

Because of its demonstrated efficacy and cost-effectiveness, the premiere self-management education intervention for osteoarthritis is the Arthritis Self-Help Course (ASHC). ASHC, developed in the early 1980s by Kate Lorig and colleagues, was adopted in the United States by the Arthritis Foundation and has been disseminated nationwide. A 20 percent reduction in pain and a 43 percent reduction in physician visits was demonstrated in four-year follow-up studies of ASHC. Early research demonstrated that each individual's belief that there was "something they could do," which Lorig labeled "self-efficacy," was more strongly correlated with positive health outcomes from ASHC than were specific health behaviors. Cost-effectiveness calculations indicated an annual savings of $189 per osteoarthritis participant due to the decreased need for physician visits.

Physical activity and weight control are important self-management strategies in osteoarthritis.

Physical Activity and Health: A Report of the Surgeon General (1996) specifically addressed osteoarthritis and stated that regular moderate exercise programs, either aerobic or resistance training, relieve symptoms and improve physical function and psychosocial status among people with osteoarthritis. Low-impact forms of exercise, such as walking, swimming, and stationary or on-the-road bicycling, are recommended to minimize the stress on affected joints. The Arthritis Foundation disseminates structured physical activity programs. Preliminary studies have shown positive health outcomes among participants in these programs. Obesity is a well-documented risk factor for the development of symptomatic osteoarthritis. A randomized controlled study showed that the amount of weight lost was strongly correlated with improvements in signs and symptoms of knee osteoarthritis.

Some persons with osteoarthritis choose to manage their condition by using various forms of complementary and alternative medicine (CAM) modalities, either along with, or in place of, medically prescribed therapies. Symptoms associated with chronic musculoskeletal conditions, including osteoarthritis, are among the most common reasons for using CAM. More information is needed, however, about the safety and efficacy of CAM modalities.

THE ROLE OF PUBLIC HEALTH IN ARTHRITIS TREATMENT AND CONTROL

Because of its large and increasing prevalence, and the large personal and societal costs, arthritis is recognized as a significant public health problem. In addition, effective management strategies are available yet underused. The *National Arthritis Action Plan: A Public Health Strategy* (NAAP) was developed under the leadership of the Centers for Disease Control and Prevention, the Arthritis Foundation, and the Association of State and Territorial Health Officials, and with the combined efforts of over ninety organizations. NAAP, released in 1999, outlines a comprehensive, systematic public health approach to decreasing the burden of arthritis for all Americans and improving the quality of life of those affected by arthritis. NAAP focuses on a population-based approach that can complement traditional medical care. Public health agencies and their partners play a role in promoting the importance of early diagnosis and appropriate management of osteoarthritis; and in assuring that persons with osteoarthritis are aware of the importance of, and have access to, effective self-management programs. Policy and system changes are needed to heighten awareness and improve access. Public health professionals are also responsible for monitoring the burden of osteoarthritis and identifying factors that influence the development or progression of osteoarthritis or disability from osteoarthritis.

JOSEPH E. SNIEZEK
TERESA J. BRADY
JAMES S. MARKS

(SEE ALSO: *Chronic Illness; Noncommunicable Disease Control; Predisposing Factors; Rheumatoid Arthritis; Self-Care Behavior; Self-Help Groups*)

BIBLIOGRAPHY

Arthritis Foundation (1997). *Arthritis 101.* Atlanta, GA: Arthritis Foundation.

Arthritis Foundation, Association of State and Territorial Health Officials, Centers for Disease Control and Prevention (1999). *National Arthritis Action Plan: A Public Health Strategy.* Atlanta, GA: Arthritis Foundation.

Felson, D. T., and Zhang, Y. (1988). "An Update on the Epidemiology of Knee and Hip Osteoarthritis with a View to Prevention." *Arthritis and Rheumatism* 41:1343–1355.

Hochberg, M. C.; Altman, R. D.; Brandt, K. D., et al. (1995). "Guidelines for Medical Management of Osteoarthritis." *Arthritis and Rheumatism* 38:1535–1546.

Hochberg, M. C. (1997). "Osteoarthritis—Clinical Features and Treatment." In *Primer on the Rheumatic Diseases,* 11th edition, ed. J. H. Klippel. Atlanta, GA: Arthritis Foundation.

Lawrence, R. C.; Helmick, C. G.; and Arnett, F. C. (1998). "Estimates of the Prevalence of Arthritis and Selected Musculoskeletal Disorders in the United States." *Arthritis and Rheumatism* 41:778–799.

Lorig, K., and Holman, H. (1993). "Arthritis Self-Management Studies: A Twelve-Year Review." *Health Education Quarterly* 20(1):17–28.

Minor, M. A. (1996). "Arthritis and Exercise: 'The Times They Are A-Changin.'" *Arthritis Care and Research* 9:9–81.

Stein, C. M.; Griffin, M. R.; and Brandt, K. D. (1996). "Osteoarthritis." In *Clinical Care in the Rheumatic Diseases,* eds. S. T. Wegener, B. L. Belza, and E. P. Gall. Atlanta, GA: American College of Rheumatology.

U.S. Department of Health and Human Services (1996). *Physical Activity and Health: A Report of the Surgeon General.* Atlanta, GA: U.S. Department of Health and Human Services, Public Health Service, Centers for Disease Control and Prevention.

—— (1999). *Handout on Health: Osteoarthritis.* Washington, DC: U.S. Department of Health and Human Services, Public Health Service, National Institute of Arthritis and Musculoskeletal and Skin Diseases.

Yelin, E., and Callahan L. F. (1995). "The Economic Cost and Social and Psychological Impact of Musculoskeletal Conditions." *Arthritis and Rheumatism* 38(10):1351–1362.

OSTEOPOROSIS

Osteoporosis (literally "porous bone") is a condition characterized by bone fragility and fracturing. The World Health Organization (WHO) defines osteoporosis as a 25 percent reduction of bone mineral density (BMD) compared to that of a healthy young adult female.

Eight million Americans have osteoporosis, and over 20 million have osteopenia (thin bones, or a loss of 10 to 25% of bone mineral density). Osteoporosis is most prevalent in Caucasians, less prevalent in Hispanics, and least prevalent in African Americans. Key predisposing factors are early menopause and a family history of osteoporosis. Other medical, psychological, and social factors may also contribute to the condition.

Osteoporosis commonly leads to fractures. Medical, social, and environmental factors that predispose people to osteoporosis-related fractures include impairment of hearing, vision, balance and cognition; debilitating illnesses; medications; postoperative conditions; and unsafe environments. In the United States, one of three females over age sixty-five will have at least one vertebral fracture. The ratio of female to male fractures of a hip is 2.5 to one. Two hundred and fifty thousand hip or wrist fractures and 500,000 vertebral fractures occur annually in the United States. Up to 15 percent of hip fractures will result in death within one year, and one of three survivors become long-term nursing home residents. The annual cost of osteoporosis in the United States is estimated to be as high as $18 million and is projected to reach $240 million by the year 2040.

There are several methods to measure bone mineral density for osteoporosis detection. The most precise is dual energy X-ray absorptiometry (DXA) of the hip. Blood and urine tests for bone resorption and formation are also used to help measure the response to therapy.

The four components of treatment are nutrition, medication, exercise, and safety. Nutritional factors are particularly important during childhood and adolescence when the bones are growing. Key components are calcium and vitamin D, supplemented by magnesium; and vitamins C and K for individuals with chronic diarrhea or on a low-vegetable diet.

Hormonal therapies—estrogens for postmenopausal females and testosterone for hypogonadal males—are widely utilized. Estrogens may be contraindicated by breast or uterine cancer or by susceptibility to vascular clotting, and prostatic disorders may preclude the use of testosterone. Bisphosphonates are potent antiresorptive drugs that can yield reductions in hip and vertebral fracturing. Use of calcitonin, another antiresorptive drug, has also shown reductions in vertebral fracturing.

Exercise and safety are essential components of fracture prevention. Vigorous weight-bearing activities are beneficial but not feasible for the elderly or infirm. Walking has not proved efficacious. Resistive exercises increase the muscle strength and bone mineral density essential to fracture prevention. Balance–enhancing activities such as dancing, careful attention to minimizing hazards in the home and work environments, and selective use of padded hip protectors for the aged and infirm all help reduce the risk of osteoporosis-related fractures.

Osteoporosis is a major and growing public health concern. Appropriate screening to identify those who are susceptible, accurate diagnosis of osteoporosis and related disorders, and prompt institution and monitoring of appropriate therapies are all essential to minimize the risks of fracture and the attendant mortality and morbidity.

ROBERT L. SWEZEY

(SEE ALSO: *Hip Fractures*)

BIBLIOGRAPHY

Melton, L. J., III (2000). "Perspective: Who Has Osteoporosis? A Conflict Between Clinical and Public Health Perspectives." *Journal of Bone and Mineral Research* 15(12):2309–2314.

Scheiber, L. B., II, and Torregrosa, L. (1988). "Evaluation and Treatment of Postmenopausal Osteoporosis." *Seminars in Arthritis and Rheumatism* 27(4):245–261.

Swezey, R. L. (2000). "Osteoporosis: Diagnosis, Pharmacological, and Rehabilitation Therapies." *Critical Reviews in Physical and Rehabilitation Medicine* 12(3):229–269.

Youm, T.; Koval, K. J.; and Zuckerman, J. D. (1999). "The Economic Impact of Geriatric Hip Fractures." *American Journal of Orthopedics* 28(7):423–428.

OVARIAN CANCER

Ovarian cancer affects 12 out of every 1,000 women in the United States over the age of forty, and only two or three of these women will ultimately be cured of their disease. The average age of onset is sixty-four. Approximately 25,500 new cases are diagnosed each year, and 14,500 women die of the disease annually. The etiology of epithelial ovarian cancer is unknown, and it is usually asymptomatic until presenting as advanced staged disease. The majority of ovarian cancers are believed to arise sporadically, however three discrete hereditary syndromes are currently recognized.

THOMAS J. RUTHERFORD

(SEE ALSO: *Cancer; Carcinogenesis*)

BIBLIOGRAPHY

Lynch, H. T., and Lynch, J. F. (1989). "Hereditary Ovarian Cancer." *Hematol Oncol Clin North Am* 6:783.

Wingo, P. A.; Tong, T.; and Bodden, S. (1992). "Cancer Statistics." *CA: A Cancer Journal for Clinicians* 45:8.

Young, R. C.; Fuks, Z.; and Hoskins, W. J. (1989). "Cancer of the Ovary." In *Cancer: Principles and Practices of Oncology*, 3rd edition, eds. V. T. DeVita, Jr., S. Hellman, and S. A. Rosenberg. Philadelphia, PA: Lippincott.

OVERWINTERING

In epidemiology, the term "overwintering" describes the process whereby vector-borne pathogens survive in cold seasons while their hosts hibernate or are otherwise dormant. This enables many dangerous pathogens—such as viruses that cause dengue and encephalitis, rickettsial species, and malaria parasites—to become active and invade new susceptible hosts when warmer weather returns. The risk of epidemic spread of a vector-borne pathogen during the hot (or wet) season commonly depends more on the successful overwintering of the pathogen during the cool, dry season than on an introduction of fresh pathogens from elsewhere.

JOHN M. LAST

(SEE ALSO: *Pathogenic Organisms; Vector-Borne Diseases*)

OZONE

See Pollution

P

PACIFIC ISLANDERS, MICRONESIANS, MELANESIANS

The populations of the Pacific are few in number, and yet they are dispersed over an area covering almost a quarter of the surface of the earth (see Figure 1). The cultures of the Pacific divide into three distinct groups. The Polynesians, including the Hawaiians, Samoans, Tongans, Maori, and Tahitians, make up the best known and largest populations in the Pacific. The other two groups are the peoples of Micronesia (little islands) and Melanesia (dark skins).

The locations of the three cultural groups are geographically distinct. With the exception of the residents of the State of Hawaii, Micronesians are in the north, Melanesians are in the south, and Polynesians are in the middle. Studies of the cultures of Micronesia and Melanesia have filled books. However, information on the public health of these peoples is much less common.

As with many indigenous cultures around the world, the concept of the human organism in these cultures is holistic—the person is seen as the amalgam of body, mind, and spirit. As such, traditional systems of healing tended to follow this concept. When the Spanish explorers of the early sixteenth century arrived in these islands, they found that spiritualists, masseuses, herbalists, and vaporists provided the basis of the healing systems.

However, the details of the nature of the health systems of both Micronesia and Melanesia have remained locked in the colonial systems of power that have dominated the region for the past four hundred years. For many of these populations, the pathway of the Spanish, followed by the Germans and then the Japanese, yielded to the Americans, Australians, French, and English after World War II. The systems of care clearly reflect this history, and the problems associated with these care systems continue to plague these young nations struggling for independence and sustainable economies.

THE AREA, THE PEOPLE, AND THEIR HEALTH

The populations of the Pacific nations, Hawaii and Papua New Guinea included, represent a small fraction of the world's people. In the area known as Micronesia, the largest centers of population are Guam (154,623), Kiribati (91,985), the Commonwealth of the Northern Mariana Islands (71,912), and the Federated States of Micronesia (133,134). Somewhat smaller are the Republic of the Marshall Islands (68,126), the Republic of Palau (18,766), and Nauru (11,845). Melanesia has somewhat larger nations, including Papua New Guinea (4,926,984), Fiji (832,494), the Solomon Islands (466,194), New Caledonia (201,816), and Vanuatu (189,618).

In general, within the region, birth and death data are somewhat unreliable. However, from the data available, the population is growing more rapidly than most other places in the world. From the high of the Republic of Marshall Islands (RMI)

Table 1

Birth and Death Data 1996-1998*				
Country	Births*	Total Fertility**	Infant Mortality***	Deaths*
Guam	2.6	3.6	8.9	4.2
Kiribati	3.2	4.4	55.3	9.0
Marshall Islands	4.5	6.6	40.9	6.4
Micronesia	2.7	3.8	33.5	5.9
Nauru	2.8	3.7	10.9	2.4
CNMI	2.9	1.7	5.8	2.0
Palau	1.9	2.5	17.1	7.4
Papua New Guinea	3.3	4.4	59.8	8.0
Fiji	2.4	2.9	14.5	5.8
Solomon Islands	3.5	4.8	25.3	4.4
New Caledonia	2.8	2.5	8.6	5.6
Vanuatu	2.6	3.3	62.5	8.5

   * per 1000 population
 ** the sum of the age-specific fertility rates over the whole range
    of reproductive ages (15-49) for a particular period (1 year) In
    essence, this represents the number of children per woman of
    child bearing age
*** deaths of infants (< 1 year) per 1000 live births

SOURCE: World Health Organization, Western Pacific Regional Office (2000).

total fertility rate (TFR) of 6.6 children per woman to the low of the Commonwealth of the Northern Mariana Islands' (CNMI), rate of 1.7 children per woman, the consistency of the growth of the region is clear. Most areas have a TFR above 3.2. The infant mortality rate (IMR) also has wild variation across the region, with Vanuatu at 62.5 and the CNMI at 5.8 deaths per 1,000 live births (see Table 1).

For the most part, the economies of this region are dependent on fishing, external government grants-in-aid, and a small tourism industry. Exceptions to this occur in Guam, which has a strong U.S. military presence, and the Commonwealth of the Northern Mariana Islands, which has a number of off-shore textile manufacturers.

The region faces an almost impossible task as it attempts to deal with the major infectious diseases of cholera, dengue, and tuberculosis at the same time that it faces an ever-increasing burden from chronic diseases, particularly diabetes and various cancers. The systems of care in place are ill-equipped to manage either of these disease patterns. As new diseases emerge in the area, including HIV/AIDS (human immunodeficiency virus/ acquired immunodeficiency disease) in Papau New

Guinea and crystal methamphetamine addiction in the Mariana Islands, the systems of care have neither the skilled providers nor the facilities and materials needed to cope with these problems.

THE PUBLIC HEALTH SYSTEMS

Throughout the colonial eras of the Spanish, the Germans, and the Japanese, the systems of public health in both Micronesia and the Melanesia were designed to assure a healthy workforce. Early records describe the "primitive" ways in which the people practiced even the most basic hygiene with water supplies contaminated by feces from animals as well as humans. Minimal available food made malnutrition a given among the population, and traditional healers practicing their trade as bone setters, herbalists, masseuses, and spiritualists, as in most indigenous populations. The establishment of the early German trading posts meant the need for local labor capable of loading and unloading ships. Thus, plantation-type medical care was made available, often from ship doctors and others with minimal training. With the movement of the Japanese into the area following World War I, the colonization of the region became more ordered, with settlers coming from Japan and local people receiving some basic education to improve the productivity of the copra (a coconut by-product) and other crops. The Japanese had physicians in all colonial outposts to address the immediate needs of the workers. Water and sewerage systems were established in the larger villages, and, in general, the public health of the population, while not excellent, was at least able to reduce the death rates from the many diseases brought to the islands over the preceding thirty years.

With World War II and the military mobilization of the Japanese colonists, the plantations became less important and the need to maintain a viable workforce was reduced. The public health system remained, as did the dispensaries and hospitals; however, as the war in the Pacific expanded, the infrastructure was destroyed.

At the end of World War II, there was no health or public health system throughout the Japanese-occupied areas. The American, Australian, and New Zealand troops dispatched to secure the various outposts brought their own medicines and providers with them and, as part of their efforts to win over the people, provided medicines

Figure 1

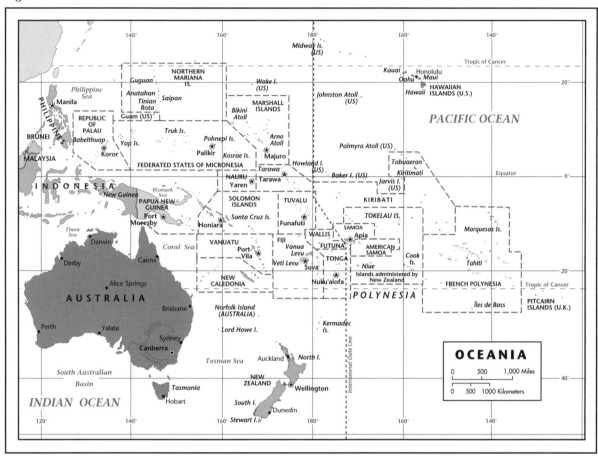

The populations of the Pacific are spread over an area that covers nearly a quarter of Earth's surface. (Maryland Cartographics)

and care to those in need. In the U.S. Pacific, an assessment of the needs of the islanders in their protection (by international mandate) was made by the USS *Whidbey* in the early 1950s. The findings were shocking, in that the people suffered from many diseases that were thought to no longer be a problem to the world. Recommendations to the U.S. government at the end of the military era established the Trust Territory of the Pacific Islands (TTPI), with headquarters in Saipan and responsibility for all aspects of life in the "American Pacific" which, with the exception of Kiribati and Nauru, encompassed all of Micronesia.

Farther south, the abundance of the U.S. treasury was not available. The Australian and New Zealand governments assisted the Melanesians (including the people from Kiribati and Nauru) in

their sphere of influence and brought public health and medical care to the southern Pacific, with the exception of New Caledonia, which remained a protectorate of France.

The modern public health and medical care systems of these two distinct regions of the Pacific have their basis in the postwar era. In the north, the U.S. government, through the TTPI, established a system of hospitals as the central points of care in all of the ten jurisdictions for which the TTPI had responsibility. In 1985 (1999 for Palau) the three areas now known as the Republic of the Marshall Islands, the Federated States of Micronesia, and Palau established a formal relationship with the U.S. government known as the Compact of Free Association. Under that compact the newly

Table 2

Leading Causes of Death, 1996-1998*

Country	Cause 1	Cause 2	Cause 3	Cause 4	Cause 5
Guam	Heart Disease 93.4	Malig Neoplasm 68.9	Diabetes 26.4	Cardiovascular 25.7	Accidents 21.9
Kiribati	Cardiovascular 55.5	Liver Disease 54.3	Gen. Debility 46.7	Gastrointestinal 28.4	Non Communicable 27.6
RMI	Malnutrition 31.9	Accidents 31.9	Sepsis 27.2	Pneumonia 19.2	Cancers 19.2
FSM	Circulatory Sys. 88.0	Endocrine/Met. 63.0	Injuries/Poison 48.0	Respiratory Sys. 41.0	Cancers 33.1
Nauru	Cardiovascular 236.9	Respiratory Sys. 198.1	Malig Neoplasm 169.8	Stillbirths 122.6	End-Stage Renal 103.8
CNMI	Cardiovascular 17.0	Diabetes 15.0	Cardiac Arrest 14.0	Myocardial Inf. 14.0	Motor Vehicle 12.0
Palau	Cardiovascular 99.4	Unknown 99.4	Circulatory Sys. 88.3	Other Injuries 77.3	Cancer 71.8
PNG	Pneumonia 20.0	Malaria 15.0	Perinatal Cond. 15.0	Tuberculosis 10.0	Heart/Pulmonary 9.0
Fiji	Circulatory Sys. 55.2	Infect/Parasitic 13.7	Respiratory Sys. 12.5	Neoplasms 11.19	Genitourinary Sys. 9.98
Solomon Is.	Respiratory Sys.	Diarrhoeal Diseases	Malaria 16.25	—	—
New Caledonia	Circulatory Sys. 124.9	Tumours 119.9	Injuries/Poisoning 77.6	Respiratory Sys. 48.8	Ill-defined 4.8
Vanuatu	Circulatory Sys. 20.7	Neonatal 18.9	Neoplasms 17.7	Respiratory Sys. 14.6	Liver Disease 5.5

* data are expressed as rate per 100,000 population

SOURCE: WHO data.

created nations were to be systematically transformed from dependencies to independent nations over a fifteen-year period. The responsibility for health services transferred to the island governments, and with it the determination of health priorities and expenditures. The period since 1985 has been spent revitalizing the public health and general health care systems. Newly trained indigenous health providers have staffed the health departments of these three nations, and reorganization of the strategies for health has come through much consultation with the World Health Organization (WHO) and the Asian Development Bank (ADB). These systems are attempting to establish primary health care centers throughout each nation, with the intent to reduce the dependence on expensive hospital-based care. However, budgets are small, needs are great, and the systems are weak.

In the southern Pacific, the transition from the post-war military care system to one operated by the national governments accompanied the independence of the various nations. The systems of care that the national governments inherited were already targeted on primary health care, and they already had a considerable investment in the use of dispensaries as a major source of care. However, the budgets have been very small in these nations as well, and the retention of trained local practitioners has been a major problem. Facilities have been built through bilateral arrangements sponsored by several foreign governments, and the basic public health infrastructure has begun to take shape through various ADB loans and other arrangements. The WHO has been very active in the southern Pacific, as has been the South Pacific Commission (now Secretariat for Pacific Communities) which has been instrumental in developing the health education focus of the region as well as the improvement of health data and general health department capacity.

In a short fifty years, the people of Micronesia and Melanesia re-created their public health systems. The water supplies are nearly all safe and sewerage is mostly disposed of in an appropriate manner. The food supply is inspected and safer, as is the supply of medicines used by the dispensaries and the hospitals. The prevalence of parasitic disease among children is remarkably reduced, as is the number of deaths from malnutrition and other nutritional deficiencies (see Table 2). However, the epidemiological transition is not over for the people of the Pacific. The future is dotted with many diseases of modernization—diabetes, substance abuse, severe mental illness, cancers, heart disease, and environmental diseases. The systems of care are not yet mature, and the need for continued support from major developed nations is obvious to any who have traveled the area.

D. WILLIAM WOOD

(SEE ALSO: *Acculturation; Cultural Anthropology; Cultural Norms; Ethnicity and Health; Geography of Disease; Indigenous Populations*)

BIBLIOGRAPHY

Carrier, J. G. (1992). *History and Tradition in Melanesian Anthropology.* Los Angeles: University of California Press.

CIA Factbook 2000. Available at http://www.odci.gov/cia/publications/factbook/.

Kiste, R. C., and Marshall, M., eds. (1999). *American Anthropology in Micronesia.* Honolulu: University of Hawaii Press.

Oliver, D. I. (1951). *The Pacific Islands.* Honolulu: University of Hawaii Press.

U.S. Department of the Interior, Office of Insular Affairs (1990). *Report on the State of the Islands, 1999.* Washington, DC: Author.

World Health Organization, Western Pacific Regional Office (2000). *Community Health Profile, 2000.* Geneva: Author.

PAN AMERICAN HEALTH ORGANIZATION

The origin of the Pan American Health Organization (PAHO) dates back to 1902 when the First International Sanitary Convention of the American Republics, meeting in Washington, DC, established the International Sanitary Bureau. The bureau was to provide a mechanism for sharing information about the occurrence of diseases and agreeing on control measures that could be applied. The fundamental purposes of PAHO, stated in its constitution, are to promote and coordinate efforts of the countries of the western hemisphere to combat diseases, lengthen life, and promote the physical and mental health of the people.

In 1924, delegates to the Seventh Pan American Sanitary Conference agreed on the first international sanitary treaty for the American States, called the Pan American Sanitary Code. The code, which is still in effect today, establishes the functions and duties of the Pan American Sanitary Bureau, which is the secretariat of the organization. One of the objectives of the code, as the first article says, is stimulation of the mutual interchange of information that may be of value in improving the public health and combating the diseases of humankind. In 1949, PAHO became, by formal agreement with the World Health Organization, its Regional Office for the Americas. A year later, a formal agreement was signed with the Organization of American States recognizing PAHO as the specialized health organization for the Inter-American System, formalizing the status that the organization had held for nearly fifty years.

All states and territories in the Americas are members of PAHO and pay a quota contribution to the organization according to a budget approved by the member states. PAHO has an office in every country, with the exception of the smaller island states of the eastern Caribbean, which are served by the Caribbean Program Coordination Office located in Barbados. PAHO's technical interests in Canada are represented by the Canadian Society for International Health. PAHO's programs are carried out through technical cooperation, which helps build the capacity of member states to address health issues that they identify as priorities. Though PAHO is not primarily a funding agency, it does mobilize external funds that supplement the regular budget to support specific projects throughout the region.

The organization operates under two basic principles: Pan-Americanism and equity. Pan-Americanism facilitates the cooperation of countries to share information and experiences and to address common goals, as envisioned in the Pan

American Sanitary Code and PAHO's constitution. For example, the member states worked together to eradicate smallpox in 1971 and poliomyelitis in 1991, and measles was targeted for eradication from the region by the end of the year 2000.

The second principle, equity, is driven by the fact that the enormous economic disparities in the Americas adversely affect the health of many of its people. The level of health status extends from that found in Canada, which has many of the best health indicators, to that found in Haiti, the least developed country in the region. Even within countries one finds enormous differences. For example, in southern parts of Brazil, health indicators may be as good as those in industrialized nations, while people living in northeastern Brazil may suffer diseases at the same rate as communities in the poorest parts of Africa. Large disparities are present in all countries of the region. They result in part from the lack of access to health services of appropriate quality, including services for health promotion and disease prevention. Disparities are not simply unjust in themselves, they impede development, including economic development. Because it is critical that countries address inequities in health and health services if they are to improve the health status of their people and their prospects for development, PAHO puts considerable emphasis on understanding, documenting, and overcoming inequities.

PAHO's work on inequities focuses on five areas: health in human development, health promotion and protection, health systems and services development, disease prevention and control, and health and environment. Each of these areas, which is addressed by a division, consists of several specific programs. All country offices and regional programs plan and evaluate their activities annually, so as to ensure the optimal use of limited resources and maximum benefit to health in the Americas.

GEORGE A. O. ALLEYNE
A. DAVID BRANDLING-BENNETT

(SEE ALSO: *International Development of Public Health; International Health; United States Agency for International Development [USAID]; World Health Organization*)

BIBLIOGRAPHY

Gwatkin, D., and Gullet, M. (1999). *The Burden of Disease Among the Poor: Current Situation, Future Trends, and Implications for Strategy*. Washington, DC: The World Bank.

Pan American Health Organization (1998). *Health in the Americas*. Washington, DC: Author.

—— (1998). *Leading Pan American Health*. Washington, DC: Author.

PAP SMEAR

The Papanicolaou (Pap) smear has been the most effective screening method developed in the prevention of cancer since the 1941 publication of *The Diagnostic Value of Vaginal Smears in Carcinoma of the Uterus* by George Papanicolaou and Herbert Traut. The Pap smear is a screening test in which a film of exfoliating cells from the lower genital tract is placed onto a slide for staining and microscopic evaluation by a qualified cytotechnologist. The advantage of the Pap smear is in the early detection and ultimate treatment of premalignant changes of the cervix. As a direct benefit of this technology, the incidence of invasive cervical cancer in the United States has been reduced 50 percent and the mortality has been decreased by more than 70 percent.

In 1999, unfortunately, 12,800 new cervical cancer cases were diagnosed in the United States resulting in 4,800 deaths. Between 50 and 60 percent of U.S. women with cervical cancer have either never had a Pap smear or have received Pap smears at irregular intervals, while almost 6,000 of the women who develop cervical cancer annually have had recent Pap smear screening. In those countries without the use of routine Pap smear screening, cervical cancer remains the primary malignancy in women that results in mortality. Since the widespread acceptance of the Pap smear, a dramatic decline in the incidence and mortality of cervical cancer has occurred. Since 1986, however, the incidence has slightly risen. This underscores the success of the Pap smear, as well as its inability to detect 100 percent of the cases.

In 1984, the American College of Obstetrics and Gynecology recommended annual screening for most women. Initial screening should begin at age eighteen, or when the individual becomes sexually active. High-risk women—those with a history of early sexual activity and multiple partners—should be screened yearly. Those with only one partner and who have two successive negative annual Pap smears might be considered low-risk and be screened every one to three years.

The inability to detect the presence of a case of disease in the screened population results in a false-negative cytologic finding. In January 1999, the Agency for Health Care Policy and Research (AHCPR) released the *Evaluation of Cervical Cytology*. The AHCPR estimated the true sensitivity of the Pap smear to be only 51 percent, which means that the test correctly identifies only half the actual cases. More alarming, from 70 to 90 percent of those Pap smear cases with false-negative cytologic findings have no cytologic abnormality even when reviewed. Therefore, the major factor in improving the reliability of the Pap smear may be adequate specimen collection, preparation, and fixation. Prior to 1988, the quality of a Pap smear was not reported. Currently, if a smear is interpretable but the quality is poor due to poor handling of the specimen, blood, infection, cellular debris, or inadequate sampling, the sample is termed "satisfactory but limited by." If the smear is uninterpretable, the sample is labeled "unsatisfactory."

Newer technologies to improve the detection of cervical disease in a premalignant state are being developed. These technologies include an automated computerized analyzer to evaluate Pap smears; liquid-based, thin-layer cytology; and tests to identify the presence of the human papillomavirus (HPV), which has been demonstrated to be a major cause of cervical abnormalities.

The automated computerized analyzer scans Pap smear slides. Cells on the slides are digitized and processed through an image interpretation algorithm that has been developed to distinguish between normal and abnormal cells. This methodology reduces the human error that occurs in the current manual cytologic interpretation. In the liquid-based, thin-layer cytologic system, cells are collected from the cervix and transferred to a liquid fixative rather than to a glass slide. Once the sample arrives at the laboratory, the cervical cells are uniformly transferred to a filter. This technology eliminates air-drying artifacts and other factors that interfere with interpretation, thereby improving the detectability of abnormalities.

Although newer technologies are aimed at reducing the false-negative rate of the Pap smear, the cytotechnologist will always find cells with no distinguishing characteristics. These cells are termed "undetermined." The management of these "atypical cells of undetermined significance" (ASCUS) is a major clinical dilemma. HPV testing has been proposed as a method to resolve this problem. HPV-positive women are at risk for cervical cancer and therefore require further clinical evaluation. HPV-negative women can be followed with a repeat Pap smear in the future. The liquid-based, thin-layer method readily allows for HPV testing, another major advantage over the standard Pap smear.

THOMAS J. RUTHERFORD

(SEE ALSO: *Cancer; Cervical Cancer; Human Papillomavirus Infection; Laboratory Services; Screening; Secondary Prevention*)

BIBLIOGRAPHY

Boyes, D. A. (1981). "The Value of Pap Smear and Suggestions for Its Implementation." *Cancer* 48:613.

Burke, L. (1997). "Evolution of Therapeutic Approaches to Cervical Intraepithelial Neoplasia." *Journal of Lower Genital Tract Disease* 4:267.

Kurman, R. I.; Henson, D. E.; Herbst, A. I. et al. (1994). "Interim Guidelines for the Management of Abnormal Cervical Cytology." *Journal of the American Medical Association* 271:1866.

Manos, M. M.; Kinney, W. K.; Hurley, L. B. et al. (1999). "Identifying Women with Cervical Neoplasia: Using Human Papillomavirus DNA Testing for Equivocal Papanicolaou Results." *Journal of the American Medical Association* 281(17):1605.

National Cancer Institute (1989). "The 1988 Bethesda System for Reporting Cervical/Vaginal Cytological Diagnosis." *Journal of the American Medical Association* 262(7):931.

Sidawy, M. K., and Tabbara, S. O. (1993). "Reactive Change and Atypical Squamous Cells of Undetermined Significance in Papanicolaou Smears: A Cytohistologic Correlation." *Diagnostic Cytopathology* 9:423.

PARASITES

See Pathogenic Organisms

PARTICIPATION IN COMMUNITY HEALTH PLANNING

The health of a community depends on many factors, including the health protection and promotion activities of local government agencies (e.g., public health, transportation, public works, parks and recreation), not-for-profit agencies (e.g., Red Cross, American Cancer Society, YMCA/ YWCA) and private sector organizations (e.g., plastic recycling firms). Because the determinants of health lie, to a great extent, outside the health sector (including socioeconomic, cultural, and working conditions), involving citizens in making decisions on issues that affect their health has long been supported by public health. Theory and practice in community health suggests that planning is best done by those individuals who will be the recipients of, or will be affected by, the resulting programs, policies, or services. Efforts to get people to change their lifestyle behaviors, their worksites (e.g., to implement a no smoking policy), or their schools (e.g., to adopt a healthier lunch menu), will be most successful if those asked to make such changes are included in the planning process. In addition to engendering positive program outcomes, participation is also thought to:

- Empower individual participants by increasing their knowledge and skill levels, their feelings of control and competence to make a difference, and their sense of self-worth and dignity.

- Nurture local planning skills and abilities.

- Build community capacity to tackle future health issues.

- Foster the overall health of the community by strengthening citizens' trust in each other and their connectedness to the community.

Opportunities for citizens to participate in health planning has often been hindered or blocked, however, by resistance from the state and from the professions, precluding citizens from making decisions and shaping policy about their own lives. Participation can be, and often is, tokenistic or consultative rather than meaningful. While it remains an attractive concept, it is one that has been realized only in a limited sense.

Community participation is often narrowly defined as simply asking community members about their health needs. Opinions are often confined to prepackaged formulas, and delegating the actual planning, implementation, and evaluation of programs is left to professional practitioners. While needs assessments and pretesting programs are crucial components of planning, participation needs to go beyond responding to surveys or opinion polls, with people actively involved in defining the issues and in all subsequent phases of the process.

It is often difficult to attract participants that reflect the diversity of a community. The participation process itself can discriminate against those in the community who are not well-educated, well-spoken, or well-off. Committee meetings and public forums can be inconvenient, inaccessible, and intimidating to all but the few who possess the requisite professional experience and educational and discretionary resources to attend. In addition to meetings being convenient and welcoming, citizens must be able to see some reflection of themselves in the participatory endeavor in order to trust the process and become involved. In the absence of broad-based participation, particularly when economy of time and problems of scale restrict participation by all, experiential participation may be a step toward achieving better representation of diverse perspectives.

Experiential participation abandons the "meeting mindset." Participation takes place in schools, worksites, churches, street corners, and coffee houses, and engages citizens in a planning process that reflects their life experiences. It also demands acknowledging and respecting the diverse and nontraditional contributions and strengths of different groups of citizens. Meaningful participation may constitute sharing experiences as recipients of services, providing input about the delivery and quality of health programs, as well as chairing meetings, interpreting statistics, and penning community health plans. A final challenge lies in maintaining the momentum of, and interest in, participatory initiatives when much of the work relies on lay volunteers with busy lives.

Examples of successful initiatives in community health planning where citizens have shared in the responsibility and decision making include the Healthy Cities/Healthy Communities projects in

Europe and North America, the Planned Approach to Community Health (PATCH) programs in the United States and Canada, and the Canadian Active Living Movement. Common to these experiences were generous timelines for accomplishing tasks; involving citizens early on in the planning process and allowing participants, rather than professionals, to define the health issues and propose solutions; participatory techniques that accommodated for and respected participants' diverse skills and contributions; and local intersectoral (e.g., education, transportation, environment, recreation) representation and collaboration on the issue.

JOAN WHARF HIGGINS

(SEE ALSO: *Citizens Advisory Boards; Community Health; Community Organization; Decentralization and Community Health; Health Promotion and Education; Healthy Communities; Nongovernmental Organizations, United States; Planned Approach to Community Health [PATCH]; Politics of Public Health; Social Assessment in Health Promotion Planning*)

BIBLIOGRAPHY

Arnstein, S. (1969). "A Ladder of Citizen Participation." *American Institute of Planners Journal* (July):216–224.

Green, L. W., and Ottoson, J. (1999). *Community and Population Health.* Boston: McGraw-Hill.

Marmot, M., and Wilkinson, R. (1999). *Social Determinants of Health.* London: Oxford University Press.

Prior, D.; Stewart, J.; and Walsh, K. (1995). *Citizenship: Rights, Community and Participation.* London: Pittman Publishing.

Putnam, R. D. (2000). *Bowling Alone, The Collapse and Revival of American Community.* New York: Simon & Schuster.

Quinney, H. A.; Gauvin, L.; and Wall, A. E. T. (1994). *Toward Active Living.* Champaign, IL: Human Kinetics.

Wharf Higgins, J. (1992). "The Healthy Communities Movement in Canada." In *Communities and Social Policy in Canada,* ed. B. Wharf. Toronto: McClelland and Stewart.

—— (1999). "Closer to Home: The Case for Experiential Participation in Health Reform." *Canadian Journal of Public Health* 90(1):30–34.

U.S. Department of Health and Human Services (1996). *Planned Approach to Community Health: Guide for the Local Coordinator.* Atlanta, GA: U.S. Department of Health and Human Services, Centers for Disease Control and Prevention, National Center for Chronic Disease Prevention and Health Promotion.

PARTICULATES

See Airborne Particles; Inhalable Particles (Sulfates); *and* Total Suspended Particles (TSP)

PASTEUR, LOUIS

Louis Pasteur (1822–1895), a French chemist and bacteriologist, was a pioneer in the fields of bacteriology and preventive medicine. He had already established an international reputation as a chemist and won the Rumford Medal of the British Royal Society for his work on the structure of crystals when he made his first foray into bacteriology in 1854. Having recently been appointed a professor of chemistry in Lille, Pasteur was invited to solve a problem in the fermentation of beer that affected its taste and rendered it undrinkable. He showed that this was caused by bacteria that could be killed by heat. In this way he invented the process for heat treatment to kill harmful bacteria, first applied to the making of beer, then to milk. This process has been known ever since as pasteurization.

He next turned his attention to two diseases of silkworms, showing these to be due to microparasites and demonstrating how these diseases could be prevented. Soon after this he suffered a stroke from which he was not expected to recover. Defying this prognosis, he went on to study and solve other bacteriological problems in both industry and animal husbandry. He showed that chicken cholera could be prevented by inoculating chickens with an attenuated vaccine and in 1881 he demonstrated that a similar attenuated vaccine could be used to control anthrax, which was then a serious threat to livestock, and occasionally to humans.

In 1880, Pasteur had begun experiments on rabies, seeking a vaccine to control this disease, which without treatment has a 100 percent death rate. Following the success of the anthrax vaccine he believed that an attenuated rabies vaccine could be made. The only way to test this vaccine would be on a human who had been bitten by a rabid dog, and this he did in July 1885. His patient was a boy,

Joseph Meister. The vaccine worked, Joseph Meister survived, and Pasteur became not just a national but an international celebrity.

Pasteur made many other important contributions to microbiology and continued to work until near his death, despite the gloomy prognosis he had been given after his stroke more than a quarter of a century earlier. Pasteur's antirabies regimen consisted of multiple injections of rabies vaccine into the skin of the abdomen. This sequence of multiple (and painful) injections was used for many years without modification to prevent the onset of rabies in anyone who had been bitten by a rabid animal. No one was brave enough to try an experiment to determine whether a less protracted and painful regimen would be as effective. Only in the 1980s did the development of genetically engineered vaccines lead to a simpler way to prevent rabies. Pasteur's name lives on in the microbiological research institute in Paris that bears his name, the Institut Pasteur, and its branches in former French colonies in Africa and Asia.

JOHN M. LAST

(SEE ALSO: *Immunizations; Rabies*)

BIBLIOGRAPHY

Dubos, R. J. (1996). *Louis Pasteur, Free Lance of Science.* San Francisco: Da Capo Press.

PATERNALISM

Consideration of paternalism involves the interactions of two principles of medical ethics—beneficence and respect for autonomy. Historically, beneficence has long retained primacy in medical ethics, and physicians have been able to rely almost exclusively on their own judgement about their patients' needs for treatment, information, and consultation. However, medicine has increasingly been confronted—especially since around 1970—with a different kind of need, namely the patient's asserted need to make an independent judgment.

The central problem in these discussions is whether the principle of respect for autonomy, which gives primary decision-making authority to patients, should have priority in medical practice over the principle of beneficence, which gives

authority to providers to implement sound principles of health care. Resolving this issue requires coming to terms with the problem of paternalism. Medical paternalism poses significant moral questions because it holds that beneficence can legitimately take precedence over respect for autonomy. From this perspective, a professional is like a parent dealing with dependent, and often ignorant and fearful, patients.

For example, suppose an incurable cancer is found in a sixty-nine-year-old man. Based on a long relationship, the man's physician knows that the patient has a history of psychiatric illness and is emotionally fragile. When the patient blurts out, "Am I OK? I don't have cancer, do I?" the physician answers, "You're as good as you were ten years ago," knowing that the response is a paternalistic lie, but also believing it justified in protecting the health and well-being of the patient.

Some leading ethicists maintain that paternalistic interventions are seldom justified, because the right of the patient to act autonomously almost always outweighs obligations of beneficence toward the autonomous patient. In the practical world, it is important to seek a balance between the demands of both beneficence and respect for autonomy. It is useful to note that this balance may be seen differently in other cultures, where there may be a stronger tilt toward beneficence.

JOHN H. BRYANT

(SEE ALSO: *Autonomy; Beneficence; Equity and Resource Allocation; Ethics of Public Health*)

BIBLIOGRAPHY

Beauchamp, T. L., and Childress, J. R. (1989). *Principles of Biomedical Ethics.* New York: Oxford University Press.

Veatch, R. M. (1989). *Medical Ethics.* Boston: Jones and Bartlett Publishers.

PATERNITY

Paternity, the state of being a father, can be legally established in several ways. When the parents of a child are married, paternity is commonly presumed. However, to determine whether a man is the father of a child born out of wedlock, a lawsuit known as a "paternity action" must be brought. In such a suit, paternity may be established if the alleged father admits paternity. If a man fails to participate in the process, then paternity may be fixed by default, or a judge may order that he provide a blood sample to compare blood types and, if necessary, DNA types with that of the mother and child.

Blood-group studies, which commonly employ the ABO system, cannot establish paternity but can conclusively exclude an alleged father from being a candidate. This is the case because a child must inherit his or her blood type (A, B, or O) from the mother or father; thus, if the child's blood type differs from both the mother's and the alleged father's types, the man could not possibly be a parent of the child. To conclusively establish paternity, DNA typing is required. Adequate samples for DNA typing can be collected from blood, semen, or body tissue such as the inside of the cheek. DNA typing compares strands of genetic material between the child and alleged father. While most courts in the United States require accuracy of 99 percent to establish paternity, comparing strands from various locations of the genetic material allows accuracy ratings of 99.9 percent. DNA typing allows an alleged father to be excluded with 100 percent certainty.

Upon the conclusion of a paternity action, the judge's order establishes paternity. Once paternity is determined, the court can consider the issues of custody, visitation, and child support. Paternity actions are also brought in cases involving family inheritances, insurance benefits, social security claims, immigration requests, and to establish the peace of mind associated with being able to determine whether the child may be at risk for any hereditary disease.

JOHN R. YORK
JEFFREY A. LINSKER

(SEE ALSO: *Child Welfare; Public Health and the Law*)

PATHOGENIC ORGANISMS

Pathogenic organisms are life forms that cause human disease. They range in size and complexity, and include molecules like proteinaceous particles (prions); viruses that are visible under an electron microscope; bacteria, fungi, and protozoan parasites that are sometimes visible to the naked eye; and multicellular parasites like tapeworms that may be many meters long. Many live in natural ecosystems, while others are commensal or parasitic on animals and/or humans. Only a few cannot survive independently of human hosts.

Pathogenic organisms can harm human health in several ways, including consuming nutriment intended for their host (tapeworms); producing poisonous metabolic products (staphylococcus, diphtheria, botulism toxin, and many others); destroying vital organs and tissues (prions, polio, rabies viruses); or interfering with body chemistry (toxic fungus). A few cause cancer (e.g. campylobacter). Their capacity to harm varies widely: The rabies virus virtually always kills its human victims, but seems to live harmlessly in many species of bats. Some obscure microorganisms that do no harm to healthy people can cause debilitating and ultimately fatal infections in persons whose immune defenses have been disrupted by the AIDS (acquired immunodeficiency syndrome) virus.

Rapid advances in microbiology, immunology, pharmacology, and other relevant sciences throughout the twentieth century have led to increasingly effective control measures against many pathogens. However, in biomass alone, microorganisms outweigh higher life forms, including humans, by several orders of magnitude, and they may number many billions of species. Eradication, or even elimination, of most pathogens from human ecosystems is thus not feasible. Humans must therefore learn to live in harmony with them as best they can. The best strategies generally are enhanced immunity and, where possible, avoidance of exposure to them and their harmful effects.

JOHN M. LAST

(SEE ALSO: *Communicable Disease Control*)

PATIENT EDUCATIONAL MEDIA

Patient educational media include a wide range of programs and materials delivered by health care organizations and designed to help patients achieve or maintain an enhanced state of health and recovery. Examples include printed materials (e.g., brochures, booklets, pamphlets), videotapes, audiotapes, and most recently, electronic programs and resources such as web sites, kiosks, or other interactive multimedia programs. While health education and the use of educational media occurs in many settings, there are at least two characteristics unique to health care settings that make it especially appropriate for such activities. First, improved health is the primary objective of activities that occur in this setting. Unlike worksites, communities, or schools, people go to a doctor's office expecting to deal with issues related to their own health. Second, health care providers are generally considered to be credible sources of health information. This combination of factors—people who are more than usually receptive and attentive to health information (e.g., patients) interacting with professionals who are trusted and respected (e.g., health care providers)—creates an environment conducive to effective patient education.

Patient educational media are typically designed to meet one of two types of objectives: (1) to inform and educate; and (2) to assist and support. Addressing the first of these objectives involves translating scientific and medical knowledge into lay terms that patients can understand. Addressing the second objective involves helping patients solve problems, cope with difficulties, or modify health-related risks and behaviors. Both types of objectives can be relevant to a broad spectrum of patient education needs, including raising awareness, changing attitudes and beliefs, motivating and supporting behavior change efforts, promoting screening, enhancing adherence to a disease prevention or treatment regimen, and guiding rehabilitation efforts.

Historically, patient educational media has consisted almost exclusively of printed pamphlets and brochures. These materials tend to use a general, rational, informational, and didactic (GRID) style of presenting health information. The GRID approach typically involves writing in the second or third person, from the perspective of one who is not personally involved in the topic of interest. It explains health-related processes and phenomena in terms that are often simplified in language, emotionally neutral, broad in scope, but short on detail. This approach seems especially well suited to meet "inform and educate" objectives like explaining risk factors, causality, biological processes, disease etiology, and surgical or other treatment procedures. Printed, mass-produced pamphlets also have the advantage of being relatively inexpensive to produce. But they have important limitations, too. Such "one-size-fits-all" materials are created for general populations, and therefore don't really consider specific characteristics of the different patients who might use them.

In order for patient educational media to stimulate changes in knowledge, attitude, or behavior, certain intermediary steps must occur. These include patients' paying attention to the materials and understanding their content. Some patient educational media are more likely to have these effects than others. For example, Petty and Cacioppo's elaboration likelihood model suggests people will process information more thoughtfully and carefully if they perceive it to be personally relevant. Information processed in this way (e.g., "elaborated" upon) tends to be retained for a longer period of time and is more likely to lead to permanent change. Thus, it can be expected that those educational programs and materials that address patients' needs most specifically will be more successful in reaching their objectives.

Targeted patient education materials are those intended to reach a specific subgroup of the general population, usually based on some set of characteristics shared by its members. For example, there are cessation programs and materials designed especially for pregnant women who smoke. Because these materials take into account the unique needs of a specific group of patients, they represent an incremental improvement over generic materials. An even more advanced approach to patient educational media is customization at the level of the individual patient. The first widespread attempt to do this began in the 1970s with the advent of computerized health-risk appraisals (HRAs). For decades since then, the HRA has been one of the most widely used health-education tools for promoting individual behavioral change in health care settings. To participate in an HRA program, individuals typically complete an assessment to provide information about their health-related behaviors (e.g., smoking, seat belt use), health-status indicators (e.g., blood pressure, cholesterol level), and other personal characteristics related to mortality risk (e.g., age, gender, weight, present disease status). This information is fed into a computer-based risk estimation algorithm that weights each of these factors according to its relative contribution to different disease states, establishes a health profile for each participant, and then looks at population mortality rates experienced by others of the same age and sex with a similar profile. HRA feedback originally appealed to patients because its quantification of personal risk status was novel and interesting. It has also appealed to health care providers, who can use its data in aggregate to help identify the patient education and health promotion needs of patients.

During the 1990s, patient educational materials began to adopt the same approach to behavioral change that HRAs use to communicate risk information. These "tailored" patient-education materials include any combination of information and behavior-change strategies intended to reach one specific person, based on characteristics that are unique to that person, that relate to the outcome of interest and that are derived from an individual assessment. The process of tailoring patient-education materials is much like the process an actual tailor uses to make custom clothing. A tailor takes a customer's measurements, asks about preferences for fabric, color, and style, and uses this information to create clothing to fit that customer. Likewise, a tailored health-communication program measures a participant's needs, interests, and concerns; and uses that information to create health messages and materials to fit that person. Studies conducted among patients in health care settings have shown that tailored messages are more effective than non-tailored messages in promoting changes in a range of health-related behaviors.

Another new approach to patient education involves multimedia strategies that may be interactive and delivered through video or electronic channels. While traditional mass media campaigns have limited effectiveness in changing behavior, the Internet and other computer-based communications have the potential to reach a very large audience with what is more like an interpersonal communication. The rapid development of technologies and the expansion of the Internet provide widely available opportunities to obtain interactive information, education, and support, tailored to individual needs and preferences.

A media-based health-education program could take the form of a web site, an interactive computer kiosk in a doctor's office, a videotape or audiotape mailed to a patient's home, telephone counseling, a printed newsletter, a self-help booklet, a brochure, or any number of other executions, either singly or in combination. Advanced technologies, such as interactive multimedia and World Wide Web programming, have several obvious advantages over printed and other traditional kinds of health education materials. First, they are less dependent on user literacy, and thus may be useful in reaching some high-risk populations. Second, they not only allow for vicarious learning through the modeling of healthy behaviors, but they can actually allow users to select a particular "model" who they feel similar to or believe to be credible. Third, because the technology is interactive, it is more engaging than one-way communication, and it can still produce a tangible product for users to take with them, such as a printed letter, behavior change plan, or even a videotape.

Nonetheless, while a number of interactive multimedia programs have been developed for health promotion purposes, there remains a dearth of rigorously designed studies assessing their effectiveness. From a more practical standpoint, it is not at all clear that a majority of health-education practitioners presently have the means to develop such programs. Furthermore, although access to electronic media, such as the World Wide Web, is growing, it is hardly universal. Unlike some of these more advanced technologies, print communication programs are widely used, have demonstrated effectiveness, and are more feasible for practitioners to produce and disseminate.

While patient educational media are available for patients in most all physicians' offices, they are seldom used on a consistent basis and in a coordinated fashion together with physician advice. Yet in one study, patients who received a physician's advice to quit smoking, eat less fat, or get more exercise prior to receiving educational materials on the same topic were more likely to remember the materials, show them to others, and perceive the materials as applying to them specifically. They were also more likely to report trying to quit smoking, quitting for at least 24 hours, and making some changes in diet and physical activity. These findings support an integrated model of patient education in which physician advice is a catalyst for patient change, and patient educational media provide the depth of detail and substance necessary for sustained change.

MATTHEW W. KREUTER
DAWN C. BUCHOLTZ

(SEE ALSO: *Assessment of Health Status; Audiotapes and Videotapes; Communications for Health; Health Promotion and Education; Health Risk Appraisal; Internet*)

BIBLIOGRAPHY

Cacioppo, J. T.; Harkins, S. G.; and Petty, R. E. (1981). "The Nature of Attitudes and Cognitive Responses and Their Relationships to Behavior." In *Cognitive Responses in Persuasion*, eds. R. E. Petty, T. M. Ostrom, and T. C. Brock. Hillsdale, NJ: Erlbaum.

Cassell, M. M.; Jackson, C.; and Cheuvront, B. (1998). "Health Communication on the Internet: An Effective Channel for Health Behavior Change?" *Journal of Health Communication* 3:71–79.

DeFriese, G. H., and Fielding, J. E. (1990). "Health Risk Appraisal in the 1990s: Opportunities, Challenges, and Expectations." *Annual Review of Public Health* 11: 401–418.

Kreuter, M. W; Chheda, S. G.; and Bull, F. C. (2000). "How Does Physician Advice Influence Patient Behavior? Evidence for a Priming Effect." *Archives of Family Medicine* 9:426–433.

Kreuter, M. W.; Farrell, D.; Olevitch, L.; and Brennan, L. (2000). *Tailoring Health Messages. Customizing Communication with Computer Technology*. Mahwah, NJ: Lawrence Erlbaum Associates, Publishers.

Kreuter, M. W.; Lezin, N. A.; Kreuter, M. W.; and Green, L. W. (1998). *Community Health Promotion Ideas That Work*. Boston, MA: Jones and Bartlett Publishers.

Kreuter, M. W.; Strecher, V. J.; and Glassman, B. (1994). "One Size Does Not Fit All: The Case for Tailoring Print Materials." *Annals of Behavioral Medicine* 21(4):1–9.

McGuire, W. J. (1991). "Theoretical Foundations of Campaigns." In *Public Communication Campaigns,* 2nd edition. eds. R. E. Rice and C. K. Atkin. Newbury Park, CA: Sage Publications.

Mullen, P. D.; Evans, D.; Forster, J.; Gottlieb, N. H.; Kreuter, M. W.; Moon, R.; O'Rourke, T.; and Strecher, V. (1995). "Settings As an Important Dimension in Health Education/Promotion Policy, Programs, and Research." *Health Education Quarterly* 22(3):329–435.

Petty, R. E., and Cacioppo, J. T. (1981). *Attitudes and Persuasion: Classical and Contemporary Approaches*. Boulder, CO: Westview Press.

Petty R. T.; Cacioppo J. T.; Strathman A. J.; and Priester J. R. (1994). "To Think or Not to Think. Exploring Two Routes to Persuasion." In *Persuasion: Psychological Insights and Perspectives,* eds. S. Shavitt and T. C. Brock. Boston, MA: Allyn and Bacon.

Skinner, C. S.; Campbell, M. K.; Rimer, B. K.; Curry, J.; and Prochaska, J. O. (1999). "How Effective Is Tailored Print Communication?" *Annals of Behavioral Medicine* 21(4):290–298.

PCBS

Polychlorinated biphenyls (PCBs) are a group of synthetic chlorinated organic compounds that are of public health concern because of their persistence in the environment and their potential cancer-causing and endocrine-disruptive effects. There are 209 individual PCB congeners of varying toxicity, but a smaller number accounts for most of the commercially distributed mixtures. PCBs usually have been sold as clear oily mixtures whose lubricating, insulating, and coolant properties have led to their being widely distributed for many industrial and commercial uses. They are relatively inert, making them particularly valuable for such uses as fireproofing, but their lack of reactivity is also responsible for environmental persistence and for bioaccumulation in the food chain.

Heavy exposure to PCBs due to contamination of cooking oil occurred in two episodes in Japan and Taiwan in which skin manifestations, including chloracne, were prominent effects. Also observed were abnormal hepatic function, neurophysiological alterations, and developmental effects in offspring.

Exposure to high levels of PCBs at the workplace can cause skin and upper respiratory tract irritation. Environmental exposure to PCBs primarily occur through ingestion of contaminated seafood, but exposure can also occur through children ingesting contaminated soil and through the skin in landfill sites. PCBs are stored in fat and are present in breast milk. Inhalation of PCBs can also occur, particularly when there are indoor sources. PCBs can be carried long distances in air, which accounts for their distribution and accumulation in food chains in otherwise pristine arctic areas.

The different PCB congeners have different rates of persistence, bioaccumulation, and toxicity. In general, as the extent of chlorination increases, the rate of metabolism and detoxification decreases. The position of the chlorine atoms on the phenyl rings also affects metabolic rate and toxicity. Contamination of commercial PCB mixtures, particularly with chlorinated dibenzofurans, may also contribute to toxicity.

Acute toxicity due to PCBs is not of concern. However, PCBs are definitely carcinogenic to laboratory animals and are considered to be carcinogenic to humans. Concern about the potential for endocrine-disruptive effects, including developmental abnormalities, is similar to the concern for other persistent chlorinated compounds. Polybrominated biphenyls (PBBs) are in many ways similar to PCBs although far lesser amounts have been produced. An episode of PBB-contaminated cattle feed in Michigan led to human consumption of contaminated meat and dairy products, resulting in evidence of immunological dysfunction.

PCBs have been among the persistent organic pollutants (POPs) that have been considered to be of particular concern in many national and international deliberations. The United States banned the manufacture of PCBs in 1977, but PCB mixtures still remain in old electrical equipment and other items manufactured before 1977. There is also substantial PCB contamination of landfills and rivers. The Hudson River has been heavily contaminated by dumping from an electrical-device manufacturing facility. There has been much controversy concerning whether dredging the Hudson River to remove PCBs may do more harm than good by causing pockets of PCBs to be stirred up and to enter the ecosystem food chain.

The United States Food and Drug Administration has established allowable tolerances for PCBs in a variety of foods, particularly dairy products and seafoods. With the possible exception of the arctic, in recent years there has been a decline in PCB levels in human fat and in the general environment.

BERNARD D. GOLDSTEIN

(SEE ALSO: *Toxicology*)

BIBLIOGRAPHY

Chen, Y. C.; Guo, Y. L.; Hsu, C. C.; and Rogen, W. J. (1997). "Cognitive Development of Yu-Cheng ("Oil Disease") Children Prenatally Exposed to Heat Degraded PCBs." *Journal of the American Medical Association* 268(22):3213–3218.

Guo, Y. L.; Hsu, P. C.; Hsu, C. C.; and Lambert, G. H. (2000). "Semen Quality after Prenatal Exposure to Polychlorinated Biphenyls and Dibenzofurans." *Lancet* 356(9237):1240–1241.

Jacobsen, J. L., and Jacobsen, S. W. (1996). "Intellectual Impairment in Children Exposed to Polychlorinated Biphenyls in Utero." *New England Journal of Medicine* 335(11):783–789.

Kimbrough, R. D. (1997). "Human Health Effects of Polychlorinated Biphenyls (PCBs) and Polybrominated Biphenyls (PBBs)." *Annual Review of Pharmacological Toxicology* 27:87.

PEER REVIEW

Peer review of health services consists of an evaluation in which practicing physicians or other health professionals assess the quality of health care delivered by another health professional. Typically, the subject and the reviewer have comparable levels of training, credentials, and experience. Care is evaluated on a case-by-case basis, and quality determination usually involves a degree of professional judgment. The process of peer review purports to measure quality, though, historically, most systematic, large-scale peer review efforts have had poor reliability. Modern methods of health care quality assessment employ objective performance indicators and statistical inference to measure practitioners' performance in comparison with evidence-based practice guidelines.

CHARLES P. SCHADE

(SEE ALSO: *Continuous Quality Assessment; Continuous Quality Improvement*)

BIBLIOGRAPHY

Nash, D. B.; Markson, L. E.; Howell, S.; and Hildreth, E. A. (1993). "Evaluating the Competence of Physicians in Practice: From Peer Review to Performance Assessment." *Academic Medicine* 68(Supp. 2):19–22.

PELVIC INFLAMMATORY DISEASE (PID)

Pelvic inflammatory disease (PID) refers to infection of the fallopian tubes and other internal reproductive organs in women. It is a common and serious complication of some sexually transmitted diseases (STDs). Douching and using an intrauterine device (IUD) are also associated with increased risk of PID. PID can damage the fallopian tubes and tissues in and near the uterus and ovaries. Untreated, PID can lead to infertility, ectopic pregnancy, and chronic pelvic pain. Each year, more than 1 million U.S. women experience an episode of acute PID. More than 100,000 women become infertile each year as a result of PID, and a large proportion of ectopic pregnancies are due to the consequences of PID. Most cases of PID are associated with gonorrhea and chlamydia; 10 to 20 percent of women with these STDs will develop PID.

PID occurs when bacteria move upward from a woman's vagina or cervix into the internal reproductive organs. Bacteria can silently invade the fallopian tubes and cause scarring that blocks or interrupts the normal movement of eggs into the uterus. Because many women have only vague or mild symptoms, PID frequently goes unrecognized. Women who do have symptoms commonly have pain in the lower or right upper abdomen, fever, unusual vaginal discharge, painful intercourse, and irregular menstrual bleeding. PID can be cured with antibiotics. Women with pelvic pain and other symptoms caused by PID should seek care immediately. The longer a woman delays treatment, the more likely she is to suffer infertility or an ectopic pregnancy in the future.

The main cause of PID is an untreated STD. Women can protect themselves from PID by taking action to prevent STDs or by getting early treatment if they do get an STD.

ALLISON L. GREENSPAN
JOEL R. GREENSPAN

(SEE ALSO: *Sexually Transmitted Diseases*)

BIBLIOGRAPHY

Centers for Disease Control and Prevention (1998). "1998 Guidelines for Treatment of Sexually Transmitted Diseases." *Morbidity and Mortality Weekly Report* 47(RR-1):79–86.

Westrom, L., and Eschenbach, D. (1999). "Pelvic Inflammatory Disease." In *Sexually Transmitted Diseases,* 3rd edition, eds. K. Holmes, P. Mardh, P. Sparling et al. New York: McGraw-Hill.

PENICILLIN

The first of the first-generation antibiotics, *Penicillium notatum* is naturally produced by a mold. It was discovered serendipitously by British bacteriologist Alexander Fleming in 1928, and later developed successfully as a powerful therapeutic weapon by Howard Florey and Ernst Chain. These three men shared the 1945 Nobel Prize in medicine for their work on penicillin. The antibiotic was initially immensely successful in curing previously fatal infections caused by common bacterial pathogens such as streptococcus, staphylococcus and pneumococcus, and in treating common sexually transmitted diseases, notably syphilis and gonorrhea.

Unfortunately, most pathogens became resistant as successive generations of microorganisms included rising proportions that had evolved an enzyme to inactivate penicillin. Also, as penicillin is a complex protein, many who receive it develop allergies that get worse with each subsequent course of treatment. Its efficacy is thereby reduced.

JOHN M. LAST

(SEE ALSO: *Antibiotics; Drug Resistance*)

PERFORMANCE STANDARDS FOR PUBLIC HEALTH

Performance standards for public health are definite and clear measures established by the public health community as a model for the measurement of the quality of public health practice. The performance standards for the National Public Health Performance Standards Program were developed by local and state public health practitioners, local board of health members, academicians, and federal public health officials to provide a common framework for measuring performance and defining the optimal level of public health practice.

The tools for measurement use the "Essential Public Health Services" as a framework. Each service is defined by indicators of performance. For each indicator, a paragraph describes the ideal level of performance. This description is followed by measures or questions to assess the system's capacity to meet this level of performance. The tools help identify strengths and weaknesses in the public health system and provide policymakers with information to help develop public health systems.

ANNETTE FEREBEE

(SEE ALSO: *Essential Public Health Services; Official U.S. Health Agencies; Performance Standards for State and Local Health Departments*)

PERFORMANCE STANDARDS FOR STATE AND LOCAL HEALTH DEPARTMENTS

Public health departments are organizations established by state and local governments to protect and promote the health and safety of the people living in or visiting the area served by a state or local government. Public health departments protect and promote health and safety by assuring delivery of the ten Essential Public Health Services which are described as:

- Monitoring community health to understand patterns of disease, injury, and environmental threats to the public's health.

- Diagnosing and investigating occurrences of disease, injury, and environmental hazards in order to control and prevent people from suffering ill health effects.

- Informing, educating, and empowering people to understand health risks and use of preventive measures to protect and promote health and safety.

- Mobilizing people in communities to take collective actions and form partnerships to solve community health problems.

- Developing policies and plans that support individual and community health improvement efforts.

- Enforcing laws and regulations that protect health and ensure safety.

- Linking people to needed personal health services and assuring the provision of health care when otherwise unavailable.

- Assuring that a competent public and personal healthcare workforce is available to people.

- Evaluating effectiveness, access, and quality of personal and population-based health services.

- Conducting research to gain new insights and develop innovative solutions to control or prevent health and safety problems.

Public health departments are not the only organizations that contribute to protecting and promoting the health and safety of state and local populations. A variety of other organizations provide services that protect and promote population health and safety. Public health departments have a leadership responsibility to work with these public health partners to assure all people are served by programs that effectively protect and promote health and safety.

The capability of state and local health departments to perform these roles varies across the United States. This difference in capability leaves some people at greater risk of experiencing a preventable health problem. Such differences in the capacity and performance of public health systems are unacceptable to public health leaders.

To assure state and local public health departments provide effective leadership in the public health system, model standards have been developed to assess the capacity and performance of public health systems and to guide improvement activities. These model standards have been established by the U.S. Centers for Disease Control and Prevention (CDC) in partnership with the Association of State and Territorial Health Officials, the National Association of County and City Health Officials, the National Association of Local Boards of Health, the American Public Health Association, and the Public Health Foundation. Similar standards have been adopted in other countries.

The model standards established by these public health organizations describe an optimal capacity and performance level necessary to effectively deliver the essential services described above. By measuring how well public health systems achieve these model standards, public health departments and their partners can identify improvement needs and take steps to enhance the quality and performance of essential public health services delivery. Improvement in performance of essential services will facilitate effective protection and promotion of everyone's health and safety.

PAUL K. HALVERSON
MICHAEL T. HATCHER

(SEE ALSO: *Association of State and Territorial Health Officials; Boards of Health; Community Health; Community Health Report Cards; Essential Public Health Services; Practice of Public Health; Practice Standards; State and Local Health Departments*)

BIBLIOGRAPHY

Corso, L. C.; Wiesner, P. J.; Halverson, P. K.; and Brown, C. K. (2000). "Using the Essential Services as a Foundation for Performance Measurement and Assessment of Local Public Health Systems." *Journal of Public Health Management and Practice* 6(5):1–18.

Halverson, P. K. (2000). "Performance Measurement and Performance Standards: Old Wine in New Bottles." *Journal of Public Health Management and Practice* 6(5):vi–x.

Harrell, J. A.; Baker, E. L. et al. (1994). *Public Health in America*. Washington, DC: U.S. Public Health Service, Public Health Functions Steering Committee.

Mays, G. P. et al. (1998). "Assessing the Performance of Local Public Systems: A Survey of State Health Agency Efforts." *Journal of Public Health Management and Practice* 4(4):63–77.

Turnock, B. J. (2000). "Can Public Health Performance Standards Improve the Quality of Public Health?" *Journal of Public Health Management and Practice* 6(5):19–25.

PERINATOLOGY

Perinatology, or maternal-fetal medicine, is the subspecialty of obstetrics and gynecology that focuses on the management of high-risk pregnancies and the assessment and treatment of the fetus. By the mid-1970s, knowledge regarding maternal and fetal physiology and disease had evolved to the point where many obstetrician/gynecologists confined their practice to these areas. In 1974, the American Board of Obstetrics and Gynecology began to offer an exam-based certification of special competency in this area. In 1977, the Society of Perinatal Obstetricians (now called the Society for Maternal-Fetal Medicine) was formed.

Modern maternal-fetal medicine specialists devote their professional practice to providing care for, and conducting research on, maternal medical disorders such as diabetes, premature labor, perinatal infectious disease, multiple gestation, and perinatal pharmacology. Additionally, they are actively involved in the assessment and treatment of the fetus. They assess fetal gestational age and growth; evaluate possible congenital anomalies; and assess the placenta and amniotic fluid and the adequacy of uteroplacental function. They employ a number of invasive techniques, such as amniocentesis, chorionic villus sampling, cordocentesis, and fetoscopy, to evaluate the fetus for genetic disorders and alloimmune disorders, evaluate fetal maturity, and treat the fetus with pharmacological agents or blood products.

JUSTIN P. LAVIN, JR.

(SEE ALSO: *Child Health Services; Maternal and Child Health; Pregnancy; Prenatal Care*)

BIBLIOGRAPHY

D'Alton, M. E.; Poole, S.; and Rinehart, R. D. (1997). *Society of Perinatal Obstetricians: The First Two Decades.* Washington, DC: Society of Perinatal Obstetricians.

PERIODIC HEALTH EXAMINATION

The purpose of the periodic health examination is to evaluate health status, screen for risk factors and disease, and provide preventive counseling interventions in an age-appropriate manner. The goal of screening and evaluation is to prevent the onset of disease or the worsening of an existing disease. For example, measurement of blood pressure is intended to detect hypertension so as to initiate treatment and prevent subsequent morbidity (e.g., stroke or renal failure) or mortality. A further goal of the periodic health examination is to educate patients about behavioral patterns or environmental exposures that pose risks for future diseases. Examples include counseling about smoking prevention and cessation to prevent lung cancer and emphysema, seat belt use to prevent motor-vehicle injuries, or modifying sexual practices to prevent the spread of sexually transmitted disease.

In the 1920s the American Medical Association first proposed a yearly, routine physical examination (check-up) for healthy patients. However, there have always been questions about exactly what to include in routine check-ups, and whether they are beneficial. An important principle of clinical medicine is to "do no harm." This is a particular concern when considering testing and counseling in well persons. In 1976, the Canadian Task Force on the Periodic Health Examination was formed to provide a systematic evaluation and recommendations about periodic health exams. The United States Preventive Services Task Force (USPSTF) was formed in 1984 to provide similar guidelines in the United States. The most recent recommendations of the USPSTF for evaluation, screening, and counseling interventions were published in 1996. Input was provided by primary-care medical societies, the U.S. Public Health Service, and the Canadian Task Force on the Periodic Health Examination. These recommendations are based on available evidence of safety and efficacy, and are tailored for patients based upon their individual age, gender, and risk-factor characteristics. Key summary findings of the USPSTF include:

1. Effective interventions that address the patient's individual health behaviors are most important for preventing the leading causes of death and disability (e.g., interventions to prevent smoking, alcohol, and other drug use; encourage use of seat belts; and encourage increased physical activity and appropriate nutrition).

2. The patient and clinician should share responsibility for weighing risks and benefits when deciding about screening and diagnostic testing and preventive interventions.

3. To maximize benefits and avoid doing harm, clinicians should be selective in choosing screening tests and other preventive services for their patients.

4. Special efforts should be taken to provide preventive services to people with less access to care.

5. Community-level public health and public-policy interventions may be more effective for some health problems than interventions delivered in the clinical setting (e.g., community educational interventions to prevent the initial onset of cigarette smoking by children, and seat belt use legislation).

Tables 1, 2, and 3 show the recommended components of the periodic health examination for children, women, and men. The clinical preventive services addressed in these tables are in the areas of immunizations, screening, and counseling. The following are some examples of preventive services offered in these categories, for specific groups.

IMMUNIZATIONS

Immunizations play an important role in the periodic health examination of young children. *Haemophilus influenzae* type B vaccine is an example of the importance of immunization for children. *Haemophilus influenzae* type B (Hib) is a bacterial organism that can cause invasive infections (such as meningitis, blood and soft tissue infections, and pneumonia) with a high risk of morbidity or mortality, particularly in infants in the first year of life, with 85 percent of disease occurring in children under five years of age. Prior

Table 1

Clinical Preventive Services for Normal Risk Children

Intervention	Birth	2 m	4 m	6 m	12 m	15 m	18 m	2 y	4-6 y	11-18 y
Immunizations										
Hepatitis B	x	x		x						
Polio		x	x	x					x	
Haemophilus influenza type B		x	x	x		x				
Diphtheria, Tetanus, Pertussis		x	x	x			x		x	
Measles, mumps, rubella					x				x	x
Varicella					x					
Screening										
Newborn screening (e.g.Hypothyroidism)	x									
Hearing	x									
Head circumference	x	x	x	x	x	x	x	x		
Height and weight	x	x	x	x	x	x	x	x	x	x
Lead					x			x		
Vision	x								x	x
Blood pressure		x			x			x	x	x
Dental health									x	x
Alcohol/Drug use										x
Counseling										
Development, nutrition, & safety	x	x	x	x	x	x	x	x	x	x
Sexually transmitted diseases										x
Tobacco, alcohol, and drug use										x

SOURCE: *Guide to Clinical Preventive Services*, 2nd ed. (1996). Alexandria, VA: Report of the U.S. Preventive Services Task Force, International Medical Publishing Inc.

to the development of effective vaccines, Hib was the leading cause of bacterial meningitis in children under five years of age, and about 500 out of every 100,000 children developed invasive Hib infections. Since the introduction of the Hib vaccine, in 1987, the incidence of invasive Hib disease has decreased by more than 95 percent, to about two per 100,000 children. Currently, immunization recommendations for children include administration of Hib vaccine at two, four, six, and fifteen months of age. Administration is clustered in the age group at highest risk for getting Hib disease, and at the youngest ages that the vaccines produce an effective immune response.

SCREENING

A careful history and a physical examination are important parts of the periodic health examination. The patient history elicits recent and current symptoms or complaints; medications being taken (and any allergies to medications); an accounting of the past medical history of the patient; the social

factors that may impact on the health of the patient (e.g., marital status, household makeup, employment); a family history of illnesses affecting family members; and a review of signs and symptoms for each of the organ systems in the body. The physical examination consists of three modalities to gather information: inspection, auscultation, and palpation. These methods are applied in a systematic way to the major systems of the body. Inspection involves observation of the body part being examined. The general appearance, color, and any other visual characteristics are noted. Auscultation involves listening, often with the aid of a stethoscope. The quality of any sound is noted, including loudness, musical tones, and effect of change in position. Palpation involves feeling both the size and texture of organs under examination. The major areas of the body to be examined are the head and neck, chest, abdomen, extremities, skin, musculoskeletal system, and nervous system. Using the three modalities in conjunction with the patient's medical history and screening tests allows an assessment of the overall health of a patient.

Table 2

Clinical Preventive Services for Normal-Risk Women

Intervention	18-35 years	40-50 years	60+ years
Immuniztions			
Tetanus-diphtheria (every 10 years)	x	x	x
Varicella (2 doses if none as a child)	x	x	x
Measles, mumps, rubella (1 dose)	x	x	
Pneumococcal (one dose)			x
Influenza (yearly)			x
Screening			
Blood pressure, height, weight, dental	x	x	x
Alcohol use	x	x	x
Pap smear (every 1-3 years)	x	x	x
Cholesterol (every 5 years)		x	x
Mammography (every 1-2 years)		x	x
Sigmoidoscopy (every 5-10 years)			x
Fecal occult blood (every year)			x
Vision and hearing (periodically)			x
Counseling			
Calcium intake	x	x	x
Folic acid	x	x	
Hormone replacement therapy		x	x
Mammography screening		x	x
Tobacco, drugs, alcohol, sexually transmitted diseases & safety	x	x	x

SOURCE: *Guide to Clinical Preventive Services*, 2nd ed. (1996). Alexandria, VA: Report of the U.S. Preventive Services Task Force, International Medical Publishing Inc.

Table 3

Clinical Preventive Services for Normal-Risk Men

Intervention	18-35 years	40-50 years	60+ years
Immunizations			
Tetanus-diphtheria (every 10 years)	x	x	x
Varicella (2 doses if none as a child)	x	x	x
Pneumococcal (one dose)			x
Influenza (yearly)			x
Screening			
Blood pressure, height, weight, dental	x	x	x
Alcohol use	x	x	x
Cholesterol (every 5 years)		x	x
Sigmoidoscopy (every 5-10 years)			x
Fecal occult blood (every year)			x
Vision and hearing (periodically)			x
Counseling			
Prostate cancer screening			x
Tobacco, drugs, alcohol, sexually transmitted diseases & safety	x	x	x

SOURCE: *Guide to Clinical Preventive Services,* 2nd ed. (1996). Alexandria, VA: Report of the U.S. Preventive Services Task Force, International Medical Publishing Inc.

pharmacologic therapy according to clinical standards of care.

Screening involves the utilization of a diagnostic procedure to check for the presence of a disease prior to the manifestation of clinical symptoms. Hypertension is a risk factor for coronary heart disease, stroke, and renal disease. Hypertension in adults is defined as having a systolic blood pressure greater than 140 mmHg (millimeters of mercury) and/or a diastolic blood pressure of greater than 90 mmHg on at least three separate occasions. It is well established that decreases in elevated blood pressure, particularly an average 5 to 6 mmHg reduction in diastolic blood pressure reduces the incidence of coronary heart disease and stroke. By measuring the blood pressure at routine health examinations for adult men and women, as shown in Tables 2 and 3, the presence of hypertension can be detected and treatment can be instituted, prior to the development of further complications of the disease. Treatments include weight and diet modification, increased physical activity, assessment for other risk factors or concomitant disease, and prescription of

COUNSELING

Counseling during the periodic health examination is also very important, for this is where physicians recommend changes in lifestyle that can affect future morbidity and mortality. One example is the recommendation that folic acid be taken by women of childbearing age (see Table 2). Folic acid supplementation has been shown to decrease the risk of neural tube defects in newborn infants, especially among women who have had a prior pregnancy with a child with a neural tube defect. The current recommendations of the United States Public Health Service, the American Academy of Pediatrics, and the Canadian Task Force on the Periodic Health Examination is that all women of childbearing age who are capable of becoming pregnant take 0.4 mg of folic acid daily. It is also recommended that women who have had a previous pregnancy affected by a neural tube defect and who are planning to become pregnant again be offered treatment with four mg of folic acid daily, beginning one to three months prior to planned conception and continuing through the first three months of pregnancy.

The periodic health examination is a vital part of health care in the United States. As new information reveals improved methods of detecting and preventing disease and risk factors for disease, and of reducing the morbidity and mortality from illness, clinicians will be able to continue to improve the effectiveness of the periodic health examination.

LEE RACHEL ATKINSON
THOMAS N. ROBINSON

(SEE ALSO: Assessment of Health Status; Blood Pressure; Canadian Task Force on Preventive Health Care; Child Health Services; Folic Acid; Haemophilus Influenzae Type B Vaccine; Immunizations; Influenza; Personal Health Services; Prevention; Preventive Medicine; Primary Care; United States Preventive Services Task Force [USPSTF])

BIBLIOGRAPHY

Canadian Task Force on the Periodic Health Examination (1994). Canadian Guide to Clinical Preventive Health Care. Ottawa: Canada Communication Group.

Committee on Infectious Diseases American Academy of Pediatrics (2000). 2000 Red Book: Report of the Committee of Infectious Diseases, 25th edition. Elk Grove Village, IL: American Academy of Pediatrics.

Green, M., ed. (1994). Bright Futures: Guidelines for Health Supervision of Infants, Children and Adolescents. Arlington, VA: National Center for Education in Maternal and Child Health.

U.S. Preventive Services Task Force (1996). Clinician's Handbook of Preventive Services, 2nd edition. Washington, DC: U.S. Department of Health and Human Services.

—— (1996). Guide to Clinical Preventive Services, 2nd edition. Washington, DC: U.S. Department of Health and Human Services.

PERSISTENT ORGANIC POLLUTANTS (POPS)

Persistent organic pollutants (POPs) are those chemicals that are not materially broken down over a reasonable period of time, usually measured in decades or more. The POPs of most concern are those that build up in the environment or are bioaccumulated and/or biomagnified in the food chain. The realization and importance of persistent environmental chemicals was first identified in the early 1960s with the publication of Rachel Carson's seminal work, Silent Spring. Carson wrote of the buildup of pesticides in birds and hypothesized that this came from direct and indirect (food chain) exposure. The magnitude of effect from Carson's work can be appreciated when one considers the breadth of environmental health sciences today and the international environmental regulations that have been promulgated.

The chemical characteristics of POPs are relatively similar. Many are polyhalogenated aromatic hydrocarbons (PHAHs), or other polycyclic aromatic hydrocarbons (PAHs) that are very slowly metabolized or otherwise degraded. The chemicals are lipid soluble; hence they are stored in the fatty tissue of all animals, and they build up in the food chain. Some classic examples of POPs are the pesticides DDT, Dieldrin, Aldrin, Heptachlor, Mirex, and Kepone. Another group of POPs are the chlorodibenzodioxins, dibenzofurans, and some PCBs. The pesticides were widely used for several years but eventually discontinued for toxicological and ecological reasons. Because of their lipid solubility, the chlorinated compounds are retained and accumulated in the lipids of insects and other invertebrates that are part of the food chain of higher-order predators, and they can eventually end up in the diets of humans and feed animals. Several of these compounds can be sequestered in soil and sediment, such as the PCBs in the Hudson River bottom sediment, where they can exist for decades.

The health effects of these chemicals, as neat compounds, have been very well studied. However, low-dose, lifetime exposure studies are lacking. Many of the organochlorine pesticides cited above are carcinogenic, teratogenic, and neurotoxic. The dioxins and benzofurans are highly toxic and are extremely persistent in the human body as well as the environment. Several of the POPs, including DDT and its metabolites, PCBs, dioxins, and some chlorobenzene, can be detected in human body fat and serum years after any known exposures. Lindane (hexachlorocyclohexane), which was used for the treatment of body lice and as a broad-spectrum insecticide, resulted in very high tissue levels, and in many cases caused acute deaths when used improperly. Lindane and some of its isomers have been identified in market-basket surveys and in human fat samples.

International efforts to minimize exposure to these compounds include the banning of their use except in emergency situations where it has been determined that no other chemical is efficacious. With the exception of DDT, few, if any, of these compounds have been authorized for use. PCBs, which were widely used in capacitors, transformers, and lubricating oils, have not been manufactured for several decades but linger in the environment. Chlorinated dibenzodioxins and dibenzofurans were never products per se, but are byproducts of products made from chlorophenols. The processes by which these final products are manufactured have been altered to minimize the unwanted dioxins. The other source of dioxins is the chlorine bleaching of paper pulp. This bleaching process has been altered to eliminate chlorine, and thereby to eliminate the possibility of dioxins. Several combustion processes also result in the formation of dioxins and benzofurans. Municipal and chemical waste incinerators can be sources of these unwanted by-products. Engineering controls have been put in place in modern facilities to minimize production. However, older and less controlled processes may continue to contaminate the environment.

Polyaromatic hydrocarbons (PAHs) are found in petroleum and petroleum derivatives. The PAHs are also found in the environment as by-products of coal gasification plants. These compounds, though usually less toxic than their chlorinated cousins, are irritants and some are carcinogenic in skin-painting studies in rodents. These compounds break down very slowly and are contaminants in soils of urban and suburban communities. PAHs will bioaccumulate and are found in fat samples of feral animals and humans.

As a broad class, the POPs are inducers of the cytochromes P450 (the so-called drug and chemical metabolizing enzymes), and in many cases the chemicals are carcinogenic. The approach being taken is to identify contaminated sites, isolate the site, remove the contaminated soil, and if possible destroy the contaminants by combustion or other means.

MICHAEL GALLO

(SEE ALSO: *Brownfields; Carson, Rachel; Dioxins; Environmental Movement; Environmental Protection Agency; PCBs; Pollution; Toxicology*)

PERSONAL HEALTH SERVICES

"Personal health services" are the services that an individual receives from others to address health problems or for health promotion and disease prevention. It is helpful to consider the meanings and implications of each of these words. "Personal" is used to connote attention to improving or maintaining an individual's health state, though that state may directly impinge upon others, either in the family or community—there are emotional attachments to sick persons; an individual illness may diminish family resources and capacities; and illnesses have direct implications for communities, such as in the transmission of communicable diseases or in alternative uses for scarce clinical-care resources. Thus, a personal illness can have a profound impact on others, and on the health and well-being of the general public.

"Health" is not an easy term to define (see the discussion elsewhere in this volume), but in the context of health services, there are important conceptual issues. One, as noted above, is the role of health promotion and disease prevention in personal health services. Since many important dimensions of prevention are related to social behaviors or environmental modifications, they are often outside the usual health care system. Another is defining the boundary of health care in terms of appropriate themes. At least in the past, various community health centers and other medical care organizations provided assistance with housing, clothing, and personal legal matters, as well as referral to religious resources. This is not an issue of worthiness, but rather the implication here is that the content of medical services varies and must be explicitly addressed and defined.

The term "services" also requires discussion. While they often connote formal professional services, the patterns and content of care that impinge on a sick individual come from a variety of sources, many of which are neither professional nor part of any organized healing system. The same might be said of the administrative connotation of the term "services," implying not only a single health practitioner, but also care received from a variety of informal sources as well as from well-developed organizations and agencies. In fact, the history and sociology of health services suggest that most sick persons receive health care from diverse sources. Based on anthropological and other studies, there is evidence that all cultures have appointed healers to deal with infirmity. In some societies, these healers may be thought of as using folk, religious, or magical methods; and the sources and content of their lore may not always be clear. In these instances, healing takes place largely in the community, and generally outside of clinics or institutional settings. Interestingly, studying the lore and practices of traditional healing systems, usually in developing countries, has become an important activity in searching for new medicinal or other preventive or therapeutic entities that might have applications in Western societies.

In other societies, healers are much more well organized, and they have generally undergone varying degrees of professionalization and administrative organization. In this case, the healing is often performed in varying types of complex clinics and institutions, usually with a great degree of subspecialization. Nonetheless, no healing system totally dominates a given culture or society, and there are always challenges from alternative healing systems. It has been shown in many countries that many individuals seek and receive health care from highly diverse types of healing systems simultaneously.

LEVELS AND DIMENSIONS OF PERSONAL HEALTH CARE

There is no widely used taxonomy for the elements of personal health services, but there are conventional terms to describe the elements of formal health services hierarchies. One example, referring to the complexity or practitioners' discipline or training, is to consider the level of care as either general, specialty, or subspecialty in nature. Another general approach to care levels is the continuum of primary, secondary, and tertiary care. "Primary care" generally refers to personal care that is broad in scope and does not usually address complex, uncommon illnesses. Primary care is generally intended to be the first contact point when a patient suspects illness, and it provides a comprehensive view of the patient, with full clinical and restorative care for a wide range of common conditions, a full regimen of health promotion and disease prevention activities, and continuity and integration of care when severe or complex illness occurs. Primary care may occur in a variety of locations, but there is a clear community emphasis.

"Secondary care" generally represents the acute general hospital and related institutional and specialty settings in the community where such care is provided; it is intermediate in complexity and intensity. It is more likely to be delivered by specialist practitioners, to be more costly than primary care, and to have few of the attributes of primary care noted above. Primary care practitioners may participate in the delivery of secondary care in certain systems.

"Tertiary care" is the most complex, expensive, and technologically intensive level of care. It is generally available in fewer locations, is extremely resource intensive, and is mostly conducted by subspecialists. Examples include the most sophisticated trauma care, burn treatment units, bone marrow and organ transplant units, and complex types of surgical procedures. Also generally included in tertiary care are rehabilitative and restorative care, which are also a major component of tertiary prevention.

Another axis for understanding personal health care is the notion of "basic health care" versus other "nonbasic" health services. Basic care is not the same as primary care, because almost all definitions of basic care in industrialized nations include access to hospital and rehabilitative care, as well as certain tertiary services. Basic health care is a complex construct that is often the subject of considerable controversy. This controversy stems from diverse moral, social, and economic values about a set of care activities to which all persons in a given society would, or should, have access, if any should be provided at all. The complexity in defining basic health care is illustrative of the nature of personal health care in general.

To begin, a basic set of services might be defined in terms of affordability to individuals and societies. Thus, for fiscal, cultural, and historical reasons, the content of a basic set of services would differ in diverse societies and countries. The content of basic health care would be very different in rural China than in the suburbs of major American cities. Even within a particular country, obtaining political and economic consensus on whether, and how much of, a society's common resources should be provided for a set of basic services is often difficult. Some of this is related to varying views on taxation and the appropriateness of helping programs; other issues relate to moral or value judgments on specific elements of the basic "benefit package." For example, there is great contentiousness about the provision of therapeutic abortion, and about applying stem cells for organogenesis.

Variant views of the content of basic health care and the service package may also occur because of judgmental differences about which services are basic and which are discretionary. Some of this stems from professional and patient competition for a relatively fixed amount of resources, and, within a particular medical system, this is often at the heart of conflicts over basic-care content. For example, cosmetic surgery is often considered to be discretionary, but not all citizens of a given society would agree. Also, there is typically conflict over whether resources should used to provide very expensive services, such as bone marrow transplant, to a few persons, or whether the resources should be used to provide comprehensive primary care to many people. No matter how expensive or rare certain medical procedures may be, it is often politically and morally difficult to explicitly deny a critically ill individual such a service, especially in a more affluent society. Yet the reality is that there are economic and societal limits on the amount of care that can be provided, and a system for rationing and allocating personal health care is always present, even if it is sometimes inconsistent, implicit, and informal.

Sometimes there are diverse opinions concerning the delivery of preventive and health-promotion services as part of a set of basic health services. Prevention is a very important part of clinical care, but preventive services can be expensive, and will thus inevitably compete with illness services for fixed resources.

SOURCES OF PERSONAL HEALTH CARE

There are many sources of personal health care for individuals. These include institutional settings; emergency departments; practitioners' offices; special clinical settings, such as ambulatory surgical centers; and less formal clinical settings in schools, workplaces, and recreational facilities. Formal health services, depending on how they are defined, can be received almost anywhere, including the modest community facilities of some developing countries, sites where nutrition advice or psychological counseling are offered, long-term care facilities, retail pharmacies, and ambulances and other medical transport units. Today, more personal health care encounters occur in the ambulatory setting than in all other settings combined. In fact, the proportion of encounters occurring in institutional settings, such as hospitals, nursing homes, chronic-care facilities, rehabilitation units, and some hospice programs, is generally declining. There are several reasons for this, including their increased geographic distance from most persons, their generally higher costs, the intense amount of requisite labor and technology, and their lesser desirability to patients.

An increasing amount of personal health care is being brought into the home; and sometimes this care can be as complex as that occurring in many ambulatory care or institutional settings. Complex treatments, various kinds of medications, physical or occupational therapy, and chore services have all been brought to the home for reasons of efficiency, quality-of-life, and convenience. Electronic technologies have also brought personal health care into the home in the form of telemedicine. This can represent a great many forms of care, including routine conversations with health professionals, educational activities with health educators or other professionals, automated educational activities or queries about health status, disease management reminders, videoconferencing, and the transmission of physiological and biochemical information relevant to medical practice. Telemedicine has also been used to provide personal health care in special remote settings, such as jobsites or in the military.

The context of care for individual illnesses or for prevention and health promotion also includes less formal health care and healing activities that are not conducted by health professionals. Two of the most important types of informal care are caregiving, which is provided by lay social networks and organizations, and self-care. The most important lay caregivers are families, but such care may also be provided by other relatives, friends, colleagues, the clergy, or representatives of charitable organizations. This source of care cannot be underestimated in terms of amount or importance, and it is an essential complement to formal caregiving within or outside the home, particularly for those with chronic illness and disability. Caregivers assist with major or minor aspects of personal care, including: (a) dispensing of medications and other treatments, (b) providing appropriate nutrition and exercise regimens, (c) assistance with basic personal hygienic activities, (d) general care of children, elders, and those with special needs, (e) transportation to medical facilities or other locations, (f) physiological monitoring, and (g) emotional support through complex illnesses. Caregiving may be extremely burdensome to the caregiver, and it may be detrimental to their emotional and health status.

Self-care is also a necessary and integral part of personal health care. It takes many forms and is often derived from experiences and education within the mainstream care system. Most persons with acute and chronic illnesses must take part in their own care. This might involve physiological and biochemical monitoring, such as blood pressure or blood sugar for diabetes mellitus; communicating a changing health status and symptom manifestations; actively complying with treatment regimens; and even modulation of specific treatments according to signs, symptoms, and other personal data. Self-care also involves health promotion and disease prevention. Much of the burden of maintaining healthful behavior falls to individuals themselves, and while there should be adequate educational and informational resources, including health professional counseling, personal attention to minimizing disease risk and maximizing health status remains critical.

As noted in the introduction, no matter how the mainstream healing system is constituted, there are often alternative healing systems and practices. In most Western societies, a substantial amount of "healing" and perceived prevention comes from alternative or complementary healers and from personal self-care practices. For example, in Western countries, there are many forms of alternative prevention or healing activities that lie outside the orthodox allopathic health care system, and these are often used simultaneously within mainstream care. A substantial proportion of persons take a variety of herbs, nutrition supplements, and other products for health purposes without instructions from mainstream sources. It is likely that all cultures, to a varying extent, indulge in multiple healing systems and practices, and conflicts among them to become dominant are often contentious.

ACCESS TO HEALTH SERVICES

Whatever the content and nature of personal health services within a society, an important dimension is access to that care. "Access" not only implies that individuals and families can easily avail themselves of necessary services for preventive and curative reasons, but also that these services will be used appropriately; and not overused. There can be many barriers to personal health care. The most important are economic barriers, and most countries have made some attempts to minimize these. However, many other actual or potential barriers exist, including poor geographic access, particularly in rural and inner city areas; cultural barriers, in both communication and treatment beliefs, between patients and professionals; inadequate transportation to care sites; and long delays in receiving care once within the care setting.

THE CONTINUING EVOLUTION OF PERSONAL HEALTH SERVICES

The nature and organization of personal health services, as with other social activities, is in constant evolution. While many of the types of services have been mentioned above, it is useful for historical and rhetorical purposes to describe their continuing evolution, beginning with the base period of the mid nineteenth century, and noting trends and forces that have shaped today's health care system. Many forces shape personal health services, and their relative roles are sometimes difficult to discern. In general, nineteenth-century prototypic Western medicine can be thought of as a loosely bound set of individual practitioners dealing with individual patients on a "retail" basis. Medicine in this period has been described as a "cottage industry." Payment for care was almost entirely the patient's and family's burden. Institutional care existed, but mostly for small numbers of patients with mental illness or communicable diseases. Hospitals were often church-operated and were largely dedicated to persons with incurable, progressive, and terminal illnesses. However, nearly all births and deaths took place in the home. Health care then began to evolve due to a variety of important forces.

Incorporation of Science and Technology. The continuing injection of scientific discoveries and technological innovations has changed health care dramatically. It has allowed a much more detailed understanding of the causes and pathogenesis of many diseases and conditions, as well as a substantial increase in illness cure and remediation—a great triumph of the twentieth century. These advances have also fostered tremendous shifts in the nature of personal health services. For example, rapidly advancing medical knowledge has led to the need for professional specialization and an elaboration and extension of professional training programs to achieve more enlightened approaches to treating specific and complex health problems. However, the injection of science and technology has had effects viewed by many as adverse, including the role of specialization in fragmenting health-services delivery, the creation of new and serious adverse effects of some therapies, such as malignancies caused by diagnostic and therapeutic radiation, and the large increase in personal health care costs, sometimes for gains viewed as marginal. There have also been environmental threats, such as those due to inadequate medical-waste disposal. Some new health care technologies, as noted above, have also caused moral and ethical dilemmas that defy easy solutions.

The continued application of science and technology has itself become more formalized. While scientific findings have always been translated into clinical practice, more recently there has been an increasing interest in, and new methods for, summarizing published scientific literature. These techniques include meta-analysis, a formal analytical combination of data from multiple studies of a given topic. Increased attention to published, peer-reviewed, scientific findings has led to evidence-based medicine, a philosophy and method of practice that emphasizes translating summarized scientific findings into clinical decision-making.

Insurance and Other Payment Systems for Clinical Care. Before the late nineteenth century, personal health care was generally paid for by patients and their families, supplemented to some extent by charity care from religious and other philanthropic organizations. Governments provided little health care except for the military and special groups in their charge. As the promise of medical care grew, private organizations, beginning with guilds and labor unions, instituted health insurance to pay for the more complex, expensive care—often related to hospitals. These programs eventually grew into the large health insurance industry that exists today. Simultaneously, governments began to fund more personal health services, often beginning with attention to maternal and child health services and indigent care. Most Western governments also began to provide direct health services, using such mechanisms as community health centers, clinics managed by public health agencies, and the provision of health professionals to communities lacking access to health services. Western governments currently fund a broad range of personal health services, ranging from the provision of nearly all health care, such as in the United Kingdom, to care for only certain segments of the population, such as in the United States, where all levels of government pay over 40 percent of national health care costs. In all cases, these funds come largely from general taxation and employer-employee taxes. Overlying these practices are the professed moral imperatives of providing basic health care to all citizens.

The Increasing Organizational Complexity of Personal Health Care Delivery. Simultaneously with advancing and diverse payment systems for care, there has been a companion growth in larger and more complex organizational forms of personal care delivery. Beginning with small groups of physicians and others joining in common administrative units (group practice), there has been a gradual development of large, complex medical-delivery organizations, ranging from nonprofit cooperatives to for-profit national and multinational corporations. These growing administrative entities may own all the service-delivery components and employ health professionals, or they may work through complex contractual arrangements with physicians, patient groups, insurers, employee/employer organizations, and government agencies. These entities usually have an explicit set of services (the "benefit package"), which are prepaid from various sources; and they may profess to emphasize preventive services (the "health maintenance organization"); but most systems have come under the heading of "health plans" or "managed care." In some situations, managed-care organizations are structured or regulated to compete with each other in an attempt to use market forces to control health care costs. Very few clinical practices are free of some form of managed care or superimposed administrative and regulatory authority.

It is difficult to summarize the effects of corporatization on personal health care, and all health care organizations are constantly reforming themselves. Conceivably, there are several salient strengths for large, tightly administrated care systems. Care costs can be more fully monitored, rationalized, and modulated, and some economies of scale may be present. Quality assurance monitoring—through large information systems, with subsequent interventions—should be facilitated more easily than in multiple, small delivery units. Similarly, the dissemination of evidence-based practice guidelines and continuing professional education programs are likely to be enhanced. Strong liaison with public health programs, such as for surveillance, communicable disease control, and public education, could conceivably enhance these activities when compared to traditional programs working wholly outside of personal care systems. However, there have been criticisms of these systems as well, including inappropriate limitations on the doctor-patient encounter; lack of responsiveness to special community needs; repeated changes in health-system contractors, which promotes discontinuity of care; a lack of competition among plans in many areas; inadequate attention to indigents and others without health insurance; and the avoidance of persons with complex and costly illnesses, such as patients with certain cancers, AIDS (acquired immunodeficiency syndrome), renal failure, or complex rehabilitation needs. Large, consolidated health systems seem to be growing and maturing,

however, and a return to small, independent care delivery units is unlikely. Thus, it is necessary for all health-delivery systems to promote continued refinement and efficiency so that societal goals for personal health care can be met.

Consumerism in Personal Health Care. As in other commercial affairs arenas, there has been a substantial impact by health care consumers on the delivery of personal care. This is not new, but the intensity of consumer participation in the care process is increasing. For example, health care organizations have become more responsive to consumer complaints and concerns, and many institutions have ombudsmen to assist patients with perceived service problems. Medical consumers often have places on steering committees or boards of directors, as well as on boards and committees reviewing research proposals for ethical concerns. Patients and others have also had an impact through participation in a variety of community-based organizations and associations, often centering on the concern for a particular illness or type of health service. These organizations work to enhance the amount and quality of patient care, and also participate in the political process to achieve particular goals. Finally, many governmental jurisdictions have laws and regulations that protect elements of consumer rights when participating in health care organizations. The degree to which consumer participation has shaped health care is a matter of dispute, but that some level of enhancement and responsiveness has occurred is clear.

Quality Assurance in the Health Care Setting. While it is likely that most health professionals have always strived for the highest quality of service attainable, modern organizational reforms have added more explicit oversight of the quality of care. These are performed by many different sources, including government-funded organizations and their institutional inspectors, health care insurers, voluntary professional organizations, and health care systems and organizations themselves. Quality assurance takes many forms, including direct monitoring of the care process through record abstraction, assessing health system administrative functions, deriving norms for utilization rates for various elements of care, selecting various index illnesses and procedures for detailed outcome measurement, tracking the health and social problems of health care professionals, monitoring adverse health events due to the care process, and, in some instances, publishing various aspects of hospital and health system performance. Quality assurance programs normally result in both organizational and technical-practice changes, which in general would be the most desired result.

An Emphasis on Prevention. With all the professional, technical, and administrative changes in the delivery of personal health services, there has also been a renewed interest in delivering evidence-based clinical preventive services. In many health care venues, detailed information on patients' prevention histories and needs are collected, and in some places manual or automated reminders assist professionals in the timely delivery of preventive care. Many quality-assurance criteria sets have minimum goals for the proportion of patients who should receive evidence-based preventive interventions. However, preventive and health-promotional services can have substantial attendant costs, and health education and counseling can consume a large amount of professional time. Thus, all health care organizations have had to find efficient and effective ways to deliver preventive care in the context of their professional practices, and this has often been challenging.

SUMMARY

Substantial organizational, technical, scientific, economic, and cultural forces have shaped the nature and content of personal health care, and for sick and disabled individuals, the sources of care have increased in breadth and sophistication. At the heart of clinical care, however, there remains a well-established process that has not materially changed, characterized by communication, education, compassion, empathy, and dignity. Successful health systems must preserve these elements as they evolve and grow.

ROBERT B. WALLACE

(SEE ALSO: *Access to Health Services; Alternative, Complementary, and Integrative Medicine; Economics of Health; Evidence-Based Medicine; Health; Health Care Financing; Inequalities in Health; Managed Care; Medicaid; Medicare;* *National Health Insurance; National Health Systems; Nurse; Physician; Preventive Medicine; Primary Care; Psychology, Health; Theories of Health and Illness; Uninsurance*)

BIBLIOGRAPHY

Jonas, S. (1998). *An Introduction to the U.S. Health Care System,* 4th edition. New York: Springer Publishing Co.

Jonas, S., and Kovner, A. R., eds. (1999). *Jonas and Kovner's Health Care Delivery in the United States,* 6th edition. New York: Springer Publishing Co.

Kohn, L. T.; Corrigan, J. M.; and Donaldson, M. S., eds. (2001). *To Err Is Human. Building a Safer Health Care System.* Washington, DC: National Academy Press.

Lighter, D. E. (2000). *Principles and Methods of Quality Management in Health Care.* Gaithersburg, MD: Aspen Publishers.

Lowe, N. K., and Ryan-Wenger, N. M. (1999). "Over-the-Counter Medications and Self-Care." *Nurse Practitioner* 24(12):34–44.

Roemer, M. I. (1991–1993). *National Health Systems of the World.* New York: Oxford University Press.

PERSONNEL

See Careers in Public Health

PERSON-TIME RATES

See Rates

PERTUSSIS

Pertussis (whooping cough) is a highly communicable infectious disease caused by the bacterium *Bordetella pertussis.* Pertussis is characterized by spasms (paroxysms) of severe coughing. The cough spasms are often followed by vomiting and by a characteristic inspiratory "whoop." The incubation period is about 7 to 20 days. Pertussis starts with symptoms similar to those of a minor upper respiratory infection and is followed by several weeks of episodes of paroxysmal coughing. Pertussis can occur among persons of any age, regardless of vaccination status, and may be relatively common among adolescents and adults in the United States, although infants less than one year old have the highest rates of reported disease. Infants with pertussis commonly require hospitalization and may die.

Between 1940 and 1945 in the United States, an average of 175,000 cases and 2,700 deaths occurred from pertussis each year. A vaccination program has been in place in the United States since 1948; in the 1990s, an average of 6,000 pertussis cases and 12 deaths are reported each year.

The U.S. vaccination schedule is five doses of diphtheria and tetanus toxoids and acellular pertussis vaccine (DtaP) for children under 7 years of age: three doses at ages 2, 4, and 6 months, a fourth dose at 15 to 18 months of age, and the fifth dose at 4 to 6 years. No pertussis vaccine is currently licensed for use in persons 7 years old or older.

Early diagnosis and antimicrobial treatment of case-patients may lessen the severity of symptoms and limit the period of communicability; treatment of close contacts can provide protection from developing pertussis.

KRISTINE M. BISGARD

(SEE ALSO: *Communicable Disease Control*)

BIBLIOGRAPHY

American Public Health Association (2000). "Pertussis." In *Control of Communicable Diseases Manual*, 17th edition, ed. A. S. Benenson. Washington, DC: Author.

Edwards, K. M.; Decker, M. D.; and Mortimer, E. A., Jr. (1999). "Pertussis Vaccine." In *Vaccines*, 3rd edition, eds. S. A. Plotkin and W. A. Orenstein. Philadelphia, PA: W. B. Saunders.

Guris, D.; Strebel, P. M.; Bardenheier, B. et al. (1999). "Changing Epidemiology of Pertussis in the United States: Increasing Reported Incidence among Adolescents and Adults, 1990–1996." *Clinical Infectious Disease* 28:1230–1237.

PESTICIDES

Pesticides are a broad class of chemicals and biological agents that are specifically designed and applied to kill a pest. Specific types of pesticides target specific types of pests: insecticides kill insects, fungicides kill fungi and bacteria, herbicides kill weeds and other unwanted plant vegetation, molluscacides kill mollusks, acaricides kill spiders, and so on. Pesticide use dates back to ancient times.

Pesticides are regulated in the United States at both the federal and state level. The primary legislation, one of the oldest environmental laws, is the Federal Insecticide, Fungicide, and Rodenticide Act (FIFRA, 1972), which is administered by the Environmental Protection Agency (EPA). Each state also has an agency responsible for carrying out FIFRA mandates. These agencies may be environmental or agricultural in nature, depending on the state. State laws can be more restrictive than the federal laws.

Pesticides are sometimes called "economic poisons." They are developed to kill something, and they are, therefore, inherently toxic. Pesticides that are less toxic are classified as "general use pesticides." These can be purchased by the average homeowner and applied without any special license or permits. More toxic compounds are called "restricted use pesticides" and their use requires a license. In some cases the restricted use materials have the same active ingredients as the general use materials, but at a higher concentration.

Anything that claims that it has pesticidal activity is, by law, a pesticide, and is subject to registration by the EPA and local state agencies. Household cleaners and bleach are legally pesticides—the pesticide registration number can be found on the product container.

Within the broad classes of products that have similar types of action (e.g., weed killers, insect killers) there are further distinctions regarding the type of chemistry. For example, among insect killers, there are synthetic pyrethroids, organophosphates, and organochlorines. The most well known are the organochlorines, such as chlordane and DDT, which became popular after World War II, and were used in agriculture, and for home and commercial use, for decades. These compounds have low acute toxicity, but are persistent in the environment and have caused a series of long-term environmental health problems. They remain in soil and tissue for a very long time, and they have been shown to have a harmful impact on animal endocrine systems. Most organochlorines were phased out of use in the 1980s. They were replaced by organophosphate materials that are less persistent, but more acutely toxic. In the beginning of the 1990s these compounds, too, were beginning to be phased out through government actions, and voluntarily by the manufacturers.

Pesticides have entered the food system in many parts of the world. Though credited with an enormous increase in food and fiber production, indiscriminate use of these products has led to acute and long-term health problems for humans and animals. There are risks associated with the application of a pesticide into a system, while at the same time there are benefits for using these materials to reduce disease, increased food production, and lessen the risk of starvation.

Pesticides have been applied in many part of the world to control vector-borne diseases such as malaria, yellow fever, dengue, and others. The most prudent way to balance the benefits with the risks is an integrated approach to pesticide use, combining all control methods—physical, biological, cultural, and chemical.

MARK G. ROBSON

(SEE ALSO: *Environmental Movement; Environmental Protection Agency; Fungicides; Toxicology*)

BIBLIOGRAPHY

Hayes, W., and Laws, E. (1991). *Handbook of Pesticide Toxicology*, Vol. 1. San Diego, CA: Academic Press.

Wallace, R., ed. (1998). *Maxcy-Rosenau-Last Public Health and Preventive Medicine*. Stamford, CT: Appleton and Lange.

PHARMACEUTICAL INDUSTRY

The pharmaceutical industry has two distinct functions: research and development (R&D), and manufacturing. Some firms are primarily engaged in R&D, while others concentrate on manufacturing. The largest and best-known pharmaceutical firms do both.

Research-oriented firms include the large, well-known drug producers, which are often multinational firms with a presence in the three largest drug markets—the United States, Europe, and Japan. Others are smaller, and usually younger, firms that are attempting to develop a narrower range of products. This grouping includes most biotechnology firms, few of which have so far succeeded in bringing the results of their research to market. Among the manufacturers are firms producing generic drugs—products that are in many ways equivalent to existing drugs whose patents have expired.

The number of pharmaceutical manufacturers is large; the Department of Commerce listed nearly 1,500 in 1997. This might suggest that the industry is highly competitive. But the number of pharmaceutical compounds is also very large. The *Physician's Desk Reference* lists 1,300 different distinct compounds. In spite of the large number of drug products, there are so many therapeutic classes that the number of products that are substitutes for one another, and hence compete with each other, is small. So though the industry as a whole is highly competitive, individual products are less so.

Another remarkable characteristic of the pharmaceutical industry is its high rate of investment in R&D, with a correspondingly rapid pace of product innovation. U.S. firms, for example, spent over $21 billion in R&D in the United States and abroad in 1998, an increase of nearly 11 percent from the year before. Expenditures in 1999 were estimated to be over $24 billion, an annual increase of 14 percent. These investments represent a 12 percent share of total revenue, a share that is nearly double that of most other industries, including office equipment, electronics, and telecommunications companies. This rate of investment has enabled the U.S. pharmaceutical industry to produce nearly half of all patented drugs that were introduced globally between 1975 and 1994.

The high rates of innovation that characterize the pharmaceutical industry result from high rates of return on investment in R&D, which create the incentives necessary to conduct this research. This implies that R&D will typically flow to clinical areas characterized by relatively large markets—either large numbers of patients; or purchasers willing to pay prices that, in the long run, cover the costs and risks of these investments. Smaller markets or markets that are unable to pay such prices will rarely attract these investments.

The Orphan Drug Act was enacted by Congress in 1984 to create incentives to encourage manufacturers to develop products for diseases affecting relatively small numbers of patients. Following the act's passage, many drugs were developed and introduced addressing these relatively rare diseases. To replicate the act's success in a broader international context, however, would require support of international organizations such as the World Health Organization or the World Bank.

STUART O. SCHWEITZER

(SEE ALSO: *Antibiotics; Drug Resistance; Economics of Health*)

BIBLIOGRAPHY

Barral, P. E. (1996). *Twenty Years of Pharmaceutical Research Results Throughout the World.* Paris: Rhone Poulenc Foundation.

Physicians Desk Reference, 54th edition (2000). Montvale, CA: Medical Economics Company.

PHENYLKETONURIA

Phenylketonuria (PKU) is an autosomal recessive disorder that results from phenylalanine hydroxylase (PAH) deficiency. If uncontrolled, PKU leads to mental retardation. The prevalence is approximately 1 in 10,000 in temperate climates and varies by race, with a frequency of 1 in 8,000 in U.S. Caucasians, and 1 in 50,000 in African Americans. Many mutant alleles are present in the population. The high frequency of defective genes suggests that there is an advantage to being a carrier, perhaps due to resistance to natural toxins. Newborn screening (with the Guthrie test) is mandated by law and is critical because the mental retardation is treatable by restricting dietary intake of phenylalanine and/or ingesting a form of phenylalanine ammonia lysase, a plant enzyme. Unfortunately, the offspring of affected mothers are typically mentally retarded, even when the child's endogenous PAH activity is adequate.

HARRY W. SCHROEDER, JR.

(SEE ALSO: *Congenital Anomalies; Genetic Disorders; Genetics and Health; Newborn Screening*)

BIBLIOGRAPHY

Scriver, C. R.; Eisensmith, R. C.; Woo, S. L. C.; and Kaufman, S. (1994). "The Hyperphenylalaninemias of Man and Mouse." *Annual Review of Genetics* 28:141–165.

PHILOSOPHICAL BASIS FOR PUBLIC HEALTH

Before embarking on a discussion of the philosophy of public health, it is important to be clear on terminology and scope. "Philosophy" means how and what people think about basic and longstanding human concerns such as knowledge, reasoning, free will, morality, objectivity and rationality, facts and values, and freedom. Although philosophy is often discussed at abstract "high ground" levels, this chapter will provide philosophy at a level much closer to everyday concerns. Call it the user-friendly "middle ground" level (Blackburn, 1999). It is important to make philosophy matter—to connect it—to how we think about and practice public health.

"Public health," like philosophy, is not easy to define. A recent definition states that "public health is the prevention of disease and premature death through organized community effort" (Beauchamp, 1995). This is a good but narrow definition, omitting prevention activities that have been historically important at the individual level, say between physician and patient. It also ignores injuries and other preventable conditions not traditionally considered diseases. However it is defined, public health is a complex force in society.

Combining philosophy and public health is like creating a giant tapestry from an inexhaustible supply of threads. Weaving philosophical concerns into the fabric of public health can look like this: knowledge is generated in the form of objective evidence from studies in biology, epidemiology, and social science; these facts provide a rational basis for undertaking interventions designed to prevent disease, injury, or death; these actions also reflect community values—some communities constrain an individual's freedom in the name of the common good. For example, U.S.-based airlines do not permit smoking, reflecting U.S. health concerns and policies. Other communities do not ask the same of their members—smoking is permitted on many international airlines.

PROBLEMS FOR THE PHILOSOPHER OF PUBLIC HEALTH

Making sense of contradictory community values is only one task for the philosopher of public health. There are conceptual problems, including ontological concerns such as defining health, disease, and causation. There are problems of knowledge, logic and scientific discovery, including epistemological concerns such as the absence of rigorous proof or disproof (underdetermination) and the nature of causal inferences. And there are problems of goodness and action; such as ethical concerns about how public health interventions reflect beneficence and how they address conditions of social and environmental justice. A central ethical problem is the extent to which individual autonomy is constrained in the name of the common good when public health interventions are implemented.

These sorts of problems can be illustrated in real-life situations, such as case studies that reflect the complex context of contemporary society. Public health, for example, is closely connected to both science and medicine.

CASE STUDY: A TRIP TO THE DOCTOR

Suppose that a few days after returning from an out-of-town trip, you feel acutely ill. You have a high fever, productive cough, and a vague sense that things will get worse before they get better. You drive to a clinic for treatment where you are examined by nurse and physician alike, who ask and probe and listen to your story and prescribe pink pills that you swallow with water from the drinking fountain. Driving home, you consider the doctor's suggestion to participate in a research study of overweight former smokers. She said that you have an increased risk of cancer and that the research will test whether that risk can be reduced by adhering to a diet high in special nutritional compounds, regular exercise, and screening tests. "Free treatment, if it comes to that," she said. "Why should I participate?" you asked. "Will it prevent cancer? Will I lose weight?" "Hard to say," she replied. "At best, we'll learn how to prevent cancer in our community. We have very high rates here. We do the science so that we know what is the best thing to do for many people."

As you experience these events, you stepped into the Venn diagram—the overlapping intersection—of public health medicine, and science. Medicine and public health both rely upon nearly identical definitions of health and disease.

Medicine and public health rely largely upon the same types of scientific studies. Medicine and public health apply scientific knowledge to individuals and populations, respectively, and thus create both opportunities for doing good and for doing harm.

There are also stark contrasts between medicine and public health. Medicine treats the sick individual; and it has the physician-patient relationship at its core. Public health prevents illness and injury in populations. The conditions under which interventions are undertaken may also be quite different. Public health actions are precautionary in nature, using available scientific evidence as a warrant. Public health involves the diffusion of information through communities empowered to help themselves, often with little input from health professionals.

Making sense out of these complex arrangements between public health and medicine and science is a major task for those who "think" about the philosophy of public health.

WHY PHILOSOPHY MATTERS

Philosophy matters because it helps us to better understand the problems of public health and how they are connected to the problems of medicine, science, and society. It can help to make clear what is meant by health and disease. Centuries ago, some conditions were believed to be the visitations of evil sprits, and today we believe them to be caused by microscopic organisms. And we "know" that our current belief is a better belief, based on using scientific tools and techniques. Philosophy, when connected to history, helps us to understand the significance of these and future changes in knowledge. What we "know" today about genes and cancer, lifestyles and heart disease, and environmental exposures and asthma will evolve, as history indicates, into something different.

What are the causes of disease? How shall we go about discovering them? These are key public health questions with important links to longstanding discussions in science and in philosophy. When is disease prevention a good thing to undertake? How can we best balance the risks and the benefits of intervening? What will society gain (and lose) from successful prevention efforts? These are central questions not only for the public health practitioner but also for the philosopher of public health. Each may start their "think" on these questions at slightly different places, but each has a compelling interest in complementary answers.

The public health practitioner examines the known causes of a disease and the impact of interventions, and then implements appropriate actions. The philosopher examines how the concepts of cause and prevention have evolved over the years, how uncertainty and the relationship between hypothesis and evidence influence the process of discovery, and may also declare a set of guiding general ethical principles that apply when implementing preventive interventions in specific cases. Yet, regardless of where the inquiries of practitioner and philosopher begin, they should be intertwined. It matters how a cause is defined and how we judge it to be present when we decide to intervene to prevent disease. It matters that an intervention designed to control disease or early death may result in harm to some exposed to it; this is a central problem in the ethics of public health screening programs. And it matters that public health relies upon the social fabric of a community—including powerful medical, legal, and political forces—to get much of its work done.

PUBLIC HEALTH'S PHILOSOPHICAL JOURNEY

Causation, ethics, science, and society are some of the signposts along public health's philosophical journey. Imagine three traveling companions— a citizen, a public health professional, and a philosopher—each asked to comment upon a government regulation requiring communitywide testing of a disease marker. The citizen may respond, "How can the government tell me what I must do with my body . . . and how do I know this screening will do me any good?!" The public health professional may respond, "What is the scientific evidence that the test finds early disease, and how certain are we that early treatment is a cost-effective way to reduce mortality in a community?" The philosopher, in turn, may ask, "What moral maxims warrant a decision requiring such screening, and how are they connected to the principles of autonomy and beneficence, theories of justice and utility, and the ever-present uncertainty of scientific knowledge?"

Public health, with its core concepts of prevention, community, methodology, disease, and health, and with its strong ties to science and the humanities, will benefit from philosophical inquiry when these three travelers find ways to help each other answer their respective questions. The precise nature of that extended conversation may include abstract "high ground" general theories, but it can also be conceived as an approach to problem-solving that connects longstanding human intellectual concerns, that connects the goals and activities of communities, that, and most importantly, affects the health of the human population.

THE PHILOSOPHICAL BASIS OF PUBLIC HEALTH

The philosophy of public health cuts across the realms of ontology, epistemology, and ethics as it strives to make sense of what public health is, what knowledge it can claim, and whether efforts to change the determinants and distribution of disease in the name of the common good are warranted. A core concern of a philosophy of public health is the balance between the interests of communities and populations and those of individuals. These interests spring from two complementary and essential public health goals: the prevention of disease and the promotion of health and well-being.

Scientific method, analysis, and synthesis play key roles in a philosophy of public health. Systems, theories, and models of disease causation are among its central explanatory themes. Public health relies upon the creative forces of scientific discovery and the accumulation of objective knowledge that rests upon a foundation of probabilistic events. Uncertainty runs through it like a river. Hypotheses ranging from the molecular constructs of biology to the dynamic forces of society will be tested by quantitative and qualitative methodologies representing distinct yet connected scientific disciplines. Despite the heavy weight of paradigmatic pressures, the methods of public health science are dynamic. Underdetermination, a fundamental state of evidentiary uncertainty, will plague strong inferences. Consensus on reasoned judgments from available scientific evidence will determine when preventive actions should be undertaken and by whom and at what cost.

Public health is soaked with values; and most often, those of the common good will be paramount. The philosophy of public health incorporates the values and traditions of communities and of relevant professions, providing an intellectual foundation for organized action to reduce suffering and promote well-being. The philosophy of public health will provide a guide for understanding how beneficent and precautionary actions can and should occur, tempered as they are by the global diversity of cultures, the complex interactions of human society with natural and constructed environments, and fundamental human rights.

Although a unique entity, the philosophy of public health is closely connected to political philosophy, economics, history, and law, just as it is connected to bioethics, and the philosophies of science, biology, and medicine.

We have a long journey ahead.

DOUGLAS L. WEED

(SEE ALSO: *Beneficence; Benefits, Ethics and Risks; Environmental Justice; Ethics of Public Health; Policy for Public Health; Screening; Social and Behavioral Sciences; Social Determinants*)

BIBLIOGRAPHY

Ayer, A. J. (1984). *Philosophy in the Twentieth Century.* New York: Vintage.

Beaglehole, R., and Bonita, R. (1997). *Public Health at the Crossroads.* Cambridge, UK: Cambridge University Press.

Beauchamp, D. E. (1995). "Philosophy of Public Health." In *Encyclopedia of Bioethics,* ed. W. T. Reich. New York: Simon & Schuster.

Blackburn, S. (1999). *Think.* Oxford, UK: Oxford University Press.

Cole, P. (1994). "The Moral Bases for Public Health Interventions." *Epidemiology* 6:78-83.

Duffy, J. (1992). *The Sanitarians: A History of American Public Health.* Urbana: University of Illinois Press.

Gillon, R. (1990). "Ethics in Health Promotion and Prevention of Disease." *Journal of Medical Ethics* 16:171-172.

Horton, R. (1998). "The *New* New Public Health of Risk and Radical Engagement." *Lancet* 352:251-252.

Last, J. M. (1991). "Ethics and Public Health Policy." In *Public Health and Preventive Medicine,* eds. J. M. Last and R. B. Wallace. Norwalk, CT: Appleton and Lange.

Nijhuis, H. G. J., and Van der Maesen, L. J. G. (1994). "The Philosophical Foundations of Public Health: An Invitation to Debate." *Journal of Epidemiology and Community Health* 48:1-3.

Raffensperger, C., and Ticker, J. (1999). *Protecting Public Health and the Environment: Implementing the Precautionary Principle.* Washington, DC: Island Press.

Rose, G. (1985). "Sick Individuals and Sick Populations." *International Journal of Epidemiology* 14:32-38.

Weed, D. L. (1995). "Epidemiology, the Humanities, and Public Health." *American Journal of Public Health* 85:914-918.

—— (1997). "Underdetermination and Incommensurability in Contemporary Epidemiology." *Kennedy Institute of Ethics Journal* 7:107-127.

—— (1999). "Towards a Philosophy of Public Health." *Journal of Epidemiology and Community Health* 53:99-104.

PHYSICAL ACTIVITY

Exercise, sport, play, games, dance—these and many other terms have been used to describe the wide variety of pursuits considered to be physical activity. "Physical activity" is a universal term defined as "bodily movement that is produced by the contraction of skeletal muscles and that substantially increases the amount of energy you expend" (USDHHS, 1996). "Exercise" is narrower in focus and is defined as "one type of physical activity conducted with the intent of developing physical fitness" (Corbin and Pangrazi, 1998). The term is typically used for calisthenics, resistance exercises, stretching exercises designed for flexibility, and aerobic exercises specifically designed to improve cardiovascular fitness. Sport, play, games, dance, and recreational activities are all different forms of physical activity, some more organized than others.

PHYSICAL ACTIVITY: A BRIEF HISTORY

Throughout history, the importance of physical activity to health and fitness has been acknowledged as an important component of life, along with work, play, and social, religious, and cultural activities. The early Greeks knew the importance of a sound body to hardy spirits and tough minds.

The Olympics exemplify the place of prominence they afforded to physical activity. Hippocrates, generally known as the father of medicine, expressed interest in the hygienic value of exercise. As early as 3000 to 1000 B.C.E. the Chinese described the principle of human harmony, a concept that valued the role of physical activity. Various Native American and African groups also have featured active lifestyles and physical activity prominently in their cultures.

Early Europeans also knew the value of regular physical activity. In the seventeenth century, John Dryden (1631–1700) wrote: "Better to hunt in fields, for health unbought, than fee the doctor for nauseous draught; the wise, for cure, on exercise depend; God never made his work for man to mend" (Paffenbarger and Hyde, 1980). By the late 1800s, the General Hygiene movement had begun. Physical activity in the United States was championed in the late 1880s by physicians—many who were greatly influenced by their European heritage—who focused on promoting exercise programs in schools with the intent of improving health. These programs, later referred to as physical education, were the principal sources of public efforts to promote physical activity in the late nineteenth and early twentieth century. From 1900 through the mid-1950s a primary reason for the promotion of physical activity (exercise) was to prepare men for war. During this same time there was an increased emphasis on school sports, with an emphasis on college athletic programs. Physical activity, as a social phenomenon, was principally an endeavor for males, however.

In 1956, President Dwight D. Eisenhower established the President's Council on Youth Fitness, a cabinet-level agency, reflecting a growing concern for the lack of fitness among American youth, specifically a concern that many youth were considered unfit for war. In 1957, the American Medical Association joined in the public effort by endorsing the president's new council. For much of the mid–twentieth century, youth fitness and physical activity were the focus of public attention.

The year 1960 is generally considered to be when the "physical fitness boom" began in the United States. It was during this period that the American College of Sports Medicine (ASCM) was founded and Dr. Kenneth Cooper's book *Aerobics* (1968) was published. These two events did much to make Americans aware of the health benefits of physical activity. In 1961, Hans Kraus and Wilhelm Raab published the book *Hypokinetic Disease*, which many consider to be a landmark publication linking disease to physical inactivity. Hypokinetic diseases (health problems associated with inactive lifestyles) became a topic for increased study by the medical and research communities. From 1950 through the 1980s the study of physical activity epidemiology led researchers to conclude that there was evidence "that the relationship between exercise and good health is more than circumstantial. If some questions are not yet answered, they are far less important than those that have been" (Paffenbarger and Hyde, 1980). In 1996, *Physical Activity and Health: A Report of the Surgeon General* synthesized the mounting evidence that physical activity and good health are inextricably linked.

PHYSICAL ACTIVITY PATTERNS IN MODERN CULTURE

The human organism is designed to be physically active. Anthropologists indicate that the need to be active is associated with our need to find food, fight predators, and to flee for safety. While the "fight or flight" response that prepares people for physical activity still exists, automation and technology have freed many from the heavy physical labor that was characteristic of previous generations. The American workweek decreased from 70 hours in 1860 to less than 40 hours in the year 2000. Baseline data for the national health goals for the year 2010 indicate that 40 percent of the adults eighteen years of age and older do no regular leisure time activity. Approximately 23 percent of adults in the United States report regular vigorous physical activity (20 minutes or more 3 days a week) and only 15 percent report moderate physical activity equal to brisk walking (30 minutes on at least 5 days a week). Health goals for 2010 outline the need to increase these proportions— by 15 to 30 percent for vigorous activity and 23 to 30 percent for moderate activity—and to reduce sedentary behaviors from 40 percent to 20 percent. Goals are also outlined for increasing participation in physical activities such as resistance training for muscle fitness and stretching for developing flexibility.

Also apparent is the decline in physical activity from childhood to adulthood. Sedentary behavior is almost nonexistent among young children (about 6 percent for boys and 8 percent for girls) but increases to more than 20 percent by age twenty (22 percent for males and 25 percent for females). Vigorous activity decreases from 71 percent for boys and 66 percent for girls at age twelve to 43 percent for males and 28 percent for females at age twenty. Moderate activity levels decrease from 39 percent for boys and 32 percent for girls at age twelve to 22 percent for males and 21 percent for females at age twenty.

Different segments of the population are more active than others. Beginning in childhood and continuing throughout life, males are more active than females, with differences varying depending on the type of activity. Disparities in activity levels are also apparent for various ethnic groups. African Americans, Hispanics, and Native Americans, for example, are typically less active than non-Hispanic whites. To some extent these differences are influenced by education and socioeconomic status. Low socioeconomic groups with low education levels are less likely to be active than middle and high socioeconomic groups with higher education levels. The fact that minority populations are underrepresented in the upper socioeconomic and upper education levels could account for some of the differences in activity levels among ethnic groups.

PHYSICAL ACTIVITY AND HEALTH

Medical progress in preventing and treating infectious disease resulted in major changes in the causes of death between 1900 and 2000. Pneumonia, tuberculosis, and diarrhea were the three most common causes of death in 1900. In 2000, in developed countries, the leading causes of death were heart disease, cancer, and stroke. Large long-term public health studies began to focus on these chronic diseases by the mid-1900s, and by the 1960s several major studies had been published establishing physical inactivity as an important contributor to chronic conditions, especially heart disease. Some of the more prominent studies showed that people in active occupations, such as bus conductors in London, postal workers who delivered the mail, and longshoreman who did hard physical labor, were less likely to have heart attacks and other related heart conditions than bus drivers, postal clerks who sorted the mail, and

white-collar workers who did little physical activity on the job.

The wealth of evidence led the Surgeon General of the United States to note: "Many Americans may be surprised at the extent and strength of the evidence linking physical activity to numerous health improvements. Most significantly, *regular physical activity greatly reduces the risk of dying of coronary heart disease*, the leading cause of death in the United States. Physical activity also reduces the risk of developing diabetes, hypertension, and colon cancer; enhances feelings of general well-being; is important for healthy bones and joints; and helps maintain function and preserves independence in older adults" (Corbin and Pangrazi, 1999). Table 1 synthesizes the findings of the research through the year 2000, as accumulated from a variety of sources.

Prior to 1960, little attention had been focused on the amount of physical activity necessary to produce health benefits. With the fitness boom in the 1960s, researchers began more intense efforts to find out "how much physical activity is enough," though the focus was primarily on how much is enough for improved fitness and physical performance, rather than on the health benefits of activity. The research, initially prompted by coaches interested in enhancing the performance of athletes, led to the development of guidelines based on the frequency, intensity, and duration of activity necessary to improve fitness for performance. By the 1970s, the focus on high intensity and short duration activity was firmly established. In 1972, the American Heart Association (AHA) published an exercise testing and training handbook and, in 1975, the American College of Sports Medicine (ACSM) published its first set of guidelines outlining the frequency, intensity, duration, and mode of exercise necessary to produce physical fitness.

The focus on exercise for fitness and performance began to change with the accumulation of public health research outlining the health benefits of activity. The evidence that accumulated in the last half of the twentieth century resulted in new guidelines in the 1990s. In July 1992, the AHA, in cooperation with ACSM, the Centers for Disease Prevention and Control (CDC), and the President's Council of Physical Fitness and Sports, issued a statement acknowledging the importance of lifestyle physical activity as a means of reducing

Table 1

Physical Activity, Health, and Disease

Overall Mortality
- Higher levels of regular physical activity are associated with lower mortality rates for both older and younger adults.
- Those who are moderately active on a regular basis have lower mortality rates than those who are least active.

Cardiovascular Diseases
- Regular physical activity or cardiorespiratory fitness decreases the risk of cardiovascular disease mortality in general and of coronary heart disease (CHD) mortality in particular. Existing data are not conclusive regarding a relationship between activity and stroke.
- The level of decreased risk of CHD attributable to regular physical activity is similar to that of other lifestyle factors, such as keeping free from cigarette smoking.
- Regular physical activity prevents or delays the development of high blood pressure, and it can reduce blood pressure in people with hypertension.

Cancer
- Regular physical activity is associated with a decreased risk of colon cancer.
- There is no association between physical activity and rectal cancer. Data are too sparse to draw conclusions regarding a relationship between physical activity and endometrial, ovarian, or testicular cancers.
- Despite numerous studies on the subject, existing data are inconsistent regarding an association between physical activity and breast or prostate cancers.

Diabetes Mellitus
- Regular physical activity lowers the risk of developing non-insulin-dependent diabetes mellitus and is associated with increased insulin sensitivity.
- Regular physical activity plays an important role in improving quality of life for both non-insulin-dependent diabetes and insulin-dependent diabetes when included as part of a well planned self-management program.

Osteoarthritis and Osteoporosis
- Regular physical activity is necessary for maintaining normal muscle strength, joint structure, and joint function. In the range recommended for health, physical activity is not associated with joint damage or development of osteoarthritis and may be beneficial for many people with arthritis.
- Competitive athletics may be associated with the development of osteoarthritis later in life, but sports-related injuries are the likely cause.
- Weight-bearing physical activity is essential for normal skeletal development during childhood and adolescence and for achieving and maintaining peak bone mass in young adults, especially females.
- It is unclear whether resistance- or endurance-type physical activity can reduce the accelerated rate of bone loss in postmenopausal women in the absence of estrogen replacement therapy.

Falling
- There is promising evidence that strength training and other forms of exercise in older adults preserve the ability to maintain independent living status and reduce the risk of falling.

Obesity
- Low levels of activity, resulting in fewer kilocalories used than consumed, contribute to the high prevalence of obesity in the United States.
- Physical activity favorably affects body fat distribution.
- Good physical fitness, associated with regular physical activity, has been shown to be a risk factor independent of body fatness. For this reason, a fit and active person who is overfat has lower risk for many chronic health problems than person of lower body fat level who is unfit and inactive.

Immune System Function
- Moderate bouts of activity tend to have an immune system boost that lasts for short periods of time after the activity has been completed.
- Regular physical activity, and associated high level physical fitness, is related to reduced incidence of upper respiratory tract infections including the common cold.
- Moderate activity can help those with some immune system disorders (e.g., HIV/AIDS) maintain body weight, muscle mass, as well as contribute to an improved quality of life.
- Extreme bouts of physical activity can result in temporary decreases in immune system function immediately after the activity (e.g., marathon).

Mental/Emotional Health
- Physical activity appears to relieve symptoms of depression and anxiety and improve mood.
- Regular physical activity may reduce the risk of developing depression, although further research is needed.

Health-Related Quality of Life
- Physical activity appears to improve health-related quality of life by enhancing psychological well-being and by improving physical functioning in people compromised by poor health.
- Cognitive functioning has been linked to good fitness and active lifestyles.

Physical Fitness
- Appropriate physical activity results in improved health related physical fitness including cardiovascular fitness, strength, muscular endurance, flexibility, and body composition.
- Good health related physical fitness is associated with reduced incidence of heart disease and other chronic diseases.
- Good health related and motor fitness improves physical performance capabilities that are associated with improved quality of life, leisure time enjoyment, and ability to work efficiently.

Adverse Effects of Physical Activity
- Serious cardiovascular events can occur with physical exertion, but the net effect of regular physical activity is a lower risk of mortality from cardiovascular disease.
- Extreme physical activity is associated with decreased immune function, some eating disorders, and overuse musculoskeletal injuries.
- Many musculoskeletal injuries related to physical activity are believed to be preventable by performing exercise properly, progressing gradually, and avoiding excessive or overtraining.

SOURCE: Adapted from various references (Corbin and Pangrazi, 1999; USDHHS, 1996; USDHHS, 2000)

disease risk. The recommendations focused on accumulating thirty minutes (or more) of moderate physical activity throughout the day over the course of most days of the week. Examples of such activities are walking up stairs (instead of taking the elevator), gardening, raking leaves, dancing, and walking all or part of the way to work. Activity can also be planned exercise or recreation such as jogging, playing tennis, swimming, and cycling.

Based on the accumulating evidence, Blair and colleagues (1993) suggested the need for a shift from the strategy of exercise for fitness to a new strategy of physical activity for public health. This new strategy, sometimes referred to as the "lifetime physical activity strategy," differs from earlier strategies in three ways. First, the new strategy focuses on the amount of physical activity necessary to produce health benefits associated with reduced morbidity and mortality rather than fitness or performance benefits. Second, the new strategy focuses on moderate activity rather than the vigorous physical activity of the old strategy designed to enhance fitness and performance. Finally, the new strategy emphasizes the value of accumulating physical activity throughout the day, as opposed to having to perform the activity in a single bout.

THE PHYSICAL ACTIVITY PYRAMID

The 2000 exercise and prescription guidelines of the ACSM acknowledged the new strategy of physical activity for health. The FIT (frequency, intensity, time or duration) formula for various types of physical activity was adjusted to include more moderate activity that results in specific health benefits. The Physical Activity Pyramid (see Figure 1) illustrates the FIT formula for six different types of physical activity, each with its own unique benefits. The Physical Activity Pyramid is modeled after the Food Guide Pyramid developed by the United States Department of Agriculture.

At the base of the pyramid (Level 1) is lifestyle physical activity. Lifestyle physical activities are those people can do as part of their regular workday or daily routine. Examples of such activities are yard work and delivering the mail. A person who works while sitting at a desk for most of the day can get lifestyle activity by walking or riding a bicycle to work rather than driving a car, or by walking up the stairs at work rather than taking an elevator. Those who are totally sedentary should focus on this level of the pyramid because moderate amounts of physical activity can provide many of the health benefits outlined in Figure 1. As the 1996 Surgeon General's Report states, "something is better than nothing," and a good start would be thirty minutes of lifestyle physical activity on most days of the week.

Level 2 of the pyramid includes active aerobic activities. Aerobic activities are those performed at a pace for which the body can supply adequate oxygen to meet the demands of the activity. Because lifestyle activities meet this criterion, they are aerobic in nature. In the pyramid, however, *active* aerobics refers to those aerobic activities that elevate the heart rate to an appropriate target heart rate. This level includes aerobic activities using the FIT formula based on target heart rate (elevating the heart rate to an appropriate intensity at least three days a week for a time of at least 20 minutes). Examples of popular moderate to vigorous active aerobics are aerobic dance, step aerobics, jogging, moderate to vigorous swimming, and biking. Because they are more vigorous than activities at Level 1, active aerobics can be performed less frequently and the time of each activity bout can be shorter.

Also on Level 2 of the pyramid are active sports and recreational activities. Some examples of active sports are basketball, tennis, hiking, racquetball, and volleyball. Like active aerobics, this type of activity is typically more vigorous than lifestyle physical activity. Sports involve vigorous bursts of activity with brief rest periods. Though they are often not truly aerobic in nature, when they are done without long rest periods they have many of the same benefits as aerobic activities. The FIT formula for active sports and recreation is similar to the formula for active aerobics.

Some sports are not vigorously active and should be considered lifestyle physical activities. For example, golf, as a physical activity, is similar to walking to work, rather than the more vigorous activity generated in tennis or basketball—it is beneficial, but not vigorous in nature. Recreational activities such as rock climbing or canoeing are not considered to be sports by some people. Nevertheless, they can be used to meet the three-day moderate to vigorous recommendation for active sports if performed vigorously. Recreational

Figure 1

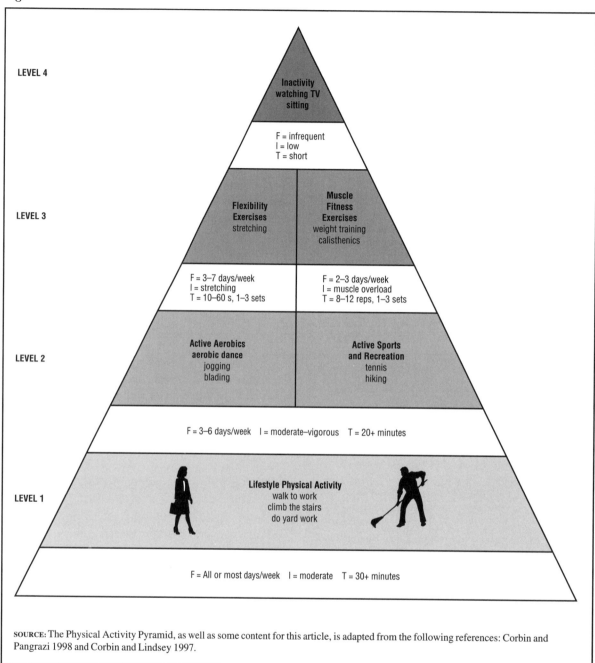

LEVEL 4

Inactivity
watching TV
sitting

F = infrequent
I = low
T = short

LEVEL 3

Flexibility
Exercises
stretching

Muscle
Fitness
Exercises
weight training
calisthenics

F = 3–7 days/week
I = stretching
T = 10–60 s, 1–3 sets

F = 2–3 days/week
I = muscle overload
T = 8–12 reps, 1–3 sets

LEVEL 2

Active Aerobics
aerobic dance
jogging
blading

Active Sports
and Recreation
tennis
hiking

F = 3–6 days/week   I = moderate–vigorous   T = 20+ minutes

LEVEL 1

Lifestyle Physical Activity
walk to work
climb the stairs
do yard work

F = All or most days/week   I = moderate   T = 30+ minutes

SOURCE: The Physical Activity Pyramid, as well as some content for this article, is adapted from the following references: Corbin and Pangrazi 1998 and Corbin and Lindsey 1997.

activities such as fishing and chess are not considered to be in this category. These activities have benefits, but are not in the moderate to vigorous physical activity category.

Flexibility exercises are included at Level 3 of the pyramid. These are referred to as exercises because they are done specifically to build the part of physical fitness called flexibility. Flexibility is the ability to use joints through a full range of motion as a result of having long muscles and elastic connective tissues. There are, no doubt, some activities from the first two levels of the pyramid that help build flexibility to some extent. Still, to develop this part of fitness, it is necessary to do special flexibility exercises that involve stretching the muscles and using the joints through their full range of normal motion. For this purpose stretching exercises are best.

Flexibility exercises should be done at least three days a week, and as often as every day. The intensity requires stretching beyond normal to a point of mild discomfort. Each exercise is performed several times for 15 to 30 seconds. It is important to perform exercises for each of the body's major muscle groups.

Muscle fitness includes strength and muscular endurance. Exercises to develop muscle fitness are included at Level 3 of the pyramid. Some of the activities from the first two levels of the pyramid can contribute to the development of muscle fitness. But most experts agree that if you want to improve muscle fitness you need to do some exercises especially designed to build it.

The ACSM recommends that muscle fitness exercises be done at least twice a week. Exercises for several different muscle groups (between 8 and 10) should be done using a percentage of the maximum weight a person can lift. The percentage (intensity) depends on the type of muscle fitness to be developed. Each exercise should be performed 8 to 12 times (a set). More frequent training and additional sets or combinations of sets and repetitions produce larger strength gains, but the additional improvement is relatively small.

At the top of the pyramid is inactivity (Level 4). Some inactivity is not necessarily bad. For example, we need adequate amounts of sleep, and after vigorous exercise rest is important. Also, there are benefits associated with activities that are fairly sedentary. Fishing can be a relaxing experience that helps people get away from the stress of daily living. Nevertheless, the Physical Activity Pyramid is meant to provide information about the benefits of regular physical activity. Sedentary living as a lifestyle is discouraged. Long periods of inactivity during the hours of the day when you are awake should be limited. People who only sit and watch television or who spend all of their free time playing video games are not getting the activity they need for good health.

Ideally, a person should do some regular physical activity from each of the first three levels of the pyramid each week. However, if doing activity at all three levels proves discouraging or seems to be too difficult, it is better to select activities from fewer categories, beginning with the bottom of the pyramid.

GENETICS, MATURATION, AGE, AND OTHER DETERMINANTS OF ACTIVITY

Studies have shown that some animals tend to be more active than others. Humans are no exception in that a genetic predisposition to be active is one of several factors that determine the daily activity levels of children and adults. While social and environmental factors account for more of the variability in human activity than genetics, there are several ways in which heredity is important.

Physical fitness is highly influenced by heredity, especially in childhood. The amount of variability in physical fitness associated with heredity ranges from 10 percent to as high as 60 percent (e.g., maximal aerobic power, 25%; muscular endurance, 21%; muscle strength, 30%; body fat, 25%; bone density, 30–60%). Evidence suggests that fit people are more likely to be active than unfit people, thus heredity influences activity levels via its relationship to fitness.

Recent evidence also indicates that all people do not respond similarly to regular physical activity. Large variations have been noted between people who have a hereditary predisposition to respond to physical activity and those who do not have this predisposition. In other words, some people have the genetic makeup to respond more favorably to physical activity than others. Given the same activity program, some show considerably greater improvements in fitness than others.

Maturation also influences physical activity and fitness. During puberty, the potential for physical activity to produce gains in fitness is enhanced. Thus, teens are more responsive to physical activity than children. The feedback from performance improvements stimulates an interest in activity among those who are more mature physically compared to those who are less mature and do not see similar benefits for the same amounts of activity. Those who mature early may be more inclined to see the benefits of regular physical activity than those who mature later.

There is an abundance of evidence to indicate that children are the most active group in society. Beginning in the early school years, activity drops consistently throughout life. The most precipitous declines occur during the teenage years. The drop in activity continues throughout life, though the drop from the teens to the early twenties is less dramatic than the drop-off from childhood to the teen years. Older adults (above 50) are typically less active than younger adults. Much of the decline with age can be attributed to decreases in dopamine levels, which are associated with decreases in motivation to be active, though social factors (influence of friends, family, and role models), psychological factors (self-efficacy, enjoyment, beliefs about activity, and barriers to activity), physical factors (weather, safety, convenience, and availability), and demographic factors (sex, education, and vocation) all play a role in adult physical activity patterns.

GUIDELINES AND APPROACHES TO INCREASING ACTIVITY LEVELS

Among the most important physical activity guidelines are those of the ACSM and the CDC, which has established guidelines for the promotion of physical activity among youth. In addition, *Healthy People 2010* (2000), a statement of national health goals, includes important national health objectives relating to physical activity and outlines priorities for changing activity patterns of Americans. Important strategies include increasing moderate and vigorous activity, as well as involvement in activities for muscle fitness and flexibility through increased school physical education, decreased television viewing, improved facilities for physical activity, and increased programs to promote walking and cycling as daily life activities. Expanded worksite health-promotion programs, improved health and wellness education, and greater public information access are other strategies that are outlined.

It is important to point out that the physical activity guidelines that are appropriate for adults are not appropriate for children. Appropriate guidelines for physical activity for children, including applications of the physical activity pyramid for younger age groups are available in *Physical Activity for Children: A Statement of Guidelines* (1998)

published by the National Association for Physical Education and Sports.

CHARLES B. CORBIN
ROBERT P. PANGRAZI

(SEE ALSO: *Behavior, Health-Related; Centers for Disease Control and Prevention; Chronic Illness; Coronary Artery Disease; Epidemiologic Transition; Foods and Diets; Healthy People 2010; Lifestyle; Nutrition*)

BIBLIOGRAPHY

American College of Sports Medicine (1975). *Guidelines for Graded Testing and Exercise Prescription.* Philadelphia: Lea and Febiger.

—— (2000). *Guidelines for Exercise Testing and Prescription,* 6th edition. Philadelphia: Lippincott, William & Wilkins.

American Heart Association (1972). *Exercise Testing and Training of Apparently Healthy Individuals: A Handbook for Physicians.* Dallas, TX: Author.

—— (1992). "Statement on Exercise: Benefits and Recommendations for Physical Activity Promotion for All Americans: A Statement for Health Professionals by the Committee on Exercise and Cardiac Rehabilitation of the Council on Clinical Cardiology." *Circulation* 86:340–344.

Blair S. N. (1993). "C. H. McCloy Research Lecture: Physical Activity, Physical Fitness, and Health." *Research Quarterly for Exercise and Sport* 64(4):365–376.

Bouchard, C. (1999). "Heredity and Health Related Fitness." In *Toward a Better Understanding of Physical Fitness and Physical Activity,* eds. C. B Corbin and R. P. Pangrazi. Scottsdale, AZ: Holcomb-Hathaway Publishers.

Caspersen, C. J.; Pereira, M. A.; and Curran, K. M. (2000). "Changes in Physical Activity Patterns in the United States, by Sex and Cross-Sectional Age." *Medicine and Science in Sports and Exercise* 32:1601–1609.

Centers for Disease Control and Prevention (1997). "Guidelines for School and Community Programs to Promote Lifelong Physical Activity among Young People." *Morbidity and Mortality Weekly Report* 46(RR-6):1–36.

Cooper, K. H. (1968). *Aerobics.* New York: M. Evans.

Corbin, C. B., and Lindsey, R. (1997). *Fitness for Life,* 4th edition. Glenview, IL: Scott, Foresman and Co.

—— (1998). *Physical Activity for Children: A Statement of Guidelines.* Reston, VA: NASPE Publications.

—— (1998). "Physical Activity Pyramid Rebuffs Peak Experience." *ACSM's Health & Fitness Journal* 2(1):12–17.

—— (1999). "What You Need to Know about the Surgeon General's Report on Physical Activity and Health." In *Toward a Better Understanding of Physical Fitness and Physical Activity,* eds. C. B. Corbin and R. P. Pangrazi. Scottsdale, AZ: Holcomb-Hathaway Publishers.

—— (2000). "Definitions: Health, Fitness and Physical Activity." *President's Council on Physical Fitness and Sports Research Digest* 3:1–8.

Kraus, H., and Raab, W. (1961). *Hypokinetic Disease.* Springfield, IL: C. C. Thomas.

National Association for Sport and Physical Education (1998). *Physical Activity for Children: A Statement of Guidelines.* Reston, VA: NASPE Publications.

Paffenbarger, R. S., and Hyde, R. T. (1980). "Exercise and Prevention against Heart Attack." *New England Journal of Medicine* 302:1026–1028.

Sallis, J. F. (1999). "Influences on Physical Activity of Children, Adolescents, and Adults." In *Toward a Better Understanding of Physical Fitness and Physical Activity,* eds. C. B. Corbin and R. P. Pangrazi. Scottsdale AZ: Holcomb-Hathaway Publishers.

—— (2000). "Age-Related Decline in Physical Activity: A Synthesis of Human and Animal Studies." *Medicine and Science in Sports and Exercise* 32: 1598–1600.

U.S. Department of Agriculture and U.S. Department of Health and Human Services (1990). *Report of the Dietary Guidelines Advisory Committee.* Washington, DC: Author.

U.S. Department of Health and Human Services (1996). *Physical Activity and Health: A Report of the Surgeon General.* Atlanta, GA: U.S. Department of Health and Human Services, Centers for Disease Control and Prevention, National Center for Chronic Disease Prevention and Health Promotion.

—— (2000). *Healthy People 2010, 2nd edition: With Understanding and Improving Health and Objectives for Improving Health.* 2 vols. Washington, DC: U.S. Government Printing Office.

PHYSICIAN

A physician working in public health focuses on diagnosing and improving the health of communities. Such physicians are dedicated to the prevention of illness, injury, and disability, and to the promotion of healthy behaviors and improved quality of life. They provide special knowledge, skills, and especially leadership to resolve public health issues. Public health physicians often have clinical and/or administrative roles in local or state health departments, federal or international health agencies, academic institutions, and not-for-profit and for-profit health and health care organizations. While physicians enter public health with different clinical backgrounds, many have formal public health training and hold specialty board certification in preventive medicine, the combined art and science of getting and keeping people healthy.

TERESA C. LONG

(SEE ALSO: *Preventive Medicine*)

PILOT STUDY

A pilot study is a small-scale methodological test intended to ensure that proposed methods and procedures will work in practice before being applied in a large, expensive investigation. Pilot studies provide an opportunity to make adjustments and revisions before investing in, and incurring, the heavy costs associated with a large study.

JOHN M. LAST

PLAGUE

Plague is a disease of rodents and their fleas that can be transmitted to humans. Throughout history, plague, often referred to as the "Black Death," has caused catastrophic pandemics resulting in deaths of tens of millions of persons. The disease is caused by a gram-negative bacterium, *Yersinia pestis.* Humans are usually infected by the bite of infective rodent fleas, but infection also occurs through handling or ingesting infectious animals or by inhaling infective respiratory droplets expelled by humans or animals.

Initial signs and symptoms of plague may be nonspecific, with fever, chills, headache, malaise, musculoskeletal pains, nausea, and weakness leading to prostration. Persons with bubonic plague, the most common form of plague, typically develop painful, swollen lymph nodes near the site of an infective flea bite. Less common forms of plague can infect the bloodstream (septicemic plague), the lungs (pneumonic plague), the throat (pharyngeal plague), or the coverings of the brain (meningeal plague). Pneumonic plague is a severe and rapidly progressive form of the disease that quickly leads to difficulty in breathing, a cough with bloody sputum, and shock.

In any of its clinical forms, plague can be fatal if not diagnosed and treated correctly early in the course of the disease. The diagnosis is made by combining information on possible infective exposures, clinical signs and symptoms, and results from laboratory tests. Treatment, which should begin as soon as the diagnosis is suspected, relies on the aminoglycoside group of antibiotics (streptomycin, gentamicin), tetracyclines (doxycycline, tetracycline, oxytetracycline), chloramphenicol, or trimethoprim-sulfamethoxazole. Laboratory diagnosis is made by direct examination of stained clinical materials, serologies, antigen-detection, isolation of culture media, and molecular-genetic characterizations.

Plague is present in wild rodent populations over large but scattered rural areas of the Americas, Africa, and Asia. Outbreaks sometimes occur among wild rodent populations and occasionally among rat populations in villages and towns, though rarely in cities. When plague involves rats living in or around homes, humans are at their highest risk of exposure. In the United States, plague occurs in the western third of the country, most often in burrowing rodents and their fleas. Plague also occurs in scattered areas of South America, especially the Andean region; in north-central, eastern, and southern Africa; in Madagascar; in several states in the Near East (Saudi Arabia, Yemen, Jordan, and Iranian Kurdistan); central and southern Asia (Georgia, Kazakhstan, Mongolia, China, and India); and Southeast Asia (Myanmar, Vietnam, and Indonesia).

Plague prevention on an individual level involves avoidance of areas of known plague activity, taking personal precautions against flea bites, avoiding sick or dead animals, and seeking medical care at the earliest signs of illness. No vaccine against plague is available in the United States. Pneumonic plague patients should be managed in isolation under respiratory droplet precautions. Postexposure antibiotics may be warranted for persons who, in the previous two days, were likely to have been exposed to infectious fleas or have

had close direct exposure to a person or animal with pneumonic plague. Routine community prevention and control of plague is achieved through sanitation and hygiene measures that limit food and harborage for rodents. In the event of a plague outbreak, flea control should be implemented before attempts are made to kill rats.

DAVID T. DENNIS

(SEE ALSO: *Black Death; Epidemics; Isolation; Universal Precautions; Vector-Borne Diseases; Zoonoses*)

BIBLIOGRAPHY

Anonymous (2000). "Plague." In *Control of Communicable Diseases Manual,* 17th edition, ed. J. Chin. Washington, DC: American Public Health Association.

Dennis, D. T., and Gage, K. G. (1999). "Plague." In *Infectious Diseases,* Vol. 2, eds. D. Armstrong and J. Cohen. London: Mosby, Armstrong, and Cohen.

Perry, R. D., and Fetherston, J. D. (1997). "Yersinia pestis—Etiologic Agent of Plague." *Clinical Microbiological Review* 10:35–66.

World Health Organization (1999). *Plague Manual: Epidemiology, Distribution, Surveillance and Control.* Geneva: Author.

PLANNED APPROACH TO COMMUNITY HEALTH (PATCH)

The Planned Approach to Community Health (PATCH) was developed in 1983 by the United States Centers for Disease Control (CDC) in partnership with state and local health departments and community groups. It was designed to provide a model to assist state and local public health agencies, in their partnerships with local communities, to plan, conduct, and evaluate health promotion and disease prevention programs. PATCH was also intended to serve as a mechanism to improve links both within communities and between communities and state health departments, universities, and other agencies and organizations. PATCH combines the principles of community participation with the diagnostic steps of applied community-level epidemiology. The development of PATCH was influenced by the theoretical assumptions underlying the PRECEDE model, by the literature on community organization and development, and by CDC's tradition of working through state health agencies in the application of health promotion and disease prevention programs.

The PATCH process guides users through five phases: (1) mobilizing the community, (2) collecting and organizing data, (3) choosing health priorities, (4) developing a comprehensive intervention plan, and (5) evaluation. Moving from the initiation to the full implementation of PATCH can take can up to a year or more. Successful implementation depends upon actively engaging community members in the process, having adequate time and resources to gather and interpret data to guide program development, and developing cohesion among stakeholder organizations. PATCH is an example of a model that has not only tested the application of theory, but has also facilitated the link between research and practice in community health education and health promotion.

PATCH is widely recognized as a practical and user-friendly model for community health promotion and disease prevention planning. It has been used in combination with other community-based planning frameworks such as Assessment Protocol for Excellence in Public Health (APEXPH) and Healthy Cities.

Public health staff in over forty states have received training in the PATCH process and it has been applied in over three hundred local communities in the United States, as well as several communities in Canada, Australia, and in the Panama Canal region by the United States military. It has also been applied in a wide variety of settings, including hospitals, managed care organizations, universities, voluntary health agencies, local health departments, agricultural extension services, and work sites. PATCH has also been employed to focus on the health needs of diverse populations to address such topics as cardiovascular disease, injury prevention, HIV/AIDS (human immunodeficiency virus/acquired immunodeficiency syndrome), teen pregnancy, and tobacco use.

Although no longer directly funded by the CDC, the PATCH process continues to be referenced and used by many organizations and agencies for community planning and for the training of new public health and health promotion professionals. Further discussion of theory, applications, and evaluation of PATCH can be found in many publications, some of which are included in the bibliography below.

BRICK LANCASTER
MARSHALL KREUTER

(SEE ALSO: *Centers for Disease Control and Prevention; Community Health; Community Organization; Epidemiology; Health Promotion and Education; Mobilizing for Action through Planning and Partnerships; PRECEDE-PROCEED Model*)

BIBLIOGRAPHY

Breckon, D.; Harvey, J.; and Lancaster, R. B. (1998). *Community Health Education: Settings, Roles, and Skills for the 21st Century*, 4th edition. Rockville, MD: Aspen Publishers.

Green, L., and Kreuter, M. (1999). *Health Promotion Planning*, 3rd edition. Mountain View, CA: Mayfield Publishers.

Journal of Health Education (1992). "Community Health Promotion: The Agenda for the '90s, PATCH." *JHE* 23, special issue.

U.S. Department of Health and Human Services. *Planned Approach to Community Health: Guide for the Local Coordinator.* Available at http://www.cdc.gov/nccdphp/patch/.

PLANNED PARENTHOOD

Planned Parenthood Federation of America, Inc. describes itself as the world's oldest and largest voluntary family planning organization. Margaret Sanger (1879–1966) started the first birth-control clinic in Brooklyn in 1916 and organizations she founded eventually merged to become the Planned Parenthood Federation of America. Women throughout the United States took up the cause and established family planning services that would became a part of the national organization. In 2000, the organization comprised 132 affiliate organizations providing reproductive health care and education in forty-seven states and the District of Columbia.

The Planned Parenthood Federation of America provides national leadership for advocacy to increase services that prevent unintended pregnancy, improve the quality of reproductive health care, and ensure access to abortion. The national organization provides family-planning services internationally through its Family Planning International Assistance program, and it supports cooperative international programs through Planned Parenthood Global Partners and the International Planned Parenthood Federation. The International Planned Parenthood Federation is headquartered in London. There are Planned Parenthood organizations in Canada and Latin America as well.

In 1998, Planned Parenthood of America affiliates operated 850 health centers and served 2,364,864 clients. Over 79 percent of these clients received contraceptive services and health assessments, including breast and cervical cancer screening. Affiliate health centers also provide testing and treatment for sexually transmitted infections, including HIV (human immunodeficiency virus) testing. Many affiliates offer abortion services, and a growing number of affiliates provide prenatal and primary care, midlife services, and expanded diagnostic and treatment services.

Planned Parenthood affiliates also provide sexuality education and risk reduction programs in their communities, and they advocate for protecting access to reproductive health services at local and state levels.

ROBERTA E. ABER

(SEE ALSO *Abortion; Abortion Laws; Contraception; Family Planning Behavior; Maternal and Child Health; Reproduction*)

BIBLIOGRAPHY

Planned Parenthood Federation of America. *Responsible Choice in Action: 1998–99 Annual Report.* New York: Author.

PLANNING FOR PUBLIC HEALTH

To "plan" means to form a scheme or method for doing or achieving something. In public health, as in most fields, planning is undertaken to determine the ways, means, and timetable by which specific goals and objectives can be achieved.

Planning in public health takes many forms. Whether within government or outside it, a planning process is employed to identify and organize the resources and actions necessary to safeguard and improve the public's health. Public health planning can occur at the municipal, state, regional, national, or international level. Goals are often defined by a specific health problem or concern (e.g., reduce heart disease, mental illness, or dental caries), and are usually coupled with specific health objectives (e.g., to reduce overall age-adjusted heart disease mortality rates by 10% over a ten-year period), service objectives (e.g., every resident of a country will be covered by health insurance for a basic set of benefits), or process objectives (e.g., develop indicators for accountability for each program area, or cut the budget by 15%).

In public health, planning can be initiated and led by a variety of public health agencies or by other health-interested organizations, although official public health agencies usually have some involvement in the planning process. Broad efforts to plan for improved population health can often benefit from involving stakeholders from other sectors whose actions influence health, such as transportation, housing, environment, economic policy, nutrition and food security, welfare, and others.

The U.S. government has established a periodic planning cycle for a comprehensive process to develop a set of national disease-prevention and health-promotion objectives. The first set of national health targets, published in 1979, was *Healthy People: The Surgeon General's Report on Health Promotion and Disease Prevention.* Goals were set to reduce mortality among infants, children, adolescents and young adults, and adults. The broad goals for the most recent decennial planning process, completed in 1999 and incorporated into the report *Healthy People 2010*, are to increase quality and years of healthy life, eliminate health disparities, and achieve access to preventive services. Goals, objectives, and specific quantifiable milestones that support each goal and objective are organized into twenty-eight topic areas by health problem, and into three select populations. There are 467 separate objectives and related indicators. Similar processes and related goals and objectives are set by states and some municipalities.

Some areas of very active public health planning include manpower resources, access to health care services, and improved structures and processes to meet the needs of specified populations, such as those with HIV/AIDS (human immunodeficiency virus/acquired immunodeficiency disease). In some circumstances, laws or regulations at the federal or state level dictate a carefully defined planning process as a condition of receipt of funds. Such is the case for the substantial funds available for care and prevention of HIV/AIDS, where an extensive community planning process with substantial participation of those affected by this condition are mandated. States and municipalities often have to submit detailed plans as a condition of receiving funds from the higher levels of government. For example, each state must submit a maternal and child health plan to receive federal block-grant money for health improvement activities for children and families.

Many tools are available to support planning. These include data and data analysis concerning the burden of disease, the distribution of available resources, and resource utilization and health outcomes. Information is also available on what interventions have been shown to be effective in practice. This information comes from a variety of sources, such as reports of the Surgeon General, the U.S. Clinical Preventive Services Task Force, and the U.S. Task Force on Community Preventive Services. Assessment of process and outcome results of planned interventions determine the effectiveness and efficiency of the plan and/or its execution.

An important movement within planning has been to involve representatives of those that will be affected by proposed plans. This participatory planning approach has significant strengths, though its influence on a specific plan and its ultimate health impact can vary.

JONATHAN E. FIELDING

(SEE ALSO: *Community Health; Community Organization; Health Goals; Healthy People 2010; Mobilization for Action through Planning and Partnerships; Regional Health Planning*)

BIBLIOGRAPHY

U.S. Department of Health, Education, and Welfare (1974). *Healthy People: Surgeon General's Report on Health Promotion and Disease Prevention.* Washington, DC: U.S. Government Printing Office.

U.S. Department of Health and Human Services (2000). *Healthy People 2010: Understanding and Improving Health,* 2nd edition. Washington, DC: U.S. Government Printing Office.

PLAQUE

Dental plaque is a biofilm that forms naturally on the tooth surface. It consists of a diverse microbial community embedded in a polymer matrix of bacterial and salivary origin. Because environmental conditions vary from place to place within the oral cavity, each tooth site with plaque represents its own distinct ecosystem, and the dominant microbial composition at each site depends on the outcome of numerous host-microbe and microbe-microbe interactions. Initial bacterial colonizers quickly become established on a clean tooth surface, and a pattern of subsequent bacterial succession has been identified. If left undisturbed, plaque reaches a maximum bulk after about seven days. Plaque deposition begins supragingivally—on the visible part of the tooth above the gum line—and if left undisturbed can progress subgingivally—into the crevice between the gum and the tooth. Microbial interactions usually keep the bacterial composition of plaque fairly stable, but when this homeostasis breaks down, the shifts in microbial balance can trigger the initiation of dental caries (tooth decay) or gingivitis (gum inflammation). Few bacteria can be isolated from around healthy gum tissue, although with gingivitis there is a considerable increase in the number and complexity of bacteria as the lesion develops. Subgingival plaque, if left undisturbed, can become a calcified matrix (calculus, or tartar) that can harbor harmful bacteria. Not surprisingly, subgingival calculus is closely associated with periodontal diseases. Specifically, *Porphyromonas gingivalis* and *Bacteroides forsythus* in subgingival plaque had been associated with both periodontal inflammation and bone loss.

Although dental plaque is commonly depicted in commercial advertising as the cause of both caries and periodontitis, dental plaque also benefits the host by helping to prevent intra-oral colonization by exogenous species. Plaque is also a repository for fluoride and other minerals that serve both to inhibit the demineralization of dental enamel—the first step in the development of a cavity—and to promote remineralization of early lesions. The fact that caries is initiated by a drop in plaque pH, following the fermentation of simple carbohydrates by certain bacteria resident in plaque, further exemplifies plaque's delicate ecology. Controlled plaque is beneficial, uncontrolled plaque can be harmful.

Prevention of plaque-related disease is geared toward plaque control rather than eradication. The goal in preventing periodontitis (diseases of the supporting structures of the tooth) is to prevent fresh plaque from becoming established enough to permit the growth of pathogenic bacteria. This goal is best achieved by thorough toothbrushing at least once per day with a fluoride-containing toothpaste, plus consistent professional prophylactic care. So long as plaque remains supragingival, it can be controlled by mechanical or chemotherapeutic means. Once plaque becomes established subgingivally, however, an individual cannot remove it and professional intervention is necessary. Carrying out personal oral hygiene with a fluoride-containing toothpaste helps maintain high fluoride levels in plaque and thus inhibits the development of caries.

BRIAN A. BURT

(SEE ALSO: *Caries Prevention; Gingivitis; Oral Health; Primary Prevention*)

BIBLIOGRAPHY

Zambon, J. J. (1997). "Principles of Evaluation of the Diagnostic Value of Subgingival Bacteria." *Annals of Periodontology* 2:138–148.

PNEUMOCOCCAL VACCINE

Pneumococcal vaccine is prepared by purifying polysaccharides (sugars) from the capsules of the most common types of *Streptococcus pneumoniae* causing human illness. The mix of types is different for adults and children. The first pneumococcal vaccines, which were administrated in a single injection, consisted of only polysaccharides and did not reliably induce protection in infants and young children, nor did they induce immunologic memory. Consequently, protection (which was only partial) lasted only for a few years. In adults these vaccines provided 50 to 80 percent protection

against severe pneumococcal disease. They were recommended for all persons sixty-five years of age or older and for younger persons with medical conditions that put them at increased risk of pneumococcal disease (such as chronic cardiovascular or pulmonary disease, diabetes mellitus, and alcoholism). Newer vaccines are prepared by conjugating the polysaccharides with some protein to induce immunologic memory and provide protection to infants as well as adults. They are administrated in a series of three injections at intervals of approximately two months. Approximately 90 percent of infants who receive the vaccine are protected from systemic disease caused by the types of pneumococci contained in the vaccine. Duration of protection and the possible need for booster doses has not yet been established. No serious adverse effects have been shown to be caused by either formulation of pneumococcal vaccine.

ALAN R. HINMAN

(SEE ALSO: *Immunizations*)

BIBLIOGRAPHY

Centers for Disease Control and Prevention (1997). "Prevention of Pneumococcal Disease: Recommendations of the Advisory Committee on Immunization Practices (ACIP)." *Morbidity and Mortality Weekly Report* 46:1–23.

PNEUMOCONIOSIS

See Occupational Lung Disease

POLICE POWERS

The term "police power" refers to the right of a government to exercise "reasonable control over persons and property" to protect the public's health and safety. Police powers are rooted in English common law, extending back at least four centuries. While police departments took their name from these powers, police departments, with their focus on crime, were not widely used until the nineteenth century. Police powers are closely related to the state's power to protect itself from outside forces. The authority derives from the notion of societal self-defense.

Police power is best understood in contrast with the *parens patria* power: the power to protect individuals for their own benefit. Confining dangerous mentally ill individuals to protect the public is a police power, while confining individuals for their own protection is a *parens patria* power. The state's authority to restrict individual liberty is much greater when it is done to protect the public. Thus, the state has considerable power to prevent the spread of tuberculosis, but not to force a person to take medication for hypertension.

Police power allows the destruction or restriction of property that poses a threat to the public, without paying compensation. It also includes the right to act without a court hearing or other due process protections, when necessary, to protect the public's health. Aggrieved persons can contest such actions through habeas corpus proceedings and other post-restriction proceedings. Some states have limited their police powers by legislation and state constitutional provisions.

EDWARD P. RICHARDS

(SEE ALSO: *Licensing; Public Health and the Law; Quarantine; Regulatory Authority*)

BIBLIOGRAPHY

Richards, E. P. (1989). "The Jurisprudence of Prevention: Society's Right of Self-Defense Against Dangerous Individuals." *Hastings Constitutional Law Quarterly* 16:329.

Richards, E. P., and Rathbun, K. C. (1999). "The Role of the Police Power in Twenty-First Century Public Health." *Journal of Sexually Transmitted Diseases* 26(6):350–357.

POLICY FOR PUBLIC HEALTH

The Institute of Medicine defines public health as "what we, as a society, do collectively to assure the conditions in which people can be healthy" (1988, p. 1). It further notes that public health is more comprehensive than the specific activities of any particular agency, organization, or sector. Public health encompasses a wide range of organized community efforts to prevent disease and promote health, and it often involves private organizations and individuals, working on their own or in partnership with the public sector. Policies for public health consist of planned activities to address health problems as they are identified and defined by a community. Thus, public health activities, including policy development, require organized community efforts as well as public involvement.

Public health practitioners typically engage in organized, interdisciplinary efforts that address the physical, mental, and environmental health concerns of communities. As defined by the Institute of Medicine, three basic public health activities are essential to the practice of public health: (1) assessing and monitoring of population and community health problems and priorities; (2) assuring that all populations have access to appropriate and cost-effective care, including health-promotion and disease-prevention services; and (3) formulating policies to resolve local, state, and national health problems in conjunction with community and government decision makers.

A public health policy is a plan or a course of action intended to influence decisions or actions made by community leaders or by private or public policy makers. Ultimately, a public health policy is intended to positively influence the health and health behavior of individuals in the population. Such policy is established through public processes involving individuals and organizations, including state and local boards of health, elected officials, community groups, public health professionals, health care providers, and private citizens. At all levels, public health policies are developed, implemented, and evaluated in a way that incorporates both quantitative and qualitative scientific information, as well as the community values that reflect the demographic, geographic, and cultural diversity of an area, region, and state.

Evaluation of public health policies is important to determine their effectiveness in achieving desired outcomes. In states where public health improvement activities are underway, two key concerns emerge in conducting an evaluation of current and planned public health policies: first, having access to timely and accurate data relevant to specific health issues, and second, establishing sound methods to meaningfully involve and inform communities, interested stakeholders, groups, and individuals most affected by the policies. The processes used to develop national health targets for the United States Public Health Service's *Healthy People* series, which began in 1979 and has continued into 2010, exemplifies public health policy development in action (e.g., examining progress and experience from an expanded scientific base and relying on a broad collaboration among government, voluntary and professional organizations, businesses, and individuals.)

PATRICIA G. FELTEN

(SEE ALSO: *Community Health; Health; Health Promotion and Education; Philosophical Basis for Public Health; Politics of Public Health*)

BIBLIOGRAPHY

California Center for Health Improvement. *Health Policy Coach*. Available at http://www.healthpolicycoach.org.

California Coalition for the Future of Public Health (1990). *The New Public Health: 1990. A Statewide Conference on the Future of Public Health in California, April 25–27, 1990*. Berkeley, CA: Author.

Institute of Medicine, National Academy of Sciences (1988). *The Future of Public Health*. Washington, DC: Author.

U.S. Department of Health and Human Services, Office of Disease Prevention and Health Promotion (1997). *Developing Objectives for Healthy People 2010*. Washington, DC: Author.

Washington Department of Health (1994). *Public Health Improvement Plan: A Progress Report. Executive Summary*. Olympia, WA: Author.

POLIOMYELITIS

Poliomyelitis, or infantile paralysis, is a highly infectious disease caused by three serotypes of polioviruses. These viruses belong to the *Enterovirsus* genus of the family Picornaviridae. The infection is transmitted from person to person and rarely produces clinical symptoms. Less than 1 percent of infections will result in paralysis. Death may result, however, especially if respiratory muscles are affected.

Although archeological findings suggest that paralytic poliomyelitis existed before the modern era, the importance of the disease was not recognized until the late nineteenth century. Annual outbreaks of poliomyelitis involving thousands of cases occurred during summer and early fall in various areas of the northern hemisphere during the first half of the twentieth century, making poliomyelitis the leading cause of permanent disability and the cause of numerous premature deaths. The Drinker respirator, also known as the "iron lung," allowed a rapid reduction of poliomyelitis mortality in the 1930s and 1940s.

A major breakthrough in poliomyelitis control took place in 1949, when John F. Enders, Frederick C. Robbins, and Thomas H. Weller developed a tissue culture system for polioviruses. The availability of cultured viruses opened the way to vaccine development. The first poliovirus vaccines were licensed for use in the United States in 1955. These vaccines, developed by Jonas Salk, consisted of formalin-inactivated viruses administered through injections. In 1963, a live oral vaccine, developed by Albert Sabin, was licensed. Within ten years of the introduction of vaccines, the number of poliomyelitis cases decreased by over 95 percent in the United States, and the last case induced by indigenous transmission of wild poliovirus in the United States was detected in 1979. Poliovirus vaccines also allowed rapid declines in disease incidence in Canada, most European countries, Australia, and New Zealand. In Cuba, a two-round mass vaccination campaign in 1962 interrupted poliovirus transmission and rendered the island free of polio.

Most developing countries did not benefit from effective poliomyelitis control before the development of national control programs in the late 1970s. Mass vaccination campaigns, introduced in the Americas during the early 1980s, proved to be an effective means of bringing poliomyelitis under control. The last case of poliomyelitis in the Americas was detected in Peru in 1991, and the western hemisphere was certified as polio-free in 1994.

In 1988, the World Health Assembly launched the Poliomyelitis Eradication Initiative, with a goal of terminating the circulation of wild polioviruses by the year 2000. This worldwide effort relies on three main strategies: high levels of vaccination through routine programs; supplementary vaccination in the form of national immunization days

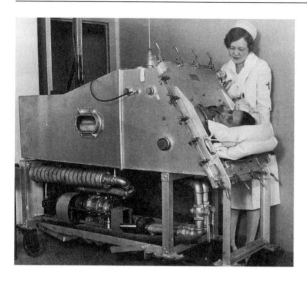

Use of the Drinker respirator (iron lung) reduced the number of deaths from poliomyelitis in the 1930s and 1940s. (© Underwood and Underwood/Corbis)

and local door-to-door immunization ("mopping-up") campaigns; and surveillance and investigation of all cases that resemble acute poliomyelitis (acute flaccid paralysis). From 1988 to 1999, the global number of estimated poliomyelitis cases decreased from 350,000 to 20,000.

An important benefit of achieving the Poliomyelitis Eradication Initiative goal will be the discontinuation of poliovirus vaccination. Stopping vaccination will require certifying all areas of the world to be free of wild poliovirus. It will also be necessary to ensure that all infectious and potentially infectious material are contained in maximum safety facilities and to stockpile enough vaccines to respond to any outbreak that might occur should poliovirus be released intentionally or unintentionally. In this way poliomyelitis eradication would follow the path pioneered by smallpox eradication.

PATRICK L. F. ZUBER

(SEE ALSO: *Communicable Disease Control; Immunizations; Smallpox*)

BIBLIOGRAPHY

Centers for Disease Control and Prevention (2000). "Poliomyelitis Prevention in the United States: Updated Recommendations of the Advisory Committee on Immunization Practices (AICP)." *Morbidity and Mortality Weekly Report* 49(RR-5):1–22.

Robbins, F. C. (1999). "The History of Polio Vaccine Development." In *Vaccine*, 3rd edition, eds. S. A. Plotkin and W. A. Orenstein. Philadelphia: W. B. Saunders.

Sutter, R. W; Cochi, S. L; and Melnick, J. L. (1999). "Live Attenuated Poliovirus Vaccines." In *Vaccine*, 3rd edition, eds. S. A. Plotkin and W. A. Orenstein. Philadelphia: W. B. Saunders.

World Health Organization. *Polio Eradication.* Available at http://www.polioeradication.org.

POLITICS OF PUBLIC HEALTH

In implementing health policy, the United States government began by taking care of its own—its armed forces and veterans. In the early years of the nation, the health of the general population was addressed only in activities aimed at the control of epidemics. The National Quarantine Service Act was passed by Congress in 1878, the year that 9,000 people died in a yellow fever epidemic in New Orleans, Louisiana, and Memphis, Tennessee. In 1890, Congress passed an appropriation bill for the National Quarantine Service, which became the United States Public Health and Marine Hospital Service in 1902, and ultimately the United States Public Health Service in 1912. In the early twentieth century, when the federal government began taking a more active interest in medicine and public health, its interest was limited to preventing or attacking epidemic diseases, through quarantine and sanitation improvement, with a very modest commitment of public funds.

Over the years, the collection of health statistics evolved as a function of state and local government, mainly in recognition of the need for vital statistics in resolving legal matters. Supported by the American Public Health Association, the National Board of Health, and the Marine Hospital Association, the Office of the Census was created in 1902, but a birth and death registration system did not cover the entire nation until 1933. Over the succeeding years, responsibility for vital statistics within the states was usually lodged within health departments, where the data were used to support maternal and child health programs, to define problems in communicable disease control, and to anticipate the problems of chronic diseases. In 1946, the federal vital statistics function was transferred from the Census Bureau to the U.S. Public Health Service.

Recognizing that records of births and deaths alone would not completely indicate the impact of illness and disease on the population, Congress, in 1893, passed a bill to collect weekly morbidity data from states and cities throughout the country, a practice that continues to this day.

In 1912, two important pieces of health legislation were enacted, one creating the Children's Bureau and inaugurating maternal and child health programs, and the other changing the name of the Marine Hospital Service to the U.S. Public Health Service (USPHS) and authorizing it to conduct field investigations and studies. These two laws have largely defined the roles of federal, state, and local jurisdiction regarding public health activities and programs. In 1915 the first statistician appointed to the USPHS began to conduct household surveys of pellagra, diet, housing, and economic status in the cotton-mill towns of South Carolina. The Great Depression of the 1930s provided the opportunity for a nationwide survey of 700,000 households in eighty-three urban areas, and the results were used over the next twenty years as baseline data for promoting public health programs. This data provided the federal government and the states with an epidemiological basis for the support of public health programs.

Health officials appointed by political leaders and government officials must define public health policy and programs within the framework of pertinent legislation and what is acceptable to the political leadership. This often leads to the politicization of public health issues and results in political debate instead of public health discourse. By contrast, Civil Service appointees, by virtue of their career protection, can more easily take independent positions on controversial public health issues without threats to their professional careers.

Another important milestone in health affairs came with the incorporation of the original Marine Service Hygienic Laboratory into the National Institutes of Health, which became the federal government's major mechanism for performing, funding, and directing medical and health research. Major disease and organ-specific institutes have developed within this framework and have contributed to major advances in our knowledge of health and disease. Some institutes have been created by political leadership from congressional leaders with a particular interest in a certain disease entity.

Interest groups that form around public health issues constitute another source of program advocacy. Many of these are organ-specific, such as the American Liver Foundation and the American Heart Association, while others are disease-specific, such as the American Cancer Society and the American Diabetes Association. These organizations raise funds in support of their interests, but they also exercise political advocacy. Groups at special risks of some diseases also participate in advocacy on their behalf. Political and public health leaders, therefore, are subject to multiple pressures for support of various programs and public health initiatives, and these pressures have the potential for creating inequities in the distribution of resources. It is fortunate when public health leaders have the credibility and stature in their communities to be perceived as sage advisors to the community and the political leadership so that such distortions in the distribution of resources are minimized.

In February 1998, the president of the United States committed the nation to eliminate health disparities among ethnic and racial groups. Following the president's lead, the Surgeon General has formally set a national goal of eliminating health disparities by the year 2010. Although not articulated as a "political" goal, its achievement will require the exercise of a political will whose magnitude has not been seen since the passage of the Social Security Act of 1935 or the Medicare and Medicaid legislation in 1965.

As late as the 1960s, public health students and preventive medicine residents were taught that as public health professionals they should stay clear of politics. Their role was seen to be protecting the public's health within the existing rules. Once those students and residents left their training and entered the world of public health practice, however, they quickly found that the important decisions affecting public health agencies' ability to protect, promote, and assure the public's health were being made in the political arena, and that those public health professionals who eschewed politics would not have the resources to carry out the mandates of public health.

It is odd to note that a nation that prides itself on its concern for human rights and that passed the Civil Rights Act of 1964 does not recognize that the existence of more than 40 million citizens and residents with no health insurance is a civil rights issue, and a human rights issue, of major proportions. Being the only major Western industrial nation that, at a time of unprecedented economic prosperity, does not guarantee its people the right to necessary and appropriate health care is not a distinction the United States should covet. Indeed, as early as 1937, Dr. Thomas Parran, the U.S. Surgeon General, declared that citizens should have an equal opportunity for health as an inherent right, along with the rights of liberty and the pursuit of happiness.

The widely praised Institute of Medicine report *The Future of Public Health* (1988), defined the role of public health in terms of three core functions, assessment, policy development, and assurance. The report also defines public health's mission as "fulfilling society's interest in creating the conditions in which people can be healthy." Thus, public health is inherently political, and society influences public health policy through the people it elects to represent it at local, state, and federal levels. Every time Congress adopts a budget that is signed by the president it is defining public health policy and determining what the nation's chief public health instrument, the U.S. Public Health Service, can do to protect the nation's health.

In every local political jurisdiction, the governing body of the local health department is a political body. Even when there is a local board of health, the local governing body usually selects its members, and by exercising those choices the political leaders influence the definition of public health policy in that jurisdiction. In one large American city, for example, all state or federal grant requests required city council approval before submission to the granting agencies. Having identified and documented an increasing incidence of deaths and injuries due to household fires in an impoverished section of the city, and

having learned from the city fire marshal that the absence of smoke detectors in those homes was contributing to the morbidity and mortality, the director of public health instructed his staff to seek a federal grant that could be used to install smoke detectors in the homes in that section of the city, especially in the homes of needy elderly citizens who, by virtue of age and disability, were at greatest risk. When that proposal was presented to the city council for approval, that city council determined that injury and death from fires was not a public health problem, but a problem for the fire marshal, and that the director of public health should stay out of such problems. In that same state, a state attorney general ruled that attending at childbirth was not a medical activity and, therefore, midwives did not need special training or licensure. The result was a high rate of obstetrical misadventures in unregulated birthing centers. These may seem extreme examples of the role of politics in defining public health policy and practice, but they underline the fact that to be successful in protecting the people's health, public health practitioners must actively enter the political environment in which public health decisions are made.

Free and low-cost school lunches have become a tradition in U.S. public schools, and Americans like to believe that this tradition represents our humanitarian concern for the proper nutrition of children from poor families. The reality is that the United States Department of Agriculture (USDA) created the program to provide a market for surplus farm products from U.S. farms. The public health goal of better nutrition for poor children was incidental. Proof of the marginal significance of a public health goal when compared to the political intent was the recent outbreak of hepatitis A among school children in a Midwestern state. When the etiology of the outbreak was traced by the Centers for Disease Control and Prevention to strawberries provided by a school lunch-program contractor who had sold the USDA strawberries purchased from a Central American country, the contractor's crime was not that he had imperiled the health and lives of dozens of U.S. schoolchildren, but that he had injured the income of U.S. farmers by selling a foreign-grown product to the school lunch program.

The determinants of the public's health are not limited to bacteria and viruses and other specific disease factors to which people are exposed.

They also include threats that can be controlled only by concerted community action, through the political process, environmental toxins, substandard housing, unsafe working environments, inadequate housing policies, the absence of universal health coverage, and personal behaviors that jeopardize people's well-being—these are all determinants of health, and none, except personal behaviors, are subject to solutions by individuals. All require community action, political responses, and political will.

At the dawn of the twenty-first century, the United States stands as the most powerful and the most wealthy nation on earth—but not the most healthy, despite the highest per capita expenditures for health services. In a study published in 1977 it was shown that "despite the increase in use of medical services by the poor, the gap in health status between the poor and nonpoor as measured by morbidity, disability, and mortality has actually widened" (Elinson, 1977). After twenty-three years, recognition of this continuing gap has led to the *Healthy People 2010* goal of eliminating these disparities.

During the period from 1910 to 1920, public discussion of national health insurance began in some of the more progressive states, and a committee of the American Medical Association made a recommendation of such a program. Only in 1943, however, was the first meaningful national health insurance bill introduced in Congress. At that time, U.S. Senators Robert Wagner, Sr. of New York State and James Murray of Montana, together with Representative John Dingell, Sr. of Michigan, proposed what became known as the Wagner-Murray-Dingell bill. Although tentative forward steps in government-financed health care had taken place in 1935 when some health care for the poor was included in the Social Security Act, the Wagner-Murray-Dingell bill was immediately labeled "socialized medicine" by the American Medical Association and others who feared government intrusion into medical practice. The bill never reached the floor of either house of Congress.

After 1965, when Congress enacted the Medicare and Medicaid legislation, it took only a few years for the costs of both programs to become a political battleground. Efforts by the Clinton administration to design a program of universal health coverage met such universal opposition from Congress that it may be a long time before another president will dare to try again. Because public-policy development is a political process, however, public opinion often sets the national agenda, and public health practitioners can take leadership in molding that public opinion.

JAMES G. HAUGHTON

(SEE ALSO: *Community Health; Conflicts of Interests; Equity and Resource Allocation; Inequalities in Health; Landmark Public Health Laws and Court Decisions; Legislation and Regulation; National Health Insurance; Official U.S. Health Agencies; Regulatory Authority; Uninsurance; United States Public Health Service [USPHS]*)

BIBLIOGRAPHY

Cohen, W. J. (1979). "Policy Planning for National Health Insurance." In *Health in America: 1776–1976.* Washington, DC: U.S. Department of Health, Education and Welfare.

Elinson, J. (1977). "Have We Narrowed the Gaps in Health Status between the Poor and the Nonpoor?" *Medical Care* 15(8):675–677.

Institute of Medicine (1988). *The Future of Public Health.* Washington, DC: National Academy Press.

Steinfeld, J. L. (1979). "The United States Public Health Service." In *Health in America: 1776–1976.* Washington, DC: U.S. Department of Health, Education and Welfare.

POLLUTION

The term "pollution," which carries with it a sense of an impurity, can be defined as a chemical or physical agent in an inappropriate location or concentration. The sources of pollution are varied. Natural sources include those that are not directly under human control, such as volcanoes, which spew forth sulfur oxides and particles; and those people could avoid, such as groundwater with naturally high levels of arsenic, which has caused poisoning in Bangladesh and Taiwan. All human activities have the possibility of polluting the environment by contaminating air, water, food, or soil, The earliest human pollution-control efforts dealt with avoidance of diseases caused by contamination of water and food by human excreta and with the control of smoke from fires used for cooking and heating. Sanitary engineering to manage human wastes remains a central public health need. Indoor air pollution due to the use of wood and fossil fuels in poorly ventilated residences also remains a major source of exposure to pollutants and a cause of respiratory disease in much of the world.

TYPES OF POLLUTION

Pollution production can be considered under the heading of the four major human activity sectors: industry, energy, transportation, and agriculture. With the marked increase in human population and the industrialization of much of the globe has come a whole new set of pollutants. Scientific advances based upon understanding the chemical and physical forces underlying nature have led to new processes and new products that have transformed society and have had a major positive impact on human health. But these industrial activities also result in air and water emissions and contamination of the soil and of food as by-products of the processes involved in manufacture. The products themselves may be the means by which pollutants are distributed to the general population, such as lead poisoning through the use of lead in house paints. In the United States and other more wealthy countries, there recently has been a marked decline in industrial pollution emissions per unit produced. This has come about through regulatory control of emissions and, in part, through the recognition by industry that emissions represent a loss of raw materials or product that is economically advantageous to retain. As developed countries move into the information era, much of the production of textiles and durable goods has shifted to developing countries, not always with the same level of pollution control or protection of the work force. In developing countries, industrial production often occurs in smaller units, such as backyard smelters, which have significant local effects and are more difficult to control.

The energy sector continues to grow rapidly worldwide. There are basically three types of energy sources: the burning of fossil fuels and biomass; nuclear power; and energy derived from natural processes such as the sun, wind, and the flow of water. Energy from fossil fuels results from the conversion of carbon to carbon dioxide, with the least efficient and most polluting fossil fuels reflecting the extent of components other than carbon and hydrogen in the fuel source. The most plentiful fossil fuel is coal, which is also among the most polluting. Coal contains mineral ashes, nitrogen, and sulfur, which produce particulates, nitrogen oxides and sulfur oxides, when coal is burned. The use of high-sulfur coal for electric power generation and for home heating was a dominant cause of major air pollution episodes in London in 1952, Donora, Pennsylvania, in 1948, and the Meuse Valley in Belgium in 1930. Much of the U.S. electric grid is powered by low-sulfur oil. Natural gas, which is a relatively pure hydrocarbon, is increasing in use and is particularly effective as a source of peak electric power during periods of high demand. The combustion of all fossil fuels produces nitrogen oxides, which are a major precursor of ozone and particulates. One form of nitrogen oxide, nitrogen dioxide, is itself a pollutant of concern. Carbon dioxide, the end product of efficient fossil fuel energy production, is a major contributor to global climate change. Reduction in carbon dioxide emissions requires more efficient production, transmission, and use of fossil fuel-derived energy. A switch to other energy sources will also help to reduce emissions.

Nuclear power has the advantage of not producing carbon dioxide or any of the sulfur oxides, nitrogen oxides, or particulates that are associated with fossil fuels. Its major disadvantages are the release of low-level radiation, the need for major water resources for cooling (with attendant ecological challenges), and, most importantly, the small but not absent risk of an uncontrolled nuclear reaction. The worst such example, and the only one in which there were substantial short-term health impacts from the civilian use of nuclear power, occurred in Chernobyl in the former Soviet Union in 1986. The extent of long-term effects due to the radiation that spread widely over Europe and globally is still being evaluated.

Wind and solar energy are expected to increase in use as the costs of fossil fuels increase and as new technology is developed. These are, in essence, free of pollution emissions. Hydroelectric power is a mainstay in some parts of the world, but dams have significant ecological implications and there is a growing movement against them. The most effective means of decreasing energy use is by lessening demand.

The transportation sector worldwide is increasingly dominated by automobile and truck emissions. In the United States there has been a marked decrease in pollutant emissions per mile driven that has been almost counterbalanced by an increase in the number of miles driven. Pollutants from gasoline-powered automobiles include the evaporation of volatile organic compounds and tailpipe emissions such as carbon monoxide, nitrogen oxides, benzene, and polycyclic aromatic hydrocarbons (PAHs). Increased engine efficiency and catalytic converters have been effective in decreasing all but nitrogen oxide emissions. Diesel engines, which in the United States are primarily used on trucks, emit high levels of particulates and PAHs. Two-cycle engines on mopeds and other smaller vehicles are relatively inefficient, with much of the fuel evaporating. This is particularly a problem in developing countries. All internal combustion engines lead to the production of carbon dioxide. Future growth in the use of personal automobiles will be a major threat to global carbon dioxide production unless new engines and power sources are developed. Control of automotive emissions is as much a function of effective planning of transportation systems, including mass transit, as it is of technology. There have been relatively few studies of airport-related pollutant emissions, a segment of transportation that is increasing rapidly.

Agriculture is also a major source of pollution. World population growth has been accompanied by increased crop yields, which have been made possible by heavy use of fertilizers and pesticides. Nitrogenous fertilizers, an important part of the increased yield, result in nitrite contamination of drinking water, to which infants are particularly vulnerable. Nitrogenous fertilizers contribute to oxygen problems in water bodies and to greenhouse gas emissions. Phosphate fertilizers are of concern because of trace amounts of cadmium and other heavy metals that sometimes are part of natural phosphates. Cadmium can be taken up into certain crops, can cause renal toxicity, and is a potential carcinogen.

There are a wide range of pesticides and herbicides that are central to modern agriculture. Each of these is chosen because of its ability to have a biological effect on a plant or insect, and there is always a possibility that the biological effect will extend to humans or to other species. Major problems have been caused by pesticides that persist in the environment, such as heptachlor. This has led to bans on persistent organic pollutants and to testing protocols to avoid developing new ones.

OTHER POLLUTION CATEGORIES

Categorizing pollution in terms of the four sectors of industry, energy, transportation, and agriculture obscures the fact that some of the most important sources of pollution are intersectorial. As just one example, the Aswan High Dam provides Egypt with an important hydroelectric source and is effective in controlling flooding and providing irrigation for agriculture. But by retaining silt it decreases the nutrient load to the Nile Delta, which leads to a much heavier requirement for chemical fertilizers for agriculture as well as loss of sardine and salmon fisheries. The lack of the flushing effect of Nile floods has led to increased salinization of the land and has optimized breeding conditions for snails that carry schistosomiasis, an ancient scourge of this area. Similarly, the use of wood for local energy in developing countries is more than just a potential source of indoor and outdoor air pollution. Loss of forests can lead to soil erosion, flooding, and desertification, and have a negative impact on global climate.

Activities that lead to human development within and across each of these major sectors have the potential for producing a pollution impact that outweighs any benefit. There is, unfortunately, one common human activity that has an enormous environmental impact with no redeeming developmental consequences: war.

Pollutants can also be characterized by chemical or physical class; by use; by industrial source; by whether they are likely to be present in air, water, food, or other media; by the organs they attack or the effects they have; by the laws that control their use; and by whether they present a local, regional, or global problem. All of these categorization schemes are valuable, but none are without its faults. Chemicals have multiple properties and uses, and are able to move across environmental boundaries. Pollution episodes have often come about through an inappropriate focus on only one aspect of a chemical. For example, the 1990 U.S. Clean Air Act required the use of oxygenated fuels, which have chemical characteristics that were thought to be beneficial in decreasing automotive emissions in polluted areas. Yet another chemical characteristics of the most commonly used oxygenate compound, methyl tertiary-butyl ether (MTBE), caused it to be a major groundwater contaminant, a problem that was not foreseen because of an inappropriately narrow focus.

A more holistic approach to environmental pollution is particularly important during the current transition period. Pollution control techniques have been largely successful in dealing with end-of-pipe emissions. Through regulatory command and control of major pollution sources there has been a steady diminution of measured emissions to air and water in developed countries, and an improvement in air and water quality. Yet major problems remain, and in some instances they are getting worse. Two interrelated categories of particular concern are global climate change and pollutants from nonpoint sources.

Our planet maintains itself through a series of feedback loops involving interconnected biological, geological, and physical processes. The science that has enhanced our understanding of these processes has also demonstrated their vulnerability to the increasing dominance of human activities, including the effect of pollutants. One example is the diminution of the stratospheric ozone layer that protects humans against the harmful effects of short-range ultraviolet light. A major source of this diminution is chlorofluorocarbons (CFCs). These compounds were seemingly ideal for refrigeration and a variety of other industrial purposes, in part because they are inert and cause little or no direct biological effects. But this lack of reactivity allows CFCs to persist and rise into the stratosphere where they enter into a reaction that decomposes ozone. An international treaty, the Montreal Protocol, has led to a decrease in this particular threat to the ozone layer. The feedback loops involved in global climate change, including the greenhouse effect which is now warming the earth, are far more complex and less well understood. Further, competitive economic and nationalistic interests have made it more difficult to deal with carbon dioxide and nitrogenous greenhouse gases.

Nonpoint source emissions refer to pollution for which there is no readily obvious target, or source. An example is damage to the Chesapeake Bay due to runoff of nitrogenous fertilizer compounds from farms along the Susquehanna River, including a heavy contribution from farms using natural fertilizing techniques. Agricultural practices and energy and transportation decisions contribute heavily to regional air and water pollution and to global warming.

UNDERSTANDING POLLUTION EFFECTS

A transition is also occurring in our understanding of the health effects of pollutants. It is now recognized that there are subtle health effects of environmental pollutants, such as endocrine disruption and neurobehavioral changes, for which newer toxicological paradigms are being developed. The unraveling of the human genome may provide a better understanding of the role of genetic susceptibility factors in response to pollution.

Understanding the effects of pollutants requires understanding how pollutants change following their release from a source, and how they can have effects many miles from their sources. For example, there are no significant direct emitters of air pollutant ozone. Rather, this major component of oxidant smog is formed in the air through the action of sunlight on a mixture of nitrogen oxides and hydrocarbons coming from many different sources, primarily automobiles. The precursors may have been emitted hundreds of miles upwind of where the ozone is eventually formed. For the northeastern United States, this means that statewide control strategies, which are the major enforcement focus of the U.S. Clean Air Act, are an inadequate approach to a regional issue. Similarly, acid rain and other forms of particulate air pollution can be derived from atmospheric reactions of gaseous sulfur dioxide and nitrogen oxides precursors occurring many hundreds of miles downwind. Agents released into water can also undergo significant changes. For example, methyl mercury, which is far more toxic than elemental mercury, is formed in water through the action of bacteria and makes its way into the food chain. The dumping of inorganic mercury from a single chloralkali plant in Minimata Bay, Japan, led to contamination of fish with methyl mercury and to over a hundred deaths and thousands of people being affected by what is known as Minimata disease. There is also a global air circulation of metals, such as mercury, and of persistent organic pollutants, such as PCBs, which tends to carry these agents toward the arctic where they often bioaccumulate.

Understanding the effects of pollutants on human health requires not only an understanding of the intrinsic hazard of the chemical or physical agent, but also the extent of human exposure. Exposure is often determined by local pathways within a community, such as whether drinking water comes from wells or from surface sources or whether individuals consume vegetables grown in their backyards or brought to market from far away. Individual activities can also alter pollutant intake; exercise, for example, increases respiratory uptake of air pollutants. Health effects due to pollutants are heavily dependent upon susceptibility factors, including age, gender, and genetic predisposition.

MANAGING POLLUTION

A variety of approaches have been developed to manage existing pollution. These include punishment of polluters through regulation, taxation, fines, toxic tort suits, and other disincentives; encouragement of nonpolluting approaches through tax and other incentives; and education of the public. The increased awareness of the potential harmful effects of pollution has had a major impact on industries and on individuals, particularly the young, who have led the way in activities such as recycling. Risk assessment has developed as a useful technique to estimate the risks of environmental pollutants and to establish priorities for environmental control and remediation efforts. These efforts to manage existing pollution are largely a form of secondary prevention in that the pollution already exists and the focus is on lessening the extent or the effects.

Primary prevention of pollution has occurred through approaches that, like any form of primary prevention, are both highly effective and difficult to quantify. The United States National Environmental Policy Act of 1969 was the first major action arising out of the new environmental movement aimed at avoiding unwanted environmental consequences. It contained the requirement that significant newly proposed federal activities have an environmental impact statement prepared in advance, the goal being the incorporation of environmental concerns into all planning processes and the avoidance of those activities that would have an adverse impact. Advances in science have had a significant primary preventive effect, in part through providing assessment tools of use in preventing the development of new harmful products by the chemical industry. As examples, a basic understanding of the role of mutation in cancer and recognition of the structural aspects resulting in the environmental persistence of chemicals have led the chemical industry to detect and quickly drop out of its development programs those new chemicals that are mutagens or are likely to persist in the environment. The Precautionary Principle is basic to public health practice, but is also now being advocated as a form of primary prevention of environmental pollution.

Control of the more challenging insidious pollutant effects related to the health of the planetary biosphere and to nonpoint sources cannot depend solely upon standard command and control regulatory approaches. Central to avoiding significant long-term consequences to health and the environment is the development of innovative pollution prevention and control strategies, including emissions trading, taxation of consumption and international compacts; better targeting of controls through improved scientific understanding of the processes involved; and a more informed public.

BERNARD D. GOLDSTEIN

(SEE ALSO: *Acid Rain; Airborne Particles; Ambient Air Quality [Air Pollution]; Ambient Water Quality; Arsenic; Automotive Emissions; Benzene; Carcinogen; Chlorofluorocarbons; Clean Air Act; Clean Water Act; Climate Change and Human Health; Ecosystems; Emissions Trading; Endocrine Disruptors; Environmental Impact Statement; Exposure Assessment; Groundwater; Human Genome Project; Lead; Mercury; National Environmental Policy Act of 1969; Nuclear Power; PCBs; Persistent*

Organic Pollutants [POPs]; Pesticides; Precautionary Principle; Radiation, Ionizing; Risk Assessment, Risk Management; Sulfur-Containing Air Pollutants [Particulates]; War)

BIBLIOGRAPHY

United Nations Environment Programme (1999). *Global Environment Outlook 2000–UNEP's Millennium Report on the Environment.* London, UK: Earthscan Publications Ltd.

World Health Organization (1992). *Report of the WHO Commission on Health and Environment.* Geneva: Author.

POLLUTION, NOISE

See Noise

POLLUTION, WATER

See Ambient Water Quality

POPULATION AT RISK

The term "population at risk" defines the denominator for the calculation of rates of incidences and prevalence. It alludes to the number of persons potentially capable of experiencing the event or outcome of interest. The number or persons who actually experience the event make up the numerator of the rate. For rates to be valid and meaningful, the population at risk must be known accurately. However, many vital statistical rates are calculated on an annual basis, and for these rates the midyear population, or an approximation based on extrapolation from a recent set of census data, is often used for the population at risk. As rates incorporate an element of time, the denominator is often expressed in person-time rather than as the population at risk.

JOHN M. LAST

(SEE ALSO: *Epidemiology; Rates; Rates: Adjusted*)

BIBLIOGRAPHY

Rothman, K. J., and Greenland, S., eds. (1998). *Modern Epidemiology,* 2nd edition. Philadelphia, PA: Lippincott-Raven.

POPULATION ATTRIBUTABLE RISK

The term "attributable risk" describes the proportion of disease that can be attributed to an exposure to risk that persons in a population have experienced. It is a general term that is usually more precisely defined by epidemiologists in one of several ways. The most widely used of these is probably the population attributable risk. This is the incidence rate of a condition in a specified population that is associated with or attributable to exposure to a specific risk. There are so many variations in the terminology of "risk" that interested readers should consult a textbook or the *Dictionary of Epidemiology* for details.

JOHN M. LAST

(SEE ALSO: *Causality, Causes, and Causal Inference; Epidemiology; Incidence and Prevalence; Risk Assessment, Risk Management*)

BIBLIOGRAPHY

Last, J. M., ed. (2000). *Dictionary of Epidemiology,* 4th edition. New York: Oxford University Press.

POPULATION DENSITY

As the term implies, "population density" refers to the number of people in a defined jurisdiction, in relation to the size of the area that they occupy. Obviously, the population density is higher in urban areas than in rural communities. In the world as a whole, the population density is very high in some nations, such as Singapore and the Netherlands, and very low in others, such as Greenland and Australia (though in Australia the density is quite high in several large cities, while the rest of the continent is sparsely settled). Tables showing the population density of the nations of the world are published by the United Nations Statistical Office. While population density is a useful measure, the proportion of people living in urban areas in relation to the area available to produce food for them might be a more meaningful statistic.

JOHN M. LAST

(SEE ALSO: *Demography; Population Growth; Rural Public Health; Urban Health*)

POPULATION FORECASTS

A population forecast provides estimates of the most likely future trends in population size and in demographic indicators such as population distribution by age and sex. A forecast is based on the current understanding of the roles played by various factors affecting population growth and on an appropriate, accepted methodology for calculating the effects of future changes in these factors. A variety of methodologies are available for making forecasts, ranging from the simple extrapolation of past trends to complex multiple-equation models involving dozens of demographic, socioeconomic, and environmental variables. In practice, most projections made in recent years rely on the so-called cohort-component method, which computes future demographic trajectories implied by assumptions (based on demographic transition theory) about future trends in birth, death, and migration rates.

The terms "forecast" and "projection" are often used synonymously, though they have slightly different technical meanings. A forecast for a population can involve more than one projection. For example, the most likely future trajectory is usually called the *medium variant*, while alternative higher and lower projections can give an indication of the uncertainty surrounding this trend. In the contemporary demographic literature, "forecast" is typically used to refer to medium variant projections.

Future population trends are of interest to a wide range of analysts, including policymakers, scientists, and planners in industry and government. Global and national trends in population size are used to estimate the future demand for food, water, and energy, as well as the environmental impact of rising consumption of natural resources. Subnational projections help planners decide where to build schools, hospitals, roads, and other infrastructure. Estimates of the number of retired people are essential to the optimal design of social security systems that provide pensions and health care. To address the needs of such a variety of potential users, projections for countries and regions within countries are usually made on a regular basis by national agencies (e.g., the Bureau of the Census in the United States). Global as well as national population projections for all countries are produced by the United Nations and the World Bank.

The projections prepared in 1998 by the Population Division of the United Nations predict the population of the world to reach 8.9 billion in 2050. This represents an increase of 2.8 billion over the 2000 population of 6.1 billion. Nearly all of this future growth will occur in the developing world—Africa, Asia (excluding Japan, Australia, and New Zealand), and Latin America—where population size is projected to rise from 4.9 to 7.8 billion between 2000 and 2050. In contrast, in the developed world—Europe, North America, Japan, Australia, and New Zealand—population size is forecast to remain virtually stable, growing from 1.19 to 1.22 billion between 2000 and 2025, followed by a decline to 1.16 billion in 2050. Trends for the two principal regions in the developed world are expected to diverge between 2000 and 2050, with an increase from 0.31 to 0.39 billion in North America and a decline from 0.73 to 0.63 billion in Europe.

JOHN BONGAARTS

(SEE ALSO: *Demographic Transition; Demography; Population Growth; Population Pyramid*)

BIBLIOGRAPHY

National Research Council, Commission on Behavioral and Social Science and Education, Committee on Population (2000). *Beyond Six Billion: Projecting the World's Population,* eds. J. Bongaarts and R. Bulatao. Washington, DC: National Academy Press.

United Nations, Department for Social and Economic Policy Analysis, Population Division (1999). *World Population Prospects: The 1998 Revision.* New York: United Nations.

POPULATION GROWTH

Populations increase as people are born or immigrate into a country, and decrease as people die or emigrate. Rates of population growth, usually expressed as a percentage, vary greatly. In the late twentieth century, growth rates in many European nations were extremely low, and in some parts of Eastern Europe and the former Soviet Union the growth rate was negative—that is, populations were declining in number. On the other hand, in some African and Latin American nations, the growth rate was around 4 percent, which is a doubling time of less than twenty years. The United

States, as of the year 2000, had a growth rate of about 1 percent per annum.

JOHN M. LAST

(SEE ALSO: *Demography; Doubling Time; Population Density; Population Forecasts; Population Policies; Zero Population Growth*)

POPULATION POLICIES

Population policy is made by national governments in an effort to either limit or expand the number of people in their country. For countries with high population growth rates, population policy generally includes programs to encourage family planning, birth spacing, and delaying the birth of a woman's first child. In the 1990s, many countries began to include improvements in women's reproductive health as part of their population policies. The national family planning programs begun in various African countries are good examples of this aspect of population policy.

Countries with very low or negative population growth rates have sometimes encouraged families to have more children through policies such as extended maternity leave with pay and family support payments. Population policy can also include measures to increase or decrease immigration.

ANNE R. PEBLEY

(SEE ALSO: *Demography; Population Growth; Population Pyramid*)

POPULATION PYRAMID

The term "population pyramid" describes the shape of a diagram showing the composition, by age and sex, of a nation's population at the time of a census. It is also called a "population profile." It is a convenient way to display in visual form the national population composition, and it is widely used by demographers, vital statisticians, public health specialists, social policy planners, and the television and print media when issues of national population are being discussed. The numbers used to construct the diagram are derived from national census returns. Because of its pyramid shape, a population pyramid is most aptly applied to a population with high birth rates and high death

rates in infancy and at all subsequent ages. The term was probably coined with this in mind, because it evokes an image of small numbers in the upper age ranges perched on top of much larger numbers of newborn infants and young children. The population pyramid of a typical developing country in the mid twentieth century had this appearance. In the Philippines and Mexico, high birth rates and high death rates in infancy and childhood preserved the pyramid shape into the 1960s.

The changes in age and sex composition of the population in many industrial nations in the twentieth century altered the shape of the population profile, sometimes dramatically. The most obvious changes are due to a decline in the number of children born, plus reduced death rates at all ages up to old age. This produces a diagram better described as a population profile rather than a pyramid. It has a narrower base, a broader middle, and a blunter apex. Sharp declines in the numbers born at times of crisis such as wars and severe depressions leave a legacy of a narrowing at the middle of the profile several decades later.

Nations that suffer severe losses of young men in major wars have a profile that shows the excess of females, and this too works its way through the age groups as the cohorts of young people grow older; this is demonstrated in the 1965 profile of the United Kingdom, with the smaller numbers of middle-aged and old men than women in the same age groups reflecting the losses of the two world wars.

The most dramatic changes in the shape of the population profile may be those that are now appearing in sub-Saharan Africa, where HIV/AIDS (human immunodeficiency virus/acquired immunodeficiency syndrome) has had a devastating effect, selectively killing young sexually active men and women and leaving nations with orphan children to be raised by aged grandparents. Other changes appear in nations where high proportions of young immigrants are rapidly absorbed, or conversely in nations where there is substantial emigration of able-bodied young adults.

Population profiles or pyramids of successive census populations are a useful tool for the visual display of the changing composition of any nation's population, such as the United States and Canada throughout the twentieth century—with changes reflecting immigration, losses in the two world wars, reduced birth rates in the depression of the 1930s, and the surging birth rates of the baby boom years.

JOHN M. LAST

(SEE ALSO: *Demography; Vital Statistics*)

POSTERS

Posters are an effective means of publicizing issues of importance to public health and serve a role in both education and intervention campaigns. In the 1980s and 1990s, antitobacco campaigns made a prominent use of posters. Among the several content analyses of health communications, one on antitobacco posters assessed the shift in the thematic content of such posters over time. There has been an evolution in antitobacco posters from an emphasis on disseminating knowledge to one on stimulating action among the public. The former approach was aimed at effecting change at the individual level, the second aims more at social action. This follows a basic tenet in social marketing theory that market segmentation is important, though many posters do not demonstrate a clear understanding of this approach.

TOM ABERNATHY

(SEE ALSO: *Communication for Health; Communication Theory; Health Promotion and Education; Mass Media and Tobacco Control*)

POTT, PERCIVALL

Percivall Pott (1713–1788) was a surgeon in London, England. Apprenticed to a surgeon at the age of sixteen, he trained at St. Bartholomew's Hospital and worked there throughout his life, eventually becoming the greatest surgeon of his time. He described the cause and appearance of a particular type of fractured wrist, known ever since as Pott's fracture, and he was the first to describe the deformity of the spine caused by collapse of a vertebra due to tuberculosis, now known as Pott's disease. He is also known among public health scientists and epidemiologists for his observations and writings on chimney sweeps' cancer. Pott correctly deduced that the prevalence of cancer of the scrotum among chimney sweeps was associated with the coal tar that accumulated in the creases of the sweeps' scrotal skin. This, and his work on tuberculosis, made Pott a memorable figure in the field of public health, as well as in surgery.

JOHN M. LAST

POVERTY AND HEALTH

People with low incomes, particularly those who live in poverty, face particular challenges in maintaining their health. They are more likely than those with higher incomes to become ill, and to die at younger ages. They are also more likely to live in poor environmental situations with limited health care resources—factors that can compromise health status and access to care. Public programs play a vital role in helping to reduce disparities in health by income by supporting health initiatives targeted at those with low incomes and maintaining a safety net of health and social services for the poor.

POVERTY IN THE UNITED STATES

The United States is one of the wealthiest nations in the world, yet a significant portion of the population still lives in poverty. Though the poverty rate declined during the 1990s due to a strong economy, 11.8 percent of Americans—over 32 million people—lived below the poverty level in 1999. Calculated to assess the cost of food and basic expenses by family size, the federal poverty level was a little over $17,000 a year for a family of four in 1999. Many of America's poor are living far below the poverty level on incomes that barely exceed $10,000. In addition to the poor, another 50 million people are "near poor" and have incomes between poverty and twice the poverty level.

The problem of poverty in America is even more alarming when looking at particularly vulnerable populations (see Figure 1). According to the Census Bureau, in 1999:

- 16.9 percent of all children and 18 percent of children under age six lived in poverty, versus 10 percent of adults.

Figure 1

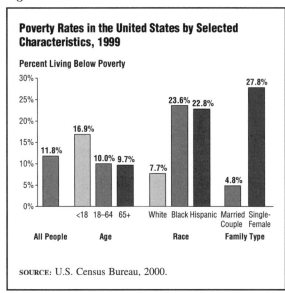

Poverty Rates in the United States by Selected Characteristics, 1999

Percent Living Below Poverty

SOURCE: U.S. Census Bureau, 2000.

• Minority racial and ethnic groups are much more likely to live in poverty—23.6 percent of blacks and 22.8 percent of Hispanics lived below the poverty level, versus 7.7 percent of whites.

• Female-headed households (with no husband present) are much more likely than married couple families to live in poverty (27.8% versus 4.8%), with black and Hispanic female-headed households having the highest poverty rates (39.3% and 38.8%, respectively).

Public assistance helps many of the lowest-income families and individuals meet their most basic financial and health needs. Social Security, for example, provides financial assistance to workers and their families in retirement, as well as to some disabled individuals, enabling those who are no longer working to maintain an income. Since its enactment in 1935, this program has helped reduce poverty among the elderly and disabled, and today less than 10 percent of the elderly live in poverty. Many low-income families have also been helped by cash assistance (also called "welfare"), formerly under the Aid to Families with Dependent Children (AFDC) program and, since 1996, under the Temporary Assistance for Needy Families (TANF) program. While this assistance is an essential source of support for millions of families, the populations that are the targets for such assistance—mainly children and single-headed households—still have some of the highest poverty rates in the nation. Poverty persists in these groups for many reasons, including low benefit levels in welfare and restrictive eligibility levels that leave most workers, even those working at minimum wage jobs, ineligible for assistance.

While the poverty statistics for the United States are alarming, the problem of poverty around the world is even more dire. According to the World Bank, the average income in the world's wealthiest countries (which includes the United States) is thirty-seven times that in the poorest nations. This differential exists because poverty in developing nations is not only more prevalent, it is also significantly deeper—2.8 billion people in the world live on less than $2 a day, and 1.2 billion live on less than $1 a day. Poverty touches all areas of the world, though the most impoverished conditions are found in South Asia, sub-Saharan Africa, and East Asia and the Pacific regions. People living in the world's poorest nations are faced not only with trying to afford food, shelter, and clothing, but also with severe malnutrition, living without basic sanitation or clean water, and a lack of access to basic education.

HEALTH AND POVERTY

The impact of poverty on health is a key focus of public health. Studies have firmly established that those with low incomes have lower health status than those with higher incomes (see Figure 2). In *Health, United States, 1998*, the United States Department of Health and Human Services highlighted many of the disparities in health status by income and documented a stairstep pattern of worsening outcomes from rich to poor that holds true for almost all risk factors, diseases, and causes of death, and persists within racial and ethnic groups. Poor Americans are significantly more likely than those with high incomes to have health risk factors that include smoking, being overweight, and having a sedentary lifestyle. However, they also use less health care than most Americans and are less likely than the nonpoor to have had a recent physician contact, receive preventive care such as immunizations or cancer screening, or to avoid hospitalization for serious conditions by receiving

Figure 2

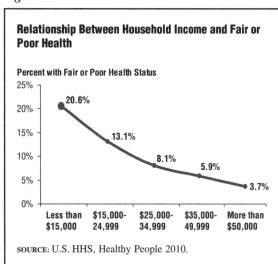

Relationship Between Household Income and Fair or Poor Health

Percent with Fair or Poor Health Status

SOURCE: U.S. HHS, Healthy People 2010.

Figure 3

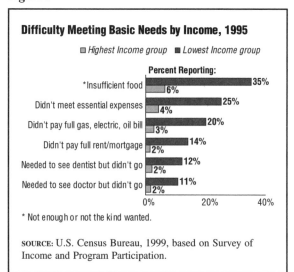

Difficulty Meeting Basic Needs by Income, 1995

* Not enough or not the kind wanted.

SOURCE: U.S. Census Bureau, 1999, based on Survey of Income and Program Participation.

preventive, office-based care. People living in poverty have a higher prevalence of disability and chronic illness and shorter life expectancy than those at higher income levels.

Internationally, the relationship between income and health is even more striking. In poor nations, up to 20 percent of children die before the age of five (versus less than 1% in richer countries), and 50 percent of children are malnourished (versus less than 5% in wealthier nations). Maternal mortality rates are also higher in poor nations. Life expectancy—one of the most revealing indicators of health status—is sixteen years shorter for men and twenty years shorter for women in poor countries than in high-income countries.

The relationship between poverty and health is complex. Many factors play into this link, including poor environmental conditions, low education levels and awareness of needed medical care, financial barriers in accessing health services, and a lack of resources necessary to maintain good health status. As Figure 3 shows, people in poverty live on very stretched incomes and have difficulty meeting day-to-day costs of living, leaving little room in their limited budget for anything beyond the essentials of food and shelter. Low-income Americans are more likely to live in older homes, which—particularly in the inner city—may expose them to lead paint, which causes developmental problems in children. People in poverty may have limited

budgets for food and may only be able to afford inexpensive foods, which tend to be processed, fatty, and lacking important nutrients. And low-income Americans may not be able to access preventive, acute, or long-term medical care when they need it.

Lack of access to medical care and insurance to help cover the costs of health care compromises the ability of many low-income individuals to maintain their health. Poor access to care stems from many factors, including lack of providers in low-income areas, transportation problems in getting to providers, discrimination by providers, and lack of financial means and health insurance to help pay for care. Poor and near-poor Americans are much more likely than higher-income Americans to lack insurance (see Figure 4) and together account for nearly two-thirds of all uninsured people in the nation. Low-income workers are less likely than those with high incomes to be offered insurance as a fringe benefit, and a typical health insurance policy—which costs on average six thousand dollars a year for a family—is often prohibitively expensive or unavailable to the poor. Medicaid provides coverage for many poor and low-income Americans, but limits on eligibility—particularly for adults—leave many outside its reach. With no coverage, the poor are forced to forgo or delay care until absolutely necessary, often seeking assistance only when their illness has progressed to a serious state.

Figure 4

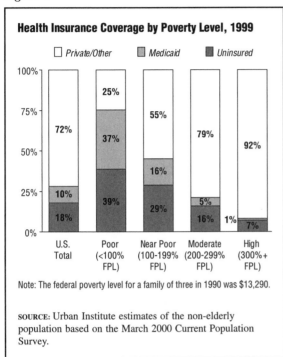

Health Insurance Coverage by Poverty Level, 1999

Note: The federal poverty level for a family of three in 1990 was $13,290.

SOURCE: Urban Institute estimates of the non-elderly population based on the March 2000 Current Population Survey.

Conditions of everyday life for the poor, such as exposure to hazardous environmental and occupational conditions (e.g., neighborhood violence or pollution) or employment in dangerous, stressful jobs that offer few fringe benefits, also influence their health care. Other "third factor" explanations look to the adverse health effects of unemployment (such as depression) or the connection between educational attainment and positive health behavior to understand why income is related to health status. In recent years, a growing body of research has looked to psychosocial factors to explain that it is not always income per se that affects health, but rather the social stratification or level of income inequality in society in general that affects health status.

ADDRESSING POVERTY AND HEALTH

Public health plays a central role in addressing the effects of poverty on health status and minimizing the disparities in health by income. Public health initiatives aimed at protecting the health of the population have been especially important in reducing communicable diseases and providing preventive health services to low-income populations.

Providing immunizations and well-baby care to children, improving sanitation and reducing environmental hazards, treating and controlling tuberculosis, and combating sexually transmitted diseases are examples of public health functions that directly affect the health and well-being of people in poverty.

Public health efforts also aim to address disparities in health by income by focusing resources in underserved areas. The U.S. federal government funds a network of community health centers, migrant and rural health centers, public housing clinics, school-based clinics, and health clinics for the homeless to provide medical care in areas with high rates of uninsurance and an undersupply of providers. Similarly, the National Health Service Corps increases access to provider services by helping to place physicians in communities with vulnerable populations. Other public health services are focused on specific diseases, particularly infectious diseases that may thrive in impoverished areas (such as tuberculosis), or increasing immunization against communicable disease. Public programs in underserved areas also provide nonmedical services that facilitate improvements in the health of low-income families, including Head Start (which provides early day care), public housing, environmental efforts aimed at cleaning up neighborhoods through lead abatement, facilities improvement, or pollution control; and nutrition programs such as school lunch assistance and the Women, Infants, and Children (WIC) feeding program.

One of the largest and most important public programs to improve access to health care for the low-income population is Medicaid, a federal-state partnership that finances health and long-term care insurance for over 40 million low-income Americans. Prior to Medicaid's passage in 1965, the poor were essentially outside mainstream medical care, relying on the charity of physicians and hospitals, or on public hospitals and clinics, for their care and often facing discrimination in their attempts to access services. Medicaid has reshaped the availability and provision of care to the poor and helped to improve health status, access to care, and satisfaction with the health care system among the poor. The value of Medicaid is underscored by the contrast in outcomes between the poor with Medicaid and the uninsured poor, where studies consistently show that the uninsured lag

Figure 5

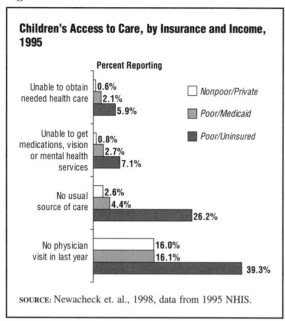

Children's Access to Care, by Insurance and Income, 1995

Percent Reporting

Unable to obtain needed health care
□ Nonpoor/Private — 0.6%
▨ Poor/Medicaid — 2.1%
■ Poor/Uninsured — 5.9%

Unable to get medications, vision or mental health services
0.8%
2.7%
7.1%

No usual source of care
2.6%
4.4%
26.2%

No physician visit in last year
16.0%
16.1%
39.3%

SOURCE: Newacheck et. al., 1998, data from 1995 NHIS.

well behind those with Medicaid, while those with Medicaid fare comparably to the privately insured (see Figure 5).

Although these programs offer valuable assistance to help low-income individuals obtain necessary medical care, the deficits in access and coverage faced by the low-income population are not easily overcome. Improvements in income can make a substantial contribution to removing health differentials by income, but supplemental efforts through insurance coverage for the uninsured and support for community-based resources in underserved areas are also important components of efforts to eliminate health disparities by income.

DIANE ROWLAND

(SEE ALSO: *Access to Health Services; Community and Migrant Health Centers; Economics of Health; Head Start Program; Healthy People 2010; Homelessness; Inequalities in Health; International Development of Public Health; Medicaid; Neighborhood Health Centers; Primary Care; Social Class; Social Determinants; Social Health; Uninsurance*)

BIBLIOGRAPHY

Dalaker, J., and Proctor, B. D. (2000). *Poverty in the United States, 1999*. U.S. Census Bureau, Current Population Reports, Series P60–210. Washington, DC: U.S. Government Printing Office.

Kennedy, B. P.; Kawachi, I.; Glass, R.; and Prothow-Smith, D. (1998). "Income Distribution, Socioeconomic Status, and Self-Rated Health in the United States: Multilevel Analysis." *British Medical Journal* 317:917–921.

Lillie-Blanton, M.; Martinez, R. M.; Lyons, B.; and Rowland, D. (2000). *Access to Health Care: Promises and Prospects for Low-Income Americans*. Washington, DC: The Kaiser Commission on Medicaid and the Uninsured.

Lynch, J. W.; Smith, G. D.; Kaplan, G. A.; and House, J. S. (2000). "Income Inequality and Mortality: Importance to Health of Individual Income, Psychosocial Environment, or Material Conditions." *British Medical Journal* 320:1200–1204.

Marmot, M. (1999). "Acting on the Evidence to Reduce Inequalities in Health." *Health Affairs* 18(3):42–44.

Pamuk, E.; Makuc, D.; Heck, K.; Rueben, C.; and Lochner, K. (1998). *Socioeconomic Status and Health Chartbook: Health, United States, 1998*. Washington, DC: U.S. Department of Health and Human Services.

Rogers, D. E., and Ginzberg, E. (1993). *Medical Care and the Health of the Poor*. Boulder, CO: Westview Press.

World Bank (2000). *World Development Report 2000–2001: Attacking Poverty*. Herndon, VA: World Bank Publications.

PRACTICE OF PUBLIC HEALTH

The phrase "practice of public health" (which will be used interchangeably with the term "public health practice") fails to evoke a single compelling image, even for public health professionals who have spent years working in the field. Unlike medicine, or law, or even engineering, both those who contribute to and those who benefit from public health practice's efforts poorly understand what it is and how it works. This article seeks to illuminate key aspects of public health practice by addressing the following basic questions:

• What is public health practice?

• Where did it come from?

• What does it do?

• How is it organized and structured?

- What challenges does it face in the twenty-first century?

WHAT IS PUBLIC HEALTH PRACTICE?

One approach to describing public health practice is to compare it to some similar activity that most people understand and appreciate. Medical practice appears to fit this bill. The major functions of medical practice are to diagnose diseases and other conditions, develop a treatment plan for those health problems, and see that the treatment regimen achieves its therapeutic goals.

Public health practice has remarkably similar functions that focus on populations rather than individual patients. Public health functions involve identifying health problems and the factors that cause them, developing a strategy to address these problems, and seeing that these strategies are implemented in a way that works. In this light, public health practice is the development and application of preventive strategies and interventions in order to promote and protect the health of populations. Public health practitioners serve the health needs of populations in very much the same ways that physicians tend to the health needs of individual patients. Medical practice focuses primarily on diseases, injuries, and other conditions while public health practice focuses at the community level on factors that contribute to higher rates of these same health problems.

The practice of public health involves both individual and collective efforts. Many different professions and disciplines contribute to public health practice, including public health nurses, nutritionists, health educators, environmental health specialists, and physicians, just to name a few. But public health practice also includes the collective efforts of public health professionals acting in concert with others, often community partners, to identify and address health problems affecting defined populations.

The need for these different disciplines and skills indicates the complexity of the factors contributing to health and disease. Various bacteria and viruses cause many infectious diseases. But other factors can cause or contribute to the development of health problems. For example, the use of tobacco and alcohol contributes to heart disease, cancer, and injuries. Behavioral choices can place an individual at risk of certain infectious diseases (sexually transmitted diseases), chronic diseases (emphysema), injuries (drug overdoses), and other conditions. There are also aspects of the physical environment that affect health (contaminated air, water, or food). The social environment can also determine health risks (low income and education levels, overcrowding, and personal safety). Other social factors related to the use of health and medical services, such as travel distance, the number of providers, and even the availability of day-care services, also influence health. With so many elements affecting health, there is no one body of scientific knowledge that guides public health practice. Instead there are many. These include epidemiology, statistics, environmental sciences, management, biological sciences, and the behavioral sciences such as anthropology, sociology, psychology, and more. Political science, economics, and law are also involved in modern public health practice. Public health is grounded in many different sciences and supported by a variety of other disciplines.

Many people think of public health practice as only those activities performed by governmental public health agencies. Public health practice certainly includes, but is not limited to, the activities of federal, state, and local health agencies (such as the federal Centers for Disease Control, state health departments, and local public health departments). But many other individuals, organizations, institutions, and collaborations contribute to public health practice—and these efforts take place in private and voluntary, as well as in public, settings. For example, hospitals and businesses are often involved in communitywide health fairs and heart and lung associations continuously promote healthy lifestyles.

With so many different participants, the practice of public health can appear to be fragmented and chaotic. But, ideally, public health practice is strategic and purposeful; it is organized (perhaps most effectively at the community level) and it is both interdisciplinary and multidisciplinary. In sum, the practice of public health embodies what a community or society does collectively in order to ensure conditions in which people can be healthy. The skills and competencies necessary for public health practice are both individual and collective.

WHERE DID PUBLIC HEALTH PRACTICE COME FROM?

Many different forces have shaped modern public health practice. These include diseases and other health threats, history, science, social values, and the role of government. Health threats have always challenged human populations; nearly all of the diseases that have wreaked havoc on society over the centuries are still with us today, including tuberculosis, cholera, malaria, yellow fever, and plague. While some diseases have disappeared due to intensive prevention and control initiatives (smallpox is a good example), there is little expectation that all diseases and illnesses can be avoided. The infectious diseases of the past have been joined by dozens of other conditions, most recently by AIDS (acquired immunodeficiency syndrome)—an infection with HIV (human immunodeficiency virus)—and by a host of chronic disease risks and environmental threats. The identification of and responses to these threats, over time and across the globe, especially responses that represent collective decisions and actions, have evolved into what we know as public health practice.

In past centuries, health risks and threats were addressed in a variety of ways. For much of recorded history, diseases were accepted as phenomena beyond human control. Acceptance and avoidance were major strategies as recently as the nineteenth century. For example, when cholera appeared in cities or neighborhoods in Europe and the United States as recently as the mid-nineteenth century, residents (if not immediately infected) could accept the risk or choose to move away until the risk subsided.

While diseases and the microorganisms that cause them have co-habited with humankind for all of history, their spread was greatly aided by industrialism, nationalism, and mercantilism in recent centuries. Industrialism brought previously agrarian societies into urban centers where the population density and unsanitary living and working conditions fostered the spread of many diseases. Nationalism and mercantilism fostered travel and trade across the globe and provided increased opportunities for diseases to be carried from one densely populated area to another. European societies that had centuries of experience with many diseases—and had developed an ecological balance with those diseases through changes in their collective immunological status—brought diseases never before seen to Native-American populations in North and South America. Small wonder that relatively tiny armies of European explorers easily conquered civilizations with much larger populations, encouraging the belief that they were indeed supernatural figures and that the diseases they brought with them were beyond human control.

It was the spread of epidemic diseases largely through seaport towns and cities that prompted the first U.S. public health responses. Boards of distinguished citizens, the first local boards of health, were appointed in cities like Philadelphia, New York, and Chicago to provide the credibility and support necessary to pursue the restrictive policies of quarantining ships and their crews, or placing notices or placards to warn citizens to avoid locations where diseases had occurred. But until the latter part of the nineteenth century, little was known about the causes and pathways of these epidemics. The work of pioneering scientists in the latter half of the nineteenth century, such as Louis Pasteur in France and Robert Koch in Germany, opened the way to the identification of specific microorganisms and eventually to the development of specific approaches to battle those germs and break the chain of transmission.

These scientific advances established that many health threats could be addressed through communitywide interventions, such as those that would ensure clean water supplies and sanitary disposal of human waste and sewage. Public health laboratories were developed to assist in diagnosing new cases so that prevention and control activities could be put in place to avoid further spread. Immunizations were developed from these scientific advances and provided to susceptible populations through massive vaccination programs. Because these efforts required both citizen support and public resources, local governments became increasingly involved in public health responses. State governments became active at a slightly later stage, primarily because infectious disease risks did not respect municipal boundaries.

The increasing involvement and expectations for governmental participation in public health responses represents an important facet of public health practice. The U.S. system of government divides duties and responsibilities between the federal government and the states. There are no specific powers related to protecting or promoting the health of its citizens identified for the national government in the U.S. Constitution. As a result, the basic responsibility for health and public health resides with the states and, as established by those states, with local governments. The federal role in health has nonetheless grown, especially over the twentieth century, as a result of its ability to pursue health goals as a power implied (though not explicitly stated) by the Constitution to promote the general welfare. With immense resources available through the federal income tax and with the ability to influence the activities of state and local governments by offering financial resources for specific programs and services through "grant in aid" mechanisms, the federal government emerged as an important player in the health field. Later its role as a major purchaser of health services through massive national programs such as Medicare and Medicaid brought the federal government even greater power and influence in the health sector. Today it maintains a substantial role in health and public health.

The extensive social and economic chaos accompanying the Great Depression in the 1930s raised public expectations that government would involve itself in protecting the health and welfare of all U.S. citizens. Prior to this time, most Americans didn't want government to have powers over their lives and welfare. Government's role as an important force in public health arose out of other needs as well. Only government can implement and enforce some of the policies and interventions necessary to battle health risks—ensuring safe public water supplies and effective municipal sewage disposal programs, for example, or investigating contacts of persons diagnosed with infectious diseases. To the extent that public resources are utilized for these ends, governmental forums are the appropriate places for these decisions. This is but one of the unique features of public health practice, its link with government. But there are several others that have come to distinguish public heath from other forms of health practice.

The public nature of public health practice means it must depend on social values and popular support for both its ends and its means. This makes public health practice inherently political in

that different values and perspectives exist in various communities as to what needs to be done about important public policy problems. These sentiments and viewpoints change over time and, as a result, the problems to be addressed by public health practice have changed over time as well. For example, infectious diseases were major concerns through the middle of the twentieth century. Chronic diseases became a major focus after the middle of the twentieth century, as did problems and gaps in the health system. Mental health and substance abuse issues became priorities in the 1970s and 1980s, while the 1990s saw violence emerge as a new problem for the public health practice agenda. The ever-changing agenda of public health practice reflects the dynamic nature of its two most influential forces: science and social values. While public health practice is grounded in science, what we choose to do with that scientific knowledge is determined by social values.

One of the most unique features of public health practice is its basis in social justice. Social justice seeks to distribute the benefits of science and technology equally among all segments of society. In the case of health benefits, this would mean eliminating disparities in mortality, disease incidence, disability, and the like. With the considerable differences in health status and outcomes between African Americans and European Americans, for example, or between rich and poor, it is clear that not all parts of the U.S. population share health benefits equally. These social links help explain why public health practitioners share an uncommon bond: the commitment to improve the health status of others.

WHAT DOES PUBLIC HEALTH DO TODAY?

The complete description for public health practice has yet to be written. The simplest and most straightforward depiction of what public health practice is all about today is best illustrated in the mission, vision, and functions outlined in the "Public Health in America" statement. This one-page document was developed to become the hymnal from which all public health practitioners would sing in the twenty-first century.

The statement articulates a vision (healthy people in healthy communities), a mission (promoting physical and mental health and preventing disease, injury, and disability), and statements of what public health practice does and how it accomplishes those ends. Six broad commitments characterize what public health does. Public health:

- Prevents epidemics and the spread of disease.

- Protects against environmental hazards.

- Prevents injuries.

- Promotes and encourages healthy behaviors.

- Responds to disasters and assists communities in recovery.

- Assures the quality and accessibility of health services.

How public health practice accomplishes these objectives and serves its mission is characterized by ten essential public health services that seek to:

1. Monitor health status to identify community health problems.

2. Diagnose and investigate health problems and health hazards in the community.

3. Inform, educate, and empower people about health issues.

4. Mobilize community partnerships to identify and solve health problems.

5. Develop policies and plans that support individual and community health efforts.

6. Enforce laws and regulations that protect health and ensure safety.

7. Link people to needed personal health services and assure the provision of health care when otherwise unavailable.

8. Assure a competent public and personal health care work force.

9. Evaluate effectiveness, accessibility, and quality of personal. and population-based health services.

10. Provide research for new insights and innovative solutions to health problems.

These statements establish a high standard for performance. But by many different measures of performance, it appears that public health practice has not fully achieved these standards. Signs of sub-optimal performance include continuing high rates of morbidity, mortality, and disability for many conditions; huge disparities among various segments of the population; and persistently unequal access to health services. Improvement in these areas requires a well organized and effectively functioning system of public health practice.

HOW IS PUBLIC HEALTH PRACTICE ORGANIZED AND STRUCTURED?

The final decades of the twentieth century witnessed a series of examinations and initiatives that changed the face of public health practice. These began with a landmark report issued by the prestigious Institute of Medicine (IOM) in 1988 entitled *The Future of Public Health*. This report examined the state of public health practice in the 1980s and concluded that the public health system was in a state of "disarray" and that it required a major re-engineering effort.

The report proposed that governmental public health organize around three broad functions: assessment, policy development, and assurance. Basically these translate into identifying what should be done (assessment), what will be done (policy development), and achieving those ends (assurance). Identifying what should be done comes from a comprehensive and broadly participatory assessment of needs and assets and involves both science and values. Determining what will be done recognizes that not all needs can be met, and that some needs are more important than others. Achieving agreed-upon ends involves evidence-based decisions about what works and what doesn't in a particular setting and about who needs to be involved in community interventions.

Some needs are identified by scientific means, such as data showing higher death rates from cardiovascular disease in a community or from reports of an increasing number of AIDS cases. However, other needs are identified by the willingness of people and organizations to mobilize over problems and issues that are important to them and their communities. In some instances, problems are identified for which there may not be convincing data. Yet these problems can be given as high or even higher priority than those advanced by the so-called experts. For example, a community may decide that leaf burning is a more important public health problem than childhood lead poisoning even when the number of reported cases of elevated blood lead levels is much greater than illnesses that are linked to leaf burning.

The IOM report also outlined a series of recommendations for strengthening the ability of the public health system to carry out its core functions. A number of these recommendations were embraced by the public health community and were reflected in initiatives appearing in the early 1990s. These initiatives closely track the core functions framework of the IOM report.

To establish a national agenda for public health and prevention, an extensive set of national health objectives to be achieved by the year 2000 was established. These *Healthy People 2000* objectives were actually the second attempt at establishing a national agenda for health in the United States. The first effort was launched in the late 1970s by then Surgeon General Julius Richmond culminating in the nation's first national health objectives targeting the year 1990. The sequel to *Healthy People 2000, Healthy People 2010*, builds on both earlier efforts but includes an expanded focus on public health practice and the public health infrastructure. *Healthy People 2010* seeks to increase the quality and years of healthy life for everyone and to eliminate health disparities by means of three strategies: promoting healthy communities, preventing and reducing diseases and disorders, and promoting healthy behaviors. Improving systems for personal and public health services is an overarching concern.

Another major public health practice initiative spawned by the IOM report was the Assessment Protocol for Excellence in Public Health (APEXPH). This was developed as a tool to facilitate the local public health leadership capacity of local public health agencies. There were two major elements of APEXPH: One was an extensive organizational self-assessment tool and the other was a framework for developing a community health action plan. Both elements of APEXPH were developed to promote greater emphasis on implementing the IOM report's core public health functions. Both elements also established a new standard of organizational and community practice for local health departments in the United States and many—but certainly not all—of the nation's 3,000 plus local health departments incorporated one or both elements.

The increased emphasis on community health planning through the development of assessments of community health needs and coordinated plans for addressing those needs evolved slowly over the 1990s. In many states and localities these were new roles for local health departments. These agencies often lacked the skilled staff, data and information resources, and links to their communities needed to carry out these duties effectively. However, there was general agreement in the public health practice community that these were necessary and appropriate roles for local health departments and initial efforts were often successful at engaging community partners.

The Institute of Medicine developed a second report on community health improvement in 1997 promoting an enhanced community health improvement process that would link community partners to specific roles in community health plans by means of specific performance measures. At the same time, a variety of other community health planning initiatives were also flourishing as hospitals, health plans, civic organizations, and health professionals began to promote similar processes. The National Turning Point Program was established in 1997 by two national foundations (Robert Wood Johnson and Kellogg) to reform the practice of public health at the state and local level through demonstration projects in fourteen states and more than forty local jurisdictions. Seven more states were added in 1999. Turning Point initiatives generally involved extensive state and local partnerships, seeking to include a wide array of partners and stakeholders from the health field and other sectors of society. For example, business, religious, educational, law enforcement, and community organization leaders joined their counterparts from public health, mental health, substance abuse, and organized medicine.

These initiatives have brought greater attention to the underlying foundation, or infrastructure, of public health practice. The infrastructure of public health can be described in at least two different ways: what it is and what it does. The first view of the infrastructure looks at the basic building blocks of the public health system, while the second looks at what those building blocks actually do. The second view correlates closely with the individual and collective practice of public health.

The most important structural elements of the public health system fall into categories such as work force, information resources, organizational relationships, and financial resources. The public health work force has been very difficult to assess in terms of its numbers, work settings, component disciplines, and skill needs. Rough estimates indicate that there are about 500,000 public health professionals in federal, state, and local public agencies, but that most lack formal training in public health. Public health workers outside these agencies may number several times that of those working for governmental health agencies. Among the largest occupational categories in the public health work force are public health nurses, environmental health specialists, health administrators, and health educators. Several national panels have identified public health competencies as essential for a wide variety of health disciplines. Universal competencies for graduate level public health workers have also been identified. These include: analytical skills, communication skills, policy development and program planning skills, cultural skills, basic public health science skills, and financial planning and management skills.

Data and information drive public health practice in terms of identifying important health problems, determining the factors causing those problems, establishing priorities, communicating with policymakers and the media, and evaluating the effectiveness of various programs and services. Increased access to information through the Internet, integrated information systems, and other collaborations could support expanded and more effective participation in planning, policy development, and assurance activities.

Local public health agencies, frequently called health departments, acting in concert with state health agencies, are often the vanguard of the public health assault on health problems. While key players, these governmental agencies require extensive collaborations and partnerships to be successful. In some instances, outdated public health laws and regulations inhibit effective action on the part of an official health agency and its potential collaborators.

The level of financial resources supporting public health practice is not precisely known. Estimates are that about 1 percent of all health expenditures, or about $40 for every man, woman and child in the United States, supports community-wide prevention programs. When all activities included in the essential public health services framework are included, the total spending for public health practice approximates $50 billion, or about $200 per capita. In comparison, nearly $4,000 per capita is spent each year on medical care services for every person in the United States. National objectives for each of these components of the public health infrastructure are included in *Healthy People 2010*.

WHAT CHALLENGES DOES PUBLIC HEALTH PRACTICE FACE IN THE YEAR 2001 AND BEYOND?

Public health practice faces many challenges. There are scores of continuing health problems (such as cancer and injuries), emerging health problems (such as AIDS and violence), and re-emerging ones (such as tuberculosis), and a slew of new issues on the public health practice agenda. While health status has never been better (as measured by life expectancy and infant mortality), the gains have not been shared equally by all segments of the population. These widening differences reflect the increasing gap between the "haves" and the "have-nots" in U.S. society and the widespread prevalence of negative social determinants of health among subpopulations in the United States and entire societies across the globe. Despite the most expensive and effective medical services in the world, health status gains have not kept pace with immense investments and the United States health system continues to focus on illness rather than health. These unacceptable realities challenge public health practitioners' core values of realizing public health's dream of social justice and creating a health system organized around health. To meet the challenges, public health practice will have to relearn the lessons of its past and move to expand its circle to include new sectors of society at every level of government—namely, more community partners and stakeholders and a more involved citizenry.

In sum, further improvements in health status that eliminate disparities in outcomes remains the greatest challenge to the practice of public health. A continuing commitment to realize the dream of social justice in health will, in all probability, continue to drive public health practice in the twenty-first century.

BERNARD J. TURNOCK

(SEE ALSO: *Assessment of Health Status; Cardiovascular Diseases; Future of Public Health; HIV/AIDS; Institute of Medicine; Koch, Robert; Malaria; Mortality Rates; Pasteur, Louis; Plague; Smallpox; Tuberculosis; Violence; Yellow Fever*)

BIBLIOGRAPHY

Core Functions Steering Committee (1994). *Public Health in America.* Washington, DC: U.S. Department of Health and Human Services, Public Health Service.

Detels, R.; Holland, W. W.; McEwen, J.; and Omen, G. S. (1997). *Oxford Textbook of Public Health,* 3rd edition. New York: Oxford University Press.

Institute of Medicine, Committee on the Future of Public Health (1988). *The Future of Public Health.* Washington, DC: National Academy Press.

Institute of Medicine, Committee on Using Performance Monitoring to Improve Community Health (1997). *Improving Health in the Community: A Role for Performance Monitoring.* Washington, DC: National Academy Press.

National Association of County and City Health Officials (1991). *Assessment Protocol for Excellence in Public Health.* Washington, DC: Author.

Scutchfield, F. D., and Keck, C. W. (1997). *Principles of Public Health Practice.* Albany, NY: Delmar.

Sorenson, A. A., and Bialek, R., eds. (1992). *The Public Health Faculty/Agency Forum.* Gainesville, FL: University of Florida Press.

Turnock, B. J. (1997). *Public Health: What It Is and How It Works.* Gaithersburg, MD: Aspen.

U.S. Department of Health and Human Services, Public Health Functions Project (1997). *The Public Health Workforce: An Agenda for the 21st Century.* Washington, DC: Author.

U.S. Department of Health and Human Services, Public Health Service (1990). *Healthy People 2000.* Washington, DC: Author.

—— (2000). *Healthy People 2010.* Washington, DC: Author.

PRACTICE STANDARDS

Practice standards are the criteria against which professional practice is measured. In 1990, the Institute of Medicine noted wide variation in usage of the term "standard," as it applies to professional practice. In some contexts standards may be minimum levels of performance or results, whereas elsewhere they represent excellence. *Minimum* standards are commonly associated with performance assessment of individual cases, resulting in identification and correction of aberrant practices. Standards of excellence may be used as targets or goals in continuous quality improvement, where the desired result is improved average performance demonstrated through reduced variation in quality measures.

CHARLES P. SCHADE

(SEE ALSO: *Accreditation of Local and State Health Departments; Continuous Quality Assessment; Continuous Quality Improvement*)

PRECAUTIONARY PRINCIPLE

The Precautionary Principle is referred to in the 1992 Rio Declaration on Environment and Development; the declaration includes the principle, "Nations shall use the precautionary approach to protect the environment. Where there are threats of serious or irreversible damage, scientific uncertainty shall not be used to postpone cost-effective measures to prevent environmental degradation." This idea is being increasingly invoked as a rationale for environmental health policy, including its formal appearance in international treaties. The Precautionary Principle, along with terms such as "sustainable development," expresses a broad approach for which there is general support and agreement. However, as with sustainable development, it is a term that is often difficult to crisply define, and its implications to specific issues are not easily agreed upon.

Three elements appear to be central to the Precautionary Principle. First, there must be some factual basis that raises a legitimate reason for concern; second, there is no certainty as to whether the concern will turn out to be justified—or whether the proposed remedy will be effective; and third, the remedy has a reasonably substantial economic or societal cost. There is some debate as to whether the Precautionary Principle is an alternative to risk assessment or whether the two approaches are mutually complementary. In retrospect, there have been many past governmental actions that clearly rank as precautionary, without the term "Precautionary Principle" being invoked. Examples include the use of maximal available control technology for hazardous air pollutants, or ALARA (as low as reasonably achievable) for radiation protection.

BERNARD D. GOLDSTEIN

(SEE ALSO: *Environmental Determinants of Health; Environmental Justice; Environmental Movement; Environmental Protection Agency; Risk Assessment, Risk Management*)

BIBLIOGRAPHY

Goldstein, B. D. (1999). "The Precautionary Principle and Scientific Research Are Not Antithetical." *Environmental Health Perspectives* 107:594–595.

O'Riordan, T., and Cameron, J., eds. (1994). *Interpreting the Precautionary Principle*. London: Earthscan Publications.

PRECEDE-PROCEED MODEL

The PRECEDE-PROCEED model provides a comprehensive structure for assessing health and quality-of-life needs and for designing, implementing, and evaluating health promotion and other public health programs to meet those needs. PRECEDE (*P*redisposing, *R*einforcing, and *E*nabling *C*onstructs in *E*ducational *D*iagnosis and *E*valuation) outlines a diagnostic planning process to assist in the development of targeted and focused public health programs. PROCEED (*P*olicy, *R*egulatory, and *O*rganizational *C*onstructs in *E*ducational and *E*nvironmental *D*evelopment) guides the implementation and evaluation of the programs designed using PRECEDE.

PRECEDE consists of five steps or phases (see Figure 1). Phase one involves determining the quality of life or social problems and needs of a given population. Phase two consists of identifying the health determinants of these problems and needs. Phase three involves analyzing the behavioral and environmental determinants of the health problems. In phase four, the factors that predispose to, reinforce, and enable the behaviors and lifestyles are identified. Phase five involves ascertaining which health promotion, health education and/or policy-related interventions would best be suited to encouraging the desired changes in the behaviors or environments and in the factors that support those behaviors and environments.

PROCEED is composed of four additional phases. In phase six, the interventions identified in phase five are implemented. Phase seven entails process evaluation of those interventions. Phase eight involves evaluating the impact of the interventions on the factors supporting behavior, and on behavior itself. The ninth and last phase comprises outcome evaluation—that is, determining the ultimate effects of the interventions on the health and quality of life of the population.

In actual practice, PRECEDE and PROCEED function in a continuous cycle. Information gathered in PRECEDE guides the development of program goals and objectives in the implementation phase of PROCEED. This same information also provides the criteria against which the success of the program is measured in the evaluation phase of PROCEED. In turn, the data gathered in the implementation and evaluation phases of PROCEED clarify the relationships examined in PRECEDE between the health or quality-of-life outcomes, the behaviors and environments that influence them, and the factors that lead to the desired behavioral and environmental changes. These data also suggest how programs may be modified to more closely reach their goals and targets.

Among the contributions of the PRECEDE-PROCEED model is that it has encouraged and facilitated more systematic and comprehensive planning of public health programs. Sometimes practitioners and researchers attempt to address a specific health or quality-of-life issue in a particular group of people without knowing whether those people consider the issue to be important. Other

Figure 1

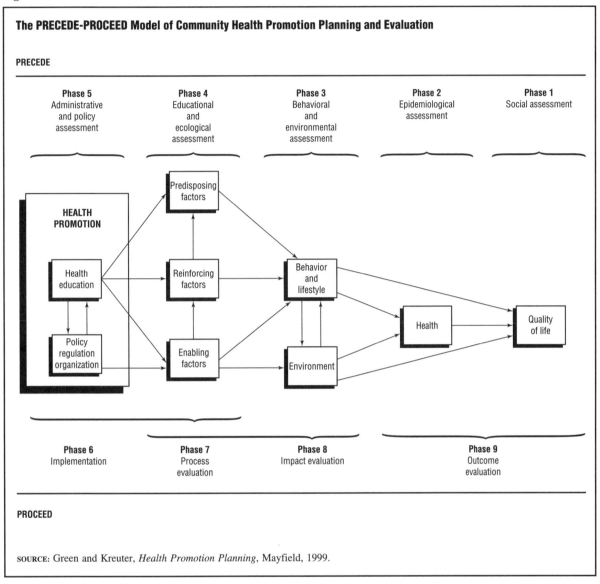

The PRECEDE-PROCEED Model of Community Health Promotion Planning and Evaluation

SOURCE: Green and Kreuter, *Health Promotion Planning*, Mayfield, 1999.

times, they choose interventions they are comfortable using rather than searching for the most appropriate intervention for a particular population. Yet, what has worked for one group of people may not necessarily work for another, given how greatly people differ in their priorities, values, and behaviors. PRECEDE-PROCEED therefore begins by engaging the population of interest themselves in a process of identifying their most important health or quality-of-life issues. Then the model guides researchers and practitioners to determine

what causes those issues—that is, what must precede them. This way, interventions can be designed based not on speculation but, rather, on a clear understanding of what factors influence the health and quality-of-life issues in that population. As well, the progression from phase to phase within PRECEDE allows the practitioner to establish priorities in each phase that help narrow the focus in each subsequent phase so as to arrive at a tightly defined subset of factors as targets for intervention. This is essential, since no single program could afford to address all the predisposing, enabling and reinforcing factors for all of the behaviors, lifestyles, and environments that influence all of the health and quality-of-life issues of interest.

Applications of the PRECEDE-PROCEED model in the public health field are myriad and varied. The model has been used to plan, design, implement, and/or evaluate programs for such diverse health and quality-of-life issues as breast, cervical, and prostate cancer screening; breast self-examination; cancer education; heart health; maternal and child health; injury prevention; weight control; increasing physical activity; tobacco control; alcohol and drug abuse; school-based nutrition; health education policy; and curriculum development and training for health care professionals. A searchable bibliography of hundreds of published applications is available on the World Wide Web (www.ihpr.ubc.ca). Also available is an interactive software training program entitled EMPOWER, which illustrates how the model can be used to plan a breast cancer detection program.

LAWRENCE W. GREEN
SHAWNA L. MERCER

(SEE ALSO: *Enabling Factors; Predisposing Factors*)

BIBLIOGRAPHY

Gold, R.; Green, L. W.; and Kreuter, M. W. (1997). *EMPOWER: Enabling Methods of Planning and Organizing within Everyone's Research.* Sudbury, MA: Jones & Bartlett. CD-ROM and manual.

Green, L. W. (1992). "Prevention and Health Education." In *Maxcy-Rosnau-Last: Public Health and Preventive Medicine*, 13th edition, eds. J. M. Last and R. B. Wallace. Norwalk, CT: Appleton & Lange.

Green, L. W., and Kreuter, M. W. (1999). *Health Promotion Planning: An Educational and Ecological Approach*, 3rd edition. Mountain View, CA: Mayfield.

PREDISPOSING FACTORS

The most common use of the term "predisposing factors" in the field of public health has been in the context of L. W. Green's PRECEDE-PROCEED model of community health promotion planning and evaluation. Years of research have shown that literally hundreds of factors have the potential to influence a given health-related behavior—either by encouraging the behavior to occur or by inhibiting it from occurring. Green's original PRECEDE model of health education planning and evaluation and the more recent PRECEDE-PROCEED model group these factors into three types: predisposing, reinforcing, and enabling factors. "Predisposing factors" are defined in these models as factors that exert their effects prior to a behavior occurring, by increasing or decreasing a person or population's motivation to undertake that particular behavior.

The term "predisposing characteristics" had initially been used in two other health-related models. J. M. Stycos employed the term in a model to predict couples' use of family planning methods. In this model, the term referred to the converging motivations of husbands and wives in making family planning decisions. R. M. Andersen then used the term in the 1960s in his behavioral model of families' use of health services. Andersen's model has been used widely in the health administration and health services research fields to explain utilization of health services. His original model postulated that people's use of health services was a function of their predisposition to use the services, the resources that enabled or impeded their use of the services, and their need for care. Predisposing characteristics were seen to include demographic factors (age and gender), social structure (education, occupation, ethnicity, and other factors measuring status in the community, as well as coping and the health of the physical environment), and health beliefs (attitudes, values, and knowledge that might influence perceptions of need and use of health services). In Andersen's behavioral model, therefore, the term "predisposing characteristics" refers broadly to everything that might predispose a person to need and use a particular service.

The initial version of the PRECEDE model adapted the concept of predisposing characteristics from Andersen and Stycos to concentrate on motivational factors subject to change through direct communication or education—that is, factors that predispose individuals or populations to want to change their behavior. The predisposing factors of importance for health education operate primarily in the psychological realm. They include people's knowledge, attitudes, beliefs, values, self-efficacy, behavioral intentions, and existing skills. All of these can be seen as targets for change in health promotion or other public health interventions. This emphasis on factors that appeal to people's motives for behavioral change has been maintained throughout the various refinements of PRECEDE and its elaboration into the full PRECEDE-PROCEED model.

As shown in Figure 1, predisposing factors that can function as targets for change in public health programs interact with each other. For example, awareness leads to cognitive learning, which, in turn, produces knowledge. Cognitive learning also amasses as experience, which generates beliefs. A change in any of these will affect the others because of the human drive for consistency. The impact of these factors, however, on behavioral change often depends on their support from enabling and reinforcing factors.

TYPES OF PREDISPOSING FACTORS

Awareness and Knowledge. Knowledge is usually a necessary but not always a sufficient cause of individual or collective behavior change. In other words, at least some awareness of a particular health or quality-of-life need and of some behavior that can be taken to address that need must exist before that behavior will occur. Usually, however, the behavior will not occur without a strong enough cue to trigger motivation to act on that knowledge and possibly also without enabling factors such as new skills or resources.

Beliefs. Beliefs are convictions that something is real or true. Statements of belief about health include such comments as "I don't believe that exercising daily will make me feel any better." The most widely used model for explaining and predicting how health beliefs relate to behavior is the health belief model. In brief, this model posits that the likelihood of taking a recommended health action is dependent on one's beliefs about the severity of the disease or health problem in question, one's susceptibility to it, and the benefits of and barriers to taking the health action—plus some kind of cue to action.

Figure 1

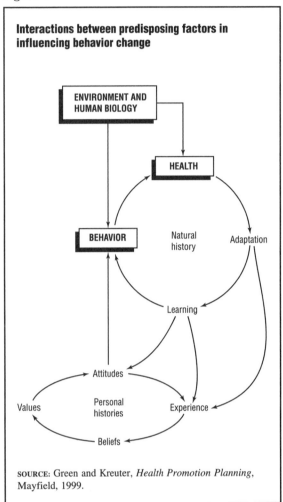

Interactions between predisposing factors in influencing behavior change

SOURCE: Green and Kreuter, *Health Promotion Planning*, Mayfield, 1999.

A potent motivator related to beliefs is fear. Fear combines an element of belief with an element of anxiety. The anxiety results from beliefs about the severity of the health threat and one's susceptibility to it, along with a feeling of hopelessness or helplessness to do anything about the threat. Such a combination can lead to a flight response, leading the person to deny that the threat is real. Health educators, therefore, usually avoid arousing fear unless they can also suggest a course of action that can be taken immediately to ease the fear.

Values. Values are the moral and ethical propositions people use to justify their actions. They determine whether people consider various health related behaviors to be right or wrong. Similar

959

values tend to be held by people who share generation, geography, history, or ethnicity. Values are considered to be more entrenched and thus less open to change than beliefs or attitudes. Of interest is the fact that people often hold conflicting values. For example, a teenage male may place a high value on living a long life; at the same time, he may engage in risky driving activities, such as speeding and driving without a seat belt, because he values the sense of power and freedom he gains through such activities. Health promotion programs often seek to help people see the conflicts in their values or between their values and their behavior.

Attitudes. Attitudes are relatively constant feelings directed toward something or someone that always contain an evaluative dimension. Attitudes can always be categorized as positive or negative. For example, a woman may feel that being overweight is unacceptable, and a young teenager may feel that taking illicit drugs is a bad thing to do. Attitudes are distinct from values in that they are directed toward specific persons, objects, or actions and are based on one or more values. They differ from beliefs in that they always include some evaluation of the person, object or action.

Self-Efficacy and Cognitive Learning Theory. Learning why particular behaviors are harmful or helpful as well as learning to modify one's behavior are prerequisites for being able to undertake or maintain behaviors that are conducive to health. Social cognitive theory (SCT) postulates a number of principles by which learning is acquired and maintained. Health education and behavioral change programs based on cognitive learning theory help a person to bring the performance of a particular behavior under his or her self-control. The most important requirement for self-regulating one's behavior is seen to be self-efficacy—that is, the person's perception of how successful he or she can be in performing a particular behavior. Self-efficacy plays a particularly important role with addictive or compulsive behaviors that are associated with a high degree of relapse, such as weight loss and smoking cessation.

Behavioral Intention. Behavioral intention is a concept fundamental to the theory of reasoned action (and the closely related theory of planned behavior), which proposes that the performance of a particular health behavior is a direct result of whether or not one intends to perform the behavior. It further assumes that all other variables that influence behavior do so through affecting one's behavioral intention. If it is to adequately predict behavior, measurement of intention must correspond as closely as possible to the measurement of behavior in terms of context, time, and outcome.

Existing Skills. If a person does not possess certain skills that are necessary for completion of a specific health behavior, then acquiring those skills would fall under the category of enabling factors. If, however, a person comes to a situation already equipped with the skills needed to successfully perform the behavior, then those skills may predispose that person to behave in a particular fashion and thus are considered predisposing factors. For example, if a teenager attended a program that taught a method of refusing illicit drugs offered by members of a peer group and has been able to refuse them on a previous occasion, then that teenager is considered to have skills that may predispose him or her to refusing drugs on a future occasion. This example reveals how existing skills may be closely related to one's behavioral intention (whether one intends to take drugs on a future occasion) and self-efficacy (regarding one's abilities to refuse drugs).

Predisposing Factors That Are Not Amenable to Change. The PRECEDE-PROCEED model views other factors such as genetic, sociodemographic, and personality characteristics as also playing a role in predisposing to health-related behavior. However, because most of these are not amenable to change through health education, they are treated as a special subcategory of predisposing factors. Some of them can be used to subdivide a population to provide focus for health education and to extend the educational component of health promotion programs to include policy and organizational changes. For example, eating nutritious breakfasts may be less prevalent among children from certain low-income immigrant families. School-based breakfast programs in inner-city schools could include nutrition education pamphlets designed for children to take home to their parents, using language and illustrations that would be especially appealing to the respective immigrant groups. Food purchasing policies might also use the information about factors predisposing the eating behavior of these immigrant groups to include selected ethnic foods in the school-based breakfast program.

Lawrence W. Green
Shawna L. Mercer

(see also: *Attitudes; Behavior, Health-Related; Enabling Factors; Health Belief Model; PRECEDE-PROCEED Model; Social Cognitive Theory; Theory of Planned Behavior; Theory of Reasoned Action; Values in Health Education*)

Bibliography

Abelson, R. P.; Aronson, E.; McGuire, W. J. et al. (1968). *Theories of Cognitive Consistency: A Sourcebook.* Chicago: Rand McNally College.

Ajzen, I. (1985). "From Intentions to Actions: A Theory of Planned Behavior." In *Action Control: From Cognition to Behavior,* eds. J. Kuhl and J. Beckman. New York: Springer-Verlag.

Andersen, R. M. (1968). *Behavioral Model of Families' Use of Health Services.* Research Series No. 25. Chicago: Center for Health Administration Studies, University of Chicago.

—— (1995). "Revisiting the Behavioral Model and Access to Medical Care: Does It Matter?" *Journal of Health and Social Behavior* 36:1–10.

Bandura, A. (1986). *Social Foundations of Thought and Action.* Englewood Cliffs, NJ: Prentice Hall.

Baranowski, T.; Perry, C. L.; and Parcel, G. S. (1997). "How Individuals, Environments, and Health Behavior Interact: Social Cognitive Theory." In *Health Behavior and Health Education: Theory, Research, and Practice,* 2nd edition, eds. K. Glanz, F. M. Lewis, and B. K. Rimer. San Francisco: Jossey Bass.

Green, L. W. (1974). "Toward Cost-Benefit Evaluations of Health Education: Some Concepts, Methods and Examples." *Health Education Monographs* 2(Supp. 1):34–64.

Green, L. W., and M. W. Kreuter. (1999). *Health Promotion Planning: An Educational and Ecological Approach,* 3rd edition. Mountain View, CA: Mayfield.

Hill, R.; Stycos, J. M.; and Back, K. W. (1959). *The Family and Population Control: A Puerto Rican Experiment in Social Change.* Chapel Hill: University of North Carolina Press.

Rokeach, M. (1970). *Beliefs, Attitudes and Values.* San Francisco: Jossey-Bass.

Rosenstock, I. M.; Strecher, V. J.; and Becker, M. H. (1988). "Social Learning Theory and the Health Belief Model." *Health Education Quarterly* 15(2):175–183.

PREGNANCY

A great deal of public health resources is spent on pregnancy. It is clear that prenatal and neonatal health play a large role in determining the health of a population, and in fact, pregnancy outcomes are often used as an indicator of a nation's health.

EPIDEMIOLOGY OF PREGNANCY

Globally, there are approximately 240 million pregnancies annually. These pregnancies result in 134 million births and 50 million induced abortions, 20 million of which are performed under unsafe conditions. Approximately 6 to 7 million of these 240 million pregnancies occur each year in the United States. These result in about 4 million liveborn babies, over 1 million induced abortions, at least 1 million spontaneous abortions (miscarriages), nearly 100,000 ectopic pregnancies (a pregnancy in which the fetus develops outside the uterus), and about 30,000 fetal deaths.

Of the 4 million babies born in the United States in 1999, 12 percent were born to women under 20 years of age. Approximately 4.5 percent of white teens (ages 15 to 19), 8.1 percent of African-American teens, and 9.3 percent of Hispanic teens gave birth. Since 1991, the teenage birth rate has been declining in the United States, particularly among African Americans, largely because of an increased use of effective contraception.

In 1999, 13 percent of the babies born in the United States were born to women 35 years old and older. The birth rate among this age group increased during the last three decades of the twentieth century, despite the fact that older women have an increased risk for having babies with chromosomal abnormalities (the risk is approximately 1 in 1,000 at age 25, 1 in 200 at age 35, and 1 in 20 at age 45).

About half of all pregnancies are unintended or unplanned, and one in three babies are born to single or unmarried mothers. (Nearly 70% of African-American babies and over 40% of Hispanic babies are born to unmarried mothers.)

Four out of five women who gave birth in 1999 started prenatal care in the first trimester, though this percentage was lower among African-American and Hispanic women. Despite an overall improvement in prenatal care utilization, the proportion of low birthweight (LBW) births and preterm births have been increasing gradually since the mid-1980s. This increase is accounted for, in part, an increase in multiple gestations and the growing number of infants born to women older than 35 years of age.

Of the 1.2 million legal induced abortions performed in 1999, 20 percent were obtained by women less than 20 years old, 60 percent by white women, and 80 percent by unmarried women.

PHYSIOLOGY OF PREGNANCY

A human pregnancy starts when the male sperm fertilizes the ovum (egg) in a woman's Fallopian tube, and it lasts, on average, 266 days. Contraception works by inhibiting the release of the ovum from the ovary (birth control pill, injectible, or subdermal implant), by impeding the release of sperm (vasectomy), by blocking sperm from entering the vagina or cervix (male or female condom, diaphragm, or cervical cap), or by blocking the Fallopian tubes (tubal ligation). Once conception takes place, the fertilized egg travels through the Fallopian tube into the uterus, where it implants about seven days later. The intrauterine device (IUD) impedes such implantation, and medications like mifepristone (RU486) causes the implanted embryo to abort.

A developing human is called an embryo between two and eight weeks after conception; thereafter it is called a fetus until delivery. Development of the major organs begins during the early embryonic period, and interference with this process may result in birth defects. Women taking harmful substances, or women with preexisting diseases like diabetes mellitus, are at increased risk for having babies with birth defects. Because the development of major organs begins during early pregnancy, often before a woman starts prenatal care or realizes that she is pregnant, preconceptional care is recommended for every woman of reproductive age.

Although most major organs are present at the end of the embryonic period, the development of their functions continues well into the fetal period, infancy, and early childhood. Interference with this process may lead to functional deficits. For example, undernutrition during this period of growth has been associated with increased risk for coronary heart disease, and maternal alcohol use during pregnancy has been linked to mental retardation and other birth defects.

Remarkable changes take place in a woman during pregnancy. The heart circulates 40 percent more blood volume to supply nutrients and oxygen to the growing baby, deeper breaths occur and an increased amount of harmful substances are cleansed through the kidneys. Digestion slows down for better absorption or nutrients, which may cause problems such as heartburn and constipation. The baby is sustained in the uterus by the placenta, which serves as the interface between maternal and fetal circulations. Hormones prepare the breasts for lactation, and the immune system is altered so that it does not reject the baby as a foreign body. While most healthy women make these adaptations readily, pregnancy can jeopardize the health, and sometimes the lives, of women who are less healthy and suffer increased stress to the system during pregnancy.

PATHOPHYSIOLOGY OF PREGNANCY

When things go wrong during pregnancy, the health of both mother and baby may be at risk of certain health problems associated with pregnancy.

Infertility. Infertility is defined as failure to conceive following a period of 12 months or longer of unprotected sexual intercourse. In 1988, over 8 million American women 15 to 44 years of age reported an impaired ability to have children. Major causes include endometriosis, poor sperm quality or low sperm count, failure to ovulate, and tubal damage.

Ectopic Pregnancy. An ectopic pregnancy is a pregnancy that has implanted outside of the uterus, most commonly in the Fallopian tubes, which may have been scarred from a previous infection, ectopic pregnancy, or tubal ligation. The growing pregnancy, if not surgically terminated, may rupture the tube, causing hemorrhage. Ectopic pregnancy is a leading cause of maternal deaths among African-American women.

Abortion. Abortion refers to the termination of pregnancy before the twentieth week of gestation (counting from the last menstrual period). Abortion can be spontaneous or induced. Most spontaneous abortions (miscarriages) involve some chromosomal abnormalities; the causes of the rest are not known, but some may be due to exposure to environmental toxins.

Birth Defects. Birth defects are the leading cause of infant death and the fifth leading cause of potential years of life lost. About 3.6 percent of all babies in the United States are born with major birth defects, the most common being cleft lip and palate, Down syndrome, neural tube defect, and congenital heart disease.

Low Birth Weight (LBW). LBW, defined as birth weight under 2,500 grams (5.5 pounds), is the second leading cause of infant death, and the leading cause of infant death among African Americans. Risk factors include short interpregnancy interval, low prepregnancy weight, inadequate weight gain during pregnancy, history of LBW or preterm birth, cigarette smoking, and socioeconomic factors.

Preterm Birth. Preterm birth, defined as delivery before 37 weeks of gestation, may result in major problems, including neurological damage from brain hemorrhage or respiratory distress from immature lungs.

Fetal Death. Fetal death refers to the death of a fetus after 20 weeks of gestation. Major causes include preexisting maternal conditions like diabetes mellitus or hypertension, and premature separation of the placenta from the uterus (placental abruption) as a result of drug use or trauma.

Infant Death. Infant death refers to death of a baby under one year of age. Major causes include birth defects, LBW, and sudden infant death syndrome (SIDS).

Maternal Death. Maternal death is defined as the death of a woman as a result of her pregnancy, from the first stages of gestation to within 42 days after the pregnancy has terminated. Risk factors include age greater than 35, unmarried status (owing to socioeconomic factors, including a lack of access to health care), and lack of prenatal care. The classic HIT triad (hemorrhage, infection, and toxemia or preelcampsia) contributes to about half of all maternal deaths. Approximately 300 women in the United States and 500,000 women in the world die every year from pregnancy-related causes. The maternal mortality ratio of 7.5 deaths per 100,000 live births in the United States did not changed significantly during the last 20 years of the twentieth century.

Preeclampsia. Preeclampsia, caused by high blood pressure during the latter part of pregnancy, is characterized by hypertension, protein in the urine, edema, and organ damage as a result of hypertension. Such organ damage may include seizure, stroke, kidney failure, liver damage, and fluid in the lungs. Preeclampsia is treated by effecting prompt delivery (and thereby ridding the body of the circulating toxin released by the placenta). Magnesium is commonly used to prevent seizure. Complications of severe preeclampsia can often be prevented with early diagnosis and appropriate treatment.

Obstetrical Hemorrhage. Obstetrical hemorrhage is characterized by excessive blood loss. It occurs prenatally as a result of premature separation (placental abruption) or abnormal location (placenta previa) of the placenta. It can also occur as a result of injury to the birth canal during delivery, retained placenta within the uterus after delivery, or the inability of the uterus to firm up (uterine atony) after delivery.

Puerperal Infection. Puerperal infections are those that occur during labor, delivery, or the postpartum period. The infection is typically caused by bacteria from the vagina ascending into the uterus. Risk factors include cesarean section, prolonged time from when the "water breaks" to delivery, poor nutrition, and maternal anemia. Prompt treatment with antibiotics can prevent significant morbidity associated with puerperal infections.

Embolism. An embolus is a clot. It could be a blood clot (thromboembolus), or a clot of fetal tissues (amniotic fluid embolus) that travels in maternal circulation. If it blocks off circulation in the lungs or the heart, the embolus could be fatal.

HEALTHY PREGNANCY

Between 1900 and 2000, infant mortality in the United States declined by 90 percent, and maternal mortality by 99 percent. This was one of the greatest achievements of public health in the twentieth century. However, the goal, established in 1994 by the International Conference on Population and Development, of every pregnancy being healthy has not been achieved. Current efforts to ensure healthy pregnancy work at three different levels of prevention.

Primary prevention involves efforts to prevent diseases from occurring during pregnancy. Examples of primary prevention during pregnancy include family planning, preconceptional care, and health promotion during prenatal care. By preventing unintended pregnancies, family planning can prevent morbidity associated with unintended pregnancies. Preconceptional care has been shown to reduce certain birth defects. Proper nutrition and cessation of tobacco, alcohol, and drug use during pregnancy can prevent low birth weight and other complications.

Secondary prevention involves efforts to facilitate early detection and treatment of diseases during pregnancy. Prenatal care provides early and continuous assessment of the pregnant woman, and includes early detection of preeclampsia, syphilis, and tuberculosis.

Tertiary prevention attempts to avert severe complications resulting from diseases during pregnancy. Examples of tertiary prevention include the administration of antibiotics in the treatment of puerperal infection, magnesium to prevent eclampsia (convulsions) in women affected by severe preeclampsia, and transfusion of blood products when obstetrical hemorrhage occurs. Regionalization of perinatal health services, so that high-risk women deliver only in hospitals equipped to deal with potential complications, plays an important role in tertiary prevention.

Much of the improvement in maternal and infant health is attributable to improved health conditions such as better sanitation, sewage control, and safer water supplies. Continued improvement is likely to come from social and behavioral changes rather than from advancement in medical care. Such developments as the expansion in the availability of legal abortions, increased education for women, and better family planning practices have all contributed to improved maternal and infant health. It is important, therefore, for public health professionals to learn how to better address social and behavioral determinants of health. For example, because smoking cigarettes during pregnancy can cause low birth weight and prematurity, it is important to find out how to stop women from smoking during pregnancy.

Because the health of a baby is tied to health of the mother, efforts to improve pregnancy outcomes must begin with women's health. Current efforts fall short by doing too little too late—to expect prenatal care to reverse all the cumulative effects of risk exposures over the course of a woman's life may be expecting too much. Future efforts should promote health not only during pregnancy, but during all of a woman's life.

MICHAEL C. LU

(SEE ALSO: *Abortion; Abortion Laws; Birthrate; Child Health Services; Child Mortality; Contraception; Family Health; Family Planning Behavior; Fecundity and Fertility; Fetal Alcohol Syndrome; Fetal Death; Folic Acid; Infant Mortality Rate; Maternal and Child Health; Newborn Screening; Planned Parenthood; Prenatal Care; Reproduction; Women's Health*)

BIBLIOGRAPHY

Barker, D. J. P. (1998). *Mothers, Babies and Health in Later Life,* 2nd edition. Edinburgh: Churchill Livingstone.

Brown, S. S, and Eisenberg, L., eds. (1995). *The Best Intentions: Unintended Pregnancy and the Well-Being of Children and Families.* Washington, DC: National Academy Press.

Centers for Disease Control and Prevention (2000). "Abortion Surveillance: Preliminary Analysis—United States, 1997." *Morbidity and Mortality Weekly Report* 48:1171–1174.

Cunningham, F. G.; MacDonald, P. C.; Gant, N. F.; Leveno, K. J.; and Gilstrap, L. C. (1997). *Williams Obstetrics,* 20th edition. Norwalk, CT: Appleton & Lange.

Curtin, S. C., and Martin, J. A. (2000). "Births: Preliminary Data for 1999." *National Vital Statistics Reports* 48:14. Hyattsville, MD: National Center for Health Statistics.

Moore, K. L. (1988). *Essentials of Human Embryology.* Toronto: Decker.

Smedley, B. D., and Syme, S. L., eds. (2000). *Promoting Health: Intervention Strategies from Social and Behavioral Research.* Washington, DC: National Academy Press.

PREJUDICE

The *American Heritage Dictionary* defines prejudice as "an adverse judgment or opinion formed beforehand or without knowledge or examination of the facts." The history of public health provides numerous examples of how irrational suspicion or hatred of a particular group, race, or religion resulted in injury to members of that group. Many of these cases of injury are owing to the differential treatment or outright medical neglect of certain groups. Human beings are a homogeneous species, and genetic data indicate that there are few biological differences between ethnic and racial populations that explain differences in health status. Discriminatory behavior by public health professionals on the basis of race, religion, or other social category jeopardizes the health care system by providing inequitable and inadequate care. In response to this threat, federal civil rights legislation proposes the rescension of federal funding to hospitals that violate civil rights laws.

STEPHEN B. THOMAS

(SEE ALSO: *Civil Rights Act of 1964; Cultural Appropriateness; Equity and Resource Allocation; Ethnicity and Health; Ethnocentrism; Inequalities in Health; Minority Rights; Segregation*)

BIBLIOGRAPHY

Krieger, N. (1999). "Embodying Inequality: A Review of Concepts, Measures, and Methods for Studying Health Consequences of Discrimination." *International Journal of Health Services* 29:295–352.

Montagu, A. (1997). *Man's Most Dangerous Myth: The Fallacy of Race,* 6th edition. Walnut Creek, CA: Alta Mira Press.

PRENATAL CARE

Prenatal care describes the health and supportive services provided to a woman during her pregnancy. Prenatal care generally consists of an ordered series of visits to health professionals, with the visits occurring monthly early in the pregnancy and weekly during the last month of pregnancy.

Comprehensive prenatal care includes the following components: (1) screening, monitoring, and testing for early identification and management of medical problems or complications (such as gestational diabetes); (2) ongoing assessment and mediation of risk factors (such as tobacco and alcohol use or domestic violence); (3) nutrition assessment and counseling; (4) health education, information, and counseling about pregnancy, labor and delivery, and baby care; and (5) assessment and care for psychosocial needs (such as stress reduction).

Prenatal care is a unique opportunity for delivering services simultaneously to a mother and her fetus. Pregnancy, and therefore prenatal care, is often the entry point for women into the health care system. The services provided during pregnancy and immediately following the delivery of an infant have significant effects on maternal and infant morbidity and mortality. Prenatal care is a window of opportunity for identifying and addressing numerous medical and behavioral health issues. For example, pregnancy may be the motivator for a woman to stop smoking or develop healthier eating habits. During prenatal care, the groundwork can be set for establishing a medical home for the infant and mother. It is an opportunity for a young family to enter into the health care system.

CAROLYN B. SLACK

(SEE ALSO: *Maternal and Child Health; Pregnancy; Reproduction; Screening*)

BIBLIOGRAPHY

Brown, S. S., ed. (1988). *Prenatal Care: Reaching Mothers, Reaching Infants.* Washington, DC: National Academy Press.

Kotch, J. B.; Blakely, C. H.; Brown, S. S.; and Wong, F. Y., eds. (1992). *A Pound of Prevention: The Case for Universal Maternity Care in the U.S.* Washington, DC: American Public Health Association.

McCormick, M., and Siegel, J., eds. (1999). *Prenatal Care Effectiveness and Implementation.* Cambridge, UK: Cambridge University Press.

PRESSURE GROUPS

Pressure groups are collections of individuals who hold a similar set of values and beliefs based on ethnicity, religion, political philosophy, or a common goal. Based on these beliefs, they take action to promote change and further their goals. For example, members of Mothers Against Drunk Driving (MADD) share a common belief that, in turn, influences the actions (e.g., advocacy, public awareness programs, policy research) they use to achieve their goals.

Pressure groups often represent viewpoints of people who are dissatisfied with the current conditions in society, and they often represent alternative viewpoints that are not well represented in the mainstream population. By forming a pressure group, people seek to express their shared beliefs and values and influence change within communities and sociopolitical structures, such as governments and corporations. Some pressure groups, such as the tobacco-control movement, have been successful at influencing change across a number of sociopolitical structures.

Pressure groups are different from political parties. Political parties seek to create change by being elected to public office, while pressure groups attempt to influence political parties. Pressure groups may be better able to focus on specialized issues, whereas political parties tend to address a wide range of issues.

Pressure groups are widely recognized as an important part of the democratic process. Some groups offer opportunities and a political voice to people who would traditionally be thought of as disadvantaged or marginalized from the mainstream population. In this way, pressure groups strengthen the democratic process by giving a voice to a variety of people. Pressure groups also offer alternatives to the political process by providing opportunities for expressing opinions and a desire for change.

While pressure groups are acknowledged as potentially beneficial to a democratic society, problems can arise when the democratic process becomes dominated by a few specific groups. In this situation, the voice of a small group of people with a particular interest can become overly influential and negatively affect the rights of other individuals. In the democratic process, there is a need for compromise in order to reach consensus regarding the common good. If pressure groups remain rigid and refuse to compromise on specific issues, they can potentially monopolize the democratic process by focusing public debate on a few specific issues.

Pressure groups may adopt a variety of strategies to achieve their goals, including lobbying elected officials, media advocacy, and direct political action (e.g., organized protests). Clearly, some pressure groups exert more influence than others. The degree to which such groups are able to achieve their goals may depend on their ability to be recognized as legitimate by the population, media, and by those in power. For example, civil rights groups, trade unions, and professional associations are more widely recognized and accepted than a newly formed, single-issue pressure group.

Significant gains in public health have been achieved because of efforts by pressure groups, including important changes and advances in public health issues such as tobacco control, occupational health and safety, air pollution, and HIV/AIDS.

Pressure groups can fulfill a valuable function within public health. They have the potential to raise the profile of previously marginalized issues and force action to improve the health of their members, as well as the health of the general population. For example, mental health service consumers have joined together to form pressure groups that have identified the issue of homelessness as an unintended consequence of deinstitutionalization. Initiatives spawned by these groups aim to improve living conditions for the homeless. These actions have provided benefits not only to the homeless, they have also positively affected the well-being of entire communities.

Individual pressure groups can form larger coalitions to advance their cause more effectively. The tobacco-control movement provides an excellent example of how a variety of pressure groups can work together across sectors and at many different levels to affect change. This movement has successfully pulled together many organizations under the umbrella of the National Center for Tobacco-Free Kids. Members include organizations from a number of sectors including health (American Public Health Association), education (American Federation of Teachers), medical (American Medical Association), civic (Americans for Nonsmokers' Rights), corporate (Adventist Health Care), youth (Girl Scouts of the USA), and religious (National Council of Churches).

JEAN SHOVELLER
TASNIM NATHOO

(SEE ALSO: *Community Organization; International Nongovernmental Organizations; Nongovernmental Organizations, United States; Politics of Public Health; Tobacco Control*)

BIBLIOGRAPHY

Libby, R. T. (1998). *Eco-Wars: Political Campaigns and Social Movements.* New York: Columbia University Press.

Mahood, H. R. (2000). *Interest Groups in American National Politics: An Overview.* Upper Saddle River, NJ: Prentice-Hall.

PREVALENCE

See Incidence and Prevalence

PREVENTION

The term "prevention" encompasses the philosophy, credo, programs, and practices that aim to defer or eliminate diseases, disability, and other forms of human suffering. Additional discussions of disease prevention, the stages of prevention (primary, secondary, and tertiary) and the issues of clinical prevention in the setting of personal health services can be found elsewhere in this encyclopedia. The notion of prevention in populations has a long history of discovering and eliminating the causes of disease. For example, in the 1840s Hungarian physician Ignaz Phillipp Semmelweis reduced the rates of puerperal sepsis among pregnant women through attendant hand washing. In the 1850s, British physician John Snow helped abort an outbreak of cholera in London that was due to a contaminated water supply. The gradual assumption of sanitary practices in public health and preventive activities in clinical practice has been in place for a long time and is increasing, although always challenging and incomplete.

THE CONTEXT OF PREVENTION: THE GENERAL CAUSES OF DISEASE AND DISABILITY

The causes of disease and disability are gradually being discovered and either removed or ameliorated due to scientific advances as well as clinical and preventive interventions. While there are many measures of health, one of the most basic, mortality rates, improved at an unprecedented rate during the twentieth century, providing a strong basis for optimism that new preventives and treatments will continue to enhance health status. However, many diseases and conditions and other causes of human suffering are of unknown or incompletely understood causes. While striving to optimize health status and minimize dysfunction and disability within populations and individuals, it is likely that there will always be a health and functional burden on societies. There are several reasons for this including: uncontrollable acts of nature, such as meteorological and climatic catastrophes; war and other forms of interpersonal violence; unanticipated adverse effects of advancing technology or occupational exposures; adverse effects of health interventions (even if the net health benefit is positive); the constant evolution of infectious organisms; naturally occurring errors in function, which will inevitably occur among complex biological systems, even in the absence of known environmental stimuli; the uncontrollability of individual behavior; and the unintended consequences of health-giving interventions, such as the development of resistance to antibiotics that once successfully cured a wide variety of life-threatening infections.

While public health and the medical sciences continue to develop new preventive and curative modalities, there are ecological factors and forces intimately related to diminished population and individual health that could be addressed even in the absence of clear causal or pathogenetic mechanisms. One of the most important is the close relation between socioeconomic status and health. Both within and among populations, those with higher levels of affluence and various social and economic resources in general have higher levels of health by almost all available indices. One particularly common finding is the relation between income inequality and mortality. There may be several explanations for the generally strong association between income levels and subsequent mortality: (1) higher income levels are a measure of a safer physical environment, including occupational exposures and the general environment; (2) higher income purchases more effective personal and family health services; (3) higher income and wealth levels are literal markers of social status, with lower levels being characterized by increased stress from social oppression and distrust; and (4) income and wealth are markers of increased education and healthy behaviors. It is also possible that the association occurs because individuals with physical or mental conditions have a lesser ability to earn higher levels of income and accumulate wealth.

Even in the absence of full explanations for the income-disease association, some possible solutions may be available, including social policies that limit large levels of income inequality, and expenditures on economic development, which might improve health status secondarily as well as increase access to personal health services. However, the evidence for the effects of these social and economic policies is incomplete, and additional intervention studies are needed.

Despite the presence of global factors that appear to be important forces for disease causation, and the likelihood that disease and disability will quite likely continue to be public health and clinical challenges, a substantial amount is known about the causes of many conditions, and preventive interventions are available to lessen, if not eliminate, their public health burden. When considering disease prevention, it is axiomatic that most important clinical illnesses have multiple causes. For example, deaths from certain viral infections may be caused by the lack of immunization facilities, the failure to handle and administer vaccines properly, household crowding, inadequate nutrition and lack of knowledge to seek early care when the infection appears, as well as biologic variability in susceptibility. Coronary artery disease is caused by several factors, including genetic contributions, high fat diets, cigarette smoking, elevated blood cholesterol levels, and inadequate exercise: Preventive action aimed at several of these factors should have a salient effect.

Thus, interventions at several critical points in disease causation—clinical, behavioral, policy, and educational—may all decrease morbidity and mortality. In many instances, multifaceted interventions may provide the best levels of prevention rather than any single approach. A corollary principle is that a preventive intervention at one locus may help prevent several conditions. An effective clinical smoking-prevention program will decrease the risk of several heart and lung diseases.

THE CONTEXT OF PREVENTION: WHERE PREVENTION TAKES PLACE

Prevention takes place at almost all important societal venues, which may be considered in a few major categories (although there is overlap among them): (1) prevention that is facilitated by a healthful environment; (2) prevention optimized by healthful personal behaviors; (3) preventive interventions delivered by health professionals—so-called clinical prevention; and (4) prevention that occurs through social actions, including political, policy, economic, educational, and other group behaviors.

Examples of each preventive venue is instructive. A healthful physical and biological environment is attained when known harmful agents are eliminated, such as lead, automotive exhaust gases, asbestos particles, and viral infectious particles. However, it is very difficult to determine the risks to health of small amounts of certain environmental agents, naturally occurring or contaminants, and risk assessment methods may be employed. Healthful personal behaviors, such as regular, appropriate exercise programs and avoiding risk-taking behaviors, such as tobacco or illicit drug use, will add measurably to positive preventive outcomes. Clinical preventive interventions, such as cancer screening, clinical health counseling, and routine immunizing practices, will add important elements of prevention to individuals and families. Finally, social and administrative activities provide some of the best prevention available in communities. Examples include providing laws that deter underage alcohol and tobacco consumption, health system policies that promote early disease detection, and taxation policies that deter purchase of harmful products such as cigarettes and firearms. All prevention activities work in concert to provide as safe and healthful an environment as possible, but, as noted below, the secondary consequences of each activity should be understood as much as possible.

DISEASE PREVENTION AND HEALTH PROMOTION

Disease prevention is often distinguished from health promotion. While the absence of important conditions is a most worthy goal, it is also useful to consider the attainment of positive health states, where not only are clinical conditions not present, but the highest levels of physical, mental and social well-being are attained. The term "health promotion" has been used to encompass interventions and behaviors that prevent diseases, but many of these same activities can be valuable for attaining the most positive functional performances, emotional attitudes, and states of well-being, irrespective of disease occurrence and risk. Some of this may be obtained by abstinence from tobacco, regular exercise programs, consumption of lower fat diets, and provision of educational opportunities. An additional term often used in public health is "health protection." This term has been used in several contexts, but often encompasses both health promotion and disease prevention, and usually refers to the programmatic and regulatory structures that are designed to limit harmful exposures and enhance health status of particular groups or the general population.

THE POSITIVE AND NEGATIVE EFFECTS OF PREVENTIVE INTERVENTIONS

The goals of prevention would be argued by few. Fundamentally, nearly all would agree that avoiding diseases, disability, and suffering would be beneficial for the health of individuals and the public. However, the methods of prevention, even if based in scientific studies of proven efficacy and effectiveness, can be contentious, and where explicit policy, practice, or programmatic interventions are instituted, there may be substantial fiscal costs to individuals and society, as well as adverse effects and moral or ethical disputes as to the appropriateness of the interventions. It is likely that all major activities and environmental exposures in all societies have both positive and adverse effects on individual and community health, and understanding the trade-offs can be a difficult but

necessary dimension of prescribing prevention programs. To elaborate this principle, examples are offered for various elements of prevention:

- Routine childhood vaccines eliminate a substantial amount of disease and death, but occasionally have important adverse effects on the health and well-being of some individuals.

- Many medications that are used for disease prevention, such as those which treat hypertension or hypercholesterolemia, will have predictable and well-established adverse drug reactions that can limit their use.

- Screening for early and asymptomatic diseases will often lead to decreased morbidity and mortality from those diseases, but the screening maneuvers may lead to occasional serious adverse effects, such as perforation of the intestine during colonoscopy. Also, since most screening tests are not perfectly accurate, it is possible that someone might be incorrectly told that a test showed no abnormality when one actually exists—this individual may take inappropriate actions based on this inadvertently false or misleading information.

- Various mechanical devices will enable some disabled individuals to extend their functional range, but the device itself might lead to occasional injuries to that individual or to others assisting him. For example, there is a real and detectable injury rate due to wheelchair use. Such use may be appropriate, but may have incumbent adverse effects.

Thus, it is important for preventive interventions not only to be effective, but also that the cost-effectiveness and benefits of these interventions be understood. Without this, the net health change may not necessarily be positive.

Some preventive interventions are controversial not because they cause some adverse effects or because they don't always work, but rather because they inadvertently promote some level of the behavior or condition they are trying to prevent. This general problem falls under a phenomenon called "harm reduction." While somewhat over-simplified, the following are examples of when and how this occurs:

- The promotion of cigarettes that may confer less exposure to certain carcinogens and other toxins may reduce the risk of some smoking-related conditions, but fail to dissuade some persons to quit smoking altogether because of the perception that the cigarette is "safer," when in fact it may not be very safe and the overall effect is negative.

- Needle exchange programs, which are intended to supply drug addicts with uncontaminated needles that would decrease the risk of blood-borne infections such as AIDS (acquired immunodeficiency syndrome) or hepatitis may be beneficial to those who avail themselves of this program, but may allow more needles to be available to others. How these needles would be used by others is sometimes uncertain. The existing evidence suggests that needle exchange programs do not promote illicit drug use.

- Similarly, the distribution of condoms to demographic or other groups at high risk of sexually transmitted diseases and unwanted pregnancies may be a preventive for some, but others are concerned that this may promote increased sexual activity, with its own health and moral dimensions.

Thus, it is possible that certain preventive interventions are helpful to those who use them, but in theory, the net benefit to the population's health may not be as great as otherwise would be anticipated. The trade-offs and secondary consequences thus should be understood for any preventive maneuver.

PREVENTIVE INTERVENTIONS: UNIVERSAL OR BASED ON SPECIAL RISK

Some preventive interventions are intended for application to high-risk or special-risk individuals. Other inventions are intended for the entire population, such as routine childhood immunizations, various educational programs in primary and secondary educational settings, and the pasteurization of milk for general distribution. Some are obviously only necessary for one gender, such as cervical cancer screening for women or prostate cancer screening for men, and some are intended only for those at risk for the unhealthy exposure of interest, such as antimalarial prophylaxis for those traveling to or residing in areas where such exposure is possible. Most authorities believe that screening infants and children for increased lead exposure, using blood levels, should be reserved for those at increased risk based on environmental exposure characteristics. Risk levels are generally defined by epidemiological studies, although in many instances the evidence necessary for precisely defining risk is often incomplete. For this and other reasons, the threshold for what constitutes "increased" risk for interventions aimed at persons with increased risk does not follow any rule as to how high the risk must be before invoking that intervention. The level chosen may be related to the risk assessment (measurement) methodology, the resources to be expended, and the amount of expected benefit. Other considerations may be of a policy nature, including decisions concerning the alternative public health or preventive uses for the intended resources.

Depending on the preventive intervention, it may be deemed that all persons in a given population are at "high" risk. One important example is coronary artery disease (heart attack, stroke, and related conditions). Here the level of risk is not only stratified within the population, but also contrasts are made with other populations. Within many Western countries, even those at lower risk according to within-population standards may be at much higher risk compared to those in some developing countries where coronary artery disease is much less common. Thus, it may be deemed that all persons in certain Western countries are at "high" risk, leading to universal and more aggressive interventions across a given population. It follows from this principle that some risk levels may be characteristic of populations and not only of individuals within those populations. Public health practice should always take that into account when providing prevention programs.

While the rhetoric defining risk status doesn't lend itself to easy quantification, as previously noted, every society has identified persons by modern public health and epidemiological methods who are at "very high" risk of certain conditions. Examples include persons in certain occupations who are exposed to high levels of environmental toxins or persons with certain genetic characteristics that define very high rates of disease onset. Such situations should be addressed by rigorous preventive interventions where possible, or in the case of genetic conditions, by at least optimally defining and minimizing risk to individuals and families. Other individuals may be at high risk of various conditions by virtue of patterns of risk-taking behaviors, and at least in some instances these can be identified and modified to some extent. Persons at very high risk of conditions, often justifiably, require levels of attention and surveillance far different from others at increased risk as well as other preventive interventions. Whether intensive attention is merited depends on the evidence that disease occurrence and human suffering can be limited.

EPIDEMIOLOGY: THE SCIENTIFIC BASIS FOR PREVENTION

While clinical prevention is aimed at individual patients and patient groups, or at those with special risks, prevention in public health is generally aimed at entire, geographically defined populations. But from a global public health perspective, clinical and population prevention are intimately linked in many ways. Patient groups sustain all of the general exposures and risks of others in a defined community, and thus require the same preventive interventions as those who are not patients. In fact, many important disease-causing factors are characteristics of communities only, and not of individuals, such as ambient air pollution levels or the availability of high-quality fire protection and health education programs in secondary schools. Conversely, many elements of population health promotion and disease prevention, such as behavioral modification programs and immunizations, are performed within the health care system, which is obviously a critical component of population health. Since nearly all citizens of communities are also health care patients at some point in their lives, reconciling the population and patient domains is necessary.

Epidemiology is the science that provides the rationale and quantitative basis for preventive interventions in both patients and communities, and in turn evaluates the effects of those interventions. This discipline describes the health characteristics and status of groups and populations, as well as their trajectories and outcomes, and quantifies the impact of various environmental exposures and personal factors on the occurrence of important health conditions. Epidemiology is largely an observational science, in that it observes disease population occurrence and environmental exposures, deduces causal pathways and mechanisms, and suggests control procedures. But it includes a strong element of randomized trials and other experimental designs where possible, such as in evaluating the efficacy of a vaccine. To do its work, epidemiology draws heavily from many other sciences and disciplines that inform health status and outcomes, such as clinical medicine, demography, behavioral science, microbiology, toxicology, administrative science, genetics, and molecular biology. As noted, this is testimony to the multifactorial nature of disease causation and the need for multidisciplinary approaches to disease prevention and health promotion. An example of cross-disciplinary activity within epidemiological disease control programs is the application of social marketing. This is an approach to communicating and disseminating health information to the community for behavioral change, using the techniques of commercial marketing. Examples of public health campaigns and programs that have used these techniques are promoting condom use among sexually active teenagers and the use of the "designated driver" in an attempt to decrease alcohol-related auto crashes and injuries.

Epidemiology's tasks usually require the calculation of disease rates, which in turn requires both a numerator (accurate disease counts), and a denominator (the population at risk for health change). Critical to both is accuracy. The population denominator, whether whole communities, important demographic segments, or groups of patients in clinical settings, must be understood. For groups defined administratively, such as patients in a hospital or clinical system, record systems will usually furnish adequate counts. For geographically defined populations, an accurate census is critical, and may not always be available. Even within industrialized nations, high levels of population migration or undocumented persons and lack of cooperation with the census in general may lead to population undercounting, often most acute for groups comprising the most important public health constituency. In many instances, effective epidemiological and public health practice requires population counts and assessments more accurate than those obtained by conventional means, employing network and other sampling or estimation techniques.

In addition to accurately determining the size of geographically defined populations, demographic trends in the United States and other industrialized countries are instructive for their effects on disease occurrence and public health. Perhaps the two most important trends are the increase in total population, although not to the extent this is occurring in developing countries, and the "aging" of populations, where the proportion of older persons is increasing relative to other age groups. Increasing population size has clear implications for environmental quality; the availability of basic resources, such as energy, transportation, and water; the transmission of infectious agents; and the nature of social interactions, which can have both negative and positive health effects. An older population similarly will have complex health effects. In general, rates for felonies and sexually transmitted diseases will be lower, but the number of cases of the chronic illnesses of older persons, such as coronary disease and stroke, cancer, diabetes, arthritis, and dementia, will likely increase. Also, since there is a progressively lower proportion of working-age persons, this may put stresses on national and regional economies, and in turn on population health status.

These demographic shifts will change the nature of prevention programs. There may be more emphasis on the prevention and early detection of the chronic conditions of older persons, and somewhat less emphasis on the conditions of younger persons, although all are important. Lower birth rates may shift resources away from maternal and child health programs toward the prevention of disability. The trend toward higher population size, improved survivorship, lower fertility rates, and a higher proportion of elders, the so-called epidemiologic transition, is occurring among many developing countries and over time will most likely shift their disease rates and prevention priorities in a similar direction to that of developed countries.

Determining the numerators for groups and defined populations (counting the diseases, conditions, and other health states in those populations) goes under the general heading of "surveillance." This takes many forms, and knowledge on disease occurrence and health status in many populations is often, at best, incomplete. For example, if a condition is never diagnosed, or if a sick individual doesn't seek medical care, then a clinical event usually remains unknown. Surveillance may be considered in two general categories: active and passive. In the former, information is collected by actively searching for disease occurrence, such as through population surveys, medical record review, and disease marker determinations in population samples. In the latter, reports are accepted from routine reporting and other voluntary sources, irrespective of whether disease reporting is a community regulation or law.

Depending on the condition, different types of surveillance techniques become most important. Historically and currently, communities have designated a set of diseases and conditions that, when medically recognized, should be reported to public health or other medical authorities. Most of these are infectious and communicable conditions, but chronic illnesses are often represented, as can any condition that might be a threat to population health. Many conditions are detected only with appropriate serological or microbiological laboratory techniques, such as many infectious and communicable conditions. Without these techniques, the infections usually would not be precisely identified and control measures executed. Thus, the public health laboratory becomes an indispensable part of a surveillance system. Laboratory ("biomarker") surveillance for some communicable diseases may be routinely performed irrespective of human clinical illness, such as by routine monitoring of sylvatic animals or patients who present to emergency rooms with any relevant clinical syndrome. Some chronic illnesses all require laboratory confirmation, such as accurate histopathology for cancer cases.

Surveillance systems may operate with other techniques, such as clinical record review. While ethical and privacy issues may deter some disease detection, this can be a very important tool for early identification of conditions with public health and preventive import. For those conditions that are not brought to medical attention or for which a diagnosis is not made, the most common approach would be population sample surveys. Here, representative samples would be interviewed or otherwise studied in an attempt to determine the prevalence and incidence of conditions not otherwise detected, or among persons not availing themselves of medical care. Population surveys also afford the opportunity to determine rates of personal behaviors and exposures that are related to disease causation, and further target disease control programs. Special studies on these population samples may reveal physical, mental, dental, or other disorders and form the basis for targeted preventive interventions. The same surveillance systems that define populations at risk and the nature and extent of preventive programs can continue to determine population disease rates as preventive interventions are invoked and applied as part of public health program evaluation.

ROBERT B. WALLACE

(SEE ALSO: *Demographic Transition; Disease Prevention; Epidemiologic Transition; Epidemiology; Notifiable Diseases; Prevention Research; Preventive Health Behavior; Preventive Medicine; Primary Prevention; Registries; Secondary Prevention; Surveillance; Tertiary Prevention*)

BIBLIOGRAPHY

Centers for Disease Control and Prevention (1999). "Framework for Program Evaluation in Public Health." *Morbidity and Mortality Weekly Report* 48(11):1–40.

Lynch, J. W.; Smith, G. D.; and Kaplan, G. A. (2000). "Income Equality and Mortality: Importance to Health of Individual Income, Physiosocial Environment or Material Conditions." *British Medical Journal* 320:1200–1204.

Teutsch, S. M., and Churchill, R. E., eds. (1999). *Principles and Practice of Public Health Surveillance,* 2nd edition. New York: Oxford University Press.

Tyler, C. W., Jr., and Last, J. M. (1998). "Epidemiology." In *Maxcy-Roseman-Last Public Health and Preventive Medicine,* 14th edition, ed. R. B. Wallace. Stamford, CT: Appleton and Lange.

PREVENTION BLOCK GRANT

The Preventive Health and Health Services Block Grant (PHHSBG) was created by Congress under Public Law 97–35, Title XIX, Block Grants, in August 1981, aimed at moving authority and responsibility for public health to states, thereby saving money on administrative costs. The original amount of available funds equaled about 75 percent of what states had been receiving for the seven categorical programs that were folded into this block grant. The funding formula was based upon what each state received from the categorical programs in Federal Fiscal Year (FFY) 1981 and their respective total population.

The PHHSBG has had a history of variable funding levels. In FFY 2000, the funding level for the core portion of the block grant was $135 million, down from $150 million in FFY 1999. Special categorical funds for rape prevention education were added to the core block grant in FFY 1996, approximately $35 million that year. States have good flexibility on what they may use core PHHSBG funds for, and no flexibility on the use of the rape prevention education funds. The core funds must be used to address the *Healthy People 2010* national health objectives for the nation that are identified by the states as priorities in their specific state. States have used core funds to provide major support for chronic disease and injury programs and emergency medical services for rural areas. Funds have also been used to support laboratory services and infectious disease prevention. Success has been seen in reducing deaths from cardiovascular disease, investigations into outbreaks of disease caused by *E. coli* bacteria, and in the development of new injury prevention programs.

FRANK S. BRIGHT

(SEE ALSO: *Block Grants for Public Health; Prevention*)

BIBLIOGRAPHY

Public Law 97–35, August 13, 1981, Title XIX: Health Services and Facilities, Subtitle A-Block Grants, 95 Stat, 535–542.

http://www.cdc.gov/nccdphp/prevbloc.

http://www.chronicdisease.org/factphb.

PREVENTION RESEARCH

Research conducted to promote prevention of illness in humans derives from all scientific disciplines, from the most basic molecular and cell biology to population sciences such as epidemiology. For example, studies of the most basic molecular cell biology and genetic mechanisms may be critical to developing a vaccine, understanding the genetic basis of disease susceptibility, or defining the adverse effects of a chemopreventive intervention. However, ultimately, all proposed preventive interventions must be evaluated in human populations, often starting with studies that define those at increased risk of the conditions of interest, proceeding to randomized, controlled intervention trials to evaluate the efficacy of the intervention. Where such trials are not feasible or ethically justifiable, epidemiological studies are needed to determine whether a net positive health benefit exists—and if so, for which populations.

ROBERT B. WALLACE

(SEE ALSO: *Prevention; Preventive Medicine; Primary Prevention; Secondary Prevention; Tertiary Prevention*)

PREVENTIVE HEALTH BEHAVIOR

In the United States and other developed countries, premature death and disability results mainly from chronic diseases such as heart disease, stroke, cancer, injury, emphysema, chronic obstructive pulmonary disease, and arthritis. Many of these illnesses have been characterized as resulting largely from "accumulated, multiple indiscretions" (Westberg and Jason 1996, p. 145) and linked to habitual, and sometimes harmful, ways of living. It follows that considerable morbidity and premature mortality could be reduced if individuals practiced certain preventive health behaviors.

PREVENTIVE HEALTH BEHAVIOR

S. V. Kasl and S. Cobb identified three types of health behavior: preventive health behavior, illness behavior, and sick-role behavior. Preventive health behavior is "any activity undertaken by an individual who believes himself to be healthy for the purpose of preventing or detecting illness in an asymptomatic state" (Kasl and Cobb 1966, p. 246). Illness behavior and sick-role behavior, on the other hand, are concepts that encompass behaviors that occur in response to specific symptoms or illness. These behaviors are aimed at minimizing the effects of illness.

Preventive health behavior generally follows from a belief that such behavior will benefit health. An obvious example is quitting smoking to reduce the chances of early morbidity and mortality. It does not follow, of course, that all beliefs on which preventive behaviors are based are well founded, nor that the resulting behaviors will have the desired outcomes. Many preventive behaviors have never been demonstrated to be effective, such as megadoses of vitamin C to prevent the common cold.

Preventive actions can reduce, but not eliminate, the chances of acquiring a disease or illness. The strength of the cause and effect relationship between a certain behavior and the health problem one is trying to prevent will determine the impact performing the behavior will have on reducing the risk. This impact is measured in terms of attributable risk. Attributable risk is a measure of the chance of acquiring a disease if the risk factors for it are eliminated or preventive health behavior is engaged in. The chances are influenced by the relationship of the preventive behavior to the etiology of the disease. Most people are aware that if you smoke you have an increased risk of getting lung cancer. Data indicate that almost 90 percent of lung cancer cases in males and 79 percent in females can be attributed to smoking, according to the Office on Smoking and Health. Some people who do not smoke get lung cancer, of course, but the numbers are small. Similarly, wearing a seat belt reduces the chance of dying in an automobile crash, yet it does not guarantee that the individual involved will not be seriously hurt.

TYPOLOGY OF PREVENTIVE HEALTH BEHAVIORS

Although individual actions contribute to a person's health behavior, preventive health behavior is not totally volitional. Sociocultural and environmental aspects of a person's life influence preventive health behavior, and these factors can have minimal to great effect in determining whether a preventive health behavior is performed.

Some preventive health-related behaviors occur for reasons unrelated to health. Cultural traditions, attitudes, and beliefs can play an important role in the ways in which people behave. In Mediterranean countries, the traditional diet has been found to be an important preventive diet. The traditional meal is often cooked in olive oil, which may help in preventing heart disease.

Social, economic, and cultural determinants of behaviors are closely linked. For many years it was unfashionable for women to smoke cigarettes. In the decades since this taboo was removed, there have been substantial gender-related changes in the overall burden of smoking-related diseases. Between 1981 and 1996 the per-person mortality burden of smoking-related diseases such as lung cancer and chronic obstructive pulmonary disease decreased by 15 percent and 16 percent, respectively, for males, but increased by 62 percent and 70 percent for females. Currently, 24.2 percent of adult men and 20.9 percent of adult women smoke cigarettes, according to the Centers for Disease Control and Prevention (CDC).

Preventive health-related behaviors are also undertaken specifically to improve or enhance health. These types of behavior include both primary prevention and early detection. Primary prevention behaviors aim to prevent the incidence of disease (the number of new cases occurring within a given time frame). Exercise to improve aerobic fitness and prevent cardiovascular disease is an example of a primary preventive behavior. People who increase their levels of physical activity have been found to have reduced levels of risk factors such as high blood pressure, high blood cholesterol, and excess body fat. Early detection (or secondary prevention) behaviors aim to prevent early forms of disease from progressing. This involves people who have already developed preclinical disease or risk factors for disease but in whom the disease has not yet become clinically apparent. Behaviors such as having a breast screen (mammogram) or a pap test for cervical cancer are intended to detect disease early so it can be treated promptly.

Some preventive health-related behaviors may, or may not, improve health outcomes. It is becoming increasingly common for people to use a range of complementary and alternative medicines to improve their health. The 1995 Australian National Health Survey estimated that almost 26 percent of the population used vitamin or mineral supplements, and over 9 percent used herbal or natural medications. Females used these therapies more than males. These behaviors are undertaken with the hope of improving health without clear evidence that the practice has beneficial effects for individuals or populations.

UNDERSTANDING PREVENTIVE HEALTH BEHAVIORS

There is no one theory or concept that explains why people perform certain behaviors. Many theories have been developed to describe, understand, explain, and influence health-related behavior. Although these theories contribute substantially to our understanding of individual behavior, they are often limited because the broader social and environmental context in which an individual lives is not taken into account. It is becoming increasingly recognized that individual unhealthful behaviors reflect the social, cultural, and environmental contexts within which they occur.

Theories, that assist our understanding of preventive health behaviors, can be divided into three categories:

1. Theories that describe the health behavior and behavior change of individuals. Commonly used theories include the health belief model; the theory of reasoned action; the transtheoretical (or stages of change) model; and social cognitive theory.

2. Theories that describe the behavior of communities and environmental changes, such as the diffusion of innovation theory and the communication-behavior change model.

3. Theories that help people understand different approaches to societal change, such as community organization theories.

These and other theories help to explain "why we do what we do when we do it." Their common thread is the belief that if a person performs a health-related behavior, the chances of acquiring a disease or an illness will decrease.

MAJOR TRENDS

Despite the general good health of people in developed countries, there is still considerable scope for improvement in preventive health behaviors. Unfortunately, the last years of the twentieth century saw only modest improvements in this area. The number of people using seat belts went from 67 percent in 1995 to 69 percent in 1997. This period also saw a reduction in the number of people reporting driving while over the blood alcohol limit and a reduction in alcohol-related motor vehicle deaths. The proportion of women aged forty years and over who received a mammogram increased from 56 percent in 1995 to almost 60 percent in 1998 (CDC). One of the most marked changes was in tobacco use among adults; the adult smoking rate in 1999 was 23 percent—the lowest it had been in forty years. In the United States, smoking rates among adolescents decreased in 1999 to 34.8 percent, equal to the adolescent smoking rate in 1995. This may be an indication of a reversal of the upward trend of the 1990s (CDC). However, this does not appear to be the case in other countries such as Australia.

Although there is a strong association between dietary behavior and many chronic illnesses, there has been little change in terms of people following dietary guidelines or eating fresh fruits and vegetables. Obesity has continued to increase, with no real change in physical activity.

CONCLUSION

It is clear that individual preventive behaviors such as eating healthful foods, exercising regularly, moderation in the use of alcohol, and the avoidance of tobacco and tobacco products can contribute greatly to a person's health. However, preventive health behavior is but one element within a complex range of influences on health. Biological, social, environmental, and economic factors also play a role. Together these influence the health outcomes for individuals as well as for populations.

JOHN B. LOWE
ALEXANDRA CLAVARINO

(SEE ALSO: *Assessment of Health Status; Behavior, Health-Related; Behavioral Determinants; Cultural Factors; Diffusion and Adoption of Innovations; Health Belief Model; Health Maintenance; Health Risk Appraisal; Illness and Sick-Role Behavior; Lifestyle; Primary Prevention; Smoking Behavior; Social Cognitive Theory; Transtheoretical Model of Stages of Change*)

BIBLIOGRAPHY

Ajzen, I., and Fishbein, M. (1980). *Understanding Attitudes and Predicting Social Behavior.* Englewood Cliffs, NJ: Prentice Hall.

Australian Institute of Health and Welfare (2000). *Australia's Health 2000: The Seventh Biennial Health Report of the Australian Institute of Health and Welfare.* Canberra: Author.

Bandura, A. (1986). *Social Foundations of Thought and Action: A Social Cognitive Theory.* Englewood Cliffs, NJ: Prentice Hall.

Glanz, K.; Lewis, F.; and Rimer, B. (1997). *Health Behavior and Health Education: Theory, Research and Practice.* San Francisco: Jossey Bass.

Kasl, S. V., and Cobb, S. (1966). "Health Behavior, Illness Behavior, and Sick Role Behavior." *Archives of Environmental Health* 12:246–266,531–541.

McGuire, W. J. (1989). "Theoretical Foundations of Campaigns." In *Public Communication Campaigns,* eds. R. E. Rice and C. Atkin. Thousand Oaks, CA: Sage.

Office on Smoking and Health (1989). *Reducing the Health Consequences of Smoking: A Report of the Surgeon General.* Washington, DC: U.S. Department of Health and Human Services.

Prochaska, J. O., and DiClimente, C. C. (1984). *The Transtheoretical Approach: Crossing Traditional Boundaries of Therapy.* Homewood, IL: Dow Jones Irwin.

Rogers, E. M. (1983). *Diffusion of Innovations,* 3rd edition. New York: Free Press.

Strecher, V. J., and Rosenstock, I. M. (1997). "The Health Belief Model." In *Health Behavior and Health Education: Theory, Research and Practice,* ed. K. Glanz et al. San Francisco: Jossey-Bass.

U.S. Department of Health and Human Services (1995). *Healthy People 2000 Review: 1994.* USDHHS publication no. PHS 95–12561. Washington, DC: U.S. Government Printing Office.

Westberg, J., and Jason, H. (1996). "Influencing Health Behavior." In *Health Promotion and Disease Prevention in Clinical Practice,* eds. S. H. Woolfe, S. Jonas, and R. Lawrence. Baltimore, MD: Williams and Wilkins.

PREVENTIVE MEDICINE

Preventive medicine is a specialty of medicine practiced by physicians devoted to health promotion and disease prevention. Physicians with expertise in preventive medicine are typically interested in health problems that have a significant impact on specific populations, such as those with multiple risk factors for cardiovascular disease, a highly prevalent condition. Conversely, a disease may become the focus of preventive medicine despite its low prevalence because it causes significant illness, disability, and death (e.g., a disease with a high case-fatality rate such as infection with the Ebola virus). Other health problems important to preventive medicine are those that disproportionately affect one narrow segment of a population, such as unintended pregnancies among urban adolescents.

Physicians who practice preventive medicine may work with individual patients in the delivery of clinical preventive services, or they may serve a defined population. In either case, the goal is to reduce the risk factors of the patient or the population that contribute to premature morbidity and mortality. Traditionally, in the United States, the medical and public health communities have assessed the diseases that cause the most mortality and have intervened to reduce their impact. Heart disease and cancers of all types remain leading causes of premature mortality. Recently, the emphasis has shifted from concentrating on diseases that are highly prevalent to a focus on the actual behaviors that cause these conditions. By approaching threats to good health in this way, behaviors such as smoking, unsafe sexual practices, dietary habits, and lack of exercise emerge as vitally important in determining disease or its absence. Preventive-medicine physicians embrace this approach to shape intervention strategies to target behaviors that cause disease.

The American Board of Medical Specialties recognizes preventive medicine as one of the twenty-four distinct medical specialties. Since 1950, the American Board of Preventive Medicine (ABPM) has certified over 7,800 physicians as specialists in preventive medicine. Of the living diplomates (physicians board certified by ABPM) in 1999, 2,752 were in public health/general preventive medicine, 2,442 were in occupational medicine, and 897 were in aerospace medicine. The American Medical Association database on physicians who designate themselves as preventive-medicine specialists reveals a decline in this specialty practice from 2.3 percent of all United States physicians in 1970 to 0.9 percent in 1997; the greatest decline has been in the area of public health and general preventive medicine. Although the needs of the public health work force have not been fully elucidated, and many factors determine physician specialty choice, the following contribute to declining participation in the field: the lack of awareness of the field of preventive medicine, the absence of requirements for certification in many public health and general preventive medicine positions, and inadequate funding during residency training. Despite their small numbers, experts in the field, as well as the collective action of professional societies that bring preventive-medicine specialists together, have been in the forefront among all medical specialties in clearly defining the knowledge and skills needed to master and the professional competencies to be used as the basis for residency training in preventive medicine.

Physicians who become diplomats of the American Board of Preventive Medicine are uniquely trained in both clinical and population-based medicine. Residency training requires a minimum of one year of training in an accredited clinical program, an academic year that almost always leads to a master's degree in public health (M.P.H.), and a practicum year that provides trainees with experience in the application of the knowledge and skills of preventive medicine in diverse settings.

The didactic component of preventive-medicine training provides the core knowledge and skills that encompass the major public health disciplines. The areas of public health in which a preventive-medicine physician must become competent are epidemiology; biostatistics; environmental and occupational health; planning, administration, and evaluation of health services; the behavioral aspects of health and disease; and the practice of preventive medicine in clinical settings. The first five areas represent the core of public health and are required of M.P.H. programs for certification by the Council on Education in Public Health. Epidemiolgy and biostatistics are the fields that define, describe, and quantify diseases and disease patterns; environmental and occupational health and the behavioral sciences cover major determinants of whether diseases flourish, diminish, or exist at all in populations; and planning, administration, and evaluation of health services encompass the competencies needed by programs and health care systems to address specific diseases and/or population-based health programs and evaluate the effectiveness of interventions.

Preventive medicine physicians must be skilled in the clinical practice of health promotion and disease prevention. They must also understand evidence-based medicine in order to know what screening tests and interventions are appropriate for their patients. Evidence-based medicine is a method for determining the content of clinical care that involves evaluating the scientific evidence supporting a particular diagnostic test or therapy and deciding whether the evidence is sufficient to establish the efficacy and effectiveness of an intervention. Preventive medicine physicians must have a good knowledge of this approach to medicine and must be able to incorporate the findings in their practices in order to evaluate their patients and provide appropriate counseling, testing, and preventive therapy.

Preventive medicine physicians have numerous employment opportunities. Many primarily practice population-based medicine and work for local, state, federal, or international health departments; the military; or large employers such as managed care organizations. Consulting opportunities exist for specialists in epidemiology; disease management systems; and program development, implementation, and evaluation. Preventive-medicine physicians also teach and conduct research in schools of public health and medicine and deliver direct patient care.

MIRIAM ALEXANDER
ROBERT S. LAWRENCE

(SEE ALSO: *Clinical Preventive Services; Evidence-Based Medicine; Health Promotion and Education; Healthy People 2010; Prevention; Preventive Health Behavior; Primary Prevention; Secondary Prevention; Tertiary Prevention*)

BIBLIOGRAPHY

Lane, D. S. (2000). "A Threat to the Public Health Workforce: Evidence from Trends in Preventive Medicine Certification and Training." *American Journal of Preventive Medicine* 18(1):87–96.

McGinnis, J. M., and Foege, W. H. (1993). "Actual Causes of Death in the United States." *Journal of the American Medical Association* 270(18):2207–12.

Woolf, S. H.; Jonas, S.; and Lawrence, R. S., eds. (1996). *Health Promotion and Disease Prevention in Clinical Practice*. Baltimore, MD: William and Wilkins.

PRIMARY CARE

The concept of primary health care was defined by the World Health Organization in 1978 as both a level of health service delivery and an approach to health care practice. Primary care, as the provision of essential health care, is the basis of a health care system. Seventy-five to eighty-five percent of the population seek primary health care yearly. It provides both the initial and the majority of health care services of a person or population. This is in contrast to secondary health care, which is consultative, short term, and disease oriented for the purpose of assisting the primary care practitioner. Tertiary care is for patients with unusual illness requiring highly specialized services. Primary care clinicians may be physicians, nurses, or various other health workers trained for the purpose. Countries with better provision of primary health care have greater patient satisfaction at lower costs and better health indicators.

While there are many definitions of primary care, the principles of accessible, comprehensive, continuous, and coordinated personal care in the context of family and community are consistent. Primary health care should be available to all people without the barriers of geography, cost, language, or culture. In primary care, all types of problems, at all ages and for both genders, are considered, including care for acute self-limited problems or injuries, the care of chronic diseases such as diabetes or AIDS (acquired immunodeficiency syndrome), the provision of preventive care services such as immunizations and family planning, and health education. Because primary health care is broad, it is information rich. Primary care clinicians coordinate care for patients among different service providers and for different patient concerns, responding to the fact that most patients have multiple problems. Continuity of care refers to the ongoing relationship between individual patients and primary care clinicians who are committed to the person, not a specific disease, body of knowledge, or specialized technique, and who recognize that physical, mental, emotional, and social concerns are related. Primary care clinicians, interested in the meaning of illness to the particular person, must negotiate care with that individual. A person's health is greatly influenced by the individual's family, culture, and community. Thus, the delivery of primary health care may be different for each individual and in different areas of the world.

The proportion of primary care physicians varies by country—for example, in Great Britain, it is 80 percent; in the United States, it is 32 percent. Primary care physicians in the United States consist of family or general practice physicians, general internists, and general pediatricians. Some primary care may be delivered by specialists, especially obstetrician-gynecologists, but it is not the focus of their practice. In the United States, primary care is also delivered by nurse practitioners and physician assistants. Considering all sources of primary care, there is still a lack of primary care providers in many areas of the country, particularly in the inner city and rural areas.

VALERIE J. GILCHRIST

(SEE ALSO: *Personal Health Services*)

BIBLIOGRAPHY

Institute of Medicine (1996). *Primary Care: America's Health in a New Era.* Washington, DC: National Academy Press.

McWhinney, I. (1986). "Are We on the Brink of a Major Transformation of Clinical Method?" *Canadian Medical Association Journal* 135:873–878.

—— (1997). *A Textbook of Family Medicine,* 2nd edition. Oxford: Oxford University Press.

Starfield, B. (1994). "Is Primary Care Essential?" *The Lancet* 344:1129–1133.

World Health Organization. *Primary Health Care.* Available at http://www.who.int/aboutwho/en/ensuring/primary.htm.

—— *Primary Health Care Concepts and Challenges in a Changing World: Alma-Ata Revisited.* Geneva. Unpublished document, WHO/SHS/CC/94.2.

PRIMARY PREVENTION

Primary prevention generally involves the prevention of diseases and conditions before their biological onset. This can be done in a variety of ways, such as preventing environmental exposures, improving human resistance to disease, or education to diminish risk-taking behaviors. Thus, general environmental and sanitary measures, such as maintaining a safe water and food supply, promoting the use of condoms to prevent sexually transmitted diseases, supplemental restraint systems in automobiles ("airbags"), and application of safe and effective vaccines are examples of primary prevention, whereby diseases and injuries do not obtain a foothold in the body.

ROBERT B. WALLACE

(SEE ALSO: *Prevention; Prevention Research; Secondary Prevention; Tertiary Prevention*)

PRIONS

Prions are infectious proteinaceous particles or, more simply, proteins that lack nucleic acid. They were discovered by Stanley Prusiner, who received the Nobel Prize in medicine in 1997 for his work on them. Prions are biologically unique, existing somewhere in the border zone between living things and nonliving matter. Although they show none of the characteristics associated with life, such as the need to metabolize and the capacity to reproduce, they are in some manner capable of replication in the body of a human or certain other mammals.

Prions apparently gain entry to the body mainly by ingestion, or else in contaminated human growth hormone, or, possibly, in contaminated blood or blood products. They selectively attack the central nervous system, causing a relentless and progressive destruction of neural tissue, leaving in its place microscopic vesicular globules. The pathological name for this is spongiform encephalopathy. Conditions in this category, all of them invariably fatal, are all transmissible. They include kuru, Creutzfeldt-Jakob disease, scrapie (a degenerative neural disease of sheep), bovine spongiform encephalopathy (mad cow disease), and variant Creutzfeldt-Jakob disease, which appears to be acquired by ingesting beef contaminated by the prions that cause mad cow disease.

As of September 2000, it remains unknown what other mammalian species are vulnerable to prions; in research laboratories they have been shown to infect rodents and primates. It is possible that all domestic farm animals are at risk, though so far only sheep, beef and dairy cattle, and wild ungulates such as deer and elk have been confirmed as vulnerable. There is no vaccine or serum to protect against infection, and no agent that can arrest or retard the progress of the spongiform degeneration once it begins.

JOHN M. LAST

(SEE ALSO: *Transmissible Spongiform Encephalopathy*)

PRISON HEALTH

In the United States, prison health care, and the study of health and medical problems of prisoners, is a recent phenomenon. Prior to 1970, medical care in jails and prisons was under the direction of county sheriffs or prison wardens. Neither public health officials nor the outside medical community showed much concern for medical services in prisons or jails or for the health status of prisoners. With the exception of the Federal Bureau of Prisons, which staffed its medical service needs with Public Health Service physicians and provided hospital care in facilities accredited under the Joint Commission for Hospital Accreditation, no general standards for medical services in prisons existed in the United States.

Health care in American correctional facilities began to improve in the 1970s. The U.S. Department of Justice provided limited funds to certain states to improve medical care in prisons, and in 1972 the American Medical Association (AMA) surveyed medical services in U.S. prisons and jails, publishing a report that documented its inadequacy. The AMA and the American Public Health Association independently began writing standards for the care of incarcerated individuals. State and federal courts, responding to legal allegations that inadequate care for prisoners was "cruel and unusual punishment" under the U.S. Constitution, began to find against many correctional facilities.

In 1983 the AMA Correctional Health Care Program evolved into the National Commission for Correctional Health Care (NCCHC), whose standards, in 1999, served more than five hundred jails, prisons, and juvenile facilities and defined the level of health services available to inmates. These voluntary standards address environmental issues, intake screening and medical examinations, access to medical care, and the need for linkages between correctional health and public health. NCCHC standards have served as a significant factor in improving correctional health services in state and local facilities and reducing the risk of adverse litigation. In addition, the National Immigration Service Bureau of Prisons follows NCCHC standards and the National Immigration Health System is accredited by NCCHC.

The first Supreme Court decision to address prison health, *Estelle v. Gamble* (1976), determined that medical care in the Texas prison system was below a constitutional level. *Estelle* and subsequent decisions established that prisoners have a constitutional right to health care equal in quality to that available in the outside community. Today, many jurisdictions meet this standard through accreditation by the NCCHC.

In 1999, over 14.5 million individuals were processed into U.S. correctional facilities. Physical and mental illness is more prevalent in this population than in the population at large, and prisoners require more primary, secondary, and tertiary care than the outside community. The number of physicians, nurses, and other health professionals serving inmates is growing, but it is still insufficient to meet medical demand. Private corporations have moved into the correctional health field to fill the service gap and meet NCCHC or other acceptable standards of care.

The burden of disease in prisoners and the quality of their care are significant public health issues. Untreated disease is a risk not only to the prisoner, but to other inmates, to correctional officers, and to the outside community. The medical care and preventive services provided to inmates reduce the burden of illness in society, lower the probability of disease transmission, and enhance the economic potential of prisoners who try to become productive members of society upon release.

JONATHAN B. WEISBUCH

(SEE ALSO: *Access to Health Services; Ethics of Public Health*)

BIBLIOGRAPHY

American Medical Association (1973). *Medical Care in U.S. Jails: A 1972 Survey.* Chicago: Author.

National Commission on Correctional Health Care (1996). *Standards for Health Services in Jails.* Chicago: Author.

—— (1996). *Standards for Health Services in Prisons.* Chicago: Author.

Poster, M. J. (1992). "The Estelle Medical Professional Judgement Standard: The Right of Those in State Custody to Receive High-Cost Medical Treatments." *American Journal of Law and Medicine* 18 (4):347–368.

PRIVACY

Any information that a person chooses to keep to himself or herself is considered "private" information. A person's right to privacy is protected under Article 12 of the United Nations (UN) Universal Declaration of Human Rights (1948): "No one shall be subjected to arbitrary interference with his privacy, family, home, or correspondence, nor to attacks upon his honor and reputation. Everyone has the right to the protection of the law against such interference or attacks." UN member countries are morally, if not legally, bound by such declarations.

Privacy relates to personal information that a person would not wish others to know without authorization, and to a person's right to be free from the attention of others. Under the ethical principle of respect for a person's autonomy, public health workers have an obligation to respect privacy. What a person regards as private is a personal choice, and it can change throughout one's life. When people disclose private information for any public health purpose, it is expected that the information will be held in the strictest

confidence. Only with this trust can public health programs succeed. One's right to privacy may, however, be superseded by legal requirements, particularly in matters pertaining to the welfare of vulnerable members of society (e.g., children) and where illegal drugs are concerned. Laws governing privacy and its limits also change over time and reflect a society's changing values.

Confidentiality and privacy are related, but distinct concepts. Privacy is a right, while confidentiality is an obligation one has to respect another's privacy. When we grant others access to ourselves, we necessarily give up some measure of privacy. However, we still retain a right over the dissemination of information in the contractual situation of informed consent. Informed consent is provided when securing a person's participation in research, or in relation to the physician-patient relationship. An infringement of confidentiality occurs when a person to whom information deemed private was disclosed in confidence fails to protect that information, or allows others access to it.

To protect privacy, agencies that compile health statistics are required to aggregate information when they tabulate subcategories of data to avoid any possible disclosure that could be inferred from small numbers of people having particular characteristics. In the context of screening people for markers of exposure to infection, researchers and practitioners have the obligation to consider the potential stigma associated with information that flows from such screening tests.

For example, in the case of HIV (human immunodeficiency virus) there is no evidence to suggest that the virus is spread through casual contact. Therefore, there is no overwhelming need for society to know a person's HIV antibody status. When government agencies implement screening programs for HIV, however, the possibility of the test results being made known could cause consternation to both the public and to individuals who test positive. Public health officials thus may implement screening programs by offering anonymous testing as a way of protecting the individual's right to privacy. There is a drawback to this, however, because the information cannot be linked to the person's record for research purposes. Nevertheless, any compulsory screening program should be done anonymously, thus avoiding any potential breach of privacy.

A voluntary screening program could be offered either anonymously or not. Generally, however, in the interest of public health, access to information is given priority over an individual's right to privacy, though it is important to give full and rational consideration to the modes of transmission and other characteristics of the pathogen of concern.

COLIN L. SOSKOLNE

LEE E. SIESWERDA

(SEE ALSO: *Benefits, Ethics, and Risks; Codes of Conduct and Ethics Guidelines; Confidentiality; Ethics of Public Health; Informed Consent*)

BIBLIOGRAPHY

Beachamp, T. L., and Childress, J. F. (1994). *Principles of Biomedical Ethics,* 4th edition. New York: Oxford University Press.

Mann, J. M.; Gruskin, S.; Grodin, M. A.; and Annas, G. J., eds. (1999). *Health and Human Rights: A Reader.* New York: Routledge.

PRIVATE FOUNDATIONS

The search for ways to improve the health of the public has been a salient goal of private foundations since their emergence as important American social institutions in the early 1900s. In 2000 there were approximately 50,000 private foundations in the United States, with assets of some $450 billion and awarded grants of $27.6 billion. Their share of total voluntary giving, however, was just above 14 percent of the $190 billion contributed by Americans that year—making foundations relatively modest participants in the annual flow of the country's philanthropic dollars. The major share (85%) came from individual charitable gifts and bequests.

Foundation giving, however, tends to be quite different from giving for general charity. The bulk of charitable dollars are devoted to the operational budgets of the churches, rescue squads, shelters, and other local agencies that depend on these funds. In economic terms, charitable dollars are largely consumption dollars. In contrast, foundation dollars are usually targeted on investment spending. They help grantee institutions explore and adopt better ways to do their work, test new ideas, and engage colleges and universities in related research and training. Activities of this type build the future capacity of foundation grantees. In this way foundations have become the largest single source of private investment capital dedicated to the progress of America's helping institutions. The record of foundation giving in public health illustrates their utility over time as public-benefit investment institutions.

Throughout most of the past century, foundations—especially Rockefeller philanthropies—have been in the forefront of infectious disease control. In combination, the Rockefeller Sanitary Commission, the Rockefeller Institute for Medical Research, the International Health Board, and the Rockefeller Foundation itself, promoted community sanitation practices and conducted laboratory research leading to the control of such scourges as hookworm, malaria, and yellow fever. Foundations were also involved in the development of the key agents (streptomycin, isoniazid) that brought tuberculosis under control. The advent of HIV (human immunodeficiency virus) infection as a major health problem has also engaged the attention and funding of many foundations. For example, the Robert Wood Johnson Foundation underwrote a series of model communitywide HIV-prevention programs.

HIV is a preventable condition calling for public education and therapeutic counseling to produce changes in population and individual behaviors. Similarly, dependence on psychoactive substances, including alcohol, requires behavioral interventions that challenge public health. The Christopher D. Smithers Foundation and the Hanley Family Foundation have worked intensively on this issue, as has the Robert Wood Johnson Foundation.

As the country enters a new century, public health surveillance has produced evidence of a changing pattern of disease—away from contagious and infectious assaults and toward chronic conditions with high levels of prevalence, mortality, and morbidity. Virtually all of these conditions (e.g., heart disease, cancer) are associated with long-term lifestyle patterns and related environmental factors that call for new and vigorous public health interventions, particularly in the areas of tobacco use and physical activity. Through state and federal agencies, particularly the Centers for Disease Control and Prevention, the public health community is addressing these issues. The Robert Wood Johnson Foundation has initiated several programs to stimulate greater private-sector participation. For example, the American Cancer Society has been a major partner in its work with states.

Over the years, foundations have provided considerable leadership to the progress of children's and family services. The Laura Spelman Rockefeller Memorial helped establish community-wide parenting education initiatives. At about the same time, the Commonwealth Fund founded child guidance clinics and funded related training in psychiatric social work, and in the 1990s it created a model form of well-child care under its Healthy Steps initiative, which brings professionals in child development into frontline pediatric practice. Many other foundations are interested in the early developmental experience of children and their transition to adolescence. Among these are the Annenberg Foundation, the Carnegie Corporation, the Charles Stewart Mott Foundation, the David and Lucile Packard Foundation, the Ewing Marion Kauffman Foundation, and the Foundation for Child Development. In concert with these and other foundations, the Robert Wood Johnson Foundation has launched initiatives to improve county-level maternal and child-care systems, establish school-based health centers, assure the completion of immunization schedules, and to institute nurse-home visiting for first-time single mothers. Also, the Johnson Foundation has partnered with other grantmakers to build statewide health and social support services for low-income families. In terms of their investments in public health, concern for the health and well-being of America's children has been a long-standing and major theme of foundation philanthropy.

Improvements in the organization and staffing of public health was accelerated in the 1920s under grants from the Commonwealth Fund to establish a twelve-state series of model county health departments. Operating standards for these projects were developed in cooperation with the American Public Health Association and were widely instituted throughout the country. Professional education for the field became solidly established in 1916 with the founding of the Johns

Hopkins School of Hygiene and Public Health under grants from the Rockefeller Foundation. Johns Hopkins formed the prototype school for the establishment by Rockefeller of 22 additional schools in 17 countries.

To assure that education would remain rooted in practice, the W.K. Kellogg Foundation funded an initiative to build formal partnerships between schools of public health, health departments, and community health service agencies. More recently, to address the learning needs of in-service public health staff at both the state and local levels, the W.K. Kellogg Foundation and the Robert Wood Johnson Foundation have formed a joint funding program called Turning Points. In addition, working with the National Governors' Association, the Robert Wood Johnson Foundation is funding a program to accelerate the development of the leadership capacity of state health officers as policymakers, administrators, and advocates for the health of the public.

Finally, public health has great needs for ascertaining the determinants of health and the health and functional status of defined communities. Epidemiology is thus one of the basic disciplines in this field, and this science of measurement has been strengthened through the grantmaking activity of the Milbank Memorial Fund.

TERRENCE KEENAN

(SEE ALSO: *Nongovernmental Organizations, United States*)

BIBLIOGRAPHY

AAFRC Trust for Philanthropy (1999). *Giving USA 2000.* New York: Author.

The Commonwealth Fund (1962). *The Commonwealth Fund Historical Sketch, 1918–1962.* New York: Author.

The Foundation Center (2000). *The Foundation Yearbook.* New York: Author.

Lageman, E. C. (1999). *Philanthropic Foundations.* Bloomington: Indiana University Press.

The Robert Wood Johnson Foundation (1992). *The Promise at Hand* Princeton, NJ: Author.

The Rockefeller Foundation (1964). *Toward the Well-Being of Mankind.* New York: Author.

PROBABILITY MODEL

A probability model, also known as a stochastic model, is a mathematical formulation that incorporates an element of randomness. This contrasts with a deterministic model, in which reliable predictions are made on the basis of observed variables. The simplest probability model is the Gaussian, or normal, distribution, of which there are many examples in biology, medicine, and public health. Variations in height, weight, blood pressure, and attack rates in outbreaks of disease are examples of Gaussian distribution.

There is an element of randomness in the distribution of many disease states, although deterministic factors also play a part. Thus, it is possible to estimate risks—such as the risk of cancer following exposure to a known carcinogen—but not to predict which individuals among the members of a high-risk group will develop cancer, or when. Many stochastic models display variation only within a relatively narrow range, however, so prediction, and therefore planning, is feasible within these limits.

JOHN M. LAST

(SEE ALSO: *Risk Assessment, Risk Management; Statistics for Public Health*)

PROSPECTIVE STUDY

See Cohort Study

PROSTATE CANCER

Prostate cancer is the most common cancer in men and the second leading cause of cancer-related death in men. An estimated 191,000 cases of prostate cancer will be diagnosed in 2001 in the United States along with 30,500 prostate cancer-related deaths. The disease is detected by a combination of abnormal serum prostate-specific antigen (PSA) and digital rectal exam (DRE), and less often as an incidental finding after prostate resection for obstructive benign disease. It is uncommon at this time to diagnose prostate cancer in association with gross urinary obstruction, bleeding, or unexplained skeletal pain.

The disease is both hereditary and sporadic with one gene (HPC2), and several gene loci recently identified. The risk for developing prostate cancer increases twofold if a first-degree relative is affected and it further increases as more family members are afflicted (first- and second-degree relatives). Although no specific cause for prostate cancer has been identified, several factors contribute to the development of the disease. This includes the level of saturated animal fat in the diet, vitamin D production, and ethnic origin. African Americans have the highest rate of prostate cancer in the world, while it is the lowest in native Asians. The disease is more commonly seen after the age of fifty.

The natural history of prostate cancer is strongly driven by the tumor grade. The risk of prostate cancer death is low (less than 10%) in patients of almost all ages with low-grade disease; however, it is substantial for patients with moderate- or high-grade disease. Metastatic disease has a very predictable natural history, with a median survival of thirty to thirty-three months after diagnosis.

Prostate cancer is generally detected by an abnormal serum PSA determination and/or an abnormal DRE. The diagnosis is generally made by an ultrasound-guided needle biopsy of the prostate. These techniques have led to a stage shift in the disease, with the majority of lesions now detected in the clinically localized state. Contemporary treatments for clinically localized disease include watchful waiting, radical prostatectomy, radiation therapy (external beam or brachytherapy), or cryosurgery. Androgen ablation (removal of testosterone-like substances from the system) can be used alone or in combination with other modalities, and is the principle form of therapy for advanced disease.

The decision whether to treat the disease or observe the patient should be based on the probability of the patient reasonably living another five to ten years, and thus takes into account the patient's age and comorbid conditions. Surgery can be very effective and is generally employed in younger men where nerve-sparing surgery can be used to preserve erectile function. The major side effect is urinary incontinence, which can be significant in a small percentage of patients. External beam radiation therapy is also a standard form of therapy which is generally performed in older patients (over age seventy). It is usually well tolerated, but a small percentage of men can develop gastrointestinal side effects related to rectal irritation.

Brachytherapy refers to the implantation of radioactive pellets in the prostate gland, usually under ultrasound guidance. This technique has been employed for approximately a decade and is an effective form of therapy in men with appropriate lesions. The major side effect from this therapy is an increase in irritative voiding symptoms. An increasing body of knowledge suggests that the addition of androgen ablation may improve the outcomes of patients receiving radiation.

Approximately 20 percent of patients treated for localized disease will experience a rise in their PSA within five years. This group of biochemical-failure patients are an enlarging cohort of patients for which exact treatment recommendations are not available. Gross loco-regional disease has become less common in the PSA era. Prostate cancer generally metastasizes to the lymph nodes and the bones, with less common involvement of the visceral organs.

Prostate tumors are classically dependent on endogenous androgens as growth factors. The removal of androgens by castration (surgical or chemical) results in a regression of symptoms and measurable disease in 80 percent of patients. Unfortunately, there are androgen-resistant clones in most tumors, which makes this form of therapy palliative. Androgen ablation can be performed by the removal of the testicles or the administration of a luteinizing hormone releasing hormone (LHRH) antagonist.

Prostate cancer relapsing after androgen ablation is designated androgen independent prostate cancer. The median survival for such patients is approximately eleven months. Although newer chemotherapy agents are displaying activity in advanced prostate cancer, treatment is generally palliative. This is an area of intense clinical investigation and protocol therapy.

S. Bruce Malkowicz

(see also: Cancer; Prostate-Specific Antigen [PSA])

Bibliography

Albertson, P. C.; Hanley, J. A.; Gleason, D. R. et al. (1998). "Competing Risk Analysis of Men Aged 55 to 74 Years at Diagnosis Managed Conservatively for Clinically Localized Prostate Cancer." *Journal of the American Medical Association* 280:975–980.

Catalona, W. J., and Smith, D. S. (1998). "Cancer Recurrence and Survival Rates after Anatomic Radical Retropubic Porstatectomy for Prostate Cancer: Intermediate-Term Results." *Journal of Urology* 160:2428–2434.

D'Amico, A. V.; Whittington, R.; Malkowicz, S. B. et al. (1998). "Biochemical Outcome after Radical Prostatectomy, External Beam Radiation Therapy or Interstitial Radiation Therapy for Clinically Localized Prostate Cancer." *Journal of the American Medical Association* 280:969–974.

Eisenberg, M. A.; Blumenstein, B. A.; Crawford, E. D. et al. (1998). "Bilateral Orchiectomy with or without Flutamide for Metastatic Prostate Cancer." *New England Journal of Medicine* 339:1036–1042.

Powel, I. J. (1998). "Prostate Cancer in the African-American: Is This a Different Disease?" *Seminars in Urologic Oncology* 16:221–226.

Ragde, H.; Blasko, J. C.; Grimm, P. D. et al. (1997). "Interstital Iodine-125 Radiation without Adjuvant Therapy in the Treatment of Clinically Localized Prostate Carcinoma." *Cancer* 80:442–453.

PROSTATE-SPECIFIC ANTIGEN (PSA)

Prostate-specific antigen (PSA) is a 32-kilodalton (kD) serine kinase that functions to liquify the ejaculate. It is technically referred to as "human kallekrin 2." Several conditions such as prostatitis, benign prostatic hyperplasia, prostate cancer, and ejaculation (mild increase) can increase serum PSA levels. Although it has been detected in other tissue, such as the breast, salivary gland, and in other tumors, it is overwhelmingly more specific for the prostate and has more organ specificity than any other existing tumor marker.

Serum PSA is measured in nanogram (ng) quantities and is very sensitive for detecting prostate cancer. After radical surgery, serum measurements should nadir to undetectable levels. The reappearance of measurable PSA is the earliest sign of therapeutic failure. While very low postoperative measurable levels may represent minimal residual benign glands, values of 0.4 ng/ml are almost always associated with disease recurrence. The first approved indication for serum PSA was for the monitoring of patients after radical prostatectomy. Levels between 4.0 and 10.0 ng/ml carry a 16 to 25 percent risk of detecting prostate cancer, while levels above 10.0 ng/ml are associated with a 60 percent risk of prostate cancer.

Although PSA is considered to be the most effective tumor marker in human oncology, its role in screening strategies for prostate cancer has not been completely established. Since its tumor specificity is low, many patients will demonstrate negative findings on a transrectal needle biopsy prompted by an elevated PSA. Earlier concerns, however, that PSA detects clinically insignificant tumors have been dispelled by multiple surgical pathology studies. It has also been repeatedly demonstrated that serum PSA and a digital rectal examination (DRE) detect more prostate cancer than either modality alone, yet prospective randomized data demonstrating a decrease in the prostate cancer deaths due to screening strategies is unavailable. Several prospective trials are in progress, but are several years from maturity. Recent trends in tumor registry data demonstrate a 12 to 16 percent decrease in prostate cancer deaths over the past five years. Most experts agree that there is some role for PSA evaluation in patients, and efforts are underway to establish reasonable guidelines for the use of this marker.

PSA evaluations should generally start at age fifty in most subjects but at age forty in African Americans and those patients with a family history of the disease. The appropriate upper age to abandon screening is problematic, yet recent data suggests that men over the age of sixty-five with an initial PSA value below one have a very small chance of ever developing prostate cancer.

Several attempts have been made to improve the test characteristics of serum PSA. PSA density accounts for the amount of PSA produced proportional to the volume of the prostate gland. A large gland with benign hyperplasia may make more PSA than a smaller gland. A smaller gland with a higher PSA may be suggestive of prostate cancer. An optimal cutoff of 0.15 has been suggested. The volume of the prostate gland cannot be precisely determined with transrectal ultrasound, making practical implementation of this concept difficult.

Age-adjusted PSA (lowering the normal value in patients younger than sixty and raising it in older patients) has been proposed to increase sensitivity in detection in younger patients. In the case of older patients this can lead to more cases of missing significant tumors, however. Some authors suggest lowering the value for young patients and keeping it at 4.0 ng/ml for older patients.

PSA levels tend to increase in men over time. The rate of increase (velocity) may provide some indication of the development of benign or malignant disease. Investigators have noticed that an increase greater than 0.75 ng/year may suggest a significant cancer risk. While this holds up with retrospective evaluations of archival serum samples, it is more difficult to calculate in patients obtaining values over short time intervals or getting evaluated by different assays over time, which may be more variable.

PSA exists as free and complex forms in the blood. Patients with prostate cancer appear to have lower amounts of free PSA in their serum, and those with benign conditions have a higher proportion of their total PSA in the free form. If the percentage of free PSA of the total is greater than 25 percent, the chance for detecting prostate cancer for overall values of 4 to 10 ng/ml is only 5 to 7 percent rather that the usual 16 to 25 percent. Since the determination of a high free-PSA fraction lowers, but does not eliminate, the risk of prostate cancer, it is often used for decisions regarding repeat biopsies rather than the initial evaluation.

S. BRUCE MALKOWICZ

(SEE ALSO: *Prostate Cancer; Screening; Secondary Prevention*)

BIBLIOGRAPHY

Carter, H. B.; Pearson, J. D.; Metter, E. J. et al. (1992). "Longitudinal Evaluation of Prostate Specific Antigen Levels in Men with and without Prostate Cancer." *Journal of the American Medical Association* 267:2215–2217.

Catalona, W. J.; Smith, D. S.; Wolfert, R. L. et al. (1995). "Evaluation of Percentage of Free Serum Prostate-Specific Antigen to Improve Specificity of Prostate Cancer Screening." *Journal of the American Medical Association* 274:1214–1219.

Morgan, T. O.; Jacobsen, S. J.; McCarthy, W. F. et al. (1996). "Age-Specific Reference Ranges for Serum Prostate-Specific Antigen in Black Men." *New England Journal of Medicine* 335:304–310.

Oesterling, J. E.; Jacobsen, S. J.; Chute, C. G. et al. (1993). "Serum Prostate-Specific Antigen in a Community-Based Population of Healthy Men. Establishment of Age-Specific Reference Ranges." *Journal of the American Medical Association* 270:860–864.

Polascik, T. J.; Oesterling, J. E.; and Partin, A. W. (1999). "Prostate Specific Antigen: A Decade of Discovery—What We Have Learned and Where We Are Going." *Journal of Urology* 162:293–306.

PROSTITUTION

Prostitution is defined as "the act or practice of engaging in sexual activity for money or its equivalent" (Garner 1999, p. 1238). Except for parts of Nevada, it is a criminal act in the United States. Prostitutes are also referred to as commercial or public sex workers. It is estimated that over 92,000 men, women, and juveniles are arrested yearly for prostitution (FBI, 2000). The number of juveniles engaging in prostitution is estimated at between 100,000 and 300,000 per year.

The greatest health consequences of prostitution are drug abuse, violence, and sexually transmitted infections, including HIV/AIDS (human immunodeficiency virus/acquired immunodeficiency syndrome), gonorrhea, pelvic inflammatory disease, and syphilis. The risk for HIV infection is increased because of multiple partners and limited safe sex practices—some customers are willing to pay more for a sexual encounter if they do not have to use a condom. Based on research conducted by the Centers for Disease Control and Prevention, the rate of HIV infection for prostitutes is three times higher if they smoke crack cocaine. Intravenous drug use also increases the risk of HIV infection for a prostitute.

Prostitutes are often victimized by the person for whom they work, and by their customers. Other health issues related to prostitution are early pregnancy for juveniles, rape, tuberculosis, post-traumatic stress disorder, assault, and other acts of violence—including murder. There are also negative consequences besides those related to

health issues. In places where it is common, prostitution lowers the value of property. It also degrades the status of women. Published research studies concerning prostitution as a public health issue in urban communities have come primarily from developing countries. It is a topic in need of more research in the United States.

KATHY AKPOM
TAMMY A. KING

(SEE ALSO: *Addiction and Habituation; Crime; HIV/AIDS; Public Health and the Law; Sexually Transmitted Diseases; Violence*)

BIBLIOGRAPHY

Baseman, J.; Ross, M.; and Williams, M. (1999). "Sale of Sex for Drugs and Drugs for Sex: an Economic Context of Sexual Risk Behavior for STDs." *Sexually Transmitted Diseases* 26(8):444–449.

Booth, R. E.; Watters, J. K.; and Chitwood, D. D. (1993). "HIV Risk-Related Sex Behaviors among Injection Drug Users, Crack Smokers, and Injection Drug Users Who Smoke Crack." *American Journal of Public Health* 83(8):1144–1148.

Federal Bureau of Investigation (2000). *Uniform Crime Reports. Preliminary Figures, 1999.* Washington, DC: United States Department of Justice. Available at www.fbi.gov/ucr/htm.

Garner, B. A., ed. (1999). *Black's Law Dictionary,* 7th edition. St. Paul, MN: West Publishing Co.

Jones, D. L.; Irwin, K. L.; Inciardi, J.; Bowser, B.; Schilling, R.; Word, C.; Evans, P.; Faruque, S.; McCoy, H. V.; and Edlin, B. R. (1998). "The High-Risk Sexual Practices of Crack-Smoking Sex Workers Recruited from the Streets of Three American Cities." *Sexually Transmitted Diseases* 25(4):187–193.

Shuter, J.; Alpert, P. L.; DeShaw, M. G.; Greenberg, B.; Chang, C. J.; and Klein, R. S. (1999). "Gender Differences in HIV Risk Behaviors in an Adult Emergency Department in New York City." *Journal of Urban Health* 76(2):237–246.

PSITTACOSIS

Psittacosis is a zoonosis, caused by bacteria of the *Chlamydia* family. It occurs naturally in many species of birds, such as domesticated parrots, and these occasionally infect humans, typically when parrots are kept in inadequately cleaned cages in a confined space frequented by their human owner.

Psittacosis is also an occupational hazard of workers in aviaries, and outbreaks have been reported among workers in poultry farms and processing plants. However, in the twenty-first century even isolated cases are uncommon, either because of improved standards of cleanliness in places where birds are kept and poultry is processed, or owing to other ecological factors. It is more likely to occur after exposure to birds imported from Latin America or Asia than those reared in the United States.

The usual mode of infection is via infected droppings or detritus on the infected bird's feathers. Psittacosis causes a feverish illness resembling pneumonia, occasionally with other manifestations, including skin rashes and inflammation of the membranes around the brain and spinal cord. It is an indolent infection that responds sluggishly to antibiotics of the tetracycline family, and can be fatal, although this is rare. Prevention depends on education of persons who are in close and continuing contact with birds, maintaining scrupulous cleanliness of bird cages, and surveillance of known or potential foci of infection such as poultry farms and shops that sell pet birds. Quarantine is applied to poultry farms and premises where infected birds have been found, and can be enforced when suspected infected birds are imported from other parts of the world.

JOHN M. LAST

(SEE ALSO: *Zoonoses*)

PSYCHOLOGY

The field of psychology plays an integral role in public health, providing treatment and education in the areas of substance abuse, addiction, and other health-related behaviors. Individuals suffering from addiction and other psychological disorders have a major impact on a community, and on the nation, causing financial loss, accidents, decreased business productivity, and numerous social and psychological effects. Therapeutic techniques for these individuals focus on development of coping skills, ego strength, improved self-esteem, and other traits needed to lead a healthy life. Assessment, community profiling, and creating

and conducting prevention and treatment programs for the public also fall within the realm of psychology. In addition, psychologists conduct research in public health problems and serve as consultants in the development of solutions to these problems.

SANDRA K. CLARKE

(SEE ALSO: *Behavior, Health-Related; Behavioral Change; Community Psychology; Psychology, Health; Substance Abuse, Definition of*)

PSYCHOLOGY, HEALTH

Psychology has various definitions, most of them stating that psychology is the study of behavior. Health psychology is the application of psychology to health-related problems and behavior. Most psychological applications in health are from the discipline of social psychology. The contribution of health psychology to public health is in such areas as psychological processes in prevention, health maintenance (e.g., not smoking), and patient education, particularly in helping people cope with an illness (e.g., mastering the use of the peak flow meter to control asthma).

HEALTH PSYCHOLOGY PERSPECTIVES

Health psychology deals with individual behavior in a social context. However, within the public health sector, behavior is not restricted to behavior of at-risk persons, but also includes behaviors of peers, parents, health professionals, employers, politicians, and others. Unfortunately, while there is a large amount of empirical data available regarding individual behavior of the at-risk person or patient, there is very little data available about behaviors at other social levels.

Health psychologists try to understand behavior by describing psychosocial determinants for individual behavior. But health psychologists also try to understand and promote behavior change. One basic assumption in health psychology is that to change people's behavior—at least through health promotion interventions—it is necessary to understand the psychosocial determinants of behavior. For example, when a smoker fails to stop smoking because of a lack of motivation, another type of intervention is required than for a smoker that fails because of a lack of social support.

The first public health applications of psychology were strongly focused on risk perception and risk taking. The best example may be the health belief model, where the perception of the severity of the risk and the susceptibility for the risk were seen as the primary determinants of health-protective behaviors. Over time, it became clear that people have many reasons for health-related behaviors, of which risk perception is often not an important one. In this multicausality approach, there is also a growing recognition of the many psychosocial and environmental influences on individual behavior. Changes in psychosocial determinants (e.g., self-efficacy) are most effective in creating behavior change when paralleled by changes in the social and physical environment (e.g., removal of barriers).

The application of psychological theories to public health is not without debate. Some professionals state that psychological theories will never be able to fully help us understand behavior and behavior change; other professionals claim that in practice there is nothing so helpful as a good theory. Both perspectives are justified. Theories are, by definition, a reduction of reality, but they do help people organize their thoughts and ask the right questions. The interesting contribution of theories is that they can generalize findings from one area of behavior to be of use in another.

PSYCHOSOCIAL DETERMINANTS OF BEHAVIOR

The most often applied theories to explain the psychosocial determinants of behavior are Icek Ajzen's theory of planned behavior and Albert Bandura's social cognitive theory. Social cognitive theory (SCT) specifies the following determinants of behavior: outcome expectations, self-efficacy expectations, behavioral capability, perceived behavior of others (modeling), and the social and physical environment.

The theory of planned behavior (TPB) is an extension of the earlier theory of reasoned action. TPB postulates that intention, the most proximal determinant of behavior, is determined by three conceptually independent constructs: attitude, subjective norms, and perceived behavioral control (or self-efficacy). The attitude towards the behavior is determined by salient beliefs, or outcome expectations, about that behavior. Beliefs are weighted by evaluations or judgments about the value or importance of the expected outcome. For example, the expected outcome of going on a low-fat diet might be a lowering of blood pressure, which could be judged to be important and worthwhile.

Subjective norms, or perceived social expectations, are beliefs that specific, important individuals or groups approve or disapprove of the behavior. These beliefs are weighted by the motivation to comply with the referent person or group—that is, how important is a friend's or group's approval or opinion. Note that Ajzen's perceived social expectations are different from Bandura's perceived behavior of others, where the social environment does not necessarily expect certain behavior. Other authors have broadened the TPB social influence construct to include perceived behavior of others, perceived expectations of others, social pressure, and social support.

Perceived behavior control or self-efficacy refers to the subjective probability that a person is capable of executing a certain action (e.g., going on a low-fat diet might be perceived to be difficult).

Since the theory of planned behavior was introduced in the 1980s, other determinants have been suggested, including: personal moral norms, anticipated regret, identity concerns, and self-evaluation. Another development is an increasing attention to the relation between intentions and behavior. Studies on implementation intention show that helping people to make plans to behave in a certain way can improve the intention-behavior link. Intentions, however, may be overruled by habits. Behaviors become habitual when performed frequently and when performed in a stable environment. Under conditions where habits conflict with intentions, intentions become poor predictors of behavior. It is possible, however, to break bad habits by replacing a habitual sequence with an alternative sequence.

TPB is most often applied at the individual level. However, it has been applied to higher ecological levels as well, such as the voting behavior of legislators regarding a cigarette tax increase, or the adoption behavior of schoolteachers and principles for HIV (human immunodeficiency virus) prevention programs.

THE PSYCHOLOGY OF BEHAVIOR CHANGE

The most prominent psychology theories of behavior change are the social cognitive theory, James Prochaska and Carlo DiClemente's transtheoretical model, Richard Petty and John Cacioppo's elaboration likelihood model, and various theories on coping and self-regulation by authors like Richard Lazarus. Social cognitive theory suggests the following methods for change: active learning, reinforcement, and modeling and guided practice (including feedback).

The transtheoretical model (TTM) has two major sets of constructs: stages of change and processes of change. In the stages of change, people are thought to move from a state of no motivation to change to one of internalization of new behavior. The first stage is "precontemplation," in which people have no intention to change their behavior. In a successful change process, people make a transition to "contemplation," in which they are thinking about changing the problem behavior. Ideally, people then move to "preparation," in which they are planning to change this behavior in the short term. People who have recently changed their behavior are in the "action stage," whereas people who have performed the behavior for a longer time are in the "maintenance stage." People in the action stage may lapse and then recycle to an earlier stage.

TTM can be used to describe and to change behavior. An important contribution of the model is the specific tailoring of educational efforts to include different models and processes of change for individuals in different stages of change. For instance, a re-evaluation of outcome expectations is used to make the change from precontemplation to contemplation; and a guided practice for skills improvement can help with the change from action to maintenance.

Social psychology has a long tradition in persuasion research. Petty and Cacioppo have a new perspective on persuasion effects with their elaboration likelihood model (ELM). The basic idea of ELM is that people differ in their ability and motivation for thoughtful information processing of persuasive messages. These authors explain two ways of information processing, central or peripheral (also called systematic versus heuristic). Central processing occurs when a message is carefully considered and compared against other messages and beliefs. Peripheral processing occurs when a message is processed without thoughtful consideration or comparison. A variable—for instance, the credibility of a sports hero as a model—may have a positive effect when the receivers process the message through the peripheral route, but a negative effect when they follow the central route, because people might realize that their behavioral capabilities are different from those of the sports hero. Research findings suggest that thoughtful information processing is related to a higher persistence of attitude change, a higher resistance to counter-persuasion, and a stronger attitude-behavior consistency. ELM suggests two ways to stimulate central processing: Make the message more personally relevant and unexpected, and repeat the message.

Self-regulatory or self-management conceptualizations, including coping theories, have to do with how individuals function to behaviorally self-correct. Various authors describe this process. The general procedure is: (a) monitoring of some aspect of behavior or health, (b) comparing one's observation with normal or desired outcomes or behavior, describing a problem or divergence from normal, and analyzing the causes of the problem, and (c) trying a behavioral correction. This entire process recycles with a return to monitoring. Self-regulatory theories are useful for the designation of health-promoting behaviors for the self-management of chronic diseases, such as asthma, diabetes, or cystic fibrosis.

GERJO KOK

(SEE ALSO: *Attitudes; Behavior, Health-Related; Health Belief Model; Social Cognitive Theory; Social Determinants; Theory of Planned Behavior; Transtheoretical Model of Stages of Change*)

BIBLIOGRAPHY

Abraham, C.; Sheeran, P.; and Johnston, M. (1998). "From Health Beliefs to Self-Regulation: Theoretical

Advances in the Psychology of Action Control." *Psychology and Health* 13:569–591.

Ajzen, I. (1991). "The Theory of Planned Behavior." *Organizational Behavior and Human Decision Processes* 50:179–211.

Ajzen, I., and Fishbein, M. (2000) "Attitudes and the Attitude-Behavior Relation: Reasoned and Automatic Processes." In *European Review of Social Psychology,* eds. W. Strebe and M. Hewstone. New York: Wiley.

Connor, M., and Norman, P., eds. (1996). *Predicting Health Behavior: Research and Practice with Social Cognition Models.* Buckingham, UK: Open University Press.

Glanz, K.; Lewis, F. M.; and Rimer, B. K., eds. (1997). *Health Behavior and Health Education: Theory, Research, and Practice,* 2nd edition. San Francisco: Jossey-Bass.

Kok, G.; Schaalma, H.; De Vries, H.; Parcel, G.; and Paulussen, T. H. (1996). "Social Psychology and Health Education." In *European Review of Social Psychology,* Vol. 7, eds. W. Strebe and M. Hewstone. New York: Wiley.

Lazarus, R. S. (1993). "Coping Theory and Research: Past, Present, and Future." *Psychosomatic Medicine* 55:234–247.

Petty, R. E., and Wegener, D. T. (1997). "Attitude Change: Multiple Roles for Persuasion Variables." In *The Handbook of Social Psychology,* 4th edition, Vol. 1, eds. D. T. Gilbert, S. T. Fiske, and G. Lindsey. Boston: McGraw-Hill.

Stroebe, W. (2000). *Social Psychology and Health,* 2nd edition. Buckingham, UK: Open University Press.

Taylor, S. E. (1995). *Health Psychology,* 3rd edition. New York: McGraw-Hill.

PSYCHOSIS

See Dementia; Depression; Mental Health; *and* Schizophrenia

PUBLIC HEALTH AND THE LAW

In *The Future of Public Health,* published by the Institute of Medicine in 1988, the mission of public health is defined as "fulfilling society's interest in assuring conditions in which people can be healthy." Public health law covers those areas of the law that advance this purpose. The reach of public health law is as broad as the reach of public health itself.

INTERRELATION OF PUBLIC HEALTH AND THE LAW: SOME DEFINITIONAL ASPECTS

Law is a body of directions or commands requiring or prohibiting certain conduct, enforceable by legal sanctions. It is also a body of directions or commands that grant authority to a public body or agency or requires such a body or agency to carry out designated powers. Thus, public health law forbids persons to engage in activities that endanger the health of others, and it specifies government agencies to carry out certain programs to advance public health and to prevent activities that are harmful to the health of individuals or of the public.

When we discuss public health, it becomes apparent that the "public" element is the legal component. Without the law (without legal authorization of public health programs, including the legal authorization and appropriation of public funds), the very existence of the field of public health is in question.

That public health law seeks to affect personal conduct is implicit in some of its common directions: Do not engage in unprotected sexual activity if you suffer from a sexually transmitted disease (STD); do not practice medicine or treat patients unless you are a licensed physician; do not operate an X-ray machine unless you have a license to do so; do not operate a restaurant unless you have a permit; do not connect the drains of a building to a sewer line unless you are a licensed plumber. So, too, examples of directions that form part of the institutional requirements of public health laws are likely to take the following form: You, commissioner or agency, are authorized or required to set standards for the practice and licensure of medicine, of dentistry, of a nurse-midwife. Other examples of institutional authorizations and requirements of public health law may include the following: You, commissioner or agency, are authorized and required to set standards for the licensure and safe operation of nuclear power plants; or, You, administrator or agency, are authorized and required to set standards for healthful ambient air quality, including standards for limits on the amount of sulfur dioxide, lead, ozone, particulate matter, and other harmful components in the ambient air.

BASIS FOR THE EXERCISE OF PUBLIC HEALTH POWERS

In the United States, governments at every level—federal, state, and local—exercise public health powers. Depending on the level of government, public health powers are based on different authorizations. States and, by delegation from the state, local governments base their authority to regulate and provide for the protection of public health on the police power to provide for the health, safety, and welfare of the people. This police power is a plenary power that the states have by virtue of being states. Governments are created so that they may exercise this power. As a plenary power, it requires no grant by the state constitution, though several states do mention the police power in their organic law. State governments are the original governments in the nation, antedating the federal government, and they hold the police power because they are sovereign governments. The police power is inherent of government, and it has been so regarded by the United States Supreme Court in the bedrock public health law case of *Jacobson v. Massachusetts*, decided in 1905. The case upheld a Massachusetts law that enabled the city of Cambridge to require all adults to be vaccinated to prevent the spread of smallpox against a claim that the law violated the defendant's right to life and liberty without due process of law. The case also demonstrates that the public health powers of local governments are derived by delegation from the state legislature, as in situations where city boards of health may pass an ordinance to prevent the spread of communicable disease.

Unlike state governments, which have the plenary police power, the federal government is a government of delegated powers, and the power of Congress to pass laws on particular subjects must be sought in the federal constitution. The federal government exercises vast public health powers, both to regulate public health and to provide for public health services.

Although other provisions of the Constitution may be drawn on, federal public health powers, in the main, rest first on "commerce power"—the power of Congress to "regulate commerce with foreign nations, and among the several states, and with the Indian tribes," under Article 1, Section 8, clause 3 of the U.S. Constitution. It also rests on the so-called "taxing and spending power"—the power to "collect taxes . . . to . . . provide for the . . . general welfare of the United States," under Article 1, Section 8, clause 1.

COMMERCE POWER

The power to regulate interstate commerce allows Congress to regulate whatever passes in commerce between the states, as well as whatever affects interstate commerce. Thus Congress has the authority to regulate not only the commercial transactions and transportation of merchandise between the states, but also all of the materials that pass in interstate commerce. A notable example of this power is the Federal Food, Drug, and Cosmetic Act (1938), which regulates the food and drugs that pass in interstate commerce, including the wholesomeness of food and the safety and efficacy of drugs and medical devices. By delegation from Congress, the Food and Drug Administration (FDA) controls and regulates what goes into the kinds and packages of food we consume (including the number of peanuts in peanut butter), and virtually everything that goes into every bottle of medicine, pills, salve, or ointment. Under the commerce power, the FDA exercises direct federal regulatory control by promulgating its own regulations and by overseeing enforcement of the law through staffs of professionals, administrators, and inspectors. Other examples of regulatory controls include the slaughtering of beef and the manufacture of beef products under the Federal Meat Inspection Act, and the production, slaughter, and sale of poultry under the analogous Poultry Products Inspection Act. Because it is difficult to tell a "local" chicken from an "interstate" chicken, the production of poultry products within a state that affects interstate commerce is also regulated.

Commerce power controls include the regulation of the production and sale of pesticides under the Federal Insecticide, Fungicide, and Rodenticide Act, as well as the sale of toxic substances—including lead paints—under the Toxic Substances Control Act, and the control of unsafe consumer products under the Consumer Product Safety Act. All of these laws have the protection of health as their major purpose, and all of them involve direct federal controls. The commerce power also provides the basis for legislation to control safety in the workplace under the Occupational Safety and Health Act, and for the Fair Labor Standards Act, because the hours people work and the wages they receive have a direct relationship to their health.

THE TAXING AND SPENDING POWER

The taxing and spending power generally does not involve direct federal regulatory controls, but instead operates through state and local governments. Federal participation in public health programs has long operated through grant-in-aid programs, which were known as categorical grants in the 1930s and 1940s. Grant programs involve grants of money by the federal government to state and local governments or instrumentalities. Such grants are conditioned on compliance by the recipients of a grant with the requirements set by Congress in the authorizing legislation. State and local governments may get federal grant money only if they meet certain conditions. These often include the provision of state or local matching grants, but more importantly the conditions may require the states and localities to undertake certain activities to meet federal requirements.

Under an early, still existing program, the federal government provided money to state and local governments for the construction of publicly owned waste treatment works in order to improve water quality through treatment of sanitary waste. To obtain these essential grants for the protection of public health, states and localities must provide matching funds and must assure that the waste treatment works meet adequate construction and public health standards, that the states and localities engage in needed planning, and that the waste treatment works are placed in appropriate locations. This grant-in-aid program was established in 1972 under the Federal Water Pollution Control Act. Grant-in-aid programs may also be encountered in the funding of hospital construction, mental health programs, newborn and maternity programs, and in many other programs. Congress, through a variety of grant-in-aid programs, has triggered numerous health initiatives, contributing significantly to new public health developments in state and local governments nationwide.

Other health-related programs based on the taxing and spending power include programs for housing and urban renewal, for school lunch programs, and for institutional services. These include health-planning services, such as preventive health-service programs, programs for the prevention of sexually transmitted diseases, community mental health programs, and alcoholism and drug addiction treatment and rehabilitation programs. Perhaps one of the most notable grant-in-aid programs is the Title 19 Medicaid program, which assists the states in providing for the medical costs of persons defined as "medically indigent."

Beginning in the 1970s, the Congress, through the grant-in-aid mechanism, supported many initiatives for environmental protection, designed not only to protect the environment, but also to protect public health. Federal water pollution and air pollution legislation initially provided the states with the funding necessary to develop programs to control environmental pollution—to create decent and healthful ambient air and water quality for the protection of public health.

Programs to protect the environment generally constitute a significant expansion of public health protection. Begun in the late 1960s, environmental programs reflect conservational as well as aesthetic concerns for the quality of the environment, but the massive regulatory system managed by the Environmental Protection Agency (EPA) is largely designed to protect the health of the human population against toxic pollutants and against the pollution of the water, the air, and the natural environment.

The vast reservoir of federal powers for the protection and enhancement of public health may be exercised both under the commerce power and under the taxing and spending power. Oftentimes, as the law develops, the federal government may get into public health matters indirectly, through the taxing and spending power, and then later take up a regulatory role under the commerce power. In the control of air pollution, for instance, early federal legislation in the 1950s simply provided grants-in-aid to states and municipalities to address their problems. Later, in regulating harmful emissions from automobiles, Congress brought the commerce power to bear in authorizing federal emission controls and their enforcement. It is notable that the protection of public health was the legislative purpose, regardless of which authorization was relied on.

PUBLIC HEALTH LAW AND LEGISLATION: EARLY BEGINNINGS

All of the public health law initiatives mentioned above, whether state or federal, originated from legislation at either the Congressional, state, or local level. Law in this country is divided into three types: (1) traditional, unwritten, or common law; (2) judge-made law, which is based on case-law decisions; and (3) the more systematic, thoroughly documented, and vastly detailed statutory law. There is hardly any federal common law, and in areas of public law such as public health law there is nearly exclusive reliance on legislation, or statutory law. In some isolated areas, such as nuisances and their abatement, there is frequent reference in the cases to an earlier non-statutory regime, but these are historical and traditional references. Today, nuisances and their abatement are addressed by state or local statutory law, and they generally fall under the jurisdiction of the lower criminal courts. In the abatement of nuisances, the statutory law may rely on injunctions, a form of equitable relief. Public health law is a field of statutory law and a field of administrative law because almost all of it operates through administrative agencies functioning under appropriate legislative delegation.

At the turn of the twentieth century, public health and its legal regulation dealt largely with the prevention of communicable disease and with environmental sanitation, including the control of the disposal of human and other wastes—with some concern for water purity and what has been referred to as the "hygiene of housing." There was some interest in food and milk sanitation and some incipient controls of health in the schools, but there was very little else. The major expansion of the field is largely a twentieth-century development. Beginning in the nineteenth century there was some state concern for public health, particularly in the control of communicable disease. Quarantine laws were not uncommon. New York had an elaborate law in the 1820s requiring ships to anchor in the harbor near Marine Hospital on

Staten Island. The law prescribed rules for clearing quarantine, requiring whitewashing and fumigation of vessels and the washing and airing of clothing and bedding. Rules were particularly strict where "yellow, bilious, malignant or other pestilential or infectious fever had existed, or if disease had broken out on board of the ship." There were also state laws allowing nuisances to be abated when they were a danger to health and allowing local governments to limit to certain restricted areas the conduct of any trade or employment offensive to the inhabitants or dangerous to the public health. The regulation of food products in the early nineteenth century was largely of an economic nature, but public health and consumer protection were at least secondary goals. Some states also gave local medical societies the power to examine and license physicians; unlicensed physicians could not use the courts to collect their fees. Other laws made the unauthorized practice of medicine the subject of a fine.

Occupational licensing of public health professions became fully established between 1890 and 1910, with licenses for practicing of medicine, dentistry, and pharmacy becoming regularly established. During this period midwives were also licensed, as were veterinarians, chiropractors and osteopaths, undertakers, embalmers, and funeral directors. It was also a time when licensure was extended to other occupations, such as plumbers, barbers, and ferriers. All of these licensing laws were based on the police power and referred to public health and safety. Though the protection of public health provided a basis for such legislation, in many instances the real motive was economic, both to collect licensing fees and to provide a protected economic position for the licensed trades and occupations.

FROM REGULATORY TO SERVICE PROGRAMS

In the nineteenth and early twentieth centuries, public health law was primarily a regulatory field, prescribing what affected persons and professionals were required or forbidden to do. In the 1930s the field added a service mission to its regulatory mission. Instead of focusing on the prevention of disease, legislation began to establish agencies to render services to the public to improve health. In addition to telling industry, businesses, and people what to do and what not to do through "command and control" regulations, modern public health programs are service-oriented. While still prohibiting harmful conduct or conditions, they provide preventive and rehabilitative services to advance the health of the population. The purpose is to create a more healthful environment, to provide the facilities and trained professionals to prevent or to limit exposure to contagion and disease, to educate people to protect themselves, and to improve people's physical and mental condition. In the area of communicable disease, for instance, governments provide immunization services for children. They provide mandatory treatment for seriously mentally ill persons who cannot take care of themselves or who may present a danger to the public, as well as providing and supporting voluntary community programs and mental health services for persons who need them. In addition to safeguarding the water supply and the healthfulness of the food, milk, and pharmaceutical needs of the people, the government also provides nutritional support, such as food stamps, and support for sound nutritional education. School health programs not only seek to prevent the spread of communicable disease in the schools, but use the schools to provide preventive services for children. In addition to school dental examinations, many states and local governments fluoridate the water supply to prevent tooth decay in young children.

DEVELOPMENTS IN THE LAST PART OF THE TWENTIETH CENTURY

In the last half of the twentieth century, the fields of public health and public health law underwent many changes. In 1965, Medicare and Medicaid were established. These health care reimbursement programs brought the government into the payment and provision of health care, introducing new regulatory controls into medical and treatment services. Government, or some other regulated third party, assumed the major cost of medical treatment for significant parts of the population. In consequence, the government has to consider what it is paying for, including the quantity and quality of health care services it subsidizes. What

had previously been a matter of private arrangement between physicians and patients became a transaction imbued with a public interest. When Medicare and Medicaid legislation became effective in 1965, the emphasis on patient care and its cost began to overshadow earlier concerns for environmental sanitation and other preventive activity.

Another significant change in public health law resulted from a 1973 decision of the Supreme Court. In *Roe v. Wade* the Court held that a pregnant woman has a choice whether to bear a child or to terminate her pregnancy. This decision involved physicians and hospitals in issues fraught with religious and moral concerns. In turn, women's freedom of choice required the availability of abortion services, and raised the question whether states were under an obligation under Medicaid to defray the cost of abortion services for the medically indigent.

Because government is involved in the provision and payment of medical care, it has also become involved in other ethical issues in health care. Both in the rendition of medical services and in the growing government responsibility for the funding of medical research, the informed consent of the patient, as well as of persons who are subjects of clinical experimentation, has involved the government in the resolution of public health-related ethical issues. Moreover, medical advances leading to the survival of severely threatened newborn infants, and the capacity of medicine to prolong the life of severely ill persons on respirators have raised ethical questions both at the beginning and at the end of life with greater frequency and greater clarity. So too, scientific breakthroughs in new reproductive technologies, including in vitro fertilization, ovum implants, and surrogate mothering, have raised ethical issues new to public health. A host of new ethical problems have also arisen from new and dramatic organ transplant techniques.

New ethical issues have followed new genetic knowledge and techniques discovered or stimulated in consequence of the federally sponsored Human Genome Project, which has begun a new diagnostic approach to the treatment of disease where not only are pathogens considered, but also individual genetic structure and inheritance. New ethical concerns are also reflected in public health law in the emphasis on the protection of privacy, which imposes new obligations on physicians, hospitals, and health agencies to protect the records and medical histories of patients.

By the end of the twentieth century the field of public health law encompassed broader and more sophisticated concerns for physical and mental health. It included a system for the medical care of the elderly and the indigent, either as a governmental system or as a system of social insurance. Public health law now also covers broad environmental concerns, including the control of air and water pollution, the control and disposal of conventional as well as toxic and hazardous waste, the control of pollution by ionizing radiation, as well as expanded concerns for the safety and wholesomeness of food and pharmaceuticals. It also covers many aspects of human reproduction, including elements of population control. It covers the control of addictive substances, such as alcohol, narcotics, and tobacco. There is an increased concern with occupational health, covering the dangers of the workplace, as well as accident prevention in the workplace, in the home, and on our highways.

THE DIVERSE CHARACTER OF PUBLIC HEALTH LAW

Public health law is a vast field and does not come in a single neat package. The many parts of the field share the common purpose of advancing the health of the population. Public health in our cities, and worldwide, depends on a reliable supply of potable water, decent sanitary provisions, sewer lines, and the sanitary disposal of human and other waste—all of which require government services and appropriations based on law. Public health also depends on adequate provisions for the disposal of toxic and industrial waste and the management of waste. What makes our cities wholesome and livable are adequate provisions, legally established and authorized, for street cleaning and the transportation and disposal of waste. Public health laws assure healthful conditions through waste disposal, housing and building codes, and codes regulating the installation of sewers and water pipes and other infrastructure facilities. Many

of these controls are found in municipal and local law. In the United States, as well as in other parts of the world, public health has been advanced not only by better medical care and the advances of modern medicine, but by the general improvements in cleanliness and physical and sanitary conditions, often left to local law and local governments. These are based on the requirements of housing legislation and building codes, which not only provide protection against the elements but prohibit overcrowding and require adequate ventilation to protect against the spread of communicable disease. Adequate housing is needed to provide a sound basis for a healthy adult life and for raising healthy children.

The future agenda for public health and public health law, both in the United States and worldwide, is to resolve the distributional inequality between the rich and the poor in health services and in the distribution of the means necessary for a wholesome life. The many ethical issues growing out of the developments in the field deal largely with so-called microethical issues, capable of resolution between physicians and patients with the assistance of an ethicist or an institutional committee. The overwhelming issue to be resolved, however, is one of macroethics and centers on the question of how to reduce the gap in the quality of care, which still depends on individual means. The difference in the number of infant deaths and the large gap in life expectancy between the most-favored and least-favored economic, racial, and ethnic groups will not yield to the efforts of ethicists, but will require changes in public policy, in public health planning, and in budgetary allocations. Changes in public health law are needed to advance distributional equity in the availability of health care through programs of insurance and subsidy. Legislation can provide for infrastructure developments in depressed neighborhoods, and for improvements in the availability of housing so as to abolish the scourge of homelessness. One of the current aims of public health must be to do away with the current reality that to be poor means to be in ill health.

FRANK P. GRAD

(SEE ALSO: *Abortion Laws; Block Grants for Public Health; Legal Liability of Public Health Officials; Legislation and Regulation; Licensing; Regulatory Authority*)

BIBLIOGRAPHY

Arras, J., and Hunt, R. (1983). *Ethical Issues in Modern Medicine,* 2nd edition. Palo Alto, CA: Mayfield.

Buchanan, A. (1989). "Health-Care Delivery and Resource Allocation." In *Medical Ethics,* ed. R. M. Veatch. Boston: Jones and Bartlett.

Fluss, S. S. (1995). "The Development of National Health Legislation in Europe: The Contribution of International Organizations." *European Journal of Health Law* 2:193–237.

Friedman, L. M. (1985). *History of American Law,* 2nd edition. New York: Simon & Schuster.

Gostin, L. O.; Burris, S.; Lazzarini, Z.; and Maguire, K. (1998). *Improving State Law to Prevent and Treat Infectious Disease.* New York: Milbank Memorial Fund.

Grad, F. P. (1986). "Public Health Law." In *Maxcy-Rosenau Public Health and Preventive Medicine: 1849–1865,* 12th edition, ed. J. M. Last. Norwalk, CT: Appleton-Century-Crofts.

—— (1990). *The Public Health Law Manual,* 2nd edition. Washington, DC: American Public Health Association.

—— (1998). "Public Health Law: Its Form, Function, Future, and Ethical Parameters." *International Digest of Health Legislation* 49:19–39.

Institute of Medicine (1988). *The Future of Public Health.* Washington, DC: National Academy of Sciences.

Lappé, M. (1986). "Ethics in Public Health." In *Maxcy-Rosenau Public Health and Preventive Medicine: 1849–1865,* 12th edition, ed. J. M. Last. Norwalk, CT: Appleton-Century-Crofts.

The President's Commission for the Study of Ethical Problems in Medicine and Biomedical and Behavioral Research (1983). *Secrecy and Counseling for Genetic Conditions: The Ethical, Social and Legal Implications of Genetic Screening, Counseling and Education Programs.* Washington, DC: U.S. Government Printing Office.

Rosen, G. (1958). *The History of Public Health.* New York: MD Publications.

PUBLIC HEALTH FOUNDATION

The Public Health Foundation (PHF) serves the public health community in the United States by providing information, data, and training on America's public health system. Through applied research, training, and technical assistance, the PHF focuses its efforts on helping strengthen and build public health agencies and systems. The PHF is an independent, nonprofit organization dedicated to supporting and advancing the efforts of local, state, and federal public health agencies and systems to promote and protect the health of people living within their respective jurisdictions. Its board of directors is composed of individuals from state and local public health agencies, boards of health, academia, and the private sector. The PHF was founded in 1970 initially as a research arm of the Association of State and Territorial Health Officials and later evolved into an independent organization focusing on overall public health system infrastructure and capacity building.

State, local, and national organizations have turned to the PHF for assistance with projects such as:

- Setting, measuring, and achieving health improvement objectives and performance standards.

- Designing tools and publications to help put science into practice.

- Tracking and planning Healthy People and other public health initiatives.

- Gathering and analyzing information about public health infrastructure.

- Interpreting data for community and professional audiences.

- Identifying "exemplary practices" and innovations.

- Designing training programs and work force development strategies.

The PHF also serves as staff to the Council on Linkages Between Academia and Public Health Practice, which is dedicated to improving the practice and teaching of public health through the creation of strong academic-practice linkages. Funding for the PHF comes from a variety of federal, state, local, foundation, and private sector sources.

Reports, tools, and descriptions of projects are available at http://www.phf.org, and PHF's online clearinghouse of distance learning offerings is available at http://www.TrainingFinder.org.

RON BIALEK

997

PUBLIC HEALTH LEADERSHIP INSTITUTE

The CDC/UC Public Health Leadership Institute (PHLI) Scholars Program is a national, year-long leadership development program for senior local, state, and federal public health officials and leaders from public health academia, the health systems, and national health organizations. It was begun in 1991 with funding from the Centers for Disease Control and Prevention (CDC) and is administered through a grant to the University of California at Los Angeles, and managed by the Public Health Institute. As of 2001, there were also 13 state or regional institutes, covering 31 states altogether. The CDC began this Institute in response to the nation's need for enhanced leadership in public health. The climate of change in public health requires the individuals who direct U.S. public health organizations not only to be good managers but also good leaders. PHLI scholars learn how to meet public health challenges and shape the future of public health by focusing on these key areas: personal growth for leadership excellence, leading organizational change, community building and collaborative leadership, and communication skills. Throughout the year, scholars participate in teleconferences, readings, electronic seminars, learning teams, an intensive on-site program, and an applied leadership initiative. They also gain support and learn from each other. The Institute's emphasis on distance learning permits scholars to continue working full-time. As of 1999, the Institute had graduated 444 scholars from across the United States. After graduating, they can join the Public Health Leadership Society (PHLS), the PHLI alumni association. As PHLS members, they continue their development as leaders through a variety of educational and networking activities.

CAROL WOLTRING
LIZ SCHWARTZ

(SEE ALSO: *Careers in Public Health; Community Organization; Leadership*)

BIBLIOGRAPHY

Fox, D.; Novick, L.; and Woltring, C. (1997). *Public Health Leaders Tell Their Stories.* Gaithersburg, MD: Aspen Publishing.

Scutchfield, D.; Spain, C. et al. (1995). "The Public Health Leadership Institute: Leadership Training for Local and State Health Officers." *Journal for Public Health Policy* 16(3):304.

PUBLIC HEALTH NURSING

Public health nursing is a specialized form of registered nursing that combines nursing and public health principles. According to the American Public Health Association, the primary focus of public health nursing is improving the health of the community as a whole rather than just that of an individual or family. Public health nursing is sometimes called a type of community health nursing. Some experts use the terms "public health nursing" and "community health nursing" interchangeably.

HISTORY

Public health nursing traces its roots to England where, in 1859, Florence Nightingale assisted in organizing district public health nursing. Each nurse was assigned a specific geographic area of London and was responsible for the health of the people living in that neighborhood. This type of organization finds its echo today in many public health departments, where public health nurses organize their work by groups of census tracts called districts and the nurse is known as the district public health nurse.

In the United States, modern public health nursing was defined by pioneering nurse Lillian Wald in the late 1800s. She established the Henry Street Settlement in New York City, where nurses lived in the neighborhoods where they worked. In the beginning, public health nursing was primarily concerned with taking care of the sick poor in their homes. Lillian Wald came to the realization that sickness found in the home had its origin in larger societal problems. She set about directing nursing efforts toward employment, sanitation, recreation, and education. It was Lillian Wald who coined the term "public health nurse." Hospital-based schools of nursing which granted nursing diplomas provided the educational preparation for nurses at this time.

In the early part of the twentieth century, Visiting Nurses Associations were formed to continue the tradition of providing care for the sick in their homes, which eventually became known as home health nursing. Public health nursing began to be practiced in both voluntary agencies such as the American Red Cross, and governmental agencies, such as local county and city health departments. Serving the needs of the poor remained a key aspect of public health nursing. In the mid twentieth century, care shifted from the home to the clinic, where nurses worked in well baby and immunization clinics for the uninsured and were active in controlling communicable diseases such as tuberculosis.

In the latter part of the twentieth century, nursing education began to move out of hospital-based programs and into community colleges and universities. Educational preparation for public health nurses varies widely in the United States with some jurisdictions requiring a bachelor's degree in nursing and others accepting a hospital diploma or associate degree from a community college. A bachelor's degree in nursing is considered a minimum requirement for public health nursing practice by many nursing professionals and professional nursing organizations. A bachelor's degree in nursing is thought to provide the background in social science and public health science such as epidemiology and environmental health that a public health nurse needs. Increasingly, public health nurses are enrolling in advanced degree programs in public health, community health nursing, and other public health specialties.

THE ROLE OF THE PUBLIC HEALTH NURSE

Ideally, the work of public health nurses is defined as "primary prevention," which means preventing disease, injury, disability and premature death. Public health nurses work as a team with other public health professionals such as environmental health specialists, health educators, epidemiologists, public health physicians, and nutritionists. As members of this team, they work with local communities to assess and prioritize the major health problems and work on a plan to alleviate or eliminate these problems and the conditions that contribute to their development.

Public health nurses are able to assist individuals and families to take action to improve their health status. Often this takes the form of teaching about healthy lifestyle choices in the home, in the workplace, and in community settings. Public health nurses assist people in applying improved health behavior choices to their everyday lives. Examples of personal behaviors that can contribute to health problems are tobacco use, improper diet, lack of physical exercise, unsafe sexual practices, and driving while intoxicated.

Public health nurses also recognize that the community and environment in which people live can affect their ability to make healthy lifestyle choices and can affect whether or not such choices exist at all. Thus, public health nurses may spend a significant portion of their time on ensuring healthy living conditions in the neighborhoods where they work and on improving the health status of the entire community, not just that of individuals. Examples of community issues on which the public health nurse may work are reducing tobacco sales to minors, fluoridation of drinking water, identifying and reducing workplace hazards, immunization of all children against communicable diseases, and reducing the risk of drowning through community education, pool safety, and construction regulation.

Public health nurses are found in a variety of settings, including schools and the workplace. Public health nurses who assist workers at the job site are called occupational health nurses. Some nurses work in local government health departments as general practice nurses in neighborhoods. In some health departments, the community intervention role of public health nurses is not well established and their work is confined to home visits and clinic work. Their primary role is that of case manager and they have a varied caseload of individuals and families whom they assist with illness-oriented concerns, such as communicable diseases and health problems of mothers and children. Sometimes, these case manager public health nurses specialize in one area, such as follow up of cases of lead poisoning or sudden infant death syndrome. Much of the funding for public health work has been fragmented, coming to local government jurisdictions from state and federal sources for a specific problem or intervention only. As a consequence, public health nursing in many settings has become more specialized and even more concentrated on caring for individuals and families, usually in the home.

Many public health nursing experts feel that this emphasis on caring for people with a disease or condition has hindered public health nurses from being full participants in public health and has diverted public health nursing away from its prevention role. Some in public health nursing would even argue that, as a result, the practice of public health nursing has lost its way and needs to refocus on the true mission of public health: to look at the health problems of a community as a whole and work with the community in alleviating those problems. They would argue that there is the mistaken perception of public health nurses as providers of personal care only. The challenge for public health nurses in the future is to apply the nursing process (assessment, diagnosis, planning, implementation, and evaluation of interventions) to improve health, not just of individuals, but also with larger segments of the population in partnership with the community.

TRENDS AND FUTURE DIRECTIONS

The practice of public health nursing has been greatly affected by sources of funding. Much of the past focus on clinic work and personal health care for the indigent and uninsured has been driven by the need to limit nursing work to what was reimbursable by a third party, such as Medicaid in the United States. Many public health nurses practice in local health departments, which are seen as the providers of last resort for care of the sick poor and the uninsured. County hospital care and out patient services have taken much of the public health funding and attention away from the primary goal of public health, that is, improving the health of the entire community. However, this is gradually changing, with a major shift in the 1990s to health plans (managed care) and the movement of Medicaid populations, in most states, into managed care programs. This has made caring for sick low-income people more financially viable for the private sector. Consequently, local health departments and their public health nursing staff have been encouraged to shift their activities back toward the primary mission of public health, which is

to work on the causes of health problems and to prevent them.

KATHLEEN N. SMITH

(SEE ALSO: *Barrier Nursing; Nurse; Practice of Public Health*)

BIBLIOGRAPHY

American Public Health Association Public Health Nursing Section (1996). *The Definition and Role of Public Health Nursing.* Washington, DC: Author.

Anderson, E. T., and McFarlane, J. (1996). *Community as Partner: Theory and Practice in Nursing,* revised edition. Philadelphia, PA: Lippincott.

Buhler-Wilkerson, K. (1993). "Bringing Care to the People: Lillian Wald's Legacy to Public Health Nursing." *American Journal of Public Health* 83(December):1778–1786.

Clark, M. J. (1996). *Nursing in the Community,* revised edition. Stanford, CT: Appleton and Lange.

Helvie, C. O. (1998). *Advanced Practice Nursing in the Community.* Thousand Oaks, CA: Sage Publications.

Keller, L. O.; Strohschein, S.; Lia-Hoagberg, B.; and Schaffer, M. (1998). "Population-Based Public Health Nursing Interventions: A Model from Practice." *Public Health Nursing* 15(June):207–215.

Kosidlak, J. G. (1999). "The Development and Implementation of a Population- Based Intervention Model for Public Health Nursing Practice." *Public Health Nursing* 16(October):311–320.

National Association of County Health Officials (1993). *Core Public Health Functions.* July.

Stanhope, M., and Lancaster, J. (2000). *Community and Public Health Nursing,* revised edition. St. Louis, MO: Mosby.

PUBLIC HEALTH PRACTICE PROGRAM OFFICE

The Public Health Practice Program Office (PHPPO) of the Centers for Disease Control and Prevention (CDC) was created in 1988 to strengthen the nation's public health system by enhancing work force capacity, building information and communications systems, improving laboratory quality, and conducting systems research. The

PHPPO is committed to strengthening the public health system and improving community-based public health practice throughout the United States and around the world. The office works closely with other CDC components to provide support for specific disease-control programs (e.g., infectious disease control, injury prevention, environmental health, and chronic disease prevention).

Work Force Development Programs. The PHPPO has pioneered the use of distance-based training through the Public Health Training Network (PHTN) as a means of improving the competency of the domestic public health work force. The PHTN is a distance-learning network that has reached over 400,000 people since its creation in 1992. The National Laboratory Training Network (NLTN) provides laboratory training courses throughout the United States. The Public Health Leadership Institute was created in 1991, and has provided training to over five hundred public health leaders and spawned a national network of state and regional leadership development programs. The Sustainable Management Development Program (SMDP) provides intensive management training for public health professionals from around the world and technical assistance to program graduates. In 1999, in cosponsorship with the Health Resources and Services Administration (HRSA), the Robert Wood Johnson Foundation, and the W. K. Kellogg Foundation, the Management Academy for Public Health, managed by the University of North Carolina at Chapel Hill, was created to provide management development experiences for managers in governmental public health agencies in four southeastern states. Finally, in 1999 the creation of a CDC Leadership and Management Institute was formed to address needs of CDC leaders and managers.

Information and Communication Systems. In 1991 the PHPPO pioneered the use of information technology in public health practice through its national award-winning program, the Information Network for Public Health Officials (INPHO). Subsequently, through support for CDC's bioterrorism program, the Health Alert Network initiative was created to further enhance information communications systems capacity, improve work force competency, and utilize performance standards to assess organizational capabilities.

Laboratory Quality. The PHPPO provides leadership in developing regulations under the Clinical Laboratory Improvement Act of 1988, working closely with partners at the Health Care Financing Administration (HCFA) to provide a comprehensive policy framework for assuring the quality of clinical laboratory services throughout the nation. Innovative activities in genetics testing, HIV (human immunodeficiency virus) testing, and tuberculosis testing have also contributed to the success of prevention programs in the United States and around the world.

Systems Research and Development. In 1990, working closely with NACCHO, PHPPO developed the APEX planning tool. Today, this is the most widely used comprehensive planning tool for local public health agencies in the United States. Further, PHPPO is leading the development of performance standards for local and state public health systems and for conducting systems research.

EDWARD L. BAKER

(SEE ALSO: *Centers for Disease Control and Prevention; Information Technology; Laboratory Services; Mobilizing for Action through Planning and Partnerships; Training for Public Health*)

PULMONARY FUNCTION

Normal individuals have a large reserve in lung function that allows breathing capacity to increase at least twenty to thirty times during periods of vigorous physical activity. It is not the ability to breathe that normally limits maximum exercise capability, nor does physical activity normally change lung function, either in the short-term or over time with training. With lung disease, however, lung function declines and can impose breathing limitations on physical activity. This may result in excessive shortness of breath with daily activities that previously could be carried out without great difficulty.

In some susceptible individuals, exercise may cause the airways ("breathing tubes") to narrow, reducing lung function and causing abnormal shortness of breath with physical activity. Such persons are thought to have "reactive" or "twitchy" airways.

This may be a manifestation of asthma, and is known as "exercise-induced asthma."

ANDREW L. RIES

(SEE ALSO *Asthma; Emphysema; Lung Cancer; Physical Activity; VO2 Max*)

BIBLIOGRAPHY

Mahler, D. A. (1993). "Exercise-Induced Asthma." *Medical Science of Sports and Exercise* 25:554–561.

Ries, A. L.; Bullock, P. J.; Larsen, C. A.; Limberg, T. M.; Myers, R.; Pfister, T.; Sassi-Dambron, D. E.; and Sheldon, J. B. (2001). *Shortness of Breath: A Guide to Better Living and Breathing*, 6th edition. St. Louis, MO: Mosby.

Q

Q FEVER

Q fever is an infectious disease caused by the bacterium *Coxiella burnetii*. The "Q" derives from "query" fever, its name before the true cause of the disease was discovered in 1937. Worldwide in occurrence, the etiologic agent is prevalent in sheep, cattle, and goats, and it is also found in ticks, rodents, birds, dogs, and rabbits. Infections in animals are usually inapparent, but the disease can cause spontaneous abortions in animals. Humans can be very susceptible and can contract the disease through inhalation of contaminated dust or particles from animal hides, excreta, and birthing materials.

Because *C. burnetii* proliferates within human white blood cells called monocytes, it is protected from part of the human immune system. A complex molecule called a lipopolysaccharide, found on the surface of the organism, further protects it from host serum defense factors. Human disease will usually present with sudden onset of headache, fever, chills, muscle soreness, and (sometimes) pneumonia. Hepatitis or endocarditis are rarer complications. Without modern detection methods, the disease is difficult to diagnose, and many human infections are probably unrecognized. It is suspected that host and microbial factors combine to determine the severity of human disease.

The antibiotic tetracycline is usually very effective in treating acute Q fever. Chronic inflammatory forms of the disease, such as Q fever endocarditis or hepatitis, require more than one year of antibiotic treatment.

Outbreaks of human Q fever are commonly reported in Asia, Australia, and parts of Europe. The disease was made reportable in the United States in 1999. Transmission from human to human is uncommon. Control of Q fever depends upon its recognition in animal populations and the culling of infected animals to prevent subsequent human exposure. A commercial vaccine, Qvax, is available in Australia.

HERB A. THOMPSON
JENNIFER MCQUISTON

(SEE ALSO: *Communicable Disease Control*)

BIBLIOGRAPHY

Centers for Disease Control and Prevention. *Q Fever.* Available at http://www.cdc.gov/ncidod/dvrd/qfever/index.htm.

Maurin, M., and Raoult, D. (1999). "Q Fever." *Clinical Microbiology Reviews* 12(4):518–553.

QUALITY OF LIFE

Before the 1970s, quality of life received little attention in the medical or public health literature, but since then the situation has been reversed. Despite its widespread use, the term "quality of life" has different meanings to different people. For some researchers and clinicians, quality of life means almost anything beyond information about death and death rates. For others quality of life is an umbrella concept that refers to all aspects of a person's life, including physical health; psychological well-being; social well-being; financial well-being; family relationships; friendships; work; leisure; and the like. In contrast, some approaches to quality of life emphasize the social and psychological aspects of life, and contrast quality of life with quality of care.

Variation is also found in measurement strategies. Some scholars believe that quality of life can be measured by objective parameters. For example, the quality of life in a city is sometimes measured by a summary of characteristics such as the schools, the cultural offerings, the aesthetic properties, the climate, the health care system, the employment possibilities, and so on. By the same token, characteristics of a person, such as income, health status, mental health status, disease profiles, educational level, and housing situation can be summed to create an overall quality-of-life measure. Others view the objective parameters that are often associated with quality of life to be indicators, whereas the actual quality of life can only be measured by a subjective appraisal made by the individual living the life. If one believes that quality of life is inherently subjective, it is then possible to test indicators by the extent to which they predict the quality of life reported by groups of people.

Why is quality of life of interest for public health? First, a good or a poor quality of life is, in some ways, the ultimate marker of the success of preventive health practices and of health care. Second, many health care regimens often seem to detract from quality of life, at least in the short run. As individuals, with the help of their physicians, make decisions about treatment choices, they may take quality of life into account, and may seek information about the likely effects on the quality of their life. Third, and related to the previous point, recent rhetoric pits quantity of life against quality of life, especially in terms of end-of-life treatments; the argument is sometimes made that some treatments are inadvisable because the quality of life likely to result for the extra time gained is too poor. Thus, quality of life has come to be seen as a gold standard for weighing the benefits and costs of life-extending treatments. Finally, in some circumstances, people are asked to change their life circumstances, perhaps forever, for the sake of their health status and care. Relocation to a nursing home would be an example of such a dramatic change. In that situation, it is incumbent on those who plan, fund, and license nursing homes to have some way of assuring that the quality of life, in so far as it is influenced by the facility, is of an acceptable standard.

In health care, the term "health-related quality of life" (HRQL) is often used. This approach narrows consideration to those aspects of quality of life that are deemed to be affected positively or negatively by medical or health care intervention. Another important distinction is between a general HRQL measure (e.g., one that asks about quality of life affected by health) in contrast to a disease-specific HRQL measure. A disease-specific approach may pose questions in relation to the effects of a particular disease (e.g., cancer, arthritis, heart disease) and its treatment with items such as "have you experienced reduction in social activities because of your condition." Other tools are comprised of objective items (for example, agree-disagree items) that are thought to be particularly relevant to the particular disease. A generic HRQL measure may simply be a general measure that attempts to tap health status using the full range of the World Health Organization's definition of health: "physical, psychological, and social well-being."

Subjective judgments of quality of life, though logically the best single source of information, are prone to be influenced by a number of factors. First, expectations influence appraised quality of life, so that an individual may become used to circumstances that could objectively be considered substandard. (This criticism also applies to measures of satisfaction.) Second, individuals may feel constrained because of courtesy or intimidation from actually expressing their views. The intimidation is more likely if the person is in vulnerable health and perceives himself or herself as dependent on care providers, a circumstance that is common for nursing home residents. Finally, lifelong personality traits may influence perceived quality of life.

Personality is generally classified according to five traits (each of which can be seen in their expression or their opposites): neuroticism, extroversion, agreeableness, conscientiousness, and openness. Although little large-scale psychological or sociological research has been done to link subjective quality-of-life results to personality, anthropologists have observed patterns that suggest underlying personality is very much related to how individuals view the quality of their life.

MEASURES OF QUALITY OF LIFE

Examples of some general HRQL measures in widespread use include the Sickness Impact Profile (SIP), which was developed by Bergner and colleagues in the 1970s, and the Medical Outcomes Studies (MOS) Short Form, known as the SF-36, developed by John Ware and colleagues. The SIP, which was developed in the 1970s, contains 136 items that tap twelve categories of well-being: sleep and rest, eating, work, home management, recreation and pastimes, ambulation, mobility, body care and movement, social interaction, alertness behavior, emotional behavior, and communication. As its name suggests the SF-36 contains thirty-six questions and generates scores in eight categories: physical functioning, role limitations due to physical problems, social functioning, bodily pain, general mental health, role limitations due to emotional problems, vitality, and general health perceptions; an SF-12 is also available that provides summary scores for physical and mental functioning.

The best known approach specifically for elderly people is the Multi-level Assessment Instrument (MIA), developed by Lawton and colleagues; this is a 152-item battery that generates scores in seven areas: physical health, cognition, activities of daily living, time use, social relations and interactions, personal adjustment, and perceived environment. More recently, Kane and colleagues have been conducting research to develop a self-report measure of the psychosocial aspects of quality of life for nursing home residents: Their eleven domains include comfort, functional competence, autonomy, dignity, individuality, privacy, relationships, meaningful activity, sense of security and safety, enjoyment, and spiritual well-being.

The Quality of Well-being (QWB) Scale, developed by Kaplan and colleagues, differs from the approaches so far described because it defines quality on twenty-four functional states on a scale ranging from 0 for death to 1 for perfect health. The scoring weights were developed based on preferences that individuals assign to the various states.

USING QUALITY OF LIFE FOR RESOURCE ALLOCATION

Some policy analysts recommend using information about quality of life under certain conditions to make decisions about the relative value of health expenditures. The term "quality-adjusted life year" (QALY) is used for approaches that try to combine the effect an intervention will have both on prolonging life and the quality of that life. For example, it would be assumed that extending life for a year for someone in a coma is not as worthwhile as adding a year of vigorous function. The QWB scale described above lends itself to a QALY approach.

Technical and ethical questions arise in applying QALY. Among the former are issues of whether those who rate the conditions have sufficient understanding to apply the judgments. It is widely known that people who do not have a particular condition devalue life with that condition more than those who actually experience the disease or health state. It is also likely that there are cultural and social class differences in how various states are valued. In a well-publicized project, the Medicaid program in the state of Oregon ambitiously applied a QALY approach to Medicaid expenditures for a wide range of conditions. A series of town meetings and phone surveys elicited public opinion about the value attached to the conditions and was combined with physicians' estimations of the magnitude and duration of effects of medical interventions. These were combined with cost information to generate a rank-ordered list of priorities. This procedure yielded results that gave a higher priority to treatment of some common conditions than to much more severe but treatable conditions affecting fewer people.

The most serious criticism of QALY measures is that, as they have been developed and applied, they seem to discount the value of the lives of people with disabilities and very elderly people. If the upper boundary of quality of life is having no functional limits, then certainly quality of life for older people is deflated. An approach called "active life expectancy" developed by gerontologists has this problem: Once the individual is dependent, he or she has no more years of active life expectancy left under the measure.

PROXY EVALUATIONS OF QUALITY OF LIFE

Even if subjective appraisal is treated as a gold standard, some people will simply be unable to communicate about the quality of their lives, and alternative sources of information must be sought. This will be particularly true of people with severe cognitive impairments such as Alzheimer's disease, or people who suffer the communication and motor problems associated with stroke (which could prevent both written or oral administration of a questionnaire). It is, of course, also true of very young children, including newborn children with disabilities that are believed to severely compromise the quality of their current and expected future lives. The hospice movement has stimulated interest in appraising quality of life at the time of death, yet many people cannot be effectively queried on the subject in the last few days of life.

Under these circumstances, the choices of information sources seem to be limited to three: family members, health professionals or paid caregivers of various types, and/or direct observations of the person, from which inferences about his or her quality of life are drawn. All of these approaches have been applied with and for people with Alzheimer's disease. Some of the work in this regard was stimulated by the growth of special care units (SCUs) for Alzheimer's disease in nursing homes, and the resulting need to determine whether residents experienced a different quality of life on those specialized units than in the general population. The direct observations include repeated systematic observation of the individual's facial expression and body language for signs of positive or negative emotion. Similar multifaceted approaches have been developed for adults with intellectual impairments due to developmental disability. However, caution is recommended in resorting to proxy informants too quickly or widely. Many seniors with Alzheimer's disease and younger people with mental retardation are, nevertheless, capable of evaluating many aspects of their lives.

Moreover, when it has been possible to get information from both the person most concerned and other informants, a growing body of studies show that family members and professionals may rate quality of life differently from the ratings of those living the life.

The growing attention to quality of life and the desire to minimize the negative effects of disease and health care on this quality reflects the highest of public health aspirations. The science of measuring quality-of-life outcomes is still under development and a matter of some controversy. Also at issue is the extent to which public health measures and health care provision can and should attempt to influence quality of life broadly, and whose values should inform the definitions of quality.

ROSALIE A. KANE

(SEE ALSO: *Assessment of Health Status; Functional Capacity; Gerontology; Health Outcomes*)

BIBLIOGRAPHY

Albert, S. M., and Logsdon, R. G., eds. (1999). "Assessing Quality of Life in Alzheimer's Disease." *Journal of Mental Health and Aging* 5(1):1–111.

Frytak, J. R. (2000). "Assessment of Quality of Life." In *Assessing Older Persons: Measures, Meaning, and Practical Applications,* eds. R. L. Kane and R. A. Kane. New York: Oxford University Press.

McDowell, I., and Newell, C. (1996). *Measuring Health: A Guide to Rating Scales and Questionnaires,* 2nd edition. New York: Oxford University Press.

Morreim, E. H. (1995). "Quality of Life in Health Care Allocation." In *Encyclopedia of Bioethics,* revised edition, ed. W. Reich. New York: Macmillan Reference.

Noelker, L. S., and Harel, Z. (2001). *Linking Quality of Long-Term Care and Quality of Life.* New York: Springer Publishing Company.

QUARANTINE

Quarantine is defined as a restriction of the activities of healthy persons or animals who have been exposed to a communicable disease. The aim is to prevent transmission of the disease from potentially infected persons to healthy persons during the incubation period. Quarantine can take two forms: absolute or complete quarantine, which consists of a limitation of freedom for a period equal to the longest usual incubation period of the disease; and modified quarantine, which involves selective or partial limitation of movement, based on known differences in susceptibility. Examples of a modified quarantine are the exclusion of children from school and the confining of military personnel to their base. Modified quarantine includes personal surveillance, medical supervision, and segregation of the individual or group; or the establishment of a cordon sanitaire (a boundary zone between uninfected and infected or exposed persons).

The word "quarantine" derives from the Italian *quaranta dei* (forty days), a reminder that the custom of segregating putatively infected persons, and the ships on which they were traveling, originated in the maritime empire of Venice in the fourteenth century. The length of time probably relates to the biblical story of the forty days Jesus spent in the wilderness, not to any real knowledge of the mode of transmission of infection. The rise of the practice, however, suggests that there was some understanding of the concept of contagion even if there was no empirical knowledge of infective periods and incubation times of the plagues that afflicted medieval Europe. Few infectious diseases have an incubation time or infective period greater than forty days. An exception is rabies, which may not declare itself for many months. That is why animals that may have been exposed to rabies are quarantined for many months when they arrive in countries where rabies does not exist.

Animal and plant quarantine procedures are often more important than human quarantine now that many of the most dangerous contagious diseases can be kept under observation without such draconian restrictions as formerly required. The economic importance of agriculture and animal husbandry in many countries makes it absolutely essential to exclude diseases that might wipe out valuable cattle herds or destroy a season's harvest. A very important human disease with an incubation time that can, and probably usually does, exceed forty days is HIV (human immunodeficiency virus) infection, but for reasons that have more to do with human rights than epidemiological insights there is no quarantine for persons exposed to HIV infection.

Quarantine as a way to control the spread of contagious diseases is an extreme form of isolation, which has several less severe variations. Bedside isolation, in which patients suffering from an infectious disease are barrier nursed to break the chain of transmission, is the mildest variation. More dangerous varieties of contagious disease, such as pulmonary tuberculosis with excretion of tubercle bacilli, diphtheria, and cholera, are preferably isolated in a special hospital or closed ward. Until recently, patients with such diseases as typhoid, paralytic poliomyelitis, and meningococcal meningitis were strictly isolated and every effort was made to preserve a cordon sanitaire around them. Their contacts were quarantined under public health laws in some jurisdictions, even though epidemiologically this made little or no sense as a means of preventing transmission of infection. Powerful antibiotics and better understanding have made quarantine unnecessary for these and many other diseases. Infected patients are now often treated in a general hospital rather than in one dedicated to infectious diseases. The practice of universal precautions is a modified form of quarantine in which patients with a contagious disease (such as HIV/AIDS [acquired immunodeficiency syndrome]) are barrier nursed and otherwise cared for so as to minimize the risk of HIV transmission.

Quarantine goes further than isolation because it includes the compulsory segregation of contacts of infectious cases. It therefore involves infringing upon the liberty of outwardly healthy people, and this has both legal and ethical implications. Any restriction of a person's freedom to move must be justified, and such a restriction sanctioned by public health laws and regulations in many nations. In the early twentieth century most industrial nations had lengthy lists of contagious diseases to which quarantine laws applied. By the 1960s most of these diseases could be controlled without such severe restrictions, and in 1969 the World Health Organization issued international health regulations for just four designated quarantinable diseases: cholera, plague, yellow fever, and smallpox. Smallpox was proclaimed eradicated by WHO in 1979, and the other diseases on the list (except cholera in some parts of the world and, occasionally, yellow fever in others) are now rarely encountered or respond well to medical treatment. The quarantine stations that were formerly a feature of large seaports around the world have been abandoned, dismantled, or turned into holiday resorts. Quarantine law and regulations still apply in many countries, however, to protect animals and plants of economic importance from exotic diseases.

Public health officials who invoke quarantine laws or regulations must justify this action ethically—on the grounds that it is in the interests of the greater good of the community. In the past, this police power of public health officials was accepted by most people as a necessary measure to control the spread of contagious disease. Community values changed in the late twentieth century, however, and there is now emotional and political resistance to restricting freedom in the interests of safeguarding the public's health. It is regarded as ethically unacceptable to quarantine promiscuous persons who are HIV-positive, even though it might be in the best interests of the general public to do so. In some places, public health officials have invoked the police power of their quarantine regulations and, sometimes with the assistance of local police forces, they have incarcerated incorrigibly promiscuous persons infected with HIV/AIDS. AIDS activists and civil rights advocates oppose this, and a debate that played out in relation to detention of polio contacts in the early twentieth century is being reprised.

JOHN M. LAST

(SEE ALSO: *Barrier Nursing; Communicable Disease Control; Ethics of Public Health; Isolation; Notifiable Diseases*)

QUININE

See Malaria

R

RABIES

Rabies is a viral disease of wild and domestic animals. It is particularly prevalent in feral dogs, while humans are occasional victims. The virus is transmitted in saliva and enters the body through puncture wounds caused by bites, or via abrasions, open cuts, or sores. The virus attacks the central nervous system by migrating up peripheral nerves from the site of entry. It can take several months to reach the central nervous system, so there can be a very long incubation period. In humans and most animals it is almost invariably fatal, but bats may be symptomless carriers. Rabies occurs almost worldwide, but it has been eliminated from Britain, Iceland, and Scandinavia through rigorously enforced animal quarantine, which has also prevented it from ever gaining entry to Australia. Because of the long incubation period, exposed animals must be quarantined for many months. In much of the world, including the United States and Canada, rabies is endemic in foxes, raccoons, skunks, bats, and other wild animals, and these occasionally infect domestic animals and humans.

The French bacteriologist Louis Pasteur developed a postexposure vaccine against rabies in 1885, using desiccated nerve tissue containing the virus. For many years, Pasteur's prolonged and painful course of injections was used to treat all persons who had been bitten by suspected rabid animals. Prophylactic immunizations for animal and human use have been much improved by the human diploid cell vaccine (HDCV), developed in the 1970s. Rabies immune globulin is used for postexposure prophylaxis. When humans are bitten by a suspected rabid animal, the animal should be killed and its brain examined for evidence of infection. Vaccination of wild animals utilizes an oral vaccine delivered in baits.

JOHN M. LAST

(SEE ALSO: *Communicable Disease Control; Immunizations; Pasteur, Louis; Veterinary Public Health*)

BIBLIOGRAPHY

National Center for Infectious Diseases. *Rabies.* Available at http://www.cdc.gov/ncidod/dvrd/rabies.

RACE AND ETHNICITY

Within public health, there is disagreement about the meaning and use of the term "race." Often, public health scientists and the general public alike mistakenly base their notions of race on the idea that the human species can be separated into distinct human races identifiable through differences in physical traits (e.g., skin color, hair texture, facial features). Furthermore these ideas frequently carry with them the notion that these physical or other distinguishing traits have a basis in a homogeneous set of genes that differentiate races from one another. These ideas originated in the fifteenth century when the ability to support such ideas using sound scientific methods was not possible. Now, scientists from many disciplines (e.g., genetics, anthropology, sociology, biology) agree that there are no distinct human races as was previously claimed.

A more recently developed concept about race is ethnicity. This concept, which emerged in the late eighteenth century, is usually conceptualized as membership in a group defined by a shared geographical origin or cultural history, including common language, religion, art, and other cultural factors. Ethnicity is distinguished from race in public health studies. In North America, the most common ethnic group designation is Hispanic, or Latino/Latina.

Historically, there are examples of extreme human rights violations justified through the notion of biologically homogeneous race and ethnic groups. Eugenics has been used to target members of racial and ethnic groups with oppressive and genocidal societal policies and actions. Just before World War II, eugenics formed the basis of Nazi genocidal policies toward Jews, and in the early twentieth century it resulted in landholding and job exclusionary policies toward European immigrants to the United States. Race as a social construction and social fact continues to figure prominently in political and ideological relations and systems of contemporary societies worldwide.

Starting in the 1970s, scientific evidence began to accumulate to support the idea that races, as distinct biologically or genetically homogeneous groups of humans, do not exist. Geneticists have shown that only a very small proportion (6% or less) of human genetic variability occurs between so-called races. Furthermore scientists within other disciplines, such as biology and anthropology, have discarded such definitions of race based upon notions of biologic or genetic homogeneity. Rather, scientists recognize that the concept of race has been socially constructed—initially in the sixteenth century to justify economic exploitation and political domination of certain populations distinguishable by physical features such as skin color—and that race is a set of economic, political, and cultural relations that result in health and social inequalities.

Public health scientists continue to use various categories of race in research. The U.S. Office of Management and Budget (OMB), setting standards for the nation, recently recommended using the categories American Indian or Alaska Native, Asian, Black or African American, Native Hawaiian or Other Pacific Islander, and White. The OMB recognizes that these categories represent a "sociopolitical construct" and "are not anthropologically or scientifically based."

In public health research, racial categories are often used to demonstrate inequalities in health status and other health-related factors such as access to and quality of health care. Unfortunately, some public health studies still interpret such inequalities as having a biologic or genetic basis. Thus, subtle and blatant forms of "scientific racism" and biological determinism are seen within the field of public health today. Public health scientists should be encouraged to use theories of race informed by current scientific evidence that so-called races are social constructs and social facts. Fortunately, public health studies have begun to identify and measure the social mechanisms (e.g., institutional and individual racism) that contribute to racial gaps rather than using race as a proxy for these exposures.

PATRICIA O'CAMPO

(SEE ALSO: *Economics of Health; Ethnicity and Health; Ethnocentrism; Eugenics; Social Determinants*)

BIBLIOGRAPHY

American Association of Anthropologists (1999). "Statement on Race." *American Anthropologist* 100(3): 712–713.

Banton, M. (1998). *Racial Theories*. Cambridge, UK: Cambridge University Press.

Bonilla, S. E. (1999). "The Essential Social Fact of Race." *American Sociological Review* 64:899–906.

Cavilis-Sforza, L. L. (2000). *Peoples and Languages,* trans. M. Seielstad. New York: North Point Press.

Lewontin, R. L.; Rose, S.; and Kamin, L. J. (1984). *Not in Our Genes: Biology, Ideology and Human Nature*. New York: Pantheon Books.

RADIATION, IONIZING

Electromagnetic waves of extremely short wavelength (X-rays and gamma rays) and accelerated atomic particles (such as electrons, protons, neutrons, and alpha particles) deposit enough localized energy in an absorbing medium to dislodge electrons from atoms with which they interact and to disrupt chemical bonds. The loss of electrons creates particles known as "ions," and these types of radiation are termed "ionizing radiation." Natural sources of such radiation, which are ubiquitous and to which all people are exposed, include cosmic rays, radioactive elements in the earth's crust, internally deposited radionuclides, and inhaled radon. Artificial sources include the use of X-rays in medical and dental diagnosis; radioactive materials in building materials, phosphate fertilizers, and crushed rock; radiation-emitting components of TV sets, smoke detectors, and other consumer products; radioactive fallout from atomic weapons; and nuclear power. Additional sources are encountered by workers in certain workplace environments.

As ionizing radiation penetrates a living cell, it collides randomly with atoms and molecules in its path, giving rise to ions, free radicals, and other molecular alterations that may injure the cell. Any molecule in the cell can be altered by radiation, but DNA is the most critical biological target because of the limited redundancy of the genetic information it contains. A dose of radiation that is large enough to kill the average dividing cell causes hundreds of lesions in the cell's DNA molecules. Most such lesions are reparable, but those produced by a densely ionizing radiation (such as a proton or an alpha particle) are generally more complex and less reparable than those produced by a sparsely ionizing radiation (such as an X-ray or a gamma ray). Any damage to DNA that remains unrepaired or is improperly repaired may result in a mutation or chromosome aberration, and both of these types of effects appear to rise in frequency in proportion to any increase in the dose in the low-dose domain.

Damage to the genetic apparatus may be lethal to cells, especially dividing cells—the depletion of which in a given organ may cause severe damage. In radiation accident victims, for example, the depletion of blood-forming cells in the bone marrow is typically a cause of early death. Although the production of an overt clinical reaction generally requires a dose that is large enough to kill many cells, smaller doses can suffice to cause malformations and other disturbances of development in an embryo. Although adverse health effects have not been demonstrated at the low exposure levels characteristically associated with natural background irradiation, it is noteworthy that at higher dose levels many of the cellular alterations that are precursors to cancer, as well as the risks of some forms of cancer themselves, appear to increase in frequency as linear-nonthreshold functions of the dose.

The risks to human health and to the environment from exposure to ionizing radiation have been reviewed repeatedly by the National Research Council, the National Council on Radiation Protection and Measurements, the International Commission on Radiological Protection, the United Nations Scientific Committee on the Effects of Atomic Radiation, and various other national and international organizations. Such organizations have generally concurred in the conclusion that the existence of a threshold for risks in the low-dose domain cannot be excluded, but that the weight of existing evidence supports the hypothesis that the genetic and carcinogenic effects of radiation increase in frequency as linear-nonthreshold functions of the dose. Assessments of the risks of low-level radiation for public health purposes are, therefore, generally based on the use of linear-nonthreshold dose-response models, their inherent uncertainties notwithstanding. In other words, there is an assumption that there is no threshold for the cancer-causing effects of ionizing radiation and that any increase in radiation exposure causes a corresponding increase in cancer risk.

ARTHUR C. UPTON

(SEE ALSO: *Carcinogenesis; Nonionizing Radiation; Nuclear Power; Radon; Ultraviolet Radiation*)

BIBLIOGRAPHY

International Commission on Radiological Protection (1991). *1990 Recommendations of the International Commission on Radiological Protection.* ICRP Publication 60. No. 1–3. New York: Pergamon.

Mettler, F. A., and Upton, A. C. (1995). *Medical Effects of Ionizing Radiation,* 2nd edition. Philadelphia, PA: W. B. Saunders.

National Research Council (1999). *Health Effects of Exposure to Radon.* Washington, DC: National Academy Press.

United Nations Scientific Committee on the Effects of Atomic Radiation (UNSCEAR) (1994). *Sources and*

Effects of Ionizing Radiation. Report to the General Assembly with Annexes. New York: United Nations.

RADIO

Radio is looked at as an important tool in educating the general public about health issues. In particular, it is believed that properly developed community radio can encourage community-driven problem solving. At the government level, radio has been used to advise the public on issues such as new health standards and seasonal food warnings.

Examples of radio's role in education and public health awareness are numerous. Sound Partners—a program run by the Benton Foundation—provides grants to public radio stations interested in developing community-oriented educational content for the good of public health. Many talk-radio stations and public broadcasters feature special call-in medical programming and general health information. Public addresses via radio, such as President Clinton's radio talk on May 6, 2000, on food safety, and the radio dissemination of automotive product recalls by the United States National Highway Traffic Safety Administration, also exhibit the effectiveness of radio as a means of informing the public.

While the above services are good for the general public, physicians need to be educated in a different manner. Internet radio involves broadcasting audio content on the Internet so it can be heard anywhere in the world through a computer or WebTV unit. Examples of Internet radio delivery systems include RealNetwork's RealPlayer and Microsoft's Windows Media Player.

Internet radio is important for the public health and medical community because it creates an opportunity for high-quality interactive distance learning and education without geographic limitations. For example, in a normal educational setting doctors would need to go to a special class or conference to educate themselves. Internet radio can provide doctors with an alternative to the traditional continuing education setting.

NEIL SCHNEIDER

(SEE ALSO: *Mass Media; Mass Media and Tobacco Control; Media Advocacy*)

RADON

Radon-222 and radon-220 (thoron) are invisible, inert, and odorless radioactive gases formed in the decay of uranium-238 and thorium-232, respectively. Uranium-238 and thorium-232 are radionuclides that are widely distributed in the earth's crust. The half-life of radon-222 is long enough (3.82 days) to enable appreciable quantities of this element to accumulate in the environment, whereas the half-life of radon-220 is so short (55 seconds) that it does not attain environmental concentrations that produce demonstrable biological effects. Radon-222, seeping out of the soil, is ubiquitous in outdoor air, where its concentration averages about 15 becquerels per cubic meter (5 Bqm^{-3} or 0.4 pCi/L). (The *becquerel* [Bq] and the *curie* [Ci] are units of radioactivity; 1 Bq = 1 disintegration per second, and 1 Ci = 3.7×10^{10} disintegrations per second. Radon is measured in picocuries per liter of air [pCi/L] or becquerels per cubic meter [Bqm^{-3}].) In indoor air, the concentration of radon tends to be much higher than in outdoor air, especially in poorly ventilated basements and underground mines, where it may exceed 1,000 Bqm^{-3} (20 pCi/L). Indoor levels may be increased substantially by the use of groundwater or well water containing elevated concentrations of radon.

The alpha particles emitted by radon outside the body do not penetrate the skin, and radon itself, like other inert gases, is breathed in and out of the lungs without interacting significantly with the surrounding tissues. Hence the biological effects of radon result from inhalation of its solid, short-lived, alpha-emitting decay products (principally polonium-218 and polonium-214), which deposit on the lining of the bronchial airway. The dose to internal organs from radon that is ingested in drinking water, even at high concentrations, is extremely low.

In humans and laboratory animals, the risk of lung cancer increases with increasing exposure to inhaled radon and its short-lived decay products. In underground miners the risk appears to increase in proportion to the total cumulative dose to cells lining the airway, and to be about two times higher in smokers than in nonsmokers. The risk from exposure to residential indoor radon at a given concentration, although yet to be defined precisely, is generally estimated to be comparable to the corresponding risk in miners. As a result, radon is thought to be the single most important cause of lung cancer in nonsmokers and to cause 10 to 15 percent of all lung cancers, or 15,000 to 20,000 lung cancer deaths each year in the United States. Hence, the U.S. Environmental Protection Agency has recommended that indoor radon concentrations not be allowed to exceed 4 pCi/L, a concentration that might be expected to double the risk of lung cancer if inhaled throughout an average lifespan.

Methods for reducing the concentration of radon and its decay products in indoor air include ventilation; air filtration; sealing of cracks in basement floors and walls; installation of a subslab exhaust system beneath the basement floor; and remediation of heavily contaminated groundwater or well water that is used for drinking, bathing, or showering. Radon can be measured in the home with a number of relatively inexpensive devices, which are available from some state and local governments as well as private firms. Pertinent information can generally be obtained from the local state radiation or the Environmental Protection Agency office.

ARTHUR C. UPTON

BIBLIOGRAPHY

Eisenbud, M., and Gesell, T. (1997). *Environmental Radioactivity: From Natural, Industrial, and Military Sources,* 4th edition. San Diego, CA: Academic Press.

Harley, N. (2000). "Radon and Daughters." In *Environmental Toxicants,* 2nd edition, ed. M. Lippmann. New York: John Wiley and Sons.

National Academy of Sciences/National Research Council (1998). *Health Effects of Exposure to Radon.* Washington, DC: National Academy Press.

U.S. Geological Survey. *The Geology of Radon.* Available at http://energy.ct.us.gov/radonhome.html.

RAMAZZINI, BERNARDINO

An Italian physician and philosopher, Bernardino Ramazzini (1633–1714) graduated with a degree in medicine from Parma in 1659, and became professor of medicine at Modena in 1682 and at Padua in 1700. He wrote many books on aspects of medicine, the most famous of which, written in 1700, is *De Morbis Artificum Diatriba* (Diseases of workers). This was the first systematic treatise on

occupational diseases, and for this achievement Ramazzini is remembered as the father of occupational medicine and hygiene. Ramazzini's book is a descriptive account of working conditions in more than fifty occupations and of the diseases of workers in these occupations. Included were miners, potters, glassblowers, painters, privy cleaners, corpse handlers, midwives, makers of wine and beer, stonecutters, standing and sedentary workers, voice trainers, singers, farmers, fisherman, and many others. Ramazzini's observations were accurate and precise, although he provided no numerical information and made statements implying rather than expressing levels of risk, so readers could not determine, for example, whether pottery was a safer occupation than knife grinding. His accounts remain a good model for occupational health, and they also provide a valuable vignette of the social history of the working classes at the time of the Renaissance.

JOHN M. LAST

(SEE ALSO: *Occupational Disease*)

RATES

A rate is a measure of the frequency of an event or phenomenon. In public health, vital statistics, epidemiology, and other aspects of the health sciences and health care, events of interest include birth, deaths (so-called vital events), outbreaks of disease, spells of sickness, hospitalizations, immunizations against infectious diseases, and many other events and phenomena. A rate is more than a number: Its aim is to compare frequencies of phenomena at different times and places, among different classes of persons. Rates are calculated by a simple arithmetical procedure:

$$\text{rate} = \frac{\substack{\text{number of events in a defined population} \\ \text{in a specified period x } 10^n}}{\text{number of persons in the population}}$$

The components of a rate are the numerator (the number of events), the denominator (the population at risk of experiencing the event), the specified period in which the events occurred, and a multiplier (a power of 10) that converts the rate from an awkward fraction to a whole number. All rates are ratios; some rates are proportions (the numerator is a portion of the denominator). For example, the "case fatality rate" is the number of fatal cases as a proportion of all cases of a condition, such as hospitalized patients with acute heart attacks. Sometimes the meaning is further restricted to mean change over time or, alternatively, the cases of a disease originating at an instant in time, known as the "instantaneous incidence rate." The customary usage refers to the ratio of cases to the population at risk of experiencing the event over a period of time, usually a year. Since the size of the population may fluctuate over this period, the denominator for this rate is arbitrarily selected to be the population midway through the year.

JOHN M. LAST

(SEE ALSO: *Incidence and Prevalence; Population at Risk; Rates: Adjusted; Rates: Age-Adjusted; Rates: Age-Specific*)

RATES: ADJUSTED

Adjustment, or standardization, is a set of summarizing procedures that are intended to remove as far as possible the effects of differences in the composition of two or more populations in which one seeks to compare and contrast health experience, for example, by examining incidence or death rates or other health indicators in these populations. When one compares health indicators among populations, several kinds of differences in their composition can distort or confound the comparison. Common variables that influence health experience include age, sex, occupation, socioeconomic status, marital status, lifestyle factors such as cigarette smoking and sedentary occupation, urban or rural location and type of residence, and ethnic background and culture. It is possible to apply adjustment procedures for each of these and other variables in such a way as to reduce or even eliminate their influence on the apparent difference in rates among several populations.

The simplest confounding factor is a difference in age composition: One population may contain much higher proportions of older persons than another. If one compares the "crude" or adjusted death rates of these two populations, the

population containing a high proportion of older people will have a higher death rate than the population containing a higher proportion of children and young adults, because older people are more likely to die than younger people.

JOHN M. LAST

(SEE ALSO: *Incidence and Prevalence: Rates; Rates: Age-Adjusted; Rates: Age-Specific*)

RATES: AGE-ADJUSTED

Two common methods of age-adjustment or standardization are the direct and indirect methods. The direct method uses weighted averages (for instance, of age-specific rates) according to a predetermined formula based on the age distributions of the populations being compared. The rates actually observed in the populations are applied to an arbitrarily chosen "standard" population, for example, the population recorded at a census in Sweden in 1940, or a "theoretical" distribution constructed by imagining what the U.S. population might have been in 1960 if certain assumptions had been correct. If numbers in some age classes are too small for stable rates to be developed, or if the numbers are unknown, the indirect method is used. In this method, the age-adjusted rates of the standard population are projected onto the population being studied, and these rates are compared to what is actually observed in the population under study. The difference between what is observed and what would be expected if the study population had the same rates as standard population is expressed as a ratio, known as the standardized mortality ratio, or standardized incidence ratio.

JOHN M. LAST

(SEE ALSO: *Incidence and Prevalence; Rates; Rates: Adjusted; Rates: Age-Specific*)

RATES: AGE-SPECIFIC

An age-specific rate is the rate measured in a particular age group. The numerator and the denominator for this rate refer to the same age group, that is, both have the same age distribution.

Thus, for instance, the age-specific death rate of persons aged 45 to 64 is:

$$\frac{\text{number of deaths among persons aged 45--64} \times 10^n}{\text{number of persons aged 45--64}}$$

Age-specific rates are normally used to display aspects of health experience, such as causes of death, for the population of a nation or of jurisdictional divisions such as states, cities, and counties within a nation; they are also used to compare the health and mortality experience among many nations. Usually, these rates are separately tabulated for males and females, to display "age-sex-specific rates," and if the number of cases or events is large enough to generate stable rates, they are further subdivided to display "age-sex-cause-specific rates." For example, trends over time in the death rates from lung cancer among both males and females aged 45 to 64 demonstrate a sharp rise in the rates since the 1950s—first among men, then among women—reflecting the trends in smoking behavior of the two sexes in the second half of the twentieth century.

JOHN M. LAST

(SEE ALSO: *Incidence and Prevalence; Rates; Rates: Adjusted; Rates: Age-Adjusted*)

RECKLESS DRIVING

According to the American Automobile Association Foundation for Traffic Safety, an average of 1,500 people are killed or injured each year as a result of aggressive driving. The National Highway Traffic and Safety Administration (NHTSA) defines "aggressive driving" as, "the operation of a motor vehicle in a manner that endangers or is likely to endanger persons or property." This behavior usually involves illegal and dangerous driving, committed with the intent to gain an advantage over the other drivers. Examples of aggressive driving include: exceeding the posted speed limit, following another vehicle too closely, passing on the shoulder of the road, failure to yield, unsafe or erratic lane changes, improper signaling, and failure to obey traffic control devices (stop signs, yield signs, traffic signals, railroad grade cross signals). Running a red light is one of the most dangerous forms of aggressive driving.

The term "road rage" differs from aggressive driving and implies a criminal offense involving "an assault with a motor vehicle or other dangerous weapon by the operator or passenger(s) of one motor vehicle on the operator or passenger(s) of another motor vehicle, or an assault precipitated by an incident that occurred on a roadway" (NHTSA). Road rage can be accompanied by behaviors such as excessive honking, yelling or making obscene gestures, flashing high beams excessively, recklessly passing or weaving in and out of traffic, speeding up when others are trying to pass, or deliberately tailgating or chasing another vehicle.

Many states have introduced or passed legislation to create specific penalties for aggressive driving offenses and for incidences of road rage. These laws create specific penalties for driving that intentionally creates a risk of harm or endangers the safety of others, involves wanton or reckless disregard for another, involves dangerous conduct contributing to the likelihood of a collision or evasive action by another, or is deliberately discourteous and shows extreme impatience.

The NHTSA has developed a guide that provides assistance in developing strategies for implementing aggressive-driving prevention programs. This guide can be found on the NHTSA web site at http://www.nhtsa.dot.gov/people.

DAVID A. SLEET
BRUCE H. JONES

(SEE ALSO: *Behavior, Health-Related; Behavioral Strategies for Reducing Traffic Crashes; Public Health and the Law*)

RECORD LINKAGE

Record linkage is the process of bringing together two or more records relating to the same entity (e.g., person, family, event, community, business, hospital, or geographical area). In 1946, H. L. Dunn of the United States National Bureau of Statistics introduced the term in this way: "Each person in the world creates a Book of Life. This Book starts with birth and ends with death. Record linkage is the name of the process of assembling the pages of this Book into a volume" (Dunn, 1946).

Computerized record linkage was first undertaken by the Canadian geneticist Howard Newcombe and his associates in 1959. Newcombe recognized the full implications of extending the principle to the arrangement of personal files and into family histories. Computerized record linkage has the advantages of quality control, speed, consistency, reproducibility of results, and the ability to handle large volumes of data. For its actual implementation, Newcombe prepared a handbook in 1988.

Sir Donald Acheson established the Oxford Record Linkage Study in Oxford, England, in 1962. This medical record linkage system connects birth, morbidity, and mortality data for an entire community. This type of system links morbidity and mortality data and provides information for studies of health care utilization and for descriptive epidemiology of disease as analyzed by characteristics of time, place, and event.

There are several different approaches to linkage. At the crudest level, linkage may be based on agreement on one or more variables—this is referred to as deterministic linkage. Decision tables, a hierarchy of rules, and a variety of different sets of matching criteria may also be used to bring record pairs together. Although a "unique numerical identifier," such as a health card number, can be used, this number may have been issued more than once, changed over time, or recorded incorrectly. Checking and verifying associated names is prudent when using numerous identifiers.

A mathematical theory of probabilistic linkage was developed by I. P. Fellegi and A. B. Sunter in 1969. In the subsequent generalized record-linking software developed, there are three main phases in linkage: searching, decision-making, and grouping. Conceptually, each record on one file is compared to each record on another file to form record pairs of all possible comparisons. In practice, in the searching phase, the files are blocked using identifiers (e.g., the phonetic code of the surname and gender code) to limit the number of potential pairs of records compared. In the decision-making phase, evidence contained in different records is compared to determine the probability, or "weight," that the records relate to the same entity. Record agreement with a rare name such as "Quigley," for example, has more weight

than agreement of a common name such as "Smith." For convenience, record pairs are commonly classified in three areas: (1) definite "linked" pairs; (2) definite "nonlinked" pairs; and (3) "possible" links, where the inference cannot be made without further evidence (see Figure 1). In the final grouping phase, a group of appropriate records relating to the same individual or entity is formed. Records may have just one link to another record, or they may have several links. Two major types of errors may be made in classifying a record pair: The pairs may be either falsely linked; or they may be incorrectly unlinked (nonlinked pairs that indeed refer to the same entity).

The potential for linkage varies greatly between countries according to how information is collected and identified. The National Death Index in the United States and the Canadian Mortality Data Base have facilitated linkages at a national level. National birth and cancer data are also available in Canada.

Agencies need to develop explicit policies and mechanisms for the review and approval process for record linkage projects so that no individual will be harmed in the linkage process, either by false linkages or by the release of confidential information. Distinctions should be made for linkages done for statistical research purposes, where only aggregate statistics are released. Where possible, informed individual consent should be obtained, and the nature of the "public good" to be served should be assessed and reviewed.

Record linkage is an important tool in creating data required for examining the health of the public and of the health care system itself. It can be used to improve data holdings, data collection, quality assessment, and the dissemination of information. Data sources can be examined to eliminate duplicate records, to identify underreporting and missing cases (e.g., census population counts), to create person-oriented health statistics, and to generate disease registries and health surveillance systems. Some cancer registries link various data sources (e.g., hospital admissions, pathology and clinical reports, and death registrations) to generate their registries.

Record linkage is also used to create health indicators. For example, fetal and infant mortality

Figure 1

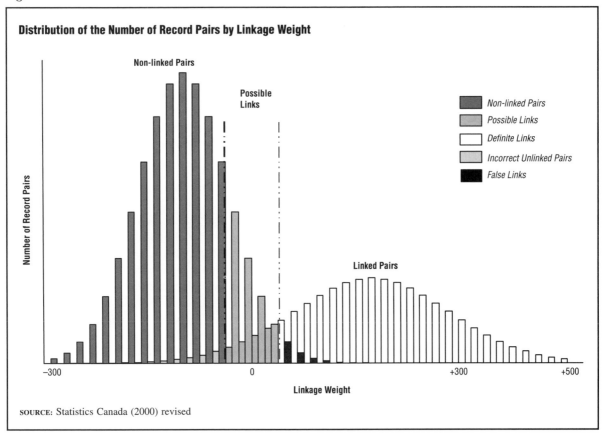

Distribution of the Number of Record Pairs by Linkage Weight

Non-linked Pairs

Possible Links

Non-linked Pairs
Possible Links
Definite Links
Incorrect Unlinked Pairs
False Links

Number of Record Pairs

Linked Pairs

−300   0   +300   +500

Linkage Weight

SOURCE: Statistics Canada (2000) revised

is a general indicator of a country's socioeconomic development, public health, and maternal and child services. If infant death records are matched to birth records, it is possible to use birth variables, such as birth weight and gestational age, along with mortality data, such as cause of death, in analyzing the data.

Linkages can help in follow-up studies of cohorts or other groups to determine factors such as vital status, residential status, or health outcomes. Tracing is often needed for follow-up of industrial cohorts, clinical trials, and longitudinal surveys to obtain the cause of death and/or cancer.

In addition, record linkage can aid in developing recommendations about regulatory standards at the national and international levels. A good example can be seen in the work of the United Nations Scientific Committee on the Effects of Atomic Radiation, which provides evaluations of the sources of ionizing radiation and the effects of

exposures. This committee assesses the consequences to human health of a wide variety of doses of ionizing radiation and estimates the dose people receive all over the world from natural and man-made radiation sources. Linkage of a variety of data sources is required, including health, exposure, and outcome information (e.g., cancer and deaths).

MARTHA E. FAIR

(SEE ALSO: *Confidentiality; Data Sources and Collection Methods; Epidemiology; Information Technology; Informed Consent; Privacy; Registries; Statistics for Public Health; Vital Statistics*)

BIBLIOGRAPHY

Baldwin, J. A.; Acheson, E. D.; and Graham, W. J., eds. (1987). *Textbook of Medical Record Linkage.* Oxford, UK: Oxford University Press.

Chong, N. (1998). "Computerized Record Linkage in Cancer Registries." In *Automated Data Collection in Cancer Registration*, eds. R. J. Black, L. Simonato, H. H. Storm, and E. Démaret. Lyon: IARC, Technical Reports No. 32:7–11.

Duncan, G. T.; Jabine, T. B.; and de Wolf, V. A., eds. (1993). *Private Lives and Public Policies: Confidentiality and Accessibility of Government Statistics.* Washington, DC: National Academy Press.

Dunn, H. L. (1946). "Record Linkage." *American Journal of Public Health* 36:1412–1416.

Federal Committee on Statistical Methodology (1997). *Record Linkage Techniques–1997 Proceedings of an International Workshop and Exposition.* Washington, DC: U.S. Office of Management and Budget.

Fellegi, I. P., and Sunter, A. B. (1969). "A Theory of Record Linkage." *Journal of the American Statistical Association* 40:1183–1210.

Howe, G. R. (1998). "Use of Computerized Record Linkage in Cohort Studies." *Epidemiologic Reviews* 20:112–121.

Newcombe, H. B. (1988). *Handbook of Record Linkage Methods for Health and Statistical Studies, Administration and Business.* Oxford, UK: Oxford University Press.

Newcombe, H. B.; Fair, M. E.; and Lalonde, P. (1992). "The Use of Names for Linking Personal Records." *Journal of the American Statistical Association* 87:1193–1208.

Newcombe, H. B.; Kennedy, J. M.; Axford, S. J.; and James, A. P. (1959). "Automatic Linkage of Vital Records." *Science* 130:954–959.

Smith, M. E., and Newcombe, H. B. (1980) "Automated Follow-up Facilities in Canada for Monitoring Delayed Health Effects." *American Journal of Public Health* 70(12):1261–1268.

Statistics Canada (2000). *Generalized Record Linkage System. Concepts, Research and General Systems.* Ottawa: Author.

RECTAL EXAMINATION

See Colorectal Cancer *and* Prostate Cancer

REED, WALTER

A native of Virginia, Walter Reed (1851–1902) received his medical education at Bellevue Medical School in New York, worked as a district physician in Brooklyn, and then joined the U.S. Army, providing basic medical services in many parts of the frontier West. Attracted by the new science of bacteriology, he was sent by the army to study with William Henry Welch at Johns Hopkins University, and was later appointed professor of bacteriology in the Army Medical School in Washington, DC in 1893. He chaired the U.S. Army typhoid fever commission of 1899, in which he, Victor C. Vaughan, and Edward O. Shakespeare established the importance of the asymptomatic typhoid carrier.

While working on this commission, he was assigned to investigate the high mortality from yellow fever in the U.S. military forces then occupying Havana in the wake of the Spanish-American War. His research there first established that, contrary to the then official position of the Surgeon General's Office, yellow fever was not caused by a gram-negative rod, the *Sanarelli bacillus.* Following this research, he and his three colleagues on the Yellow Fever Commission, Aristides Agramonte, James Carroll, and Jesse Lazear, undertook to test, in experiments with human volunteers, Carlos Finlay's hypothesis that yellow fever could be transmitted by the bite of the *Aedes Aegypti* (then known as *Stegomyia fasciata* or *Culex fasciatus*) mosquito. A key feature of Reed's experiments was the long interval—about twelve to eighteen days—between the infecting of mosquitoes via their feeding on yellow fever patients and the exposure of human volunteers to the bites of the infected mosquitoes. Reed had been impressed by the observation of U.S. Army surgeon Henry Rose Carter that yellow fever epidemics were characterized by a two- to three-week interval between the first case and the next set of cases. Reed correctly surmised that this represented the period of incubation of the infective agent in the mosquito.

Reed's procedure successfully transmitted yellow fever to several volunteers, confirmed that *Aedes Aegypti* was the essential vector of the disease, and was followed immediately by a mosquito eradication program led by Major William Gorgas (1854–1920) that virtually eradicated yellow fever in Havana for the first time in recorded history. Gorgas (who attained the rank of Major General during World War I), also led the mosquito eradication program that permitted construction of the Panama Canal. Happily, all of Reed's volunteers recovered from their experimental yellow fever infections, but Jesse Lazear died after being bitten by an infected mosquito that he allowed to feed on his arm.

NIGEL PANETH

(SEE ALSO: *Communicable Disease Control; Finlay, Carlos; Vector-Borne Diseases; Yellow Fever*)

BIBLIOGRAPHY

Kelly, H. A. (1907). *Walter Reed and Yellow Fever.* New York: McLure, Phillips.

REFERENCE LABORATORY

The completion of the laboratory analysis on a sample or specimen may require methods and procedures that the laboratory does not have. Also, standards of medical practice or legal requirements may dictate the completion of testing by another laboratory. In these cases, the first laboratory may send the specimen, some part of the specimen, or something derived from the initial examination of the specimen to another laboratory that can complete the examination. In these instances, the sending of the material to be analyzed is considered a referral, and the second laboratory is the "reference laboratory." In general, this term is applied to any laboratory that does additional analysis or testing on a sample or specimen sent from another laboratory.

ERIC C. BLANK

(SEE ALSO: *Assurance of Laboratory Testing Quality; Laboratory Services; Laboratory Technician; Practice Standards*)

REFUGEE COMMUNITIES

In recent decades, the world has experienced unprecedented levels of human migration due to globalization, changing international economic patterns, and ethnic conflict. Between 1980 and 1997 the worldwide refugee population increased from 9 million to over 41 million persons. Approximately 20 million of these individuals are formally classified by the United Nations as "refugees," meaning they have been forced to flee across their own international borders. The others are classified as "internally displaced persons," meaning they have fled their homes but have not been able to leave their countries. These numbers do not include the millions of voluntary economic migrants who leave their homes in impoverished rural communities in developing countries in order to take manufacturing and related jobs in larger cities or foreign countries.

Forced human migration is a significant public health challenge. The United Nations High Commissioner for Refugees estimates that one in every thirty persons in the world will be a formal or informal refugee at some point in his or her life. Furthermore, 95 percent of all refugees are estimated to come from, and reside in, developing countries in Asia, Latin America, and Africa, where health status is already compromised. Refugee health is also a critical mother-and-child issue, as approximately 80 percent of all refugee populations around the world are comprised of women and children, with children accounting for 50 percent of these groups.

A HISTORY OF REFUGEEISM

While refugees have existed throughout human history, the term was first formally used in 1573 to describe Calvinists fleeing political repression in the Spanish-controlled Netherlands. Refugees were not only defined as victims of persecution, but were also seen as individuals with political, religious, economic, or other affiliations that aroused solidarity.

Providing aid and protection to refugees has increasingly become the collective duty of the international community. After the end of World War I and the creation of the League of Nations, refugee assistance began to be institutionalized. At the end of World War II, the United Nations superceded the League of Nations and created the International Refugee Organization (IRO) in 1946. In 1950, the IRO was replaced by the office of the United Nations High Commissioner for Refugees (UNHCR), which was mandated to encourage countries to receive refugees, prevent them from being forcibly returned, and provide assistance and protection to them.

The 1951 United Nations Convention on Refugees has been ratified by almost 120 countries. It defines a refugee as "any person who, owing to a well-founded fear of being persecuted for reasons of race, religion, nationality, membership in a particular social group, or political opinion, is outside the country of his nationality, and is unable to or, owing to such fear, is unwilling to avail himself of the protection of that country" (Médecins Sans Frontières, 1997). This definition reflects the reality of postwar Europe, but has since been found inadequate in dealing with the special situations faced by refugees from other continents. Therefore, in 1967, this protocol abolished geographic restrictions on the scope of the convention.

National wars of liberation and post-independence conflicts in both Africa and Asia greatly contributed to the problem of mass refugee movements in the early 1960s. During this period, the UNHCR began to give more attention to the new reality of refugees in developing countries due to war and insecurity, and it expanded its definition of refugees to include those who fled general danger rather than just those who feared persecution. In 1969, due to significant refugee problems in Africa, the UNHCR definition was formalized by the Organization of African Unity (OAU) to include those refugees who were forced to leave their native countries not only because of persecution, but also aggression, occupation by an outside force, foreign domination, or disturbance of peace by the country of origin. In 1984, the Cartagena Declaration was added to the OAU definition to include victims of massive human-rights violations.

Significant legal and socioeconomic differences exist between formally recognized "refugees," "internally displaced persons," and "economic migrants." Refugees that have been officially recognized by the United Nations and other international political bodies are generally entitled to a number of legal benefits and to humanitarian assistance. In general, these refugees are individuals that did not want to flee their homes, but were forced to do so. However, once resettled or repatriated, many of these families are reunited to some extent. The protection and services that can be offered to internally displaced persons is generally much more limited because they are still located in what might be defined as "enemy territory." Their health status is usually even lower than that of refugees because they do not have access to humanitarian assistance.

Millions of people around the world, though, leave their homes more willingly, particularly in impoverished rural areas in developing nations, in order to migrate to larger urban centers or even other countries in search of a better standard of living. While these "economic migrants" may not be facing violence or persecution, they nonetheless are generally experiencing extreme levels of poverty. Many of these economic migrants must move into larger cities in their own countries in order to survive, and they often take up residence in dangerous, crowded shantytowns and work in menial jobs. Indeed, for the first time in human history, more people on earth will soon be living in cities rather than in rural areas due to these new migration patterns. Some economic migrants seek work and better opportunities in foreign countries, sometimes entering these countries illegally. However, many others are recruited legally by developed nations to work in low-paying, dangerous, and mundane jobs in agriculture, manufacturing, meatpacking, and other fields. In general, economic migrants are entitled to fewer formal benefits than refugees when moving to a new country, particularly if they are there illegally. They typically have experienced far less trauma and violence during their flight than refugees, but nonetheless can suffer from acculturation stress and depression due to their resettlement. Economic migrants are often younger men who may send much of their salaries back home to their families.

CAUSES OF MIGRATION

Refugeeism, as well as migration in general, is not a new problem, but rather one that dates back to the earliest human times. There are many reasons beyond those in the UNHCR and OHR definitions to explain widespread forced human migration. G. Loescher and A. D. Loescher (1994) suggest that external aggression, internal civil strife, and massive violation of human rights are also reasons for migration. Similarly, the International Committee of the Red Cross and the Johns Hopkins School of Public Health indicate that political and ethnic conflicts are currently among the most important reasons for refugeeism.

Political persecution is a major cause of forced migration, and this often depends on what group controls a nation and its resources. Violence tends to decrease as per capita income rises, which means that weak states are prone to internal violence. Similarly, population displacement is associated with economic tension. Again, when economic tensions rise, poverty may increase as well, which can lead to ethnic conflict. These kinds of tensions can easily interact with other factors that lead to population displacement and prolonged conflicts. As discussed previously, people who leave their country willingly because of economic hardships do not qualify for UNHCR protection or assistance, except in cases when their situations are exacerbated by political violence. However, in reality, there are millions of people worldwide who are forced to leave their homes annually due to severe economic hardships.

Environmental and ecological factors can also be root causes of migration. For instance, migration occurs as food supplies dwindle due to overgrazing, topsoil erosion, deforestation, conversion from food crops to cash crops, inadequate reserves, water deficits, overpopulation, and related issues. If natural disasters occur on top of these existing problems, they may then have an impact on existing tensions, which may ultimately turn into armed conflicts.

Ethnic tensions, based on race, language, culture, and religion, are also among the reasons people seek refuge. Examples of ethnic conflicts in recent years include those in Yugoslavia, Somalia, Burundi, and Rwanda. Ethnic conflict increasingly affects civilians, rather than military troops. Ethnic tensions may cause displacement for two reasons. First, when ethnicity is highly susceptible to political exploitation, some groups seek community support by fanning ethnic antagonism, reactivating tensions that may have been dormant for a long time. This is more likely to happen when one ethnic group captures control of a given state. Second, when a sense of oneness starts to disintegrate, those groups that have become disenfranchised may be seen as obstacles to nation building. However, many ethnic conflicts are not truly about cultural identity, but rather about the control of resources.

Finally, human rights abuses are another cause of refugeeism and international migration. Research indicates that human rights violations do not occur in a vacuum. As mentioned earlier, they coexist with economic constraints, disruptions in food supplies, political weakness and instability, ethnic conflicts, traditional violence, and ecological deterioration. Human rights are usually at the core of humanitarian emergencies, and they become international responsibilities when states fail to respond.

THE REFUGEE AND IMMIGRANT EXPERIENCE

There are three phases of the refugee experience: preflight, flight, and settlement. During these phases, refugees go through common experiences. During the preflight phase, refugees may encounter economic hardship, social disruption, political oppression, and physical violence, triggering a need to leave their home. Hazards include imprisonment, death or disappearance of family members, loss of property and livelihood, physical assaults, witnessing assaults or murders of loved ones, fear of the unexpected, famine, and starvation.

In the second phase, the flight period, refugees face many dangers, including physical hardships such as rape, witnessing others being beaten or killed, anxiety about forced repatriation, family separation, robbery, illness and injuries, and malnutrition. They must also go through a difficult formal process to qualify for final resettlement in a third country. Economic migrants usually have less urgency in their need to flee, and may experience fewer traumatic events.

Refugees ultimately either repatriate to their home country, reside permanently in a second neighboring community, or move to a third country of asylum. Repatriation to their home country is the best solution if it is safe to do so, but millions of refugees and migrants around the world are unable to return home and must remain in second or third countries of asylum. During the resettlement phase, significant sources of stress come from feelings of loss, social isolation, culture shock, accelerated modernization, and minority status. The experience of economic migrants that resettle in a third country will vary dramatically, in part based on whether they are there legally or illegally. They generally do not garner the same level of sympathy and humanitarianism from the host community that may be shown to newly arrived refugees fleeing a war.

The time it takes to adjust to a new culture varies with each migrant, influenced by the stability of life before becoming a migrant, personality, level of trauma experienced, skills possessed, and the amount of support and resources available. There are a number of phases of adjustment that refugees experience as they resettle in the United States: the arrival phase; the reality phase; the negotiation or alienation phase; and the integration or marginalization phase. During the arrival phase, immigrants typically have very high expectations and are filled with hopes about the future. During the reality phase, migrants may realize that what they expected is not necessarily what they are experiencing, and they recognize that there are many obstacles to achieving their expectations. Many experience stress as a result of any trauma and cultural bereavement they may have experienced. If they receive enough support during this phase, they can often cope well and make a smooth move to the next stage.

The third phase of refugee resettlement consists of either negotiation or alienation. During this stage, refugees start making moves toward cultural and physiological integration. However, if adequate support is not available for them during this stage, the stresses of their new lives, combined with the consequences of their past trauma, may move them into alienation rather than integration, and they may experience serious psychological, social, and legal problems. This stage is characterized by apathy, isolation, and dysfunctional attitudes, which leads refugees to become marginalized.

However, if refugees receive early support, they may move into the stage of integration rather than marginalization. In this stage, refugees find satisfactory long-term adaptation to their new society and start to settle into routine lives. A very early network of support is critical to help refugees achieve integration. Economic migrants can experience each of these phases as well.

REFUGEE AND IMMIGRANT RESETTLEMENT IN THE UNITED STATES

Since World War II, more refugees have found permanent homes in the United States than in any other country. In order to be designated as refugees by the United States, they must have a well-founded fear of persecution in their countries of origin because of race, region, nationality, membership in a particular social group, or political opinion.

The U.S. government works closely with the UNHCR, other international and nongovernmental organizations, and other governments to protect refugees, displaced persons, and victims of conflicts. According to the U.S. Committee for Refugees, the United States resettled up to 76,554 refugees in fiscal year 1998. The United States spends millions of dollars each year in order to ensure that the survival needs—such as food, health care, and shelter—of these refugees are met.

According to the U.S. Committee for Refugees, the United States is ranked first among the top twenty donor nations that contribute funding for programs that assist refugees. The U.S. government provided $364 million in 1999 to the UNHCR, the International Organization for Migration (IOM), and the United Nations Relief and Works Agency for Palestine Refugees in the Near East (UNRWA).

There are four refugee-processing priorities that have been established and are used to process refugee cases during resettlement programs. These priorities are as follows:

Priority One. UNHCR or U.S. embassy identified cases, including persons facing compelling security concerns in countries of first asylum; persons in need of legal protection because of the danger of refoulement; those in danger due to threats of armed attack in an area where they are located; persons who have experienced recent persecution because of their political, religious, or human rights activities (prisoners of conscience); women-at-risk; victims of torture or violence; physically or mentally disabled persons; persons in urgent need of medical treatment not available in the first asylum country; and persons for whom other durable solutions are not feasible and whose status in the place of asylum does not present a satisfactory long-term solution. All nationalities are eligible for this processing priority.

Priority Two. Groups of special humanitarian concern to the United States.

Priority Three. Spouses, unmarried sons and daughters, and parents of persons lawfully admitted to the United States as permanent resident aliens, refugees, asylees, conditional residents, and certain parolees; over-21-year-old unmarried sons and daughters of U.S. citizens; and parents of U.S. citizens under 21 years of age. (Spouses and unmarried sons and daughters under 21 of U.S. citizens; and the parents of U.S. citizens who have attained the age of 21 are required by regulation to be admitted as immigrants rather than as refugees.)

Priority Four. Grandparents, grandchildren, married sons and daughters, and siblings of U.S. citizens and persons lawfully admitted to the United States as permanent resident aliens, refugees, asylees, conditional residents, and certain parolees.

Most decisions on refugee admission ceilings, adjustments, and appropriations to refugee agencies are made by the United States Congress. However, the State Department, the attorney general, and the president's office can help decide special cases.

Each year the United States admits large numbers of legal immigrants from around the world to join family members or to work in jobs with labor shortages or special needs. Millions of illegal immigrants are also believed to live in the United States. While some of these individuals have entered the country illegally, many of them have simply overstayed their tourist visas for employment reasons. These economic migrants, particularly those from developing nations in Africa, Asia, and Latin America, have traditionally been concentrated in large metropolitan areas in the United States, particularly along the southern border and coastal areas. However, in recent years, this diversity has spread to rural Midwestern regions, particularly where meat processing or agricultural jobs exist. Many of these communities in rural states are now experiencing a "rapid ethnic diversification" due to a sudden influx of refugees and economic migrants.

REFUGEE AND IMMIGRANT HEALTH CHALLENGES

Refugees are among the most at-risk populations for poor health status in the world. Most of them flee countries where their health status was already compromised. When refugees and some economic migrants first leave their homes, they often spend an initial period of time in a temporary camp or squatter settlement where their health status can be seriously compromised. During the emergency phase following the initial arrival of a large number of migrants to these camps, mortality rates are very high due to crowded conditions, trauma, limited medical care, poor sanitation and drinking water resources, and other factors. The diseases that are highly prevalent during the emergency phase typically include measles, malnutrition, diarrhea, respiratory infections, malaria, meningitis, and hypothermia. Most of these conditions develop because of the rapid nature in which emergency housing is established, often by the refugees themselves. Many of these "camps" consist of nothing more than temporary tents made from blankets, and they often spring up directly on the other side of the border from the country the people fled.

Military units from their own country may periodically conduct illegal raids on the refugees. Young children and women, who often leave the refugee camps to get water and firewood, are frequent targets of sniper fire or victims of landmines of enemy forces. Many of these emergency camps are also built in poor conditions, such as near swamps or wetlands where mosquitoes and other insect vectors are common.

During the postemergency or consolidation phase in refugee camps, the mortality rates decline to the level of the surrounding host population. Specific health issues that need to be addressed during this phase include curative health care, reproductive health care, child health, sexually transmitted diseases, tuberculosis, and psychosocial and mental health needs. In order to reduce mortality and morbidity rates, general public health measures must include the following: initial assessment, immunizations, water and sanitation, food provision, shelter and site planning, emergency medicine, control of communicable diseases and epidemics, public health surveillance, human resources and training, and coordination of services.

The United Nations feels that the most desired solution, where possible, is to assist refugees in returning to their own countries. However, many millions are unable to ever go home due to continuing political unrest and other factors. Therefore, refugees and immigrants experience health problems not only during their departure phase, but also at the time of their resettlement in a host country. Such problems vary depending on immigration status and area of origin. For example, refugees from developing countries in Africa may have not experienced Western medicine, whereas those who come from countries such as Cuba, Bosnia, and Russia have some familiarity with Western-style health care. Similarly, immigrants who come from tropical areas could present with conditions that Western physicians might not recognize immediately, such as malaria and schistosomiasis.

However, despite their different backgrounds, most refugees share common experiences related to wars, extreme poverty, and other disruptions—such as physical and psychological health problems prior to and during their resettlement. T. Gavagan and L. Brodyaga recommend physical examinations and laboratory tests, as well as screenings for nutritional status, mental health, and infectious diseases. Within thirty to ninety days of arriving in their resettlement country, all refugees should have a domestic health assessment for the purpose of reducing health-related barriers to successful resettlement while protecting the health of the general population. Similarly, L. K. Ackerman emphasizes that a health assessment done in the resettlement country can detect important medical conditions and protect the health of the host population. In the United States, these programs are typically managed by refugee health offices, which vary from state to state. Components generally include a health history, physical examination, immunization updates, and screenings for anemia, hepatitis B, parasitic infections, pregnancy, tuberculosis, vision, hearing, and dental abnormalities. Mental health challenges such as depression, post-traumatic stress disorder, and acculturation shock are among the most frequently seen conditions among refugees from around the world.

Some research done specifically on the health status of Bosnian and other refugees that have resettled in the United States indicates that they initially tend to have a poorer health status than other people in the host community. This can be characterized by poor appetite, high smoking rates, poor dental health, decreased memory, limited leisure time, mood swings, sleep problems, and decreased energy and patience. According to Ackerman, some refugees that resettle in the United States may suffer from malnutrition, tuberculosis, low immunization rates, depression, hepatitis B, poor dental health, and war-related injuries. Some of the most significant psychological conditions may be experienced by many refugees who are victims of ethnic cleansing. For example, Ackerman states that 65 percent of Bosnian refugees in the United States were found to have post-traumatic stress disorder, and 35 percent suffered from depression.

There is a need for ongoing health assessments to explore more fully not only the medical and psychological problems of refugees, but also their health beliefs. Findings from a complete health history and physical examination, awareness of the physical and mental health problems encountered by migrants, and familiarity with their cultural beliefs will enable health care providers to provide complete and compassionate care to this very high-risk population.

MICHELE YEHIELI
CLEMENTINE MUKESHIMANA

(SEE ALSO: *Ethnicity and Health; Famine; Genocide; Immigrants, Immigration; Natural Disasters; Terrorism; United Nations High Commissioner for Refugees; War*)

BIBLIOGRAPHY

Ackerman, L. K. (1997). "Health Problems of Refugees." *Journal of the American Board of Family Practice* 10(5):337–348.

Bloom, S. (2000). *Postville: A Clash of Cultures in Heartland America.* New York: Harcourt Publishers, Inc.

Bureau of Immigration, Refugees and Migration. Information available at http://www.state.gov/www/global/prm.

"Coming Here: Pioneers and Immigrants Who Made Iowa Home" (2000). *The Iowan Magazine* (September-October Spec. Issue).

Gavagan, T., and Brodyaga, L. (1997). "Medical Care for Immigrants and Refugees." *American Family Physicians* 57(5):1061–1068.

Geiger, H. J., and Cook-Deegan, R. M. (1993). "The Role of Physicians in Conflicts and Humanitarian Crises: Cases Studies from the Field Missions of Physicians for Human Rights, 1988 to 1993." *Journal of American Medical Association* 270(5):616–620.

Kaufman, J. (1995). "American's Heartland Turns to Hot Location for the Melting Pot." *The Wall Street Journal* (October 31).

Kemp, C. (1999). *Refugee Health Problems and Issues.* Available at http://www.baylor.edu/~charleskemp/refugeehealthproblems.htm.

Loescher, G., and Loescher, A. D. (1994). *The Global Refugee Crisis: A Reference Handbook.* Santa Barbara, CA: ABC-Clio.

Médicins Sans Frontières (1997). *Refugee Health: An Approach to Emergency Situations.* Brussels: Author.

National Alliance for the Multicultural Mental Health (2001). "Refugee Adaptation in Resettlement Roles." *Lessons from the Field: Issues and Resources in Refugee Mental Health.* Available at http://www.ifsa-user.org/help_ref/lessons_field_manual.pdf.

Riedlmayer, A. J. (1993). *A Brief History of Bosnian-Herzegovina.* The Bosnian Manuscript Ingathering Project. Available at http://www.kakarigi.net/manualbriefhis.htm.

Rogge, J. R. (1987). *Refugees: A Third World Dilemma.* Totowa, NJ: Rawman & Littlefield.

Smyser, W. R. (1987). *Refugees: Extended Exile.* Washington, DC: The Center for Strategic and International Studies.

U.S. Committee for Refugees (1999). *World Refugee Survey.* Immigration and Refugee Services of America. Washington, DC: Author.

U.S. Department of Health and Human Services (1994). "World Health Day, April 7, 1994." *Morbidity and Mortality Weekly Report* 43(11):197.

Yehieli, M.; Joslyn, S.; Mukeshimana, C.; Dobie, S.; Gonnerman, M.; and Lutz, G. (2001). *Assessing the Health Status of Newcomers: A Report on Bosnians and Latinos in Black Hawk County, Iowa.* Cedar Falls, IA: Center for Social and Behavioral Research, University of Northern Iowa.

REGIONAL HEALTH PLANNING

The National Health Planning and Resources Development Act of 1974 created a network of U.S. regional agencies to develop health plans that would result in a health care system that met the health needs of individuals while also containing costs. These health systems agencies (HSAs) were empowered to implement their plans by using mechanisms such as Certificate of Need (CON) and Appropriateness reviews. CON review requires hospitals, nursing homes, and clinics to submit an application for proposed capital expenditure and service expansion projects to a regionally based board of trustees. The board evaluates each project to determine whether it meets the criteria established through the plan development process and whether the applicant should be permitted to proceed. Appropriateness review would have enabled the HSAs to consider existing services to determine if they were needed. Appropriateness review was never fully implemented, however.

From the start, HSAs were controversial—some physicians and health care facilities didn't believe this type of oversight was necessary. The composition of voluntary regional boards of trustees was prescribed by the law to include a majority of consumers (reflecting the area's demographics) and certain providers. Local board composition was sometimes challenged; and although the boards reported directly to the national Health Care Financing Administration (HCFA), HSAs sometimes found themselves at odds with state and local political agendas.

In the mid-1980s, federal funding for HSAs was discontinued. The HSAs that remained were created by state legislatures with less ambitious goals and usually a stronger focus on CON review than on plan development. As the 1990s evolved and the backlash against regulation grew, the federal and state governments, along with the private sector, expanded their reliance on the health care market to control health care costs and to force a rational delivery system to develop. Corporate "shopping" and health maintenance organizations were expected to afford incentives to providers to deliver quality health care at a reasonable price. The focus of government intervention changed to providing information to purchasers and users of health care to help them become better consumers. Although there are some areas where local health planning and Certificate of Need review continue on a limited basis, a federal role in the process is gone, and state funding for this purpose continues to decline.

NANCY J. ROTH

(SEE ALSO: *Health Care Financing Administration; Health Maintenance Organization [HMO]; Planning for Public Health*)

REGISTRIES

Registries have been used by public health departments for many years to record cases of diseases of public health importance. In many countries, tuberculosis was the first condition for which registries were established, as many people who suffered from this contagious disease were living in their community. These people often had to remain in their jobs because there were no invalid pensions to support them. If they were excreting sputum containing tubercle bacilli with every cough, it was important for the chest physicians who cared for them, and for public health specialists, to remain in touch with them to ensure that as much as possible was being done for them—and to limit the spread of the disease. When the public health problem of tuberculosis declined in the late 1950s, other troubling diseases were surfacing.

The most important of these diseases was cancer. Many jurisdictions (counties, states, and even nations) established cancer registries, some of which were population-based (covering the entire population of a defined political jurisdiction). This is an important feature of a cancer registry, because it permits the calculation of rates. If cancer registration is prompt and complete, cancer registries are a valuable epidemiological resource that can be used to calculate incidence rates and risks, as well as to maintain surveillance and monitor trends in cancer incidence and mortality.

Cancer registries endeavor to use every available source of information to establish and confirm cancer diagnoses. These sources include clinical reports, reports of surgical operations, reports of biopsies and pathological specimens, radiological investigations, and autopsies. In many jurisdictions, reporting of all these ways in which cancer may present is routine and mandatory. Moreover, it is discrete, so cancer patients may not even know that the information about them and their diagnosis is recorded in a cancer registry. Informed consent is not usually part of the process. The information in a cancer registry is, however, carefully safeguarded.

When individuals with cancer become aware that personal details about them are recorded in a cancer registry, they object very rarely, and they can usually be reassured that the registry serves a valuable public health purpose. The issue of informed consent has been widely discussed by elected politicians as well as by cancer registry staff. In almost all jurisdictions, other than some European nations with a totalitarian past, it is accepted that the need for complete registration overrides the niceties and logistical problems of informed consent. In addition, a certain number of people will withhold their informed consent, which can invalidate the entire registry, especially with rare cancers.

Registries have also been used to record patients taking certain kinds of medication, and for various other purposes. Attempts to establish registries for persons with substance abuse and for sex offenders have not been successful because such persons are often elusive and evade contacts with authorities and relevant specialists.

JOHN M. LAST

(SEE ALSO: *Agency for Toxic Substances and Disease Registry; Informed Consent*)

BIBLIOGRAPHY

Menck, H., and Smart, C. (1994). *Central Cancer Registries: Design, Management and Use.* Langhorne, PA: Harwood Academic Publishers.

World Health Organizations (1976). *WHO Handbook for Standardized Cancer Registries.* Geneva: Author.

REGULATIONS AFFECTING HOUSING

Regulations affecting housing are enacted to assure decent, safe, and sanitary conditions for occupancy and habitation. They are enacted as codes through government ordinance and are usually administered by a local zoning, building, or health department. (A state may adapt standards to be enforced by a state agency where no local enforcement is available.) Code provisions may address new construction, improvements, or general property maintenance.

Most local codes are based on standards developed by professional organizations, such as the Building Officials and Code Administrators (BOCA) and the National Fire Protection Association (NFPA), with input from engineers, architects, technicians, builders, contractors, materials producers, and trade associations. Local housing and building codes include standards for occupied dwellings with regard to heating, ventilation and air conditioning, electrical wiring systems, plumbing, structural components, light, maximum occupancy, and fire safety. They also specify the requirements under which repairs or improvements are completed. Most major improvements and new construction require prior approval through a formal permit process that establishes the scope of the work and provides for review by a certified inspector to ensure that all work complies with established codes. Routine maintenance generally does not require formal review.

The agency responsible for enforcing a code may also require repairs or improvements of structures due to damage, deterioration, or the existence of a hazard. In these instances, the local agency must issue "orders-to-comply" to the titled owner or person in control of the premises specifying the nature of the violation and providing a minimum time for completion of repairs. Dilapidated structures may also be condemned and vacated. Provisions for razing dilapidated structures may be outlined in the codes. The administrative appeal process, which is subject to subsequent judicial review, is also included in the codes.

A code may provide for civil and criminal penalties for noncompliance. Civil penalties include administrative fines or completion of repairs at the owner's expense. Unpaid penalties may be assessed as liens against the real estate at issue. A code violation may also be prosecuted as a misdemeanor criminal offense, with penalties of court-imposed fines or incarceration.

A number of factors affect the ability of a community to adopt and adequately enforce a housing code. The willingness and ability of local elected representatives to provide the necessary financial and political support is essential for effective enforcement, as is the cooperation of the local courts in prosecuting violators. Civil remedies such as making necessary repairs and levying a property tax lien may prove prohibitive to less affluent communities. The age and general condition of the local housing stock also affects the ability of local agencies to enforce codes. The prevalence of older deteriorated housing serves as a serious impediment in some areas. Organized efforts by local contractors, property owners, and housing

advocates can influence enforcement efforts, as can the availability of state or federal funds for rehabilitation and demolition.

The enforcement of local codes is intended to assure a decent, safe, and sanitary housing stock, to enhance residential property values, to further local political objectives, and to eliminate blighting influences in a community. Although the manner and method of code enforcement varies from community to community, the minimum basic requirements for occupied housing are fairly consistent.

MICHAEL G. SMYLIE

(SEE ALSO: *Community Health; Environmental Determinants of Health; Regulatory Authority*)

REGULATIONS AFFECTING RESTAURANTS

A restaurant, or food establishment, is a place that prepares or serves food for human consumption. For the purposes of health regulations, this definition includes mobile food service operations, catering operations, and vending machine locations. In the United States, a license from the local health department is generally required to operate a food establishment. To reduce the risk of food-borne illness, local food codes contain certain standard requirements. These requirements will be checked by a sanitarian or health inspector during an inspection of a food establishment.

Source/Labeling. All food must be properly labeled, wholesome, safe for human consumption, and from an approved source.

Temperature. The danger zone for potentially hazardous foods is between 41°F and 140°F. Potentially hazardous foods (those capable of supporting the growth of disease-causing microorganisms) should be held at an internal temperature of 41°F or below during cold holding and 140°F or above during hot holding.

Cooking. Poultry, exotic meats, stuffed fish, and meat must be cooked to an internal temperature of 165°F or above. Pork, ground fish and meats, injected meats, and unpasteurized eggs must be cooked to an internal temperature of 155°F or above. All other potentially hazardous food (except beef roasts, for which temperature and cooking time depend on weight) are to be cooked to an internal temperature of 145°F or above.

Cooling. Potentially hazardous cooked foods should be cooled from 140°F to 41°F within four hours, using methods such as placing the food in shallow pans, ice baths, or blast chillers.

Thawing. Food should be thawed either in a refrigerated unit at 41°F or below, under cold running water, in a microwave for immediate cooking, or as part of the cooking process.

Employee Health. Food-service employees should be excluded from a food establishment if diagnosed with salmonellosis, shigellosis, *E. coli* infection, or hepatitis A. In addition, food-service employees should be restricted from working with exposed food; clean equipment, utensils, or linens; or unwrapped single-use items if the employee has symptoms associated with acute gastrointestinal illness, such as diarrhea, fever, vomiting, jaundice, or sore throat with a fever.

Handwashing/Gloves. Food-service employees must wash their hands and exposed portions of their arms with soap for at least twenty seconds, thoroughly rinse with clean water, and dry with a paper towel, sanitary towel, or a heated air hand-drying device before starting work; after using the restroom; after touching their nose, mouth, or hair; after coughing or sneezing, after tobacco use, eating, or drinking; when switching between working with raw foods and working with ready-to-eat foods; after handling garbage, soiled tableware, or soiled kitchenware; after handling animals; and as often as necessary during work to keep them clean. They must avoid contact with exposed, ready-to-eat food with their bare hands, using only suitable utensils such as spatulas, tongs, or single-use gloves.

Cross-Contamination. Food should be protected from cross-contamination during storage, preparation, holding, and display. Ready-to-eat foods must be stored above raw meats and seafood. Raw poultry must be stored below all other foods. During preparation, separate equipment for each type of raw animal food can be used. All food-contact surfaces should be washed, rinsed, and sanitized after each use.

JAMES E. KUDER

(SEE ALSO: *Food-Borne Diseases; Licensing, Regulatory Authority; Salmonellosis; Shigellosis*)

BIBLIOGRAPHY

Berenson, A. S., ed. (1995). *Control of Communicable Diseases Manual,* 16th edition. Washington, DC: American Public Health Association.

Educational Foundation of the National Restaurant Association (1992). "The Safe Foodhandler." In *Applied Foodservice Sanitation,* 4th edition. New York: John Wiley and Sons.

U.S. Department of Health & Human Services (1999). *The Food Code.* Washington, DC: U.S. Public Health Service.

REGULATORY AUTHORITY

Regulatory authority is the power that the legislature gives an agency to enforce statutes, to develop regulations that have the force of law, and to assist the public in complying with laws and regulations. The power that can be delegated and the method of delegation are determined by the state or federal constitution. Some agencies are charged with enforcing specific statutes passed by a legislative body and given little discretion in their actions. Public health agencies are generally delegated broad authority and wide discretion to develop regulations and enforcement policies based on their expertise. When these regulations are published and adopted by the agency, they have the force of law unless they exceed the agency's statutory authority.

The most important regulatory authority delegated to public health agencies is the power to act quickly and flexibly—without promulgating formal regulations and without judicial hearings—when necessary to respond to exigent circumstances. To prevent abuse, hearings and other review proceedings are available after the action has been taken. More commonly, however, public health agencies promulgate specific regulations or adopt national codes as binding in their jurisdiction. These are enforced through licensing and other mechanisms that require regulated entities to adhere to the regulations. This provides clear guidance for the regulated entities and simplifies enforcement. Deviation from the standards is easily documented, preventing lengthy legal challenges to enforcement actions.

EDWARD P. RICHARDS

(SEE ALSO: *Licensing; Police Powers; Public Health and the Law*)

BIBLIOGRAPHY

Grad, F. (1990). *The Public Health Law Manual.* Washington, DC: APHA Press.

Richards, E. P., and Rathbun, K. C. (1998). "Public Health Law." In *Maxcy-Rosenau-Last Public Health and Preventive Medicine,* ed. R. B. Wallace. Stamford, CT: Appleton and Lange.

RELAPSING FEVER

Relapsing fever is an acute relapsing systemic illness caused by infection with spirochetal bacteria in the genus *Borrelia*. Louse-borne (epidemic) relapsing fever (LBRF) is caused by *Borrelia recurrentis*, and tick-borne (endemic) relapsing fever (TBRF) by several closely related species of *Borrelia*. Louse-borne relapsing fever is transmitted by the human body louse, *Pediculus humanus*; TBRF is transmitted by the bite of various soft-bodied ticks of the genus *Ornithodorus*. LBRF has, for the past several decades, been reported only in Ethiopia and several surrounding countries. It especially affects populations that are crowded, impoverished, and displaced by war or famine—all factors associated with poor hygiene and lice infestation. TBRF occurs in scattered temperate and tropical areas worldwide; in the United States it occurs almost exclusively in the western states, especially in forested, mountainous areas. TBRF typically occurs in small, often familial, clusters, and it is associated with sleeping in rodent- and tick-infested homes or cabins.

Following a usual incubation period of four to seven days, illness begins with the abrupt onset of fever, aches and pains in muscles and joints, headache, shaking chills, sweats, loss of appetite, weakness, and prostration. Periods of fever usually last for several days, typically ending with a crisis characterized by rigors and rising temperature, followed by an abrupt fall in temperature, profuse sweating, and hypotension. Untreated, relapses may recur after intervals of several days to a week or more. An average of three, and as many as ten, relapses may occur in TBRF, while only one to three relapses occur in LBRF. Relapses are associated with antigenic changes in bacterial outer-surface proteins.

The diagnosis of borrelial fevers is made by eliciting a history of possible infective exposure, by the typical relapsing character of the illness, and by identifying borreliae in the patient's blood. Relapsing fever is readily cured with any of several antibiotics—tetracyclines, erythromycin, and chloramphenicol are recommended choices. Control and prevention of LBRF relies on basic sanitation and hygiene to prevent or rid clothing and bedclothes of body lice, early case detection, and treatment. TBRF is prevented by removing rodent nests from buildings, rodent-proofing homes and cabins, and treating suspected tick harborage with chemical acaricides.

DAVID T. DENNIS

(SEE ALSO: *Communicable Disease Control; Environmental Determinants of Health; Vector-Borne Diseases*)

BIBLIOGRAPHY

Anonymous (2000). "Relapsing Fever." In *Control of Communicable Diseases Manual,* 17th edition, ed. I. Chin. Washington, DC: American Public Health Association.

Dworkin, M. S. et al. (1998). "Tick-Borne Relapsing Fever in the Northwestern United States and Southwestern Canada." *Clinical Infectious Diseases* 26: 122–131.

RELATIVE RISK

The epidemiological term "relative risk" can confuse the uninitiated. Risks are the same as chances, and are derived from rates. The risk of an event, such as the occurrence of a specified disease or a death from a specified cause, is calculated from the incidence or death rate of the specified disease. For example, if the infant mortality rate in a given population is ten per one thousand live births, this means that a newborn infant has a one in one hundred chance, or risk, of dying in its first year of life. About one in every five persons dies eventually of cancer; thus the lifetime risk of dying of cancer is about one in five, or 20 percent; about one in every four of us gets cancer at some time during life; so the lifetime risk of getting cancer is about 25 percent. The concept of relative risk is more complex, and it is not made easier by the fact that the term has more than one meaning—although its different usages are similar. The three common meanings are:

1. The ratio of the risk of a disease or death among those exposed to a specified risk to those not exposed to this risk. This meaning of the term is commonly called the "risk ratio."

2. The ratio of the cumulative incidence rate in those exposed to a specified risk to the cumulative incidence rate in those not exposed to a specified risk. This is called the "cumulative incidence ratio."

3. Relative risk is probably most often equated with the "odds ratio" that is calculated from the results of analyzing the data obtained in a case-control study. Although the odds ratio is not a rate, if the condition being studied is relatively rare—say occurring less often than one in one thousand members of a population—it approximates to what the rate would be if the numbers studied were large enough. Thus, in published epidemiological papers (and media reports of them) relative risk is often used as a synonym for the odds ratio. Again, an example may help to clarify this: In a case control study of 50 cases and 50 controls, 20 cases and 12 controls were exposed to the risk factor; the odds ratio therefore is $(20 \times 38) \div (12 \times 30) = 2.1:1$ (usually expressed as 2.1).

Note that the correct technical name for this is the "odds ratio approximation of relative risk," though this is often abbreviated to "relative risk" and is cited as such in media reports. It is a valid approximation only if the numbers and the differences between exposed and unexposed groups are large enough to exceed the limits of chance variation, and if the case-control study abides by the assumption that the condition under study is relatively rare. Mathematically inclined epidemiologists have written voluminously and in abstruse detail about the arcane details involved in the "rare disease assumption" and in the proper and improper uses of the odds ratio approximation of relative risk.

JOHN M. LAST

(SEE ALSO: *Case-Control Study; Odds Ratio; Risk Assessment, Risk Management*)

BIBLIOGRAPHY

Breslow, N. E., and Day, N. E. (1980). *Statistical Methods in Cancer Research*, Vol 1: *The Analysis of Case-Control Studies.* Lyon: IARC Publications.

Schlesselman, J. J. (1982). *Case-Control Studies–Design, Conduct, Analysis.* New York: Oxford University Press.

REPORTABLE DISEASES

See Notifiable Diseases

REPORTING, MANDATORY

A fundamental role of public health agencies is the collection and analysis of data that facilitate the identification, control, and further prevention of the spread of infectious diseases. All states require the reporting of certain diseases to either the local or state health department. Physicians are required to report all notifiable diseases. In some states laboratories, hospitals, and others are also required to report. The method and timing of the report may range from a weekly card via mail to an immediate phone call. The data from the states are then forwarded to the Centers for Disease Control and Prevention. There are a few disease conditions that are then reported to the World Health Organization.

State governments have realized the value of mandating the reporting of certain conditions other than infectious diseases. Incidents of gunshot wounds, child and domestic abuse, assaults, homicide, and some intentional and unintentional injuries require reporting to agencies such as the courts and child and adult protection, police, and health departments. Local agencies use this information for monitoring, investigation, and prevention. Additionally, there is sometimes a requirement to report these occurrences to those state and federal agencies that monitor the incidence and prevalence of various conditions and events, including specific conditions such as cancer and congenital defects.

Mandatory reporting at the local level of government is generally most effective when immediate response to an issue is necessary. State- and national-level reporting is important for tracking issues over time.

FRANK HOLTZHAUER

(SEE ALSO: *Centers for Disease Control and Prevention; Communicable Disease Control; Homicide; Notifiable Diseases; Violence; World Health Organization*)

BIBLIOGRAPHY

Benenson, A. S., ed. (1995). *Control of Communicable Diseases Manual,* 16th edition. Washington, DC: American Public Health Association.

REPRODUCTION

Reproduction is the process by which offspring are formed and genetic material is passed on from one generation to the next. In humans, reproduction is sexual.

FERTILIZATION

Gametes are produced by the reproductive glands, or gonads. Female gonads (ovaries) produce ova and male gonads (testes) produce sperm. Both ovum and sperm are haploid, which means that they contain half the normal (diploid) amount of genetic material (DNA) of the adult. During coitus, about 100 million sperm are deposited in the vagina, but only a few hundred reach the site of fertilization in the fallopian tube. One sperm penetrates the ovum during a process that leads to the fusion of the sperm and ovum nuclei, which contain the DNA. This fusion restores the diploid chromosome number, so that offspring inherit about half of their genes from each parent.

The fertilized ovum, now called the zygote, undergoes repeated cell divisions as it moves toward the uterus and implants in the endometrium. Only 20 to 25 percent of fertilized ova result in successful pregnancies. The rest fail to divide, fail to implant, or miscarry. Many of these unsuccessful pregnancies are genetically abnormal.

PREGNANCY

During the first trimester of pregnancy, the conceptus differentiates various specialized structures and organs, a process called embryogenesis. At the completion of this period, the embryo becomes a fetus. During the second and third trimesters, the fetus continues to grow and mature. By the ninth month, the fetus should be able to breathe on its own and maintain a normal body temperature. Survival rates are greater than 99 percent for babies born in most developed countries. Infant mortality is an important measure of public health and is influenced by many factors, including the proportion of births that occur prematurely or with birthweight that is too low. Other factors, such as the availability of services to ensure safe delivery and good health for mother and fetus, also influence infant mortality.

About 3 percent of infants have major congenital anomalies that are apparent in the first year of life. Such birth defects are the most frequent causes of infant mortality in many developed countries. Some congenital anomalies result from chromosomal abnormalities or mutations of single genes or gene pairs, but the cause of most birth defects is unknown. Many congenital anomalies appear to result from combinations of genetic and nongenetic factors that have not yet been identified.

Supplementation of the mother's diet with folic acid around the time of conception reduces the occurrence of neural tube defects and certain other birth defects. Reducing the occurrence of birth defects by folic acid dietary supplementation or food fortification is an important but largely unfulfilled public health opportunity.

Teratogenic exposures are thought to be responsible for about 10 percent of congenital anomalies. A variety of infections, medications, alcohol, and other agents can adversely affect embryonic or fetal development under certain exposure conditions. The embryo is most sensitive to damage from most teratogenic exposures between two and ten weeks after conception. Teratogenic exposures are an especially important cause of birth defects because they are potentially preventable.

CONTRACEPTION

Contraception is the process or means used to prevent pregnancy. Contraceptive options include abstinence, spermicide, male condoms, female condoms, hormonal methods, diaphragm, intra-uterine devices (IUDs), and surgical sterilization. Different methods of birth control have different degrees of effectiveness against pregnancy and of protection against sexually transmitted diseases (STDs). Each method has specific advantages, risks, and limitations.

The most effective method of birth control is abstinence. This method is 100 percent effective against pregnancy and has a decreased risk of contracting STDs. For sexually active people, the effectiveness for pregnancy prevention by surgical sterilization or hormonal contraceptive methods, when properly used, is about 99 percent. IUDs and condoms with spermicide can provide protection against pregnancy that is almost as good, although inconsistent use is often a limiting factor in practice with methods such as condoms. Condoms can also provide protection against STDs.

The use of effective contraceptive methods has led to fewer unwanted pregnancies and possibly a decrease in the spread of STDs in industrialized countries. Declining infant mortality has produced a growing population and a greater need for family planning measures in most of the world, but the overall reproductive health of women has often received less attention. This is evidenced by high rates of maternal mortality and STDs. It is estimated that about 600,000 maternal deaths occur each year, with the overwhelming majority in developing countries. Close to 80 percent of these deaths are direct results of complications rising during pregnancy, delivery, or the post-partum period. The remaining 20 percent are due to pre-existing maternal conditions that worsen during pregnancy, such as HIV/AIDS (human immunodeficiency virus/acquired immunodeficiency syndrome), malaria, heart disease, or hepatitis. Maternal mortality is highest in south and southeast Asia, sub-Saharan Africa, and Latin America.

One possible consequence of STDs is pelvic inflammatory disease (PID), a major cause of damage to female reproductive organs that can lead to death if untreated. Barrier contraceptive methods that decrease the risk of contracting STDs may also protect against PID. Oral contraceptive use is also associated with a decreased risk of PID, although the mechanism of this protection is unknown. IUDs are believed to increase the risk of PID, especially in women who are at an increased risk for STDs. PID currently affects about 1 million American women, most of whom are from lower socioeconomic classes.

Since no method of birth control except for complete abstinence is 100 percent effective, unwanted pregnancies do occur. In these cases, induced abortion may be used to terminate the pregnancy. Induced abortion has important ethical, psychological, and medical drawbacks when used as a substitute for contraception. Physical complications are frequent when abortions are done without proper sterile technique or by individuals who lack the necessary training and skills. Complications may include severe pain, infection, uterine perforation, hemorrhage, and death. Unsafe abortion is a major cause of death and illness for women of childbearing age. It is estimated that complications of unsafe abortions are responsible for 13 percent of maternal deaths. In some parts of the world, one-third or more of all maternal deaths are associated with unsafe abortions.

INFERTILITY

Infertility is an inability to have children. In medical practice, infertility is diagnosed when a couple has been unable to conceive after one year of unprotected intercourse timed to coincide with ovulation. If the woman is over thirty-five years of age or has been unable to carry a pregnancy to term, this time is reduced to six months. Infertility affects 5.3 million Americans. Approximately 40 percent of infertility is due to female factors, 40 percent to male factors, and 20 percent to either combined or unknown factors. STDs and PID are two conditions that can lead to infertility in women. Therefore, educating the public about the risks of these infections is important in preventing infertility and improving women's health.

Conventional treatments for infertility depend on the cause and may include hormonal therapy and surgical procedures. In cases in which conventional methods fail, more advanced assisted reproductive technologies (ARTs) may be used. Current use of ARTs other than artificial insemination by donor is restricted because of limited availability, expense, and relatively low success rates.

PRENATAL DIAGNOSIS AND SCREENING

A variety of prenatal diagnostic techniques are available for couples at increased risk of having a child with certain genetic or developmental abnormalities. These tests include amniocentesis and chorionic villous sampling (CVS). Such invasive techniques are associated with small risks of inducing pregnancy loss or fetal damage and require skilled operators and sophisticated ultrasonography equipment. Ultrasound examination and maternal serum screening tests, which are not associated with any known fetal risks, are used for routine pregnancy screening in some jurisdictions. These techniques can identify many, but not all, fetuses with Down syndrome or serious structural abnormalities such as spina bifida. Because very few fetal abnormalities can be treated effectively before delivery, prenatal screening or diagnosis may raise serious ethical and social issues related to the abortion of fetuses considered to be less than perfect.

Increased availability and public support of reproductive medical care and related educational and prevention initiatives in most developed countries have had an important beneficial effect on the health of women and young children. However, such services are not readily available in all parts of the world, and maternal and infant mortality as well as death and illness from STDs are far too frequent. Providing public health interventions to deal with these problems in an appropriate cultural, social, and religious context remains an urgent and often very challenging priority.

JAN M. FRIEDMAN
ROXANA MOSLEHI

(SEE ALSO: *Abortion Laws; Contraception; Maternal and Child Health; Population Growth; Population Policies; Pregnancy; Prenatal Care; Sexually Transmitted Diseases; Teratogens; Women's Health*)

BIBLIOGRAPHY

Carr, B. R., and Blackwell, R. E. (1998). *Textbook of Reproductive Medicine.* Stamford, CT: Appleton & Lange.

Enkin, M.; Keirse, M.; Neilson, J. et al. (2000). *A Guide to Effective Care in Pregnancy and Childbirth,* 3rd edition. New York: Oxford University Press.

Evans, A. T., and Niswander, K. R. (2000). *Manual of Obstetrics,* 6th edition. Philadelphia, PA: Lippincott Williams and Wilkins.

Frederiksen, M. C. (2000). *Rypins' Intensive Reviews: Obstetrics and Gynecology.* Philadelphia, PA: Lippincott Williams and Wilkins.

Friedman, J. M.; Dill, F. J.; Hayden, M. R.; and McGillivray, B. C. (1996). *National Medical Series for Independent Study: Genetics.* Philadelphia, PA: Lippincott Williams & Wilkins.

Hildt, E., and Graumann, S., eds. (1999). *Genetics in Human Reproduction.* Burlington, VT: Ashgate Publishing.

Killick, S. R. (2000). *Contraception in Practice.* London: Martin Dunitz Publishers.

Lambeau, N. C.; Morse, A. N.; and Wallach, E. E. (1999). *The Johns Hopkins Manual of Obstetrics and Gynecology.* Philadelphia, PA: Lippincott Williams and Wilkins.

World Health Organization (1999). *AIDS Epidemic Updated: December 1999.* Geneva: Author.

—— (1999). *Reduction of Maternal Mobility.* Geneva: Author.

RESEARCH IN HEALTH DEPARTMENTS

The *Dictionary of Epidemiology* defines research as "the organized quest for new knowledge, based on curiosity or on perceived needs. Research may consist of systematic empirical observation or hypothesis testing and the use of a preplanned research design such as an experiment." Research can take many forms but the basic goal is the discovery of new knowledge.

Some state health departments have been extensively involved in research, especially New York, Massachusetts, and California. However, the majority of local health departments are part of municipal or county governments and do not have the resources, trained personnel, or incentive to do research. Most local health department research has been limited to epidemiological studies in communicable disease outbreaks or community assessments to determine community health profiles. However, research is increasingly becoming an item on health departments' agendas. In 1994 the National Association of County Health Officials published ten essential elements needed for any community trying to achieve the highest level of health possible. To "research new insights and innovative solutions to problems" is on that list. In the 1990s the Centers for Disease Control and Prevention, the Association of Teachers of Preventive Medicine, and the Association of Schools of Public Health began developing cooperative agreements to encourage the development of public health collaborative research ventures. This connection between public health agencies, which can identify problems and issues needing more data, and academic institutions with trained and experienced research personnel should lead to improved knowledge that can be translated into improved practice.

Both state and local health departments can benefit from joining with academic institutions for public health research. There are many who can collaborate on research. From universities the partners may include epidemiologists, occupational medicine specialists, social scientists, and health-behavior clinicians. From the public health side, practitioners in health education, environmental health, communicable and chronic disease control, and program planning and implementation can be involved.

Since health departments are involved with the practice of public health and have the responsibility to protect the public from potential health hazards, their communities may benefit most from prevention research. This type of research would allow health departments to identify at-risk populations, to identify potentially dangerous environmental and other hazards, to develop communication strategies that promote appropriate health behavior and effective means of reducing the level or impact of these hazards, and to evaluate the effects of their interventions.

Prevention research can investigate how and why people utilize different preventive services such as cancer screenings and vaccinations. It can develop monitoring systems that follow disease trends and identify emerging problems. It can study better ways to discourage health-harming behaviors and encourage health-enhancing ones.

It can look at methods that better educate the public health work force to meet future challenges.

Linkages between public health agencies and academic institutions are beginning to materialize. These collaborations have produced results that can be introduced into public health practice, where they can then provide benefits to communities. Continued cooperative ventures have the potential to use resources more efficiently, bring together disciplines that have traditionally been separate, and create innovative solutions to problems.

MARGUERITE A. ERME

(SEE ALSO: *Essential Public Health Services; Laboratories Services*)

BIBLIOGRAPHY

The Institute of Medicine (1998). *The Future of Public Health.* Washington, DC: National Academy Press.

Lane, D. S. (1999). "Research Linkages Between Academia and Public Health Practice—Building a Prevention Research Agenda." *American Journal of Preventive Medicine* 16(3S):7–9.

Lasker, R. D., and the Committee on Medicine and Public Health (1997). *Medicine and Public Health: The Power of Collaborators.* New York: New York Academy of Medicine.

Last, John M., ed. (1995). *A Dictionary of Epidemiology,* 3rd edition. New York: Oxford Press.

Scutchfield, F. D., and Keck, C. W. (1996). *Principles of Public Health Practice.* Albany, NY: Delmar Publishers.

RESIDENTIAL HOUSING

Residential housing provides room and food in exchange for pay for persons with physical, mental, or emotional conditions. These include the frail elderly, who are not able to live independently. Residential housing facilities are often referred to by the following terms: residential care facility, personal care home, domiciliary care facility, board and care home, adult foster care, adult family homes, or assisted living facilities.

Homes may be operated by for-profit or non-profit corporations, by the government, or by sole proprietors. The number of residents can vary considerably, from one to several hundred. Funding for this type of care is usually private pay, with residents relying on Veteran's Administration contracts, SSI, Social Security, special state funds, or provider subsidies from a variety of sources.

These facilities have the capacity to deliver 24-hour care to residents, as needed. Typical available care includes room and board (meals), supervision or hands-on assistance with personal care needs, reminding residents to take their medications on time, laundry and housekeeping services, and social activities. Most states prohibit these facilities from providing nursing care services, including administration of topical or oral medications, except on a short-term basis as delivered by a visiting nurse.

There is no federal system of licensing or certification for these facilities. States and local jurisdictions generally share responsibility for their licensure; for example, local jurisdictions get involved with ensuring the safety of physical buildings for residents and workers.

RACHEL JEAN-BAPTISTE
DUNCAN NEUHAUSER

(SEE ALSO: *Regulations Affecting Housing*)

BIBLIOGRAPHY

Pynoos, J., and Golant, S. (1995). "Housing and Living Arrangements for the Elderly." In *Handbook of Aging and the Social Sciences,* eds. R. H. Binstock and L. K. George. San Diego, CA: Academic Press.

RESTAURANTS

See Regulations Affecting Restaurants

RETAIL SALES OF TOBACCO

See Enforcement of Retail Sales of Tobacco

RETIREMENT

Aging is associated with an increased likelihood of major life transitions, such as onset of disease and disability and of widowhood. In contrast to these "unplanned" changes, retirement is a major transition that is often contemplated, anticipated, and planned for a number of years before the actual event. Retirement at the end of one's career has been described as "a fixture of the American social ethos and political economy" (Hayward et al., 1998). Much research has focused on the economic aspects of retirement, particularly income security, while other research has tried to describe and understand the potential negative impact of retirement on health and well-being.

Many reviews of the evidence have concluded that a negative impact on physical and mental health of retirees has not been demonstrated. This conclusion is based on convergent evidence showing an absence of an adverse impact, rather than confusing evidence that does not permit any broad generalizations.

Older studies tended to show neither adverse effects nor benefits associated with retirement. Some specific variables, such as subjective evaluations of the health of retirees, sometimes showed health improvement, but this was seen as a function of reinterpreting one's health in the absence of the physical demands of a job. More recent studies have tended to show some benefits of retirement, primarily in the psychological domain and in health behaviors. One longitudinal study did show modest adverse effects on blood pressure and serum cholesterol, but these were deemed clinically insignificant. Retirement could also lead to a higher propensity to seek care, which might be misinterpreted as more episodes of illness. A 1991 study of older steel workers who were forced to retire early because of downsizing did not show any adverse effects on their health. Thus, loss of a job close to normal retirement age may have only small negative effects.

In addition to the broad conclusion of no adverse impact on health and functioning, the following points can be made on the basis of accumulated evidence:

1. Variations in postretirement outcomes are most convincingly seen as reflecting a continuation of pre-retirement status, particularly in the areas of physical health, social and leisure activities, and general well-being and satisfaction.

2. Certain predictors of outcome, such as prior attitudes toward the process of retirement and expectations about post-retirement outcomes, appear to make their contribution primarily via their association with underlying variables, such as prior health status and financial aspects of retirement. Consequently, they do not indicate the differential impact of retirement but rather reflect, once again, a continuation of pre-retirement attitudes and status.

3. Variables reflecting aspects of a person's work role (e.g., job satisfaction, work commitment) do not appear to be powerful or consistent predictors of outcomes. This conclusion may be viewed as somewhat of a surprise, and it can be argued that the cumulative evidence on this point is not yet very compelling.

There is no question that poor health leads to "early" or "involuntary" retirement. This makes it difficult to test the proposition that planned ("on schedule") retirement does not have a negative impact, but unplanned and involuntary ("off schedule") retirement does. The difficulty is that the downward health-status trajectory that precipitated the retirement will manifest itself as poorer health status after retirement.

Those who choose to continue to work well beyond conventional retirement age are an unusual group, made up of people in good health and with a strong commitment to work. It is in this group that the effects of "mandatory" retirement need to be studied, not among blue-collar workers who usually prefer to retire early, and do so if retirement benefits are adequate. But, unfortunately, people in such occupational groups as doctors, judges, and farmers, who often continue working beyond normal retirement, are not easily recruited into a study of "mandatory" retirement.

Phyllis Moen, a sociologist, has argued that the relationship between retirement and health is a very complex one and that most designs do not capture this complexity. She has developed a life-course model that may lead to a more sophisticated research agenda for the future. In spite of this complexity, the accumulated evidence so far leads to the conclusion that no adverse effects of retirement have been documented.

STANSILAV KASL
BETH A. JONES

(SEE ALSO: *AARP; Aging of Population; Behavior, Health-Related; Widowhood*)

BIBLIOGRAPHY

Gall, T. L.; Evans, D. R.; and Howard, J. (1997). "The Retirement Adjustment Process: Changes in the Well-Being of Male Retirees Across Time." *Journals of Gerontology: Psychological Sciences* 52B:P110–P117.

Gillanders, W. R.; Buss, T. F.; Wingard, E.; and Gemmel, D. (1991). "Long-Term Health Impacts of Forced Early Retirement among Steelworkers." *Journal of Family Practice* 32:401–405.

Hanushek, E. A., and Maritato, N. L., eds. (1996). *Assessing Knowledge of Retirement Behavior.* Washington, DC: National Academy Press.

Hayward, M. D.; Friedman, S.; and Chen, H. (1998). "Career Trajectories and Older Men's Retirement." *Journals of Gerontology: Social Sciences* 52B:S91–S103.

Kasl, S. V., and Jones, B. A. (2000). "The Impact of Job Loss and Retirement on Health." In *Social Epidemiology*, eds. L. Berkman and I. Kawachi. Oxford, UK: Oxford University Press.

McGoldrick, E. A. (1989). "Stress, Early Retirement, and Health." In *Aging, Stress, and Health*, eds. K. S. Markides and C. L. Cooper. Chichester, Sussex: John Wiley.

Moen, P. (1996). "A Life Course Perspective on Retirement, Gender, and Well-Being." *Journal of Occupational Health Psychology* 1:131–144.

Palmore, E. G.; Fillenbaum, G. G.; and George, L. K. (1984). "Consequences of Retirement." *Journal of Gerontology* 39:109–116.

Parnes, H. S., and Sommers, D. G. (1994). "Shunning Retirement: Work Experience of Men in Their Seventies and Early Eighties." *Journals of Gerontology: Social Sciences* 49:S117–S124.

RETROVIRUS

Retroviruses replicate inside cells they have invaded, using an enzyme called "reverse transcriptase" to transcribe RNA into DNA. In this way they can evade the body's natural immune defense mechanisms as they make new copies of themselves. The most important retrovirus is the human immunodefeciency virus (HIV). HIV invades and destroys host cells, particularly T-helper lymphocytes, which are crucially important in maintaining the body's immune defense mechanisms. Disruption of immune defense mechanisms following the destruction of T-helper lymphocytes is the main way in which HIV leads to AIDS.

JOHN M. LAST

(SEE ALSO: *HIV/AIDS; Pathogenic Organisms*)

RHEUMATOID ARTHRITIS

Rheumatoid arthritis (RA) is an inflammatory disease of the joints, the cause of which is still unknown. Infectious factors are being studied, including bacterial and viral organisms, but no definite involvement of any agent has been proven. There are indications that some genetic patterns are present in higher frequencies in patients with rheumatoid arthritis. This seems related to an increased frequency in some families, but not beyond a fairly weak association.

The disease can start at any age, with the childhood type of inflammatory arthritis peaking at around age two. In adults it predominates in women (the prevalence being 2.5 times greater in women) and appears more often during the childbearing years. Studies done around the world show a frequency of 1 to 5 percent in most populations. Historically, some recognizable forms of arthritis have been found in Egyptian mummies, though rheumatoid arthritis is not one of them. Its major descriptions in the medical literature roughly coincide with the start of the industrial revolution.

The main feature of the disease is an inflammation of the synovial tissues inside the joints. Synovium is usually present as a thin specialized tissue responsible for the production of the fluid that lubricates the joint. In RA, the synovium becomes swollen and shows the presence of many inflammatory cells. There is an excessive production of fluid and joints become swollen, warm, painful, and difficult to move—both because of the pain and because of the presence of the fluid, whose volume in the confined space of the joint restricts motion. RA mainly involves peripheral joints and does not usually involve the spine. The small joints of the fingers (except for the terminal joints) and the bones of the wrist are typically involved.

Inflammation in the joints causes the release of destructive enzymes from the inflammatory cells that have been attracted to the synovial tissue. The enzymes also collect in the fluid. These enzymes, which are usually part of the body's defense against bacteria, find the tissues in the joint to be grist for their destructive activity, and they also attack the cartilage covering the joint surfaces. This destruction can continue into the bone, and the joint can be so damaged as to render it incapable of normal function.

In about 85 percent of patients with RA a protein is found in the blood called *rheumatoid factor*. Although it is present in high frequency and concentration in RA, it can be found in other diseases, and even occasionally in normal individuals. RA is not simply a joint disease but can involve many other organs and tissues, including the eye, skin, lungs, heart, and blood vessels throughout the body.

Although some children, mostly girls in their teens, can have RA, the disease in the very young usually involves only a few large joints (knees and ankles). There is, however, an unusual form that afflicts children with high intermittent fevers and an extensive rash.

Treatment of RA has changed drastically (for the good) in the past few years. Aspirin was the original analgesic, anti-inflammatory drug, and it has been used for RA for over one hundred years. Aspirin is a versatile drug, but the high doses required for inflammatory arthritis frequently lead to gastric irritation. Gold compounds were the initial disease-modifying anti-rheumatic drugs (DMARDs) and have been in use for about seventy years.

The next development, starting in the early 1960s, was a rapid surge of nonsteroidal anti-inflammatory analgesic drugs (NSAIDs), which provided more prolonged activity and less gastric irritation than aspirin. The latest type of NSAIDs have even fewer gastric irritating properties but are still potent. The DMARDs that came after gold were hydroxychloroquine, an antimalarial agent that is mildly anti-inflammatory, and sulfasalazine, also mildly anti-inflammatory.

More recently, the drug methotrexate, which has been used in cancer chemotherapy, was found to be anti-inflammatory, and it has been successfully used in the treatment of RA. A major advance came with the development of biologic compounds that specifically block a link in the inflammatory "cascade" of cell-stimulating proteins. One of these is an antibody to an early product in this cascade. It is given intravenously and is effective when given at six- to eight-week intervals. Another is a "blocking" agent given by subcutaneous injection twice a week. An antibody to the B-lymphocyte involved in inflammation is also being developed. These new therapies are based on a new understanding of inflammation, even though the cause of RA still eludes researchers.

JOHN BAUM

(SEE ALSO: *Osteoarthritis*)

BIBLIOGRAPHY

Klippel, J. H., ed. (1997). *Primer on the Rheumatic Diseases,* 11th edition. Atlanta, GA: Arthritis Foundation.

RICKETTS, HOWARD

Howard Taylor Ricketts (1871–1910) was born in Findley, Ohio. He received an undergraduate degree in zoology from the University of Nebraska and then completed his medical degree at Northwestern University in 1898. After continuing his studies at Rush Medical College and in Europe, Ricketts became an associate professor of pathology at the University of Chicago in 1902. That same year, the state of Montana began funding medical research into the etiology of Rocky Mountain spotted fever. While this disease rarely claimed more than a dozen lives in a year, it was particularly virulent in Bitterroot Valley, an increasingly prosperous and influential community. After three years of research and surveys, however, scientists disagreed on its origin and its process of transmission.

Ricketts initiated a new study of spotted fever in 1906. By using laboratory animals, Ricketts was able to demonstrate that ticks transmitted the disease and this finding led to a public health campaign that targeted the elimination of ticks. Although Ricketts observed a very small bacillus,

he was unable to isolate and culture the causal agent using contemporary laboratory techniques. Nonetheless, his work suggested that bacterial diseases could be biologically transmitted from pests to people. He published his findings in the *Journal of the American Medical Association* under the title "A Micro-Organism Which Apparently Has a Specific Relationship to Rocky Mountain Spotted Fever: A Preliminary Report" in 1909.

The following year a lack of funding prevented Ricketts from returning to Montana, and, instead, he traveled to Mexico City to study a disease that provided a similar puzzle, typhus fever. Ricketts again discovered that arthropods, in this case lice, carried the disease and transmitted it to humans. At the same time, he was also frustrated in his attempts to culture the bacillus. While conducting this study, Ricketts contracted typhus fever and died, but his belief that both diseases were due to microorganisms was proven in the next decade. The disease-causing genus of bacteria *Rickettsia* is named after Howard Ricketts.

JENNIFER KOSLOW

(SEE ALSO: *Rickettsial Diseases; Typhus, Epidemic; Vector-Borne Diseases*)

BIBLIOGRAPHY

Harden, V A. (1985). "Rocky Mountain Spotted Fever Research and the Development of the Insect Vector Theory, 1900–1930." *Bulletin of the History of Medicine* 59(4):449–466.

—— (1990). *Rocky Mountain Spotted Fever: History of a Twentieth Century Disease.* Baltimore, MD: Johns Hopkins University Press.

RICKETTSIAL DISEASES

The term "Rickettsial diseases" is loosely applied to a variety of infectious diseases caused by gram-negative fastidious bacteria belonging to the genera *Rickettsia, Orientia, Ehrlichia,* and *Coxiella.* This grouping is justified by historical aspects of the discovery of each microorganism, by similarities in their microbiological and ecological characteristics, and by their association with arthropod vectors (lice, fleas, ticks, and mites). Rickettsial diseases described in this section include both classical

Table 1

Rickettsial Diseases of Humans

Disease[1]	Organism	Invertebrate vector	Reservoir/Mammalian host	Typical mode of transmission to humans	Natural cycle	Geographic distribution
Typhus group:						
Epidemic typhus	*R. prowazekii*[2]	Human body louse	Human	Infected lice and their feces	Human-louse	Worldwide
Endemic (Murine) typhus	*R. typhi*	Flea, louse	Rodents	Infected flea feces	Rat-flea cycle	Worldwide
*Murine-typhus like infection	*R. Felis* (ELB agent)	Cat flea	Opossum, rats	Unknown	Transovarian in cat fleas and opossum-flea cycle	Worldwide
Spotted fever group:						
Rickettsialpox	*R. akari*	Mouse mite	Mite/mice	Mouse mite bite	Transovarian in mites and mite-mouse cycle	Worldwide
Rocky Mountain spotted fever	*R. rickettsii*	Dog, wood tick	Tick, rodents, lagomorphs, canines	Tick bite	Transovarian in ticks and tick-rodent cycle	Western Hemisphere
Boutonneuse fever, Mediterranean SF[3]	*R. conorii*	Ixodid tick	Ticks, rodents, dogs	Tick-infested terrain, houses, dogs, tick bite	Transovarian in ticks	Africa, Southern Europe to India
*Astrakhan SF	Unnamed rickettsia	Ixodid tick	Dogs, hedgehog, ticks	Tick bite, aerosol	Unknown	Europe
North Asian tick typhus	*R. sibirica*	Ixodid tick	Rodents, canines	Tick bites	Transovarian in ticks and tick-rodent cycle	Europe, Asia
*African tick bite fever	*R. africae*	Ixodid tick	Ruminants	Tick bites	Transovarian in ticks	Sub-Saharan Africa
Queensland tick typhus	*R. australis*	Ixodid tick	Rodents, marsupials	Tick bite	Circulation in tick population	Australia
*Flinders Island SF	*R. honei*	Ixodid tick	Rodents, dogs	Tick bite	Unknown	Australia
*Oriental SF	*R. japonica*	Ixodid tick	Rodents	Tick bite	Unknown	Japan
Israeli tick typhus	*R. sharonii*	Ixodid tick	Dogs, rodents, hedgehog	Tick bite	Unknown	Israel
Scrub typhus group:						
Scrub typhus (tsutsugamushi fever)	*Orientia tsutsugamushi*	Trombilicud mite	Rodents, marsupials	Chigger bite	Transovarian in mites	Southern Asia, Australia
Ehrlichioses:						
*Human monocytic ehrlichiosis	*Ehrlichia chaffeensis*	Ixodid tick	Deer?	Tick bite	Tick-white deer	USA, Europe / Worldwide
*Human granulocytic ehrlichiosis	HGE agent	Ixodid tick	Horse, deer, cattle	Unknown	Tick- horse, deer, cattle	Northern USA, Europe
*Unknown disease	*E. ewingii*	Ixodid tick?	Dogs?	Unknown	Tick-dog?	USA
Sennetsu ehrlichiosis	*E. sennetsu*	Fluke?	Raw fish?	Unknown	Unknown	Japan, Malaysia

[1] Newly emerging diseases are indicated with a star (*)
[2] More details on epidemic typhus and *R. prowazekii* -associated infections can be found in the section: "Typhus."
[3] SF – Spotted fever.

SOURCE: Courtesy of author.

and newly emerging rickettsioses and ehrlichioses (see Table 1).

RICKETTSIOSES

The classical rickettsioses have been divided traditionally into several groups: louse- and flea-borne typhus group rickettsial diseases; tick- and mite-borne spotted fever group (SFG) rickettsial diseases, and chigger-borne scrub typhus. Epidemic typhus, murine typhus, spotted fevers, and scrub typhus share one dominant feature: widespread microvascular injury, which develops as a result of the invasion of, and multiplication of, rickettsiae in the cytoplasm of endothelial cells. Rickettsioses typically begin with an acute onset of symptoms one to two weeks after exposure to rickettsiae. Common symptoms include fever, severe headache, malaise, and myalgia. A rash often appears a few days after the onset of fever, the appearance of

Figure 1

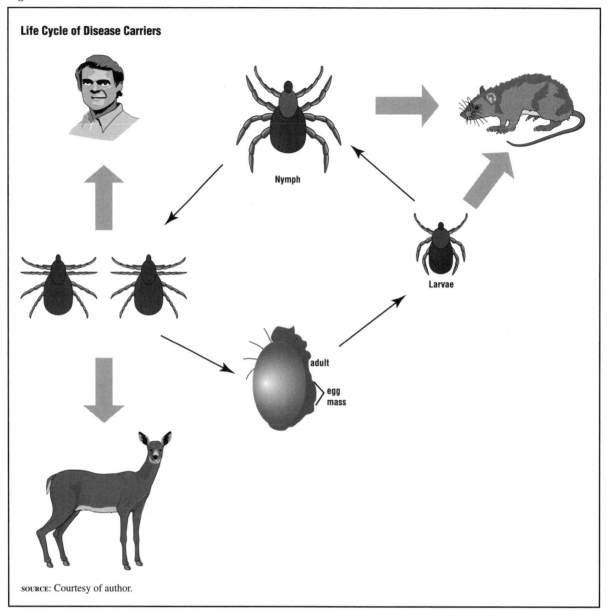

Life Cycle of Disease Carriers

Nymph

Larvae

adult

egg mass

SOURCE: Courtesy of author.

which varies depending upon the type of disease. In scrub typhus, tick typhus, and rickettsialpox a specific skin lesion develops at the site of the infecting arthropod bite (see Figure 1).

Rocky Mountain spotted fever (RMSF), epidemic typhus, and scrub typhus are frequently life-threatening illnesses when left untreated. Murine typhus and the other spotted fever infections are typically milder, but they may have fatal outcomes in weakened patients.

Epidemic and recrudescent typhus, caused by *R. prowazekii*, are fatal to their infective louse hosts. Other forms, however, do not kill their arthropod hosts, increasing the possibilities of transmission. Pathogenic species of *Rickettsia* are also transmitted through their mammalian hosts. Humans get infected when they enter areas infested with infected arthropods. RMSF, endemic typhus, rickettsialpox, sylvatic epidemic typhus, and cat-flea transmitted *R. felis* infection are indigenous to the United States. Epidemic typhus

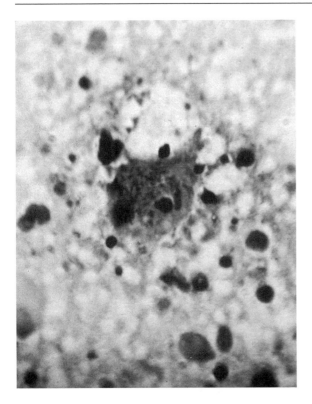

A slide showing cells infected with Rocky Mountain spotted fever, which can be fatal if left untreated. (Photo Researchers, Inc.)

and endemic typhus occur worldwide. Mediterranean spotted fever, African tick bite fever, North Asian tick typhus, Flinders Island spotted fever, Oriental spotted fever, Queensland tick typhus and scrub typhus infections all have a specific geographical distribution, which is determined by the distribution of the specific arthropod that carries each disease. Travelers are often infected in one country but exhibit symptoms in another because of the lengthy incubation period for rickettsial diseases.

The specific diagnosis of rickettsioses is most often based on the indirect detection of specific antibodies in the patient's serum, or by detection of rickettsiae in skin biopsy samples. A history of travel, camping, and arthropod bites is particularly important for diagnostic purposes. Doxycycline, tetracycline, and chloramphenicol are the recommended drugs used in the treatment of rickettsioses. Preventive measures include avoiding contact with infected ticks, mites, fleas, lice, and chiggers, and

their removal from skin and clothing before transmission of the rickettsia occurs. There is no effective commercial vaccine to prevent these diseases, but several promising experimental vaccines have been developed.

EHRLICHIOSES

Intracellular bacteria in the genus *Ehrlichia* are the cause of four human diseases that emerged in the later half of the twentieth century (see Table 1). *Ehrlichia chaffeensis* infects mainly macrophage and monocyte cells, and it causes human monocytic ehrlichiosis (HME). Another isolate, which is not yet officially named, invades human granulocytes and causes human granulocytic ehrlichiosis (HGE). It is closely related to *E. ewingii* and *E. phagocytophila*. *E ewingii*, an organism first associated with illness in dogs, has recently been found to also cause disease in humans. *E. sennetsu*, the agent of sennetsu ehrlichiosis in humans, is unusual because it is not transmitted by ticks. It appears to be associated with the consumption of raw fish. Several other closely related species of *Ehrlichia* cause illnesses in dogs, horses, and other animals. In contrast to *Rickettsia* and *Orientia*, which grow directly in the cytoplasm of their host cells, ehrlichiae grow in phagosomes where they form clustered, mulberry-like microcolonies called *morulae*.

Monocytic ehrlichiosis occurs widely in the southern United States. Human granulocytic ehrlichiosis occurs in the United States, Europe, and Africa. Ehrlichiae are transmitted by tick bites, and ticks acquire the bacteria by feeding on infected animals. The American lone star tick is the vector of *E. chaffeensis*, while the blacklegged tick (deer tick) and western blacklegged ticks are vectors for HGE. The incidence of ehrlichioses correlates with the season of greatest tick activity, peaking from May to July, but the diseases may occur throughout the year in conjunction with human exposure to ticks.

Clinical manifestations of HME and HGE appear after a one- to three-week incubation period and may persist for three to eleven weeks if the diseases are untreated. Ehrlichioses present as a wide range of nonspecific symptoms, including fever, headache, myalgia, gastroenteric dysfunctions, and inflammation of the lymph nodes. Severe cases may be complicated by respiratory insufficiency, neurological symptoms, renal failure, gastrointestinal hemorrhage, and opportunistic viral or fungal infections. Fifty-six to 62 percent of patients require hospitalization, and 2 to 5 percent of patients die.

Clinical diagnoses of ehrlichioses are based on the presence of persisting fever and exposure to ticks in endemic areas. Laboratory diagnosis during the acute stage is achieved by identification of ehrlichial DNA from patient blood samples or detection of cells containing mulberry-like clusters of organisms in peripheral blood smears.

Ehrlichial infections generally respond well to treatment with doxycycline. Ehrlichioses may be prevented by avoidance of tick bites, wearing protective clothing, use of repellents, and prompt removal of attached ticks. Vaccines are not yet available.

MARINA E. EREMEEVA

(SEE ALSO: *Q Fever; Ricketts, Howard; Typhus, Epidemic; Vector-Borne Diseases; Zoonoses*)

BIBLIOGRAPHY

National Center for Infectious Diseases. "Rocky Mountain Spotted Fever." Available at http://www.cdc.gov/ncidod/dvrd/rmsf/index.htm.

—— "Ehrlichia Infection (Ehrlichiosis)." Available at http://www.cdc.gov/ncidod/dvrd/ehrlichia/index.htm.

Raoult, D., and Roux, V. (1997). "Rickettsioses as Paradigms of New or Emerging Infectious Diseases." *Clinical Microbiological Reviews* 10:694–719.

RIGHT TO HEALTH

The phrase "right to health" is not a familiar one, although the constitution of the World Health Organization and a number of international human rights treaties recognize the right to the "highest attainable standard" of health. Although enunciated in these international documents, the scope and meaning of the "right to health" as a human right is only gradually being clarified.

Approaching health issues through a rights perspective adds an important dimension to consideration of health status, emphasizing the link of health status to issues of dignity, nondiscrimination, justice, and participation, as these aspects are embodied in principles underlying all international human rights.

A rights-based perspective on health can be seen as reflecting the following elements of all rights and applying them to health status issues:

- Conceptualizing something as a right emphasizes its exceptional importance as a social or public goal.

- Rights concepts focus on the dignity of persons.

- Equality or nondiscrimination is a fundamental principle of human rights.

- Participation of individuals and groups is an essential aspect of human rights.

- The concept of rights implies entitlement.

- Rights are interdependent.

- Rights are almost never absolute and may be limited, but such limitations should be subject to strict scrutiny.

- The dignity of all must be respected, in particular the dignity of society's most vulnerable: the poor, racial and ethnic minorities, disabled persons, and the mentally handicapped.

While it is difficult to provide evidence that there should be a right to health, more practical would be the right to the opportunity to achieve good health. But even that is complex—attaining good health requires social, economic, and environmental support, which in turn provide the opportunity for good health. A key factor in realizing the opportunity for health is the right to health care.

JOHN H. BRYANT

(SEE ALSO: *Access to Health Services; Equity and Resource Allocation; Ethics of Public Health*)

BIBLIOGRAPHY

Gostin, L., and Mann, J. (1994). "Towards Development of a Human Rights Impact Assessment for the Formulation and Evaluation of Public Health Policies." *Health and Human Rights* 1:59.

Leary, V. (1994). "The Right to Health in International Human Rights Law." *Health and Human Rights* 1:28.

RINGWORM

See Fungal Infections

RISK ASSESSMENT, RISK MANAGEMENT

During the last two decades of the twentieth century, risk science evolved into an important academic and applied discipline. The U.S. National Research Council issued a pioneering report in 1983, titled *Risk Assessment in the Federal Government: Managing the Process*. This report represented the first formalized effort to describe the health-risk assessment and management process in a structured way. It consolidated earlier efforts at developing a comprehensive framework, and it has been widely endorsed throughout the world.

The framework consists of three components: research, risk assessment, and risk management. Research refers to the collection, analysis, and interpretation of biological, chemical, and physical data from laboratory and other scientific studies, including studies on human populations, where possible. Risk assessment is defined as the characterization of the potential adverse health effects of human exposures to environmental hazards. Risk assessment consists of four steps: hazard identification (the process of determining whether exposure to an agent can lead to adverse health outcomes), dose-response assessment (characterizing the relation between the dose of an agent administered or received and the occurrence of adverse health effects in exposed populations), exposure assessment (measuring or estimating the intensity, frequency, and duration of human exposures to an agent currently present in the environment), and risk characterization (estimating the risk of adverse health effects under specific conditions of human exposure).

At the risk-management stage, alternative regulatory options are developed and evaluated. Selection of a particular regulatory option involves consideration of the public health, economic, social, and political consequences of implementation. Other factors of significance include the technical feasibility of the proposed solution, the desired level of control, the ability to enforce regulations, uncertainty in scientific data and the corresponding inferential bridges used to fill gaps in knowledge, and the public perception and level of information. The implementation of a specific course of action should be accompanied by the communication of information concerning the basis of the decision to affected parties.

Catalyzed in part by the guidance provided by the U.S. National Research Council, risk science evolved rapidly. In Canada, Health Canada developed a comprehensive framework for the assessment and management of population health risks, which served to identify the critical steps involved in health-risk assessment and management in further detail. The Canadian Standards Association also issued a national standard for risk assessment. An important feature of this standard was its broad applicability, providing general risk-assessment guidelines for health, environmental, and engineering applications. This was followed by a similar standard focusing on principles for risk-management decision making. The Canadian Public Health Association used the Health Canada risk-determination framework to establish a benefit/risk/cost determination framework to describe and evaluate risk/benefit methodology as it is applicable to the field of prescription drug use, including the use of quality adjusted life years (QUALYs) to measure risks and benefits.

The most recent contribution to the field of health-risk assessment is the 1997 report of the U.S. Presidential/Congressional Commission on Risk Assessment and Risk Management, based on a dynamic process involving the ongoing engagement of stakeholders. The Commission's *Framework for Environmental Health Risk Management* is designed to help all types of risk managers—including government officials, private-sector businesses, and individual members of the public—make good risk-management decisions when dealing with any type of environmental health risk. The framework is general enough to work in a wide variety of situations, with the level and effort invested being scaled to the importance of the problem, the potential severity and economic impact of the risk, the level of controversy surrounding the risk, and resource constraints. The framework is intended primarily for risk decisions related to setting standards, controlling pollution, protecting health, and cleaning up the environment. The framework consists of six steps: (1) define the problem and put it into context, (2) analyze the risks associated with the problem in context, (3) examine options for addressing the risks, (4) make decisions about which options to implement, (5) take actions to implement the decisions, and (6) conduct an evaluation of the results of the action. All stages of the process are implemented with the involvement of interested and affected parties.

The three key principles underpinning this framework include adopting a broad context for risk assessment (instead of evaluating single risks associated with single agents in single environmental mediums, the framework puts health and environmental problems in their larger real-world contexts); involvement of stakeholders at all phases of the process; and adopting an iterative approach, so that any new information or perspectives that may emerge may be taken into account by revisiting early stages of the process.

In addition to the overall frameworks for risk assessment and risk management described here, progress has also been made in many areas, including the use of scientific data to characterize health risks; the principles underlying risk-management decision making; understanding public perception of risk (and differences between public and expert opinion); and the communication of information on risk, and its potential influence on perceived risk.

The development of these frameworks and associated principles and guidelines have brought an element of clarity to the field of risk assessment and risk management. Principles such as fairness, equity, utility, honesty, and autonomy encourage consistency, transparency, and completeness in decision making. Risk-management principles can be of value in assigning priorities to important risk issues competing for attention and resources, in reaching decisions in the face of scientific uncertainty about the level of risk associated with health hazards, in balancing benefits and risks, and in acknowledging social and cultural considerations

in risk management. Without such guidance, risk-management decision making can be highly complex, raising difficult questions to which there are often no easy answers.

DANIEL KREWSKI

(SEE ALSO: *Benefits, Ethics, and Risks; Environmental Determinants of Health; Exposure Assessment; Risk Communication; Toxicology*)

BIBLIOGRAPHY

Benett, P., and Calman, C., eds. (1999). *Risk Communication and Public Health.* Oxford, UK: Oxford Medical Publications.

Canadian Standards Association (1997). *Risk Management: Guideline for Decision-Makers.* Toronto: Author.

Hattis, D. (1996). "Drawing the Line: Quantitative Criteria for Risk Management." *Environment* 38:11–15, 35–39.

Health Canada (1990, revised 1993). *Health Risk Determination: The Challenge of Health Protection.* Ottawa: Author.

Krewski, D.; Slovic, P.; Bartlett, S.; Flynn, J.; and Mertz, C. K. (1995). "Health Risk Perception in Canada II: Worldviews, Attitudes, and Opinions." *Human and Ecological Risk Assessment* 1:53–70.

Presidential/Congressional Commission on Risk Assessment and Risk Management (1997). *Framework for Environmental Health Risk Management.* Final Report, Vol. 1. Washington, DC: U.S. Government Printing Office.

U.S. National Research Council (1983). *Risk Assessment in the Federal Government: Managing the Process.* Washington, DC: National Academy Press.

—— (1994). *Science and Judgement in Risk Assessment.* Washington, DC: National Academy Press.

—— (2000). *Scientific Issues in Developmental Toxicity Risk Assessment.* Washington, DC: National Academy Press.

RISK COMMUNICATION

Communicating environmental risk is central to the successful management of environmental hazards. The field of risk communication is rapidly evolving due to a better understanding of the importance of effective communication in the maintenance of a healthy environment, and due to social and technological changes that affect how risk is communicated and understood. Not surprisingly in a democracy, there has been an almost complete failure of authoritative models of risk communication. Informing people about risks at the same time as or after a risk-management decision is made is not acceptable to the public. Distrust by the modern environmental movement of government and industry has been fueled by heavy-handed attempts to communicate risk that have led to public outrage rather than to public understanding. In recent decades there has been an attempt to better appreciate how the public perceives risk and how best to accurately inform the public about risks so that appropriate environmental management can proceed.

A gap exists between the priority assigned to different forms of environmental risk by the public and the priority assigned by technical experts. For example, experts believe that the health risk posed by hazardous waste sites is far less than that of indoor air pollution, yet the public consistently ranks the former as a much higher risk. Studies of risk perception have shown that the public response cannot simply be attributed to ignorance or to irrationality. Instead, there are a variety of dimensions to public risk perception that extend beyond that of the technical data. These include factors such as who is benefiting from the risk and whether the risk is familiar or unfamiliar, voluntary or involuntary, controllable or uncontrollable. The potential for catastrophe and the risk to children or to future generations also affects the extent of risk perceived by the public. There are also social, economic, and cultural dimensions to risk perception. For example, the risk of radionuclide contamination of salmon by atom-bomb production activities in the Columbia River Valley will be perceived differently by Native Americans, for whom salmon fishing is not simply a source of food but an integral part of their culture. Risk perception is thus not a straightforward probability calculation based upon exposure and dose-response measurements, but is complex, subjective, and value-laden. Effective risk communication requires the negotiation of a set of rules for each specific problem and with each specific public.

The theoretical basis for environmental risk communication arises in large part from advances in the understanding and the practice of public health education. A number of models have been developed for promoting the healthful behavior of individuals and communities. Classical diffusion theory, in which an expert resource system provides knowledge to a user community, is inadequate to explain the persistent gaps between experts and the public in the level of concern for different environmental threats. The health belief model, based upon stimulus-response and cognitive theories of behavior, explains behavioral change on the basis of patients' beliefs in their own susceptibility to a disease or condition. Under this model, the seemingly ubiquitous presence of environmental contaminants in air and water, and the possibility of serious and frightening endpoints such as cancer, lead to a high level of perceived threat. Control of these threats is accomplished through empowerment of the individual or community. Communications about risk are better understood in a context in which the hearer has the ability to control the risks and to make decisions about them. Social learning theory explains health behaviors in terms of a reciprocal determinism with personal factors and external influences, including physical and social influences. Emphasis is placed on the individual's locus of control and on observational learning as a means to develop behaviors and responses to potential threats.

Behavioral psychologists and others involved in environmental risk communication have employed and transcended health-education theory to provide many insights into the particular problems involved in environmental risk communication. A driving force in much of the research has been the "not in my backyard" (NIMBY) problem. This refers to the difficulty that government and industries have in siting any facility that seems to provide an environmental threat to the local public. NIMBY is not uncommon in other health-related circumstances, such as the siting of methadone clinics or halfway houses for those recovering from psychiatric illness. However, the depth of public opposition to environmental threats has been particularly effective in overturning siting plans based upon concerns that might otherwise seem irrational to experts in risk assessment and risk management.

Analysis of NIMBY and related situations has made it clear that trust is a factor of central importance in risk communication. The extent of distrust for institutions involved in environmental risk management has been strongly linked to the perception of high risks and to the willingness of the public to actively oppose, rather than passively accept, institutional plans.

Efforts to improve risk communication have extended across multiple facets of the problem. Effective risk communication begins with getting the numbers right. As an example, in response to public concern about a perceived increased level of birth defects in a community, a state health department performed a risk assessment that led them to the reassuring statement that levels of birth defects were within the expected range. However, when a local citizens group was able to demonstrate that the health department's survey had missed at least a few cases of birth defects, further communications from the health department were not believed.

It is also of value to perform a risk characterization, the last formal step of a risk assessment, which can make a risk more understandable to the public. This includes abandoning the use of logarithms; providing information as to who is at risk under what circumstances; and, rather than as a numerical abstraction, expressing the risk in terms of the time period during which an additional adverse event would be expected to occur in a specific population. There is also general agreement that as part of a risk characterization the uncertainties inherent in a specific risk-assessment need to be explained to the public and to decision makers. But it is preferable that uncertainty be expressed descriptively and semi-quantitatively instead of by mathematical notation. As a general rule, an expert who takes the time to try to explain the meaning of a risk probability in lay terms will be able to communicate more believably, and hence more effectively. Similarly, effective risk communication may require the expert to focus on which of the many numbers sometimes generated in a risk assessment are most pertinent to the stakeholder. The source of information is also important, with academics generally ranking higher in credibility than industry or government experts.

Risk comparisons are often used in risk communication to fashion a conceptual metric stick for the stakeholder. It seems reasonable to compare a risk of a new technology or a pollutant to that of an existing risk, such as dying in an automobile accident. But, in fact, risk comparisons are highly problematic. Because they often seem unfair, they can lead to a loss in credibility of those who use them carelessly. Automobile travel is of value to the individual, while exposure from a chemical waste site or a new industry may be of no personal value whatsoever, except to those who expect to profit by it monetarily. Automobile travel is also voluntary, as is cigarette smoking, while exposure to toxic emissions is often unavoidably forced upon people. Further, most people do not believe that the statistical risk assigned to driving is pertinent because they drive safely as compared to "those other drivers." There are situations, however, in which a carefully chosen risk comparison can be helpful in communicating the extent of risk. A related approach is to compare the potential for risk reduction from alternative uses of the same expenditure, an approach that can be helpful if, in fact, the money can be moved among choices and the benefits can be accurately calculated.

In recent years the emphasis in risk communication has been on involvement of the stakeholders as early as possible in all of the steps of the risk analysis. Building on theoretical and practical advances in risk communication, the Presidential/Congressional Commission on Risk Assessment and Risk Management advocated stakeholder participation in the entire process of risk assessment and risk management. Their six-step framework begins with a first step of evaluating a risk problem in its local context, and continues through succeeding steps of risk assessment, presentation of options, making of decisions, performing actions, and evaluating outcomes. All of these steps are to be done in an open, transparent, and iterative process that involves stakeholders throughout.

Nevertheless, there are no simple and obvious approaches to successfully communicating technical information about risk to the public. Enhanced public education in science and technology would be helpful in the long term, but by itself is not a solution, as most of the problem lies with the communicators and with the inherent complexity of our modern society. Two "laws" seem to typify environmental risk communication to the community. The first concerns sincerity. If a government or industry has already made its risk-management decision, pretending that it is consulting with the community will lead to a backlash likely to prevent it from carrying forward the decision. The second law is that there are no applicable laws—each community is different, as is each risk situation. But there are general principles related to clarity, respect, openness, and responsiveness that are of value in effective risk communication.

The increasing international pressure for harmonizing risk-assessment processes, particularly in relation to trade issues, has led to a number of interesting efforts to understand apparent international differences in risk perception. For example, one contentious subject is whether the greater unwillingness of the European public to accept genetically modified food sources or beef from cattle previously treated with growth hormone represents a difference in risk perception, or is simply a means to erect a trade barrier against products from the United States. Understanding the broader cultural issues in risk perception and communication will be of importance in an increasingly globalized world.

BERNARD D. GOLDSTEIN

(SEE ALSO: *Communication for Health; Communication Theory; Environmental Movement; Health Belief Model; Health Promotion and Education; Not In My Backyard [NIMBY]; Risk Assessment, Risk Management; Social Cognitive Theory*)

BIBLIOGRAPHY

Fischhoff, B. (1994). "Acceptable Risk: A Conceptual Proposal." *Risk: Health, Safety and the Environment* 5:1–28.

Goldstein, B. D., and Gotsch, A. R. (1994). "Risk Communication." In *Clinical Occupational and Environmental Medicine*. Orlando, FL: W. B. Saunders Company.

National Research Council (1989). *Improving Risk Communication*. Washington, DC: National Academy Press.

—— (1996). *Understanding Risk-Informing Decisions in a Democratic Society*. Washington, DC: National Academy Press.

Slovic, P. (1987). "Perception of Risk." *Science* 236: 280–285.

Tinker, T. L.; Pavlova, M. T.; Gotsch, A. R.; and Arkin, E. B. (1998). *Communicating Risk in a Changing World*. Beverly Farms, MA: OEM Press.

ROSS, RONALD

Ronald Ross (1857–1932) was a British medical scientist, entomologist, and epidemiologist. Born in India, he studied medicine at St. Bartholomew's Hospital in London and then went to India to embark upon a career in the Indian Medical Service, where he focused his attention on malaria. On a return visit to Britain he met the tropical disease specialist Patrick Manson, discoverer of the mosquito-borne transmission of filariasis (parasitic worms), who urged him to concentrate on the quest for the mechanism of mosquito transmission of malaria.

Ross worked in the south of India around Madras, where malaria was highly endemic and often fatal. After much careful and painstaking work, he discovered that only the small, inconspicuous female anopheline mosquitoes carried the malaria parasite. The males lived entirely on fluids from succulent plants, and culicine mosquitoes did not carry malaria parasites. During later work in Sierra Leone and in Ismailia, Egypt, Ross did microdissections to show the development of the parasite in the female mosquito's stomach and its migration to the salivary glands, publishing his findings in a series of papers and monographs.

In addition to laboratory-based and microscopic studies of mosquitoes, Ross developed the first mathematical models of malaria epidemiology, factoring into these models all the relevant variables relating to the life cycles of the malaria parasite in humans and mosquitoes. His models allowed for variations in ambient temperatures and other factors that influenced both the mosquito's breeding period and the time taken for parasites to mature. He received the Nobel Prize in medicine in 1902 for his work on malaria. The Ross Institute and Hospital for Tropical Diseases, later absorbed into the London School of Hygiene and Tropical Medicine, was established to house his work in his later years in England. In his spare time, Ross wrote poetry, plays, and an autobiography. He received many other honor besides the Nobel Prize, including a knighthood.

JOHN M. LAST

(SEE ALSO: *Malaria; Manson, Patrick*)

RPR TEST

The rapid plasma reagin (RPR) test has several useful purposes. It is used to screen asymptomatic individuals for syphilis, diagnose symptomatic infection, and monitor disease activity and response to treatment. Unlike the fluorescent treponemal antibody absorption (FTA-ABS) test, which measures specific antibodies to the syphilis bacterium, the RPR test measures nonspecific antibodies that are produced when *Treponema pallidum* interacts with human tissue. These antibodies also cross-react with a purified mixture of lipids (cardiolipin, lecithin, and cholesterol), known as "reagin," which is used as the substrate in the RPR test.

The RPR is a simplified version of the other nonspecific screening test for syphilis, the VDRL test. The RPR card test uses a mixture of reagin and carbon particles to which a patient's serum is added. Flocculation, or clumping, of the particles is read as a "reactive" or positive test. The test can be quantitated by examining serial dilutions of serum. A difference of two dilutions is required to demonstrate a significant difference between two tests.

JUDITH E. WOLF

(SEE ALSO: *Antibody, Antigen; Fluorescent Treponemal Antibody Absorption; Syphilis; VDRL Test*)

BIBLIOGRAPHY

Hook, E., and Marra, C. (1992). "Acquired Syphilis in Adults." *New England Journal of Medicine* 326:1060–1069.

Wolf, J. (1997). "Syphilis." In *Current Diagnosis,* 9th edition, eds. R. Conn, W. Borer, and J. Snyder. Philadelphia, PA: W. B. Saunders.

RUBELLA

Rubella, also known as German measles or three-day measles, is a mild, self-limited viral disease. Humans are the only known natural host. In up to 50 percent of persons who are not immune, a diffuse maculopapular red rash develops in two to three weeks after contact with secretions from the mouth or nose of an infected person. From 20 to 50 percent of those infected do not develop symptoms, however. Along with the rash, infected persons may experience enlarged lymph glands, conjunctivitis, and runny nose. Adult women may also experience joint pain or swelling.

When infection occurs early in pregnancy, the risk of the fetus being infected may be as high as 90 percent. Consequences of fetal infection include miscarriages, stillbirths, and severe birth defects, known as congenital rubella syndrome (CRS). Known defects include cataracts, heart defects, and hearing impairment. Up to 20 percent of the infants born to mothers infected during the first half of their pregnancy have CRS.

Because many people with rubella do not have symptoms, and because many rash illnesses look similar to rubella, a laboratory test is required to confirm rubella infection. A blood test can be used to detect rubella antibodies, and the virus can be cultured and isolated from a sample of blood, nasal or throat secretion, urine, spinal fluid, or body tissues such as cataracts.

Rubella circulates year-round, with a regular seasonal peak during springtime. Before the rubella vaccine was used in the United States, major epidemics occurred every six to nine years. The last major U.S. rubella epidemic occurred in 1964–1965 and caused an estimated 12.5 million cases of rubella and 20,000 cases of CRS in live-born infants. Prior to vaccine use, rubella occurred mainly among children. With the success of the U.S. rubella immunization program, the incidence of rubella has decreased by 99 percent to a reported 267 cases of rubella and six cases of CRS in 1999. In the United States, most cases of rubella now occur mainly among adults who were born in countries that do not have a long history of widespread vaccination.

In 1969, three rubella vaccines were licensed for use in the United States. In 1979, the currently used vaccine—called RA27/3—was introduced, replacing the other three. More than 95 percent of those vaccinated develop lifelong immunity. In the United States, one dose of rubella vaccine is recommended for all susceptible persons twelve months of age and older, unless vaccination is contraindicated.

Side effects following vaccination include low-grade fever, rash, joint pain and swelling, and lymphadenopathy. Joint pain and transient joint swelling tend to be more severe in vaccinated women than in men or children. Overall, joint pain and swelling tend to be more severe and last longer in persons who have the natural rubella disease than those who receive the rubella vaccine.

Although use of rubella vaccine is contraindicated in pregnant women or women planning pregnancy within three months, the U.S. registry on inadvertent vaccination in pregnancy has documented that all infants listed in the registry were free of defects associated with CRS. These data are consistent with results reported from other countries. Other groups that should not be given the vaccine include persons with immunodeficiency diseases or compromised immune systems and those who have recently received immunoglobulin or have severe fever.

SUSAN E. REEF

(SEE ALSO: *Communicable Disease Control; Contagion; Immunizations*)

BIBLIOGRAPHY

Cooper, L. Z., and Alford, C. A., Jr. (2001). "Rubella." In *Infectious Diseases of the Fetus and Newborn Infant,* 5th edition, eds. J. S. Remington and J. O. Klein. Philadelphia, PA: W. B. Saunders.

"Measles, Mumps, and Rubella—Vaccine Use and Strategies for Elimination of Measles, Rubella, and Congenital Rubella Syndrome and Control of Mumps: Recommendations of the Advisory Committee on Immunization Practices (ACIP)." *Mortality and Morbidity Weekly Report* 47(RR-8):1–57.

Plotkin, S. A. (1999). "Rubella Vaccine." In *Vaccines,* 3rd edition, eds. S. A. Plotkin and W. A. Orenstein. Philadelphia, PA: W. B. Saunders Company.

RURAL PUBLIC HEALTH

There are two common methods used to determine if an area may be properly defined as "rural." The first is based on population density and defines a community of under 2,500 people as rural. The other approach involves the designation of counties as being either "metropolitan" or "nonmetropolitan." The principal criterion for considering a county metropolitan is the presence of a city with 50,000 or more inhabitants within the county. Using this definition, which is more popular with organizational and planning groups due

to a greater availability of data, nearly one-fourth of the residents of the United States live in nonmetropolitan counties, and the number of nonmetropolitan counties is much greater than the number of metropolitan counties. In 1998, this translated to approximately 54 million people living in rural America.

Rural communities may be at greater public health risk because of certain geographic and demographic characteristics. Compared to urban and suburban areas, residents of rural communities have lower average total incomes, higher unemployment rates, lower educational levels, poorer housing, increased levels of poverty, and a greater proportion of elderly in their midst. Rural economies are more likely to be dependent upon a single industry. The lack of other industry to take up the slack when the singular principal economic activity is stressed can lead to abrupt shifts in economic well-being and to population migration away from the area.

The lower population density in rural areas plays a prime role in the breadth and scope of health systems that are developed there. Access to health care is often problematic. The relative paucity of health professionals in these areas makes it difficult for residents to reach health care providers, particularly medical and dental specialists, physical therapists, and a variety of other practitioners. There are few health care facilities that can manage acute or chronic health conditions, and at times even primary care is difficult to access. The loss of a physician or a health care facility may cause a major disruption in a rural community's health care system.

A number of financial factors can create barriers to health care in rural settings. Medicaid eligibility is often more restricted by rural states; the percentage of uninsured individuals in rural areas is growing; and income for rural family physicians is 15 percent lower than for their urban counterparts, though they tend to see more patients and work longer hours.

Rural minorities lag behind rural whites and urban minorities on many crucial economic and social measures. These disparities, in addition to inadequate community organizational and network resources supportive of minorities, are formidable barriers to rural minorities seeking to access and utilize the already limited health system.

RURAL HEALTH RISKS, NEEDS, AND ISSUES

Rural areas often have a distinct set of health problems. These may be more complex or need to be addressed in a different way, than health problems in metropolitan areas. Farming, mining, and lumbering accidents; environmental hazards; migratory populations; managed-care barriers; and health screening underutilization—these all add complications to rural health practice. In addition, certain problems are unique to certain areas. Farming communities may have greater encounters with zoonotic diseases, insecticide and pesticide contamination, farm machinery accidents, and farmers' lung disease, while rural areas in West Virginia have health problems such as black lung disease, that are unique to coal miners.

Injury is of particular concern in rural areas, not only because of its higher incidence but also because of the higher per capita trauma death rate and the limited resources available to treat injury. Delayed discovery of injury, long transportation times, rudimentary training of prehospital personnel, fewer available physicians, and less experience with trauma patients all result in a poorer prognosis for rural injury patients than those injured in urban settings. Many rural areas rely on volunteer emergency medical technicians with limited equipment and training to provide prehospital care. As a result, trauma patients may be less likely to receive potentially lifesaving interventions such as intravenous fluids or an artificial airway. Volunteer personnel may also be delayed in responding to emergencies.

Environmental hazards of concern in rural areas include pesticides, toxic waste products from factories and chemical plants, and the growing disposal of nuclear waste in these areas. Although regulations have been developed to cope with many environmental hazards, there are many gaps in oversight and monitoring mechanisms. In addition, the potential health hazards of many environmental agents are not fully understood.

The underutilization of common health screening procedures is a serious problem in rural areas. Women in rural parts of the United States are less likely to use breast cancer, cervical cancer, and osteoporosis screening than other major population groups, and higher rates of breast cancer and

late-stage disease have been found in some surveys. Migrant populations, principally minority migrant farm workers, tend to lack any form of regular health care. While they are the targets of a variety of federal and state public health programs, their disproportionately increased disease burden persists.

A variety of diseases and health problems are newly emerging or reemerging in rural communities. While HIV/AIDS (human immunodeficiency virus/acquired immunodeficiency syndrome) infection has been slowing in homosexual populations, its relative frequency is increasing significantly among minorities, women, drug abusers, and rural residents. In contrast to the early 1980s, the twenty-five U.S. counties with the highest rates of increase in HIV infection during the 1990s were mostly rural counties with an average population of 73,000. One of the reasons for this may be due to the increased migration of AIDS patients to rural settings. A higher frequency of heterosexual activity is also noted among rural patients with HIV infections. This expansion of the AIDS epidemic to rural areas is worrisome because rural communities have fewer adequate health care facilities and services than urban areas, particularly for the care of such a complex and multifaceted disease as AIDS. Rural areas have also experienced an increase in other sexually transmitted diseases.

Drug abuse continues to be a significant health problem in rural communities. Rural adolescents and adults have an equal or higher prevalence of alcohol, marijuana, and tobacco use (lifetime and current use) in comparison with national samples. A 1999 report by the National Center on Addiction and Substance Abuse at Columbia University indicated that the increased use of illegal drugs in students may be increasing at an appreciably greater rate in rural youth than urban youth. Adult drug usage was found to be about equal across communities of all sizes. Another study in a grade school population in New Hampshire showed that for all grades and both genders, alcohol is the preferred drug, followed by cigarettes. Marijuana is the third choice for female children while chewing tobacco is third for male children. The use of inhalants, cocaine, downers, uppers, psychedelics, quaaludes, tranquilizers, and heroin was comparatively low.

The prevalence of mental health disorders, particularly mild disorders or early phases of more serious disorders, is not adequately delineated in rural populations. However, the scarcity of mental health professionals and mental health services in rural areas is clear—fewer than one in five rural hospitals has treatment service for these conditions.

Drug-resistant tuberculosis is increasingly affecting rural populations. This is due in large part to infected migrant populations that have received erratic treatment, leading to the growth of drug-resistance within these populations. Resistant strains from HIV/AIDS patients in rural areas may also be playing a role in this increase.

Evidence suggests that rural residents also suffer from more chronic illness—including visual and hearing impairments; ulcers; thyroid, kidney, and heart disease; hypertension; emphysema; and arthritis—than do urban residents. Rural residents also report more activity restrictions from these health conditions.

There is growing information that homelessness is a significant problem in rural areas. Homeless families, in particular, are a growing segment of the homeless population, including the subsector of the rural homeless. This group has a high prevalence of single family heads, unimmunized and developmentally delayed children, and behavioral problems among children and mothers.

Other health problems, such as domestic violence, exist in rural areas, but the significance is difficult to determine, however, because of insufficient data.

HEALTH SYSTEMS IN RURAL SETTINGS

Rural health care is characterized by a relative paucity of available health services, facilities, and health professionals. This is particularly true for health problems that require specialized and tertiary care. Many small rural hospitals closed during the 1990s, and many health care facilities are in serious financial straits. Transportation problems further aggravate other barriers to accessing the health systems in rural settings.

The Balanced Budget Act of 1997 had a serious adverse consequence on the ability of many rural health care providers and facilities to maintain the services they provided to rural Medicare and Medicaid beneficiaries. The mandated Medicare prospective payments systems and other Medicare payment changes caused some rural hospitals, already struggling financially, to reduce their services or close completely. The more recent Medicare, Medicaid, and SCHIP Balanced Budget Refinement Act of 1999 addressed many issues that resulted from the implementation of the Balanced Budget Act of 1997. It is estimated that the net impact of the 1999 act was to restore approximately $17 billion, over five years, of the reduction anticipated from the 1997 act. However, these budgets still create a variety of responses to meet the health care needs of rural populations, rather than promoting a policy that strengthens a more integrated and coordinated rural health system. It is quite apparent that more comprehensive financial incentives that can support system integration through reduced duplication of services and increased health care efficiencies remain elusive.

During the last decade of the twentieth century, the private sector in urban areas moved to embrace managed care as a way to decrease costs while attempting to maintain, or even improve, access and quality of care. Managed care structures have developed much more slowly in rural areas because of the relative scarcity of health professionals and a lower population density—with the attendant deficiency in dependable transportation. To gain the same efficiencies that were anticipated in the private sector, the use of waivers has been used to bring managed care to the Medicaid environment in metropolitan areas, including some contiguous rural areas. The transition to Medicaid managed care has been fraught with difficulties in client enrollment, access to services, and provider reimbursement. Because of the uncertainties in providing managed care to rural Medicaid populations, coupled with the potential of decreased profits or even financial losses, managed care organizations are not eager to expand Medicaid waivers into rural areas. The failure to expand managed care in rural areas may not necessarily be a negative phenomenon, however, because of the variable success that managed care systems have had in urban settings.

The public health infrastructure of rural areas is also being assaulted by financial problems and the lack of adequately trained personnel. In many areas, a single public health authority, often with no public health training of the personnel, is the operational unit for the community or county. However, dramatic changes are unfolding in local and county public health departments. In 1998, for example, the Texas Legislature approved a bill (HB 1444) for restructuring the state's local public health departments and aligning their responsibilities with the ten essential public health services. The Texas Department of Health; academic, public, and private health organizations; and community partnerships are all working together—with some support from tobacco lawsuit dollars—to bring this public health restructuring to fruition.

A number of efforts are also in place or being developed to improve rural health care services. Some regions have established ambulance or helicopter services for transporting serious, acute, or chronically ill residents to larger, more appropriate health facilities. In other instances, small clinics and secondary care installations (e.g., community health centers, rural health clinics) have been developed through sponsorship and collaboration by rural hospitals, private medical groups, and federal or state programs. These smaller clinics or care centers may be staffed by nurse practitioners or physician assistants, often with needed backup by rural physicians. In other models, specialists from urban areas or larger communities travel to rural areas on a regular basis, providing more specialized health services.

Home health care is reaching rural residents, although there are some differences compared to home care in urban settings. Rural residents are less likely to receive home health care than urban dwellers, and while urban patients typically have long-term illnesses and are physically dependent, rural patients are more likely to be recipients of post-acute care, often recovering from heart attacks.

An important model for addressing rural health systems is the consolidated or integrated system developed by the Marshfield Clinic in a rural region of central Wisconsin. This six-hundred-physician multispecialty group medical practice runs thirty-seven regional centers and provides all levels of care, both outpatient and inpatient, from primary care through highly specialized tertiary care. Computerized information systems are extensively used for patient care and administrative functions. This has provided opportunities for rural health research and public health surveillance.

Another ongoing collaborative model is that of an obstetrical service (supervised by Columbia University) woven into a system of fourteen satellite clinics providing primary health care in rural upstate New York and linked to a referral rural hospital, the Mary Imogene Bassett Hospital. A team of nurses, nurse-midwives, and obstetricians in this practice model have demonstrated the feasibility of providing effective care for women and their families living in rural communities.

Urban-based health maintenance organizations and hospitals have also organized private satellite rural group practices, and universities have sponsored rural medical practices, particularly as related to their resident and student training programs (some of these are related to the federally supported Area Health Education Centers).

Finally, rural residents, perhaps mainly through necessity, tend to exhibit greater reliance on self-care, with the principal role as caregiver usually occupied by rural women. With further health education and health promotion awareness, these women could be major forces in improving the health of their families and the communities.

HEALTH PROFESSIONALS

Obtaining a quality professional health care workforce has been a long-term, unresolved problem in many rural areas. Not only is the number of primary-care physicians practicing in rural areas often inadequate, but many such practitioners are also in older age brackets. In addition to physicians, shortages of health professionals include midlevel practitioners such as nurse practitioners, nurse-midwives, physician assistants, and nurse anesthetists. Dentists, social workers, allied health personnel, pharmacists, and mental health personnel, are also in short supply. In addition, health professionals, particularly medical specialists, are needed to manage the special needs of mothers and children, the elderly, those with complex and chronic illnesses such as AIDS, and minority populations. Midlevel health professionals or practitioners (e.g., nurse practitioners, certified nurse-midwives, physician assistants) are quite useful in providing needed primary care services to rural communities. Their role in rural health centers, in particular, as well as related governmental efforts to establish a more adequate reimbursement mechanism under Medicare and Medicaid for the services of midlevel practitioners (Rural Health Clinic Services Act), enhances their outreach to rural residents. The American Academy of Family Practitioners has released guidelines in the supervision of these practitioners to direct, coordinate, and review such care. A greater liberalization of health professions practice acts in individual states to expand the scope and autonomy of clinical practice by these midlevel professionals, a highly controversial issue, could potentially reduce even further the unmet primary health care needs of rural communities. Reform of payment systems to favor rural and primary care clinicians as a whole would be beneficial to counter the specialty and geographic differential in incomes among physicians and other health professionals.

Unfortunately, the principal factors (e.g., education and training, reimbursement, regulation) that influence the recruitment and retention of needed health professionals in rural America are not given sufficient attention by educational institutions, governmental programs, and policymakers. To adequately meet the needs of rural communities it is vital that effective interventions take place in the health profession education system, which is predominantly geared to urban areas in recruitment, orientation, and training.

On the positive side, there are a number of programs, such as the Area Health Education Centers, Interdisciplinary Rural Health Training Grants, and other rural initiatives sponsored by the Health Resources and Services Administration, that provide support for the education and training of health professionals for rural areas. The placement of, and increased access to, health professionals and facilities in rural areas is promoted by the National Health Service Corps, the Community and Migrant Health Center Program, and through telecommunications and health support efforts from the Office of Rural Health Policy. Likewise, there are educational institutions that promote efforts to improve the health workforce in rural communities. A study of these institutional efforts by the National Rural Health Association (1992) revealed some quite successful academic programs that feature specific characteristics such as targeted recruitment efforts, rural-oriented didactic and clinical instruction, effective preceptors

at rural practice sites, and availability of sociocultural or ethnographic information about rural populations for students. Selected successful rural-oriented academic programs include the following characteristics:

- Recruitment efforts target students from nonmetropolitan areas.

- A specific program or tract is rural-oriented in both didactic and clinical instruction, with faculty that are knowledgeable of and committed to rural health.

- Preceptors at rural practices sites are fully qualified to teach/evaluate students and are integrated into the faculty.

- Students learn sociocultural and ethnographic information about the rural population.

- Academic programs tailored to allow students to remain in their own community are developed.

- Administrative support for the academic program, including technology maintenance, and faculty and student travel and lodging is provided.

In 1995, Texas A&M University opened the School of Rural Public Health, which is intended to provide a strong academic resource to educate students and future leaders, develop research on important issues, and provide service and outreach to benefit the health of rural communities and residents. The school is also making a concerted effort to provide public health education to the large proportion (estimated at over 80%) of individuals assuming public health responsibilities who have had little formal education in public health. This effort is being made through a graduate education program, and it could be of special significance to rural communities and counties where no public health department exists and the only public health resource is a single health professional with minimal public health education.

In spite of these and other excellent programs and activities, the problem of an inadequate health professions workforce in rural areas persists. It is clear that additional innovative, effective measures and a more determined commitment to address this national problem are required.

RESEARCH ON RURAL HEALTH ISSUES

Research on rural health issues is also plagued by a research and institutional structure and bias that favors urban areas. Yet, there is a substantial need for research efforts to identify and analyze significant rural health problems. Research is needed on attitudes about family planning services among adolescents and young adults, access to health care for rural Medicaid populations, the health of rural homeless families, and incidence and management of domestic violence and mental health disorders.

It is also important to develop and monitor health policies that take consequences for rural communities into account. At the beginning of the twenty-first century, much health policy activity revolved around cost containment issues rather than access to services. Access is, of course, a crucial issue for rural communities and needs to be addressed. The policy implications of ongoing and future demographic changes—such as the increase in rural elderly residents and minority populations and the frequency of chronic diseases, which place significant stresses on rural health systems—also require attention. Policy development will need to address the emergence and increase of diseases such as HIV/AIDS, sexually transmitted diseases, drug-resistant tuberculosis, and substance abuse in rural populations. Effective environmental interventions in farms, including the allocation of more resources to farm safety programs and a revision of current farm safety legislation, is also necessary.

CIRO V. SUMAYA

(SEE ALSO: *Economics of Health; Environmental Determinants of Health; Equity and Resource Allocation; Essential Public Health Services; Farm Injuries; Inequalities in Health; Migrant Workers; Regional Health Planning; Urban Health Planning; United States Department of Agriculture [USDA]*)

BIBLIOGRAPHY

Calle, E. E.; Flanders, W. D.; Thun, M. J.; and Martin, L. M. (1993). "Demographic Predictors of Mammography and Pap Smear Screening in U.S. Women." *American Journal of Public Health* 83(1):53–60.

Davis, K., and Stapleton, J. (1991). "Migration to Rural Areas by HIV Patients: Impact on HIV-Related Health Care Use." *Infection Control and Hospital Epidemiology* 12:540–543.

DeStefano, F.; Eaker, E. D.; Broste, S. K.; Nordstrom, D. L.; Peissig, P. L.; Vierkant, R. A.; Konitzer, K. A.; Gruber, R. L.; and Layde, P. M. (1996). "Epidemiologic Research in an Integrated Regional Medical Care System: The Marshfield Epidemiologic Study Area." *Journal of Clinical Epidemiology* 49(6):643–652.

First, R. J.; Rife, J. C.; and Toomey, B. G. (1994). "Homelessness in Rural Areas: Causes, Patterns, and Trend." *Social Work* 39(1):97–108.

Flowe, K. M.; Cunningham, P. R.; and Foil, B. (1995). "Rural Trauma Systems in Evolution." *Surgery Annual* 27:29–39.

Gesler, W. M., and Ricketts, T. C., eds. (1992). *Health in Rural North America*. News Brunswick, NJ: Rutgers University Press.

Grossman, D. C.; Kim, A.; Macdonald, S. C.; Klein, P.; Copass, M. K.; and Maier, R. V. (1997). "Urban-Rural Differences in Prehospital Care of Major Trauma." *Journal Trauma: Injury, Infection, and Critical Care* 42(4):723–729.

Hahn, B., and Flood, A. (1995). "No Insurance, Public Insurance and Private Insurance: Do These Options Contribute to Differences in General Health?" *Journal of Health Care for the Poor and Underserved* 6(1): 41–59.

Lam, N. S., and Liu, K. B. (1994). "Spread of AIDS in Rural America, 1982–1990." *Journal of Acquired Immune Deficiency Syndromes* 7(5):485–490.

Monroe, A. C.; Ricketts, T. C; and Savitz, L. A. (1992). "Cancer in Rural Versus Urban Populations: A Review." *Journal of Rural Health* 8(3):212–220.

Mueller, K. (1999). *Rural Implications of the Balanced Budget Retirement Act of 1999*. Columbia, MO: Rural Policy Research Institute.

National Rural Health Association (1992). *A Rural Health Agenda for the Future. Report to Health Resources and Services Administration*. Rockville, MD: Author.

Nyman, J. A; Sen, A.; Chan, B. Y.; and Commins, P. P. (1991). "Urban/Rural Differences in Home Health Patients and Services." *Gerontologist* 31(4):457–466.

"Rural Health: A Challenge for Medical Education" (1990). Proceedings of the 1990 Invitational Symposium. *Academic Medicine* 65(12)Supp.

Stevens, M., and Youells, F. (1995). "Drug Use Prevalence in a Rural School-Age Population: The New Hampshire Survey." *American Journal of Preventive Medicine* 11:105–113.

Stone, S. E.; Bron, P. M.; and Westcott, J. P. (1996). "Nurse-Midwifery Service in a Rural Setting." *Journal of Nurse-Midwifery* 41(5):377–382.

Swanson, L. L. (1996). *Racial/Ethnic Minorities in Rural Areas: Progress and Stagnation, 1980–90*. Agricultural Economic Report No. 731. Washington, DC: U.S. Department of Agriculture.

U.S. Department of Health and Human Services (1992). *Vital and Health Statistics: Current Estimates from the National Health Interview Survey, 1991*. Hyattsville, MD: Author.

RUSH, BENJAMIN

Benjamin Rush was born in 1745 in Byberry, Pennsylvania, approximately twelve miles from Philadelphia, where he died in 1813. In 1761, Rush began a medical apprenticeship with a distinguished physician, Dr. John Redman in Philadelphia, and he completed his training at the University of Edinburgh, where he studied with William Cullen and was exposed to the philosophies of the Enlightenment. Upon obtaining his degree, Rush returned to Philadelphia in 1769 and became a professor of Chemistry at the College of Philadelphia's medical school, where he instructed approximately three thousand American students between 1779 and 1812. Being very determined to advance the human condition, Rush formed the first dispensary for medical relief for the poor in the United States. Later in his life, he focused on diseases of the mind. He approached mental illness as a disease as significant as those that attacked the body. While his theory of causation was representative of the limitations of medical theory of the time, his advocacy of humane facilities, his use of occupational therapy, and his belief that mental illness could be understood through systematic study have led him to become known as the father of American psychiatry.

At times, Rush found himself embroiled in controversy. During a yellow fever epidemic that raged through Philadelphia in 1793, Rush advocated numerous and generous bloodlettings, which many of his colleagues viewed as extreme and dangerous.

During the American Revolution, Rush served as surgeon general of the Continental army. He deplored the squalid conditions of the encampments and, undiplomatically, blamed George Washington for their condition. Rush advocated personal cleanliness, a better diet, and resisting the temptation of distilled liquors, accurately identifying the health-related hazards of whisky and gin. After the war, Rush led the campaign to tax whiskey and use the tax money to finance the new government of the United States.

Rush's seminal works include: *A Syllabus of a Course of Lectures on Chemistry* (1770); *Directions for the Preserving the Health of Soldiers* (1778); *An Enquiry into the Effects of Spirituous Liquors upon the Human Body, and Their Influence upon the Happiness of Society* (1784); and *Medical Inquiries and Observations Upon the Disease of the Mind* (1812).

JENNIFER KOSLOW

(SEE ALSO: *Alcohol Use and Abuse; History of Public Health; Mental Health*)

BIBLIOGRAPHY

Binger, C. (1966). *Revolutionary Doctor Benjamin Rush, 1746–1813*. New York: W.W. Norton & Company.

Farr, C. B. (1994). "Benjamin Rush and American Psychiatry." *American Journal of Psychiatry* 151(6):64–73.

King, L. S. (1991). *Transformations in American Medicine: From Benjamin Rush to William Osler*. Baltimore, MD: Johns Hopkins University Press.

ISBN 0-02-865352-1

90000

9 780028 653525

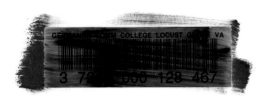
Ref.
RA
423
.E53
2002

For Reference

Not to be taken from this room

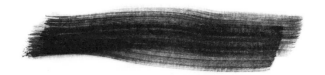